D1239188

# Uveitis

Fundamentals and Clinical Practice

# UVEITIS

## Fundamentals and Clinical Practice

**Robert B. Nussenblatt, M.D.**
Scientific Director
Head, Laboratory of Immunology
National Eye Institute
National Institutes of Health
Bethesda, Maryland

**Scott M. Whitcup, M.D.**
Clinical Director
National Eye Institute
National Institutes of Health
Bethesda, Maryland

**Alan G. Palestine, M.D.**
Associate Clinical Professor of Ophthalmology
Georgetown University School of Medicine
Washington, District of Columbia

**Second Edition**

*With 254 illustrations and 51 color plates*

Mosby

St. Louis Baltimore Boston Carlsbad Chicago Naples New York Philadelphia Portland
London Madrid Mexico City Singapore Sydney Tokyo Toronto Wiesbaden

Mosby
Dedicated to Publishing Excellence

A Times Mirror Company

*Publisher:* Anne S. Patterson
*Editor:* Laurel Craven
*Associate Developmental Editor:* Wendy Buckwalter
*Project Manager:* Mark Spann
*Production Editor:* Steve Hetager
*Manufacturing Supervisor:* Tony McCallister
*Editing/Project Management:* Top Graphics
*Designer:* David Zielinski

SECOND EDITION
**Copyright © 1996 by Mosby–Year Book, Inc.**

Previous edition copyrighted 1989

A NOTE TO THE READER
The authors and publisher have made every attempt to check dosages for accuracy. Because the science of pharmacology is continually advancing, our knowledge base continues to expand. Therefore, we recommend that the reader always check product information for changes in dosage or administration before administering any medication. This is particularly important with new or rarely used drugs.

All rights reserved. No part of this publication may be reproduced, stored in a retrieval system, or transmitted, in any form or by any means, electronic, mechanical, photocopying, recording, or otherwise, without prior written permission from the publisher.

Permission to photocopy or reproduce solely for internal or personal use is permitted for libraries or other users registered with the Copyright Clearance Center, provided that the base fee of $4.00 per chapter plus $.10 per page is paid directly to the Copyright Clearance Center, 27 Congress Street, Salem, MA 01970. This consent does not extend to other kinds of copying, such as copying for general distribution, for advertising or promotional purposes, for creating new collected works, or for resale.

Printed in the United States of America
Composition by Graphic World, Inc.
Printing/binding by Maple-Vail Press
Color separation by Desktop Graphics Systems

Mosby–Year Book, Inc.
11830 Westline Industrial Drive
St. Louis, Missouri 63146

**Library of Congress Cataloging in Publication Data**

Nussenblatt, Robert B.
Uveitis: fundamentals and clinical practice / Robert B. Nussenblatt, Scott M. Whitcup, Alan G. Palestine.—2nd ed.
p. cm.
Includes bibliographical references and index.
ISBN 0-8151-6446-7
1. Uveitis. I. Whitcup, Scott M. II. Palestine, Alan G. III. Title.
[DNLM: 1. Uveitis—therapy. 2. Uveitis—immunology. 3. Uveitis—diagnosis. WW 240 N975u 1996]
RE351.N87 1996
617.7′2—dc20
DNLM/DLC
for Library of Congress 95-33363
CIP

96 97 98 99 00 / 9 8 7 6 5 4 3 2 1

To our families,
friends,
fellows,
and patients

APR - 5 1996 C.I. Login # 84.15

# Foreword

Patients with intraocular inflammatory disease continue to provide some of the greatest intellectual challenges in our specialty. Although most cases of uveitis were previously attributed to tuberculosis and syphilis, it is now known that hundreds of conditions cause uveitis. Unfortunately, the difficulty in managing the patient with uveitis does not stop with accurate diagnosis. Appropriate treatment requires that the physician consider a number of issues, including the choice of medications, management of side effects, and surgical intervention when warranted. Furthermore, knowing when *not* to treat is often as important as knowing when to treat.

*Uveitis: Fundamentals and Clinical Practice* is an indispensable reference and guide to the physician treating patients with uveitis. Drs. Nussenblatt, Whitcup, and Palestine not only provide readers with the basic fundamentals of ocular immunology but also delineate their practical approach to the diagnosis and treatment of patients with uveitis. In large part the book is based on experience with patients seen at the National Eye Institute. I have had the opportunity to spend time with the authors at the NIH and have attended their case conferences. The practicality of their book follows from incorporating relevant patient case studies into the text.

I found the first edition of the book to be extremely helpful in my care of patients. However, the field of uveitis has changed dramatically over the last 6 years. Therefore the second edition has been completely updated. The authors have added many new clinical photographs, fluorescein angiograms, tables, and diagrams to supplement the text. More than 50 color plates also have been included. I am sure that the second edition of *Uveitis: Fundamentals and Clinical Practice* will be an invaluable reference to any professional faced with the challenge of caring for patients with intraocular inflammatory disease.

**J. Donald M. Gass, M.D.**
Professor of Ophthalmology
Bascom Palmer Eye Institute
University of Miami School of Medicine
Miami, Florida

# Preface

Accurate diagnosis of uveitis and successful treatment of the patient with this condition remain a difficult challenge for the practicing ophthalmologist. Plutarch said, "Medicine, to produce health, has to examine disease." The inflamed eye has been studied for hundreds of years, but before 1950 effective therapy for uveitis did not exist. Many physicians treated patients with uveitis by inducing hyperpyrexia—raising the patient's body temperature to 41° C—by placing them in steam baths, or by injecting them with typhoid toxin! Even Sir Stewart Duke-Elder commented that such treatment, although occasionally successful, was poorly tolerated and dangerous for the patient. In 1949 Philip Hench and colleagues reported the successful use of corticosteroids for the treatment of rheumatoid arthritis. Thus the modern age of treatment of inflammatory disease was born.

The field of uveitis has been revolutionized over the past 50 years. Our understanding of the pathogenesis of ocular inflammatory disease has progressed rapidly. We can now more accurately diagnose diseases that we did not even know existed just years before. Additionally, the practicing physician now can choose from a wide array of antiinflammatory medications. Basic science research in immunology has led to new therapeutic approaches to the patient with uveitis, including induction of oral tolerance and monoclonal antibody therapy against cytokines and cell adhesion molecules. However, immunosuppressive therapy is a two-edged sword, and as Francis Bacon said, one must be careful not to "cure the disease and kill the patient."

The goal of this second edition of *Uveitis: Fundamentals and Clinical Practice* remains the same as that of the first—to provide the practicing ophthalmologist and the resident in ophthalmology with a comprehensive text that presents both the immunologic fundamentals of uveitis and a practical approach to the diagnosis and treatment of the various forms of the disease. Although the book has been written primarily for ophthalmologists, two of us have completed training in internal medicine in addition to ophthalmology, and we hope that physicians treating patients with systemic disease associated with ocular inflammation will also benefit from this book. Again, we have chosen to limit the number of authors of this book—three for this edition—rather than to solicit single chapters from a multitude of authors. We believe that this approach has allowed us to present the subject in a cohesive fashion.

We have tried to build on the strengths of the first edition, and, most important, to make specific improvements. We have added new illustrations and improved the overall quality of the illustrations. More than 50 of the illustrations are now presented in color. We have included additional fluorescein angiograms, indocyanine green angiograms, and tables. Chapters on our diagnostic and therapeutic approach to patients with uveitis also have been expanded. Therefore this book is a bit longer than the first edition. However, we have again refrained from presenting an encyclopedic dissertation but rather have tried to write a highly readable text. Although the chapters are arranged in what we consider to be a logical order, they can be read independently. We have also chosen to include what we think are the most useful references for the practicing physician rather than to list every known reference on any given topic.

This book is divided into five parts. Part 1 deals with the basic concepts of the immune system and the pathogenesis of uveitis. Part 2 focuses on our diagnostic approach to patients with uveitis, and Part 3 presents the medical and surgical treatment of the disease. Uveitis caused by infection is discussed in Part 4, and the noninfectious causes of uveitis are included in Part 5. All the chapters have been updated, and many of them have been completely rewritten. We hope that the reader finds this second edition as useful as the first edition, but new and improved.

We have based this book, to a large extent, on our experience with the patients we have examined and treated at the National Eye Institute and on the discussions we have had with our colleagues. We especially would like to thank the Director, Dr. Carl Kupfer, for his continued support; Dr. Chi-Chao Chan, our ocular pathologist, for her friendship, support, expertise, and enthusiasm; and Dr. Igal Gery and Dr. Rachel Caspi, whose knowledge, friendship, and advice have been of immeasurable help. We also wish to thank the ophthalmic photographers, Ernie Kuehl, Pat Ciatto, Marilois Chicca, and Anthony Conoway, who have labored after hours through secluded pupils and hazy vitreous. We also need to thank our colleagues, the physicians who refer patients to us; our clinic coordinators, who assist us with our studies and patient care; and especially our fellows, who are indispensable to the program and contribute greatly to our advances in the field. A special thanks goes to our patients, many of whom travel great distances to obtain care and who contribute to our understanding of the disease in an attempt to help others.

Finally, we thank our families and friends, whose support and tolerance allowed this second edition to become a reality.

**Robert B. Nussenblatt, M.D.**
**Scott M. Whitcup, M.D.**
**Alan G. Palestine, M.D.**

# Preface to the First Edition

Concepts in intraocular inflammatory disease (uveitis) have evolved rapidly over the past few years. Basic and clinical observations have begun to place at least some of these disorders into perspective. The concept of this book is to provide the resident in ophthalmology and the practicing ophthalmologist with a comprehensive volume that presents both immunologic fundamentals as they relate to uveitis and the practical approach to the treatment of these diseases. We have written this book reflecting our views as to basic mechanisms and approaches to therapy, with the hope that other points of view are fairly presented as well. In order to provide a coherent and consistent framework, we chose to coauthor this book rather than solicit individual chapters from many authors. The basic and clinical concepts presented here evolved from the Tuesday and Thursday conferences our group has had for several years, in which we discuss the patients with uveitis examined that day at the National Eye Institute. Those who have attended these free-wheeling meetings have found them profoundly stimulating for all.

We have divided the book into several sections. The first deals with basic immune concepts that we feel are relevant to understanding intraocular inflammatory disease. This is followed by a discussion of concepts related to the examination of the uveitis patient, as well as to the philosophy of therapy and the concepts behind clinical trials. Finally, disease entities are discussed with an attempt to cover three major areas for each disorder: clinical appearance, tests and immune factors, and therapy. Though the chapters are arranged in what we feel is a logical order, they can be read independently. The reader is referred to relevant other chapters in the text. Two other points need to be stressed. We have not included an encyclopedic list of references for all the entities discussed. Rather, we have chosen articles that we felt would be useful for the reader who wishes to further delve into a specific subject. Secondly, the stress of some chapters is not necessarily related to the prevalence of an entity. Diseases for which newer approaches to therapy or newer immune concepts have been developed, or for which information is difficult to find in one clinical text, have been discussed in greater detail.

We hope that this book will prove to be a practical, useful text. We believe it will help the practitioner better understand the various uveitic entities and help as well in preparing a rational therapy. We sincerely hope that the text stimulates the intellectual excitement in the reader that our conferences have stimulated for us. We would like to look back on this book in the years to come as a benchmark, appreciating at that time how much more we have advanced since it was written.

Over the past years, we have been able to evaluate large numbers of patients with uveitis who have entered into a variety of clinical studies at the NIH. We wish to thank the staff of the National Eye Institute, in particular the Scientific Director, Dr. Jin Kinoshita, and the Director, Dr. Carl Kupfer, for creating an environment conducive to such studies. Special note must be paid to Dr. Igal Gery, whose support, help, teaching, and friendship are so precious; and to Dr. Chi Chan, whose innovative immunohistologic techniques have helped us in beginning to understand these disorders as never before. We are grateful for the expertise of the NEI ophthalmic photographers, who have labored through many a small pupil. The NIH itself provides an atmosphere so special that one needs to experience it to appreciate it. Thanks as well must be extended to our fellows, whose devotion and hard work helped us in expanding our knowledge. A special thanks goes to the many ophthalmologists who have steadfastly supported our endeavors. Finally, a special debt of gratitude goes to our patients, these wonderful souls with whom we have experienced so much.

We cannot end this note without thanking our families, particularly our wives, who put up with so much during the preparation of this book.

**Robert B. Nussenblatt, M.D.**
**Alan G. Palestine, M.D.**

# Contents

**PART 1 Fundamentals**

1 *Elements of the Immune System, 3*
Immune Cells and Their Products, 3
Cellular Interactions: Hypersensitivity Reactions, 15

2 *Concepts of Disease Pathogenesis, 18*
Immune Characteristics of Eye, 18
Immunogenetics, 22
Immune Complex–Mediated Disease, 26
T-Cell Responses and Autoimmunity, 29
Ocular Autoimmunity, 32
Cell-Adhesion Molecules, 38
Immune Responses to Invading Viruses and Parasites, 41

**PART 2 Diagnosis**

3 *History Taking in the Patient With Uveitis, 51*
Sample Uveitis Questionnaire, 53

4 *Examination of the Patient With Uveitis, 58*
Visual Acuity, 58
External Examination, 59
Pupils and Extraocular Muscles, 59
Intraocular Pressure Measurement, 59
Slit-Lamp Biomicroscopy, 60
Vitreous, 64
Retina and Choroid, 65
Optic Nerve, 68

5 *Development of a Differential Diagnosis, 69*
Classifying Uveitis, 69

6 *Diagnostic Testing, 79*
Pretest Likelihood of Disease, 79
Diagnostic Tests for Uveitis, 81
New Diagnostic Tests, 88

7 *Evaluation of the Uveitis Literature, 91*
Clinical Trials in Uveitis, 93

**PART 3 Medical Therapy and Surgical Intervention**

8 *Philosophy, Goals, and Approaches to Medical Therapy, 97*
Goals and Philosophy, 97
Nonsurgical Therapeutic Options, 99
FK506, 118

9 *Role of Surgery in the Patient With Uveitis, 135*
Considerations, 135
Removal of Band Keratopathy, 136
Corneal Transplantation, 137
Cataract Surgery, 137
Glaucoma Surgery, 142
Treatment of Vitreoretinal Disease, 144
Laser Treatment, 145
Diagnostic Surgery, 146

## PART 4 Infectious Uveitic Conditions

*10 Bacterial and Fungal Diseases, 155*

Leprosy, 156
Tuberculosis, 158
Spirochetal Disease, 160
Chronic Granulomatous Disease, 178
Fungal Disease, 179

*11 Acquired Immunodeficiency Syndrome, 186*

Human Immunodeficiency Virus, 186
Cytomegalovirus Retinitis, 188
Herpes Zoster, 194
*Pneumocystis Carinii* Choroiditis, 194
*Mycobacterium Avium-Intracellulare* Choroiditis, 195
Other Diseases, 195
Drug-Related Ocular Inflammation, 196

*12 Acute Retinal Necrosis and Progressive Outer Retinal Necrosis, 198*

Acute Retinal Necrosis, 198
Progressive Outer Retinal Necrosis, 203

*13 Other Viral Diseases, 207*

Herpes Simplex Virus Infection, 207
Herpes Zoster Virus Infection, 208
Other Viral Infections, 209

*14 Ocular Toxoplasmosis, 211*

Organism, 211
Clinical Manifestations, 213
Histopathology and Immune Factors, 218
Therapy, 223

*15 Ocular Histoplasmosis, 229*

Systemic Findings, 229
Ocular Appearance, 229
Etiology and Immunology, 232
Therapy, 233

*16 Toxocara Canis, 238*

Ocular Manifestations, 239
Histopathology and Immune Factors, 239
Treatment, 241

*17 Onchocerciasis and Other Parasitic Diseases, 244*

Onchocerciasis, 244
Giardiasis, 248
Ophthalmomyiasis, 249
Cysticercosis, 250
Caterpillar Hairs, 250
Amebiasis, 251
Diffuse Unilateral Subacute Neuroretinitis, 251
Seasonal Hyperacute Panuveitis, 252

*18 Postsurgical Uveitis, 256*

Acute Bacterial Endophthalmitis, 256
Chronic Bacterial Endophthalmitis, 257
Fungal Endophthalmitis, 258
Lens-Induced Uveitis, 259
Inflammation From an Intraocular Lens, 259
Laser-Induced Uveitis, 260

## PART 5 Noninfectious Uveitic Conditions

*19 Anterior Uveitis, 265*

Epidemiology, 265
Clinical Description, 265
Idiopathic Anterior Uveitis, 266
HLA-B27–Associated Anterior Uveitis, 267
HLA-B27–Associated Anterior Uveitis With Systemic Disease, 268
Disease Associations, 273

*20 Intermediate Uveitis, 279*

Epidemiology, 279
Clinical Manifestations, 280
Prognosis, 282
Differential Diagnosis, 282
Etiology, 284
Treatment, 285

*21 Sarcoidosis, 289*

Epidemiology, 289
Etiology, 289
Clinical Manifestations, 290
Pathology, 294
Diagnosis, 295
Treatment, 296

*22 Sympathetic Ophthalmia, 299*
Clinical Appearance, 299
Tests and Immunologic Characteristics, 302
Therapy, 307

*23 Vogt-Koyanagi-Harada Syndrome, 312*
Clinical Aspects, 312
Laboratory Tests, Etiology, and Histopathology, 317
Therapy, 321

*24 Birdshot Retinochoroidopathy, 325*
Clinical Manifestations, 325
Tests, Histology, and Etiology, 329
Therapy, 330

*25 Behçet's Disease, 334*
Clinical Manifestations, 335
Immunologic and Histologic Considerations, 344
Therapy, 347

*26 Retinal Vasculitis, 354*
Clinical Characteristics, 354
Ocular Vasculitic Disorders Without Systemic Disease, 355
Ocular Vasculitic Disorders With Systemic Disease, 358

*27 Serpiginous Choroidopathy, 364*
Clinical Features, 364
Pathology, 366
Etiology, 367
Differential Diagnosis, 367
Therapy, 368

*28 White-Dot Syndromes, 371*
Multiple Evanescent White-Dot Syndrome, 371
Multifocal Choroiditis and Panuveitis, 373
Acute Retinal Pigment Epitheliitis, 375
Acute Posterior Multifocal Placoid Pigment Epitheliopathy, 376
Subretinal Fibrosis and Uveitis Syndrome, 379
Acute Zonal Occult Outer Retinopathy, 381

*29 Masquerade Syndromes, 385*
Intraocular Lymphoma, 385
Lymphoid Hyperplasia of Uvea, 390
Other Malignant Processes Manifesting as Uveitis, 391
Multiple Sclerosis, 392
Other Nonmalignant Conditions, 392

COLOR PLATES FOLLOW P. 47

# PART 1

# FUNDAMENTALS

# CHAPTER 1

# Elements of the Immune System

In an ever-changing field, a review of the immune system is the subject of numerous books, courses, and scientific articles. However, certain principles have been established that, in the main, have survived the test of time and rigorous scrutiny. This chapter aims to prepare the reader with the basic essentials needed to follow a discussion concerning the mechanisms proposed for intraocular inflammatory disease; therefore it is weighted in the direction of topics that appear relevant to the understanding of that subject. It is clear to any observer of immunology that a detailed description of immune events would be far beyond the scope of this book. For those well versed in this field, this chapter may be somewhat superfluous. Additional suggested reading materials are included at the end of the chapter to help those so inclined to further solidify their understanding of this area or to cover other topics that have not been described.

## IMMUNE CELLS AND THEIR PRODUCTS

The immune system is the result of several cell types, including lymphocytes (T cells, B cells), macrophages, and polymorphonuclear cells. However, additional cells, such as dendritic cells in the skin and spleen, and ocular resident cells in the eye, also should be included. These components add up to a complex immune circuitry, which in the vast number of cases responds in a way that is beneficial to the organism. A review of the normal functions of some of the major players of the immune response should help in understanding the factors that may lead to disease.

### Macrophages/monocytes

Phagocytic cells originate in the bone marrow. The concept that phagocytosis was important for the immunologic defense of the organism was proposed by Ilya Metchnikoff at the end of the nineteenth century. The macrophage, which is relatively large (15 μm), has an abundant smooth and rough endoplasmic reticulum. Lysosomal granules and a well-developed Golgi apparatus are also found. Several functional, histochemical, and morphologic characteristics of these cells can be noted (Table 1-1). In addition to the phagocytic characteristics already alluded to, these cells contain esterases and peroxidases, and they bear membrane markers that are typical of their cell line (i.e., OKM1 antigen). Other cell surface markers are also present, such as class II antigens (see Chapter 2), Fc receptors (for antibody), and receptors for complement. These enzymes and cell markers help to identify this class of cells, as well as their state of activation. The presence of esterase is a useful marker to distinguish macrophages from granulocytes and lymphocytes. Further, 5′-nucleotidase is present in "resident" tissue macrophages, but it is actively degraded with activation of the macrophage and is no longer detectable. Monocytes will leave the blood

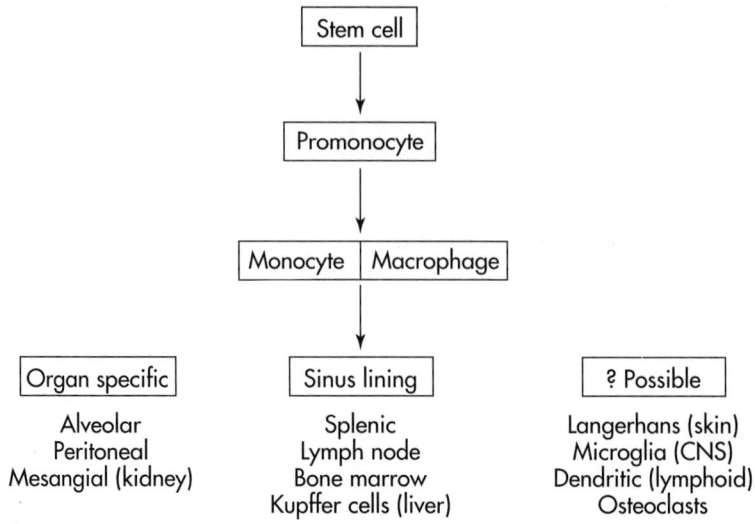


**Fig. 1-1.** Macrophage differentiation.

**Table 1-1.** Macrophage characteristics

| Histochemical | Surface antigens | Receptors | Functions |
|---|---|---|---|
| 5′-Nucleotidase | OKM1 | Fc | Phagocytosis |
| Esterase | Class II antigens | IgM | Pinocytosis |
| Alkaline phosphodiesterase | | Lymphokine | Immune activation |
| Aminopeptidase | | Lactoferrin | Secretory |
| | | Insulin | Microbicidal |
| | | C3b | Tumoricidal |
| | | Fibrinogen | |
| | | Lipoprotein | |

stream either because of a predetermined maturational process or induced migration into an area as a result of chemotactic substances, often produced during inflammatory events. Once taking up residence in various tissues, they become macrophages that frequently are known by other names (Fig. 1-1).

Macrophages play at least three major roles within the immune system. The first is to directly destroy foreign pathogens as well as dying or diseased tissue. Killing of invading microbes is in part mediated by a burst of hydrogen peroxide ($H_2O_2$) activity by the activated macrophage. An example with ocular import is the engulfment of the toxoplasmosis organism, with the macrophage often being a repository for this parasite if killing is inadequate (see Chapter 14). The second is to activate the immune system. Macrophages or other cells with similar characteristics are mandatory for antigen-specific activation of T lymphocytes. Internalizing and processing of the antigen by the macrophage are thought to be integral parts of this mechanism, and the macrophage is often described as an antigen-presenting cell (APC). It should be noted that other cells such as dendritic cells in the skin and B cells can act as APCs as well. The macrophage and lymphocyte usually need to be in close contact with one another for this transfer to occur. Another requirement is for the cells to have in common a significant portion of their major histocompatibility complex (MHC), genes that express various cell surface membranes that are essential for cellular communication and function (see Chapter 2). Thus this MHC-restricted transfer of information leads to an initiation of an immune response, ultimately with both T and B cells potentially participating. Other cell surface markers are needed for activation. This "two signal" theory has centered around other cell surface antigens such as the B7/CD28 complex. The engagement of B7 (on the macrophage side) with CD28 initiates the transcription of cytokine genes. Third, the macrophage is a potent secretory cell. Proteases can be released in abundance, which can degrade vessel surfaces and perivascular areas. Degradation products that result from these reactions are chemotactic and further enhance an immune response. Interleukin-1 (IL-1), a monokine with a molecular weight of 15 kilodaltons (kd), is produced by the macrophage (as well as other cells) after interaction with exogenous pathogens or internal stimuli, such as immune complexes or T cells. IL-1 release directly affects T-cell growth and aids this cell in releasing its own secretory products. IL-1 is noted to act directly on the central nervous system with a by-product being the induction of fever. Still other macrophage products stimulate fibroblast migration and division, all of these with potentially important consequences in the eye. Subgroups of mature macrophages have been defined by monoclonal antibodies, by their being observed as residing in specific tissues and having somewhat different functional properties.

### T cells

T cells are found in large numbers in the systemic circulation. Lymphocytes are broadly divided into two major categories, T cells and B cells (discussed later). These appelations are based on initial observations of chickens, in which a subgroup of lymphocytes homed to the thymus where they underwent a maturational process leading to the heterogeneous population now recognized as "thymus-dependent" or T cells. The thymus, the first lymphoid organ to develop, has essentially two compartments, the cortex and the medulla. Within the thymus are found epithelial cells, thymocytes (immature lymphocytes), occasional macrophages, and more mature lymphocytes. The highly cellular cortex is the center of mitoses, with large numbers of immature thymocytes and epithelial cells adhering to each other. As the thymocytes mature to T cells, they migrate to the medulla and are ultimately released into the systemic circulation. Extracts from thymic preparations have been studied in vitro and have led to the concept of thymic hormones, such as thymopoietin, necessary for the normal maturation of T cells. Although an intimate understanding of the mechanisms involved is lacking, major alterations occur to the thymocyte during this maturational process. There is the activation of specific genes needed for only this portion of the life cycle of the cells. There are, in addition, lifelong characteristics that are acquired. These include the development of specific receptors that recognize particular antigens, the acquisition of MHC restriction needed for proper immune interactions, and the acquisition of various T-cell functions, such as "killing" and "helping" other cells.

A most important quality that these cells possess is their immunologic recall or anamnestic capacity, as well as the capacity to produce lymphokines (cytokines) (Table 1-2). A T cell previously sensitized to a particular antigen can retain this immunologic memory for essentially its lifetime. With a repeat encounter, this memory response leads to an immune response, more rapid and more pronounced than the first. Such an example is the positive skin response seen after purified protein derivative (PPD) testing.

The central role of the T cell in the immune system cannot be overemphasized. T cells function as pivotal modulators of the immune response, particularly by helping B-cell production of antibody and augmenting cell-mediated reactions through further recruitment of immunoreactive cells. T cells also may downregulate or prevent immune reactions through active suppression. In addition to these "managerial" types of roles, some T-cell subsets are known to be cytotoxic and are recognized as belonging to the predominant cells in transplantation rejection crises. The accumulated evidence supports the importance of T cells in many aspects of the intraocular inflammatory process—from the propagation of disease to its subsequent downregulation.

**Major subsets.** The functions that have been briefly described are now thought to be carried out by at least three major subsets of T cells. The identification of these major subsets and their subgroups has been made immeasurably easier with the development of monoclonal antibody technology (see B-cell discussion in next section). It was observed early on that T cells (as well as other cells) manifest a myriad of different molecules on their cell-surface membranes, some expressed uniquely at certain periods of cell activation or function. It was noted that certain monoclonal antibodies directed against these unique proteins bound to specific subsets of cells, thereby permitting a

**Table 1-2.** Cytokines

| Type | Source | Target and effect |
|---|---|---|
| Interferon-γ | T cells | Antiviral effects; promotes expression of MHC II Antigens on cell surfaces; increases MØ tumor killing; inhibits some T-cell proliferation |
| Transforming growth factor–β | T cells, resident ocular cells | Suppresses generation of certain T cells; involved in ACAID and oral tolerance |
| Interleukin | | |
| IL-1 | Many nucleated cells, high levels of MØ keratinocyte, endothelial cells, some T and B cells | T- and B-cells proliferation; fibroblasts—proliferation, prostaglandin production; CNS—fever; bone and cartilage resorption; adhesion-molecule expression on endothelium |
| IL-2 | Activated T cells | Activates T cells, B cells MØ NK cells |
| IL-3 | T cells | Affects hemopoietic lineage that is nonlymphoid eosinophil regulator; similar function to IL-5 GM-CSF |
| IL-4 | T cells | Regulates many aspects of B-cell development, affects T cells, mast cells, and MØ |
| IL-5 | T cells, eosinophils | Affects hemopoietic lineage that is nonlymphoid, eosinophil regulator: similar function to IL-3 GM-CSF; induces B-cell differentiation into IgG and IgM secreting plasma cells |
| IL-6 | MØ T cells fibroblasts; endothelial cells, RPE | B cells—cofactor for Ig production; T cells–comitogen; proinflammatory in eye |
| IL-7 | Stromal cells in bone marrow and thymus | Stimulates early B-cell progenitors; affects immature T cells |
| IL-8 | NK cells, T cells | Chemoattractant of neutrophils, basophils, and some T cells; aids in neutrophils adhering to endothelia; induced by IL-1, TNF-α and endotoxin |
| IL-9 | T cells | Supports growth of helper T cells; may be enhancing factor for hematopoiesis in presence of other cytokines |
| IL-10 | T cells, B cells, stimulated MØ | Inhibits production of lymphokines by Th1 T cells |
| Il-11 | Bone marrow stromal cells (fibroblasts) | Stimulates cells of myeloid, lymphoid, erythroid, and megakaryocytic lines; induces osteoclast formation; enhances erythrocytopoiesis, antigen-specific antibodies, acute-phase proteins, fever |
| IL-12 | B cells, T cells | Induces IFN-γ synthesis: augments T-cell cytotoxic activity with IL-2; is chemotactic for NK cells and stimulates interaction with vascular endothelium; promotes lytic activity of NK cells; antitumor effects regulate proliferation of Th1 T cells but not Th2 or Th0 |
| IL-13 | T cells | Antiinflammatory activity as IL-4 and IL-10; downregulates IL-12 and IFN-α production and thus favors Th2 T cell responses; inhibits proliferation of normal and leukemic human B-cell precursors; monocyte chemoattractant |
| IL-14 | T cells | Induces B cell proliferation, malignant B cells; inhibits immunoglobulin secretion |
| IL-15 | Variety of cells | Stimulates proliferation of T cells; shares bioactivity of IL-2 and uses components of IL-2 receptor |

*ACAID,* Anterior chamber–acquired immune deviation; *GM-CSF,* granulocyte-macrophage colony-stimulating factor; *IFN,* interferon *MØ,* macrophage; *NK,* natural killer; *RPE,* retinal pigment epithelium; *TNF,* tumor necrosis factor.

way to identify them (Tables 1-3 and 1-4). The antibodies to the CD3 antigen (e.g., Leu-1) are directed against an antigen found on all mature human T cells in the circulation; approximately 70% to 80% of lymphocytes in the systemic circulation bear this marker. Antibodies to the CD4 antigen (e.g., OKT4 and Leu-3) define the helper subgroup of human T cells (about 60% to 80% of the total T cells). These cells are not cytotoxic but rather aid in the regulation of B-cell responses and in cell-mediated reactions. These $CD4^+$ cells respond to antigens complexed to MHCs of the class II type. It is the $CD4^+$ subgroup of cells that is particularly susceptible to the human immunodeficiency virus of the acquired immunodeficiency syndrome (see Chapters 2 and 11), with the percentage of this subset decreasing dramatically as this disease progresses. Further, these helper cells are necessary components of the autoimmune response seen in the experimental models of ocular inflammatory disease induced with retinal antigens (see discussion of autoimmunity in Chapter 2).

Antibodies to the CD4 antigen (i.e., OKT8 and Leu-4 antibodies) distinguish a suppressor/cytotoxic T cell, making up about 20% to 30% of the total number of T cells. This marker identifies either one cell with the very different roles of suppression or cytotoxicity depending on yet poorly understood mechanisms, or it identifies at least two different cells sharing this particular cell surface antigen. $CD8^+$ cells will react to antigens complexed with MHC class I molecules. Antibodies directed against the CD8 antigen block class I histocompatibility–associated reactions. A list of presently available antisera to human T-cell subsets or distinctive

**Table 1-3.** Monoclonal antisera for human immune cells

| Monoclonal antibody | CD | Specificity | Source* |
|---|---|---|---|
| OKT3 | 3 | All mature T cells | 1 |
| Leu-1 | 5 | All mature T cells, B cells, neoplasm | 2 |
| Leu-4 | 3 | All mature T cells | 2 |
| OKT4 | 4 | Helper/inducer T cells | 1 |
| Leu-3a | 4 | Helper/inducer T cells | 2 |
| Leu-8 | | Inducer T cells | 2 |
| OKT8 | 8 | Suppressor/cytotoxic T cells | 1 |
| Leu-2a | 8 | Suppressor/cytotoxic T cells | 2 |
| Leu-15 | 11b | Suppressor T cells | 2 |
| Leu-7 | – | NK cell | 2 |
| Leu-14 | 22 | B cells | 2 |
| OKM1 | 11 | Macrophages, NK cells | 1 |
| MS | 11 | Histiocytes, epithelioid cells, macrophages | 2 |
| OKla | – | HLA-DR | 1 |
| HLA-DR | – | HLA-DR | 2 |

*CD,* Cluster differentiation; *HLA,* human leukocyte antigen; *NK,* natural killer.
**1,* Ortho Diagnostics, Raritan N.J.; *2,* Becton Dickinson, Sunnyvale, Calif.

**Table 1-4.** Selected human leukocyte differentiation antigens

| Cluster designation | Main cellular distribution | Associated functions |
|---|---|---|
| CD3 | T cells, thymocytes | Signal transduction |
| CD4 | Helper T cells | MHC class II coreceptor |
| CD8 | Suppressor T cells, cytotoxic T cells | MHC class I receptor |
| CD11a | Leukocytes | LFA-1, adhesion molecule |
| CD11b | Granulocytes, MØ | Mac-1 adhesion molecule |
| CD11c | Granulocytes, MØ, T cells, B cells | α-Integrin, adhesion molecule |
| CD19 | B cells | B-cell activation |
| CD20 | B cells | B-cell activation |
| CD25 | T cells, B cells | Il-2 receptor (Tac), activation |
| CD45 | Leukocytes | Maturation |
| CD54 | Endothelial, dendritic, and epithelial cells; activated T and B cells | ICAM-1, adhesion molecule; ligand of LFA-1 and Mac-1 |
| CD56 | NK cells | N-CAM, adhesion molecule |
| CD68 | Macrophages | |

*ICAM,* Intercellular-adhesion molecule; *IL,* interleukin; *LFA,* lymphocyte function-associated molecule; *MHC,* major histocompatibility complex; *N-CAM,* neural cell adhesion molecule.

**Table 1-5.** Comparison of T-cell markers in human, mouse, and rat

| Class | Human | Mouse | Rat |
|---|---|---|---|
| Pan T | OKT3, Leu-1 | | |
| Helper/ sup- pressor (effector) | OKT4, Leu-3a<br>OKT8, Leu-2a | Ly-1<br>Ly-2 | W25<br>QX8 |
| Suppressor (inducer) | – | Ly-1, I-J, Qa-1 | – |
| Cytotoxic OKT8 | OKT8 | Ly-2 | OX8 |
| Class II antigen | OKla, HLA-DR | la | la |

cell-surface antigens, as well as their rough equivalent in the mouse and rat, can be seen in Table 1-5.

Intercellular communication is in large part mediated by cytokines. Cytokines are produced by lymphocytes (lymphokines) and macrophages (monokines), as well as other cells. They are hormonelike proteins capable of amplifying an immune response as well as suppressing it. With the activation of a T lymphocyte, the production and release of various lymphokines will occur. One of the most important is interleukin-2 (IL-2), with a molecular weight of 15,000 in humans. The release of this lymphokine has the capacity to stimulate lymphocyte growth and amplify or augment specific immune responses. Another lymphokine is interferon (IFN)-γ, an important immunoregulator with the potent capacity to induce class II antigen expression on cells. Transforming growth factor–β (TGF-β) is a ubiquitous material produced by many cells, including platelets and T cells, with the distinct ability to downgrade immune responses initially augmented by IL-2 production; it appears to play an important role in anterior chamber–acquired immune deviation (ACAID) and oral tolerance (see Chapter 2). A large number of lymphokines have been purified and their effects described (see Table 1-2).

Much interest has centered around the T-cell receptor (TCR) (Fig. 1-2). T cells need to produce the TCR on their cell surface to correctly "receive" information transmitted to it by peptides presented on the APC. This complex interaction involves the MHC antigen on the APC surface, the peptide, either the CD4 or CD8 antigen, and the TCR. The TCR is similar in structure to an immunoglobulin, having both an alpha and a beta chain. The more distal ends of these chains are variable, and the hypervariable regions are termed *V* (variable) and *J* (joining) on the alpha chain and *V, J,* and *D* (diversity) on the beta chain. Compared with the number of immunoglobulin genes, there are a smaller number of V genes and more J genes in the TCR repertoire. It is logically assumed that the peptide, which is special in shape and therefore fits specifically in a lock-and-key fashion into the groove between the MHC and TCR, would be the "cement" of this union. In general that would be true, but "superantigens," which can bind to the sides of these molecules, can also bring them together and, under the right circumstances, initiate cellular responses. These superantigens are glycoproteins and can be bacterial products such as enterotoxins or viral products. It has been suggested that of all the possible combinations of gene arrangements that could possibly happen to produce the variable region that is believed to cradle the peptide, certain genes within a family seem to be noted more frequently in autoimmune disease. One such group is the Vβ family, with Vβ8.2 receiving much attention. A very small number of cells have a TCR made up not of alpha and beta chains, but rather gamma and delta chains. These cells are usually CD4 and CD8 negative, and their ability to interact with APCs is not great. They appear to be highly reactive to heat-shock proteins.

Helper T cells have been further subdivided, based on their functional characteristics, into two groups. The first is that of the Th1 cell (Fig. 1-3). These cells show a cytokine profile of IL-2 and IFN-γ. The cytokine profile of Th2 cells comprises IL-4, TGF-β, and IL-10. In many animal models of human disease, Th1 cells are associated with the initiation of disease, whereas Th2 cells are related to disease suppression.

### B cells

B cells make up the second broad arm of the lymphocyte immune response. Originating from the same pluripotential stem cell in the bone marrow as the T cell, the maturational process and role of the B cell are quite different. The term *B cell* originates from observations obtained from work with chickens, where it was noted that antibody-producing cells would not develop if the bursa of Fabricius, a uniquely avian structure, was removed. The human equivalent appears to be the bone marrow.

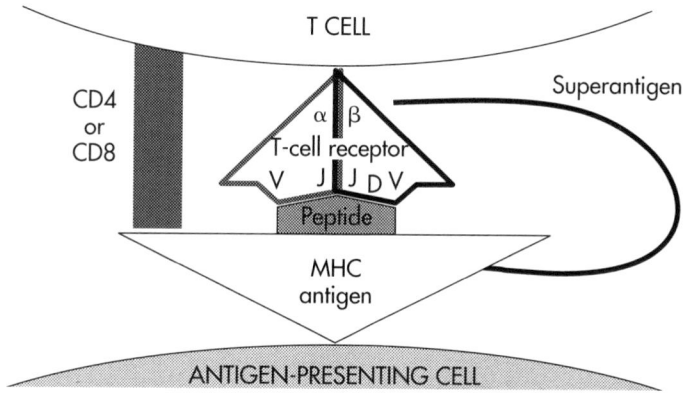


**Fig. 1-2.** Structure of T-cell receptor *(TCR)* and its interactions.

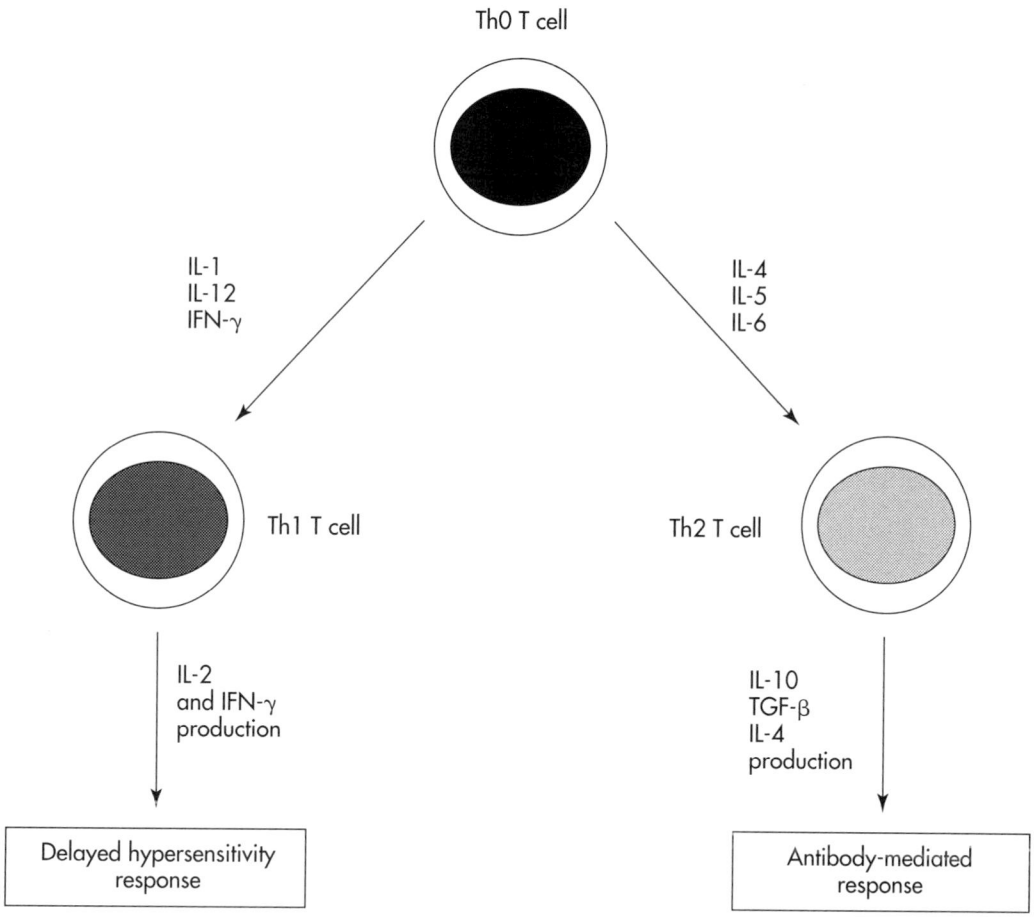


**Fig. 1-3.** Subtypes of T helper cells and their products.

The B cell, under proper conditions, will develop into a plasma cell that is capable of secreting immunoglobulin. Therefore the role of the B cell is to function as the effector cell in humoral immunity. The unique characteristic of these cells is the presence of surface immunoglobulin on their cell membranes.

At least two distinct subgroups of B cells have been described. The first type, memory B cells, live for long periods, are readily activated, and will produce Ig isotypes other than IgM (see next section). These cells presumably play an important role in the anamnestic response of the organism. This is the very rapid antigen-

**Table 1-6.** Characterisitics of human immunoglobulins

| | IgG | IgA | IgM | IgE | IgD |
|---|---|---|---|---|---|
| Molecular weight ($10^3$) | 150 | 150-300 | 900 | 190 | 180 |
| Heavy chain | γ | α | μ | ϵ | δ |
| Subclass | 1, 2, 3, 4 | 1, 2 | 1, 2 | – | – |
| J chain | | + | + | | |
| Crosses placenta | + | – | – | – | – |
| Serum half-life (days) | 21 | 6 | 5 | 2 | 3 |
| Complement activation | + | – | + | – | – |
| Serum concentration (mg/dl) | 110 | 25 | 10 | 0.001 | .3 |
| **IN EYE** | | | | | |
| Conjunctiva | Rich | Rich | Varies | Varies | Varies |
| Cornea | Moderate | Moderate | 0 | ? | 0 |
| Aqueous | Low | Low | Low | ? | 0 |
| Iris | Low | Low | Low | Varies | Varies |
| Choroid | Rich | Rich | Rich | Varies | Varies |
| Retina | Low | Low | Low | 0 | 0 |
| Vitreous | – | – | – | – | – |

From Allansmith M: Unpublished data, 1987. Used by permission.

specific immune response that occurs when the immune system encounters an antigen to which it has already been sensitized. Another subgroup consists of B1 ($CD5^+$) lymphocytes, whose characteristics overlap with other B cells, but they appear to be derived from a separate lineage and they are very long-lived. These cells produce IL-10, and they have been associated with autoantibody production. Chronic lymphocytic leukemias often derive from B1 cells.

B cells initially express surface immunoglobulins M and D (IgM, IgD) simultaneously, with differentiation occurring only after appropriate activation. Five major classes of immunoglobulins are identified on the basis of the structure of their heavy chains, which are alpha, gamma, mu, delta, and episilon, corresponding to immunoglobulins A, G, M, D, and E (Table 1-6). The structure of the immunoglobulin demonstrates a symmetry with two heavy and two light chains uniformly seen in all classes (Fig. 1-4). The production of immunoglobulin usually requires T-cell participation. Most "relevant" antigens are T-cell dependent, meaning that the addition of antigen to a culture of pure B cells will not induce immunoglobulin production. However, polyclonal B-cell activators, such as pneumococcus cell wall lipopolysaccharide, pokeweed mitogen, dextran, and the Epstein-Barr virus, have the capacity to directly induce B-cell proliferation and immunoglobulin production. Interleukin-4 (IL-4, B cell–stimulatory factor 1), a lymphokine produced by some T cells, plays an important role in B-cell activation. Sometimes in conjunction with costimulants, IL-4 will cause resting B cells to express large numbers of class II antigens on their surface and helps them switch to produce IgG1 on subsequent stimulation with lipopolysaccharide. Another lymphokine playing a role in B cell maturation is IL-5 or B cell–growth factor 2. IL-7 also plays a role in the early maturation process of pre–B cells.

An important need of the B-cell system is to rapidly respond to immunoglobulin needs as the demands change, that is, to switch from one Ig type to another. This Ig class switching, which requires a gene rearrangement, is inherent to the B cell and is in part controlled by lymphokines. IL-4 has been associated with a switch to express IgG and IgE, whereas IFN-γ controls a switch to IgG2a and TGF-β to IgA.

**Classes of immunoglobulins.** Immunoglobulin G (IgG) is the major immunoglobulin class found in the human being, making up three quarters of the total immunoglobulin produced. Plasma cells that produce IgG are found mainly in the spleen and the lymph nodes. Four subclasses of IgG have been identified in human beings (G1-G4). G1 and G3 fix complement readily and can be transmitted to the fetus.

Immunoglobulin M (IgM) consists as a pentamer made up of the typical antibody structure linked by disulfide bonds and J chains (Fig. 1-5).

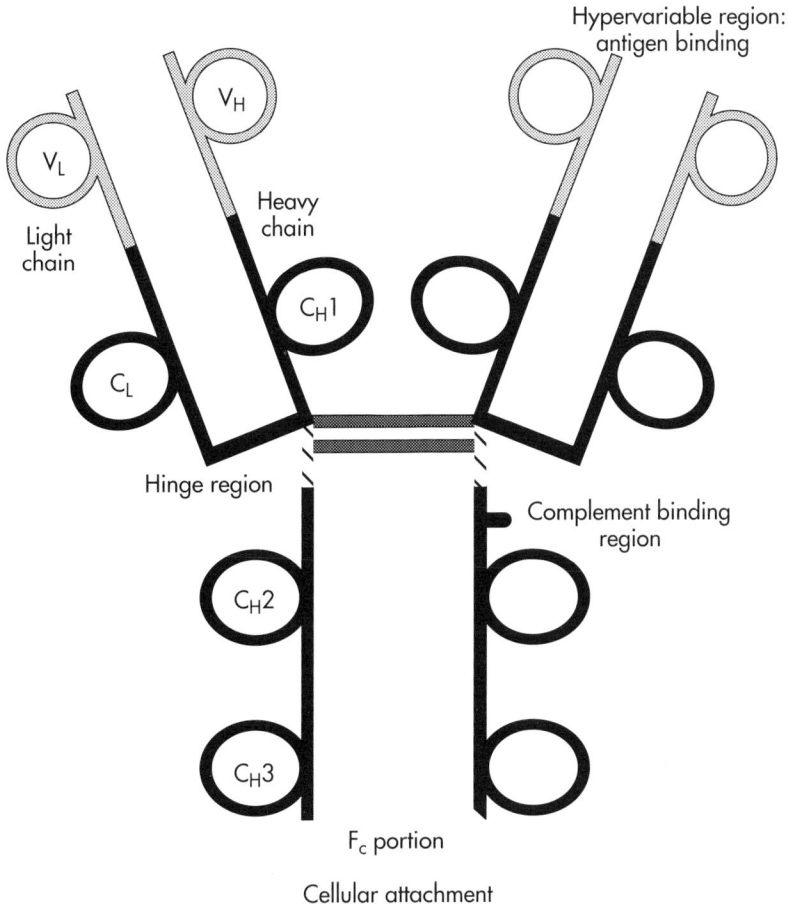


**Fig. 1-4.** Structure of human IgG molecule.

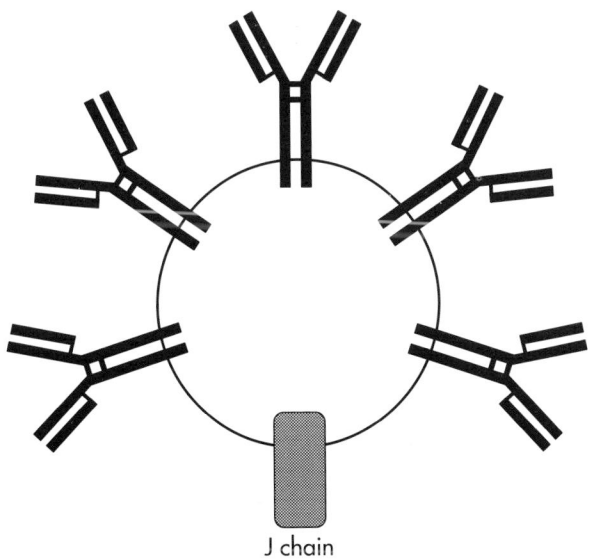


**Fig. 1-5.** IgM pentamer with J chain.

Only about one fifteenth as much IgM is produced as compared with IgG. Because of its size, it generally stays within the systemic circulation and, unlike IgG, will not cross the blood-brain barrier or the placenta. This antibody is expressed early on the surface of B cells. Therefore, initial antibody responses to exogenous pathogens, such as *Toxoplasma gondii,* are of this class. The observation of an IgM-specific antibody response helps to confirm a recent, newly acquired infection. IgM has a complement binding site. It can mediate phagocytosis by fixing C3a, a component of the complement system.

One major role of both IgG and IgM is to interact with both effector cells and the complement system to limit the invasion of exogenous organisms. These immunoglobulins aid effector cells through opsonization, which occurs by the antibody coating an invading organism and assisting the phagocytic process. The Fc portion of the antibody molecule then can readily interact with effector cells, such as macrophages (or T cells), thereby helping effectively clear the infection. Persons with deficiencies in IgG and IgM are particularly prone to infection by pyogenic organisms such as *Streptococcus* and *Neisseria spp.* In addition, both of these antibodies will activate the complement pathway, inducing lysing cells by that mechanism as well.

Immunoglobulin A (IgA) is the major extravascular immunoglobulin although it comprises only about 10% to 15% of the intravascular total. Two isotypes of IgA are noted, with IgA1 more commonly seen intravascularly, whereas IgA2 is somewhat more prevalent in the extravascular space. The IgA-secreting plasma cells are found in the subepithelial spaces of the gut, respiratory tract, tonsils, and the salivary and lacrimal glands. IgA is an important component to the ocular surface's defense mechanism, being found in a dimer linked by a J chain, a polypeptide needed for polymerization. In addition, a secretory component, a unique protein with parts of its molecule having no homology to other proteins, is needed for the IgA to appear in the extravascular space. The secretory component is produced locally by epithelial cells that then complex with the IgA dimer/J chain (Fig. 1-6). This new complex is internalized by mucosal cells and then is released on the apical surface of the cell through a proteolytic process. The amount of IgA within the eye is quite small. IgA

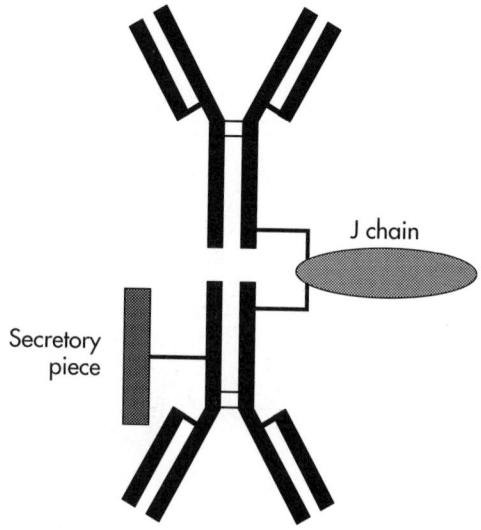


**Fig. 1-6.** IgA dimer with J chain and secretory piece.

can fix complement through the alternate pathway, and it can serve as an opsinin for phagocytosis. IgA appears to exert its major role by preventing entry of pathogens into the internal environment of the organism by binding with the infectious agent. It may also impede the absorption of potential toxins and allergens into the body as well. Further, it can induce eosinophil degranulation.

Immunoglobulin E (IgE) is slightly heavier than IgG because its heavy chain has an additional constant domain. IgE has the shortest half-life of the immunoglobulin classes except perhaps for secreted IgD. Mast cells and basophils have Fc receptors for IgE, and IgE is thought to be one of the major mediators of the allergic or anaphylactoid reaction (see next section). It appears to be an important defense mechanism against parasites; one way IgE accomplishes this is to prime basophils and mast cells. Although its role in ocular surface disease has been well recognized, this has not been the case for intraocular inflammation.

Immunoglobulin D (IgD) is found in minute quantities in the serum (0.5% of serum Ig). It is found simultaneously with IgM on B cells before specific stimulation. Little more is known about this antibody other than it is a major B cell membrane receptor for antigen.

Antibodies directed toward specific antigens, particularly cell-surface antigens of the immune system, have provided the clinical and basic investigator with a powerful tool with which to identify various components of the immune system as was described in the T-cell section. The development of monoclonal antibodies

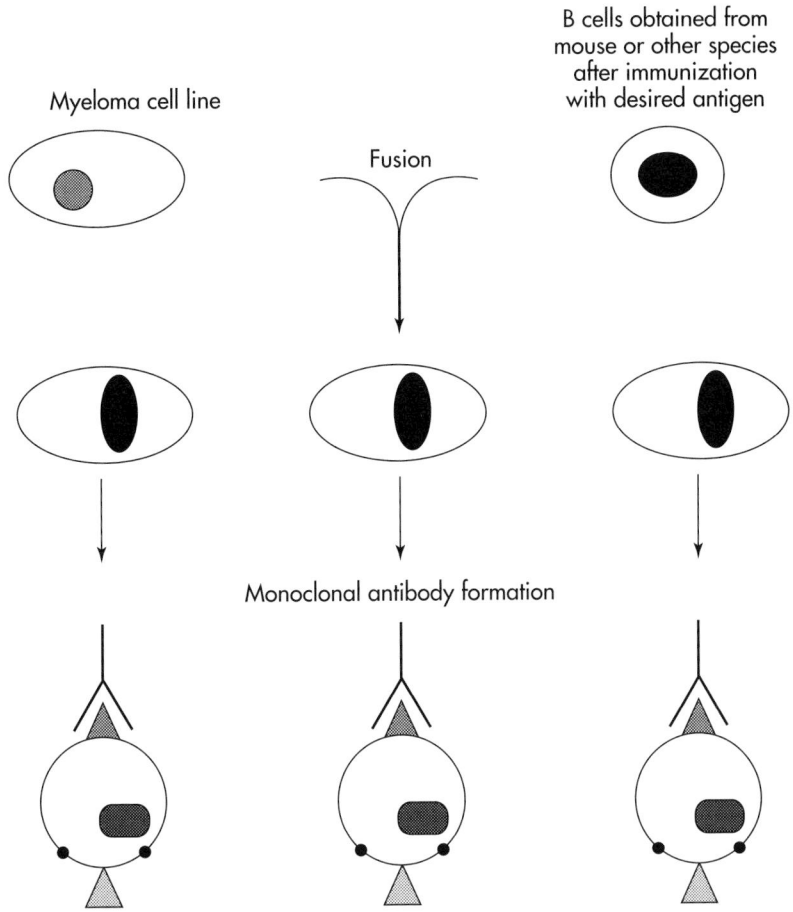


**Fig. 1-7.** Monoclonal antibody formation. B cells capable of secreting desired antibody are fused with myeloma cell. These fused cells are grown in medium that permits only fused cells to divide. These cells are then screened for production of desired antibody.

using hybridoma technology has permitted the production of these immune probes in almost unlimited quantity (Fig. 1-7). Immortalized myeloma cells can be fused with a B cell committed to the production of an antibody directed toward a relevant antigen. This is usually accomplished with the use of polyethylene glycol, which promotes cell membrane fusion. By careful screening, clones of these fused cells (i.e., hybrid cells or hybridomas) can be identified as producing the antibody needed. These can be isolated and grown, yielding essentially an unlimited source of the antibody, derived from one clone of cells and directed against one specific determinant. Monoclonal antibodies have been raised against cell markers of virtually all cellular components of the immune system (see Table 1-3). Antibodies can now be "humanized" so that only the variable end remains of mouse origin. The advantage to this is the decreased probability of an immune response to a foreign protein.

### Other cells

**Mast cells.** This large cell (15-20 μm) is intimately involved with type I hypersensitivity reactions (see next section). Its most characteristic feature is the presence of large granules in the cytoplasm. Mast cells, which contain a large number of biologically active agents, include histamine, serotonin, prostaglandins, leukotrienes, and chemotactic factors of anaphylaxis. Histamine is stored within the mast-cell granules. Once released into the environment, histamine can cause smooth muscle to contract and can increase small vessel permeability, giving the typical "wheal and flare" response noted in skin tests. Serotonin, in human beings, appears to have a major effect on vasoconstriction and blood pressure, whereas in rodents it may also affect vascular permeability. Prostaglandins, a family of lipids, are capable of stimulating a variety of biologic activities, including vasoconstriction and vasodilation. Leukotrienes are compounds produced de novo with antigen stimulation. Leukotriene $B_4$ is a potent chemotactic factor for both neutrophils and eosinophils, whereas leukotriene $C_4$ and $D_4$, for example, enhance vascular permeability. At least two chemotactic factors of anaphylaxis attract eosinophils to a site of mast-cell degranulation, whereas other factors attract and immobilize neutrophils.

Mast-cell involvement in several external ocular conditions has been established. However, it is not yet clear what role this cell may play in intraocular inflammatory disorders. Mast cells are present in abundance in the choroid, and they appear to be related to the susceptibility of at least one experimental model for uveitis (see discussion of autoimmunity in Chapter 2). Further, the control of mast-cell degranulation has been ascribed to certain T cell produced IgE–like molecules in mice, and if corroborated in humans, would broaden the role for this cell considerably.

**Eosinophils.** This bilobed nucleated cell, about 10 to 15 μm in size, is closer to the lymphoid series than are neutrophils. The most morphologically unique characteristic of these cells is the some 200 granules that are highly acidophilic (taking up eosin in standard staining procedures) and that are found in the cytoplasm. They are almost entirely made up of major basic protein (molecular weight [mol. wt.] 9000), but other toxic cationic granules include eosinophil-derived neurotoxia, eosinophil cationic protein, and eosinophil peroxidase. A minor percentage of these cells (5%-25%) have IgG receptors, and about half may have complement receptors on their cell-surface membranes, although it is not clear whether receptors for IgE are present. Eosinophils contain an abundant number of enzymes, which are quite similar in nature to those contained in neutrophils. Both cells contain a peroxidase and catalase, both of which can be antimicrobial, but eosinophils lack lysozymes and neutrophils lack the major basic protein. Eosinophils also contain several antiinflammatory enzymes, such as kininase, arylsulfatase, and histaminase.

The eosinophil arises in the bone marrow, probably from a separate stem cell than that of neutrophils. The time spent in the systemic circulation is probably quite short, and the number seen on a routine blood smear is usually very low (1% or less of nucleated cells). These cells can be attracted to an area in the body by the release of mast-cell products and, once localized to an inflammatory site, the cell is capable of performing several functions. The eosinophil may play an immunomodulatory role in the presence of mast-cell and basophil activation.

As mentioned, the cell contains the antiinflammatory agents histaminase and arylsulfatase, capable of neutralizing the effect of histamine release and slow-reacting substance, both products of mast cells. Further, basophil function may be inhibited by prostaglandins ($PGE_1$, $PGE_2$), both produced by eosinophils. An additional immunomodulatory mechanism is the capacity of the eosinophil to ingest immunoreactive granules released by mast cells. An extremely important role played by these cells is in the immune system's response to parasitic organisms. Eosinophils are seen in high numbers at the site of a parasitic infiltration and are known to bind tightly to the organism through receptors. Further, the release of the major basic protein granules or an eosinophil-produced peroxidase complexed with $H_2O_2$ and deposited on the parasite's surface membrane will lead to the death of the invading organism. Major basic protein may play a role in corneal ulceration in severe cases of allergy.

**Resident ocular cells.** The interaction of the resident ocular cells with those of the immune system is a most provocative concept. It is clear that several cells of the eye, including the retinal pigment epithelium and the Müller cell, have either functions similar to cells within the immune system or can be induced to bear markers that potentially permit them to participate in immune-mediated events. It may be that the initial priming of the immune system may occur through this interchange or that the continued recruitment of immune cells may be mediated through these mechanisms. The effect of immune cells and their products may also be important for certain ocular conditions, inasmuch as macrophage, as well as T-cell products, have a profound effect on fibrocyte growth and division, and the retinal pigment epithelium and Müller cell may respond in like fashion. The retinal pigment epithelium, when activated, can act as efficient antigen-presenting cells. Numerous lymphokines are found in the eye, many of them produced by ocular resident cells.

### Complement system

The complement system is a cascade of soluble proteins that "complement" the function of antibodies in the immune system. Each complement protein is a proteolytic enzyme that acts as substrate for the enzymes which precede it in the cascade and that then acts as a part of a proteolytic complex for the next protein in the cascade. The classic complement pathway begins when C1q, C1r, and C1s (parts of the first component of complement) interact with membrane bound antigen–antibody complexes to form an enzyme that cleaves C4 into C4a and C4b. C4b binds to the cell membrane, followed by C2, which is then split by C1s to yield a complex called C4b,2b. This complex splits C3 into C3a and C3b, which then joins the complex to make C4b,2b,3b. This complex cleaves C5 into C5a and C5b. C5b then binds to the cell membrane, and C6, C7, and C8 bind to it. The resulting C5b,6,7,8 complex then leads to C9 polymerization into the membrane.

The alternate pathway of complement does not require antibody, but it can be activated directly by bacterial cell walls and is therefore a nonspecific defense mechanism. In this pathway a small amount of preexisting C3b cleaves factor B into Ba and Bb. The bacterial cell wall or other membranes assist in the step. The resulting C3b,Bb complex then cleaves more C3, forming a C3b,Bb,3b complex, which can then cleave C5, and the pathway proceeds as already described.

The end result is the generation of chemotactic protein fragments (C5a), protein fragments that cause smooth muscle contraction (C3a and C5a), protein fragments that cause mast-cell degranulation (C5a), molecules that assist in neutrophil phagocytosis (C3b), and molecules that are capable of promoting cell lysis (C5b,6,7,8,9). The complement system therefore is involved in many of the effectors of the inflammatory response.

## CELLULAR INTERACTIONS: HYPERSENSITIVITY REACTIONS

### Interactions of immune components

Fig. 1-8 is a simplified version of the myriad number of interactions that have been

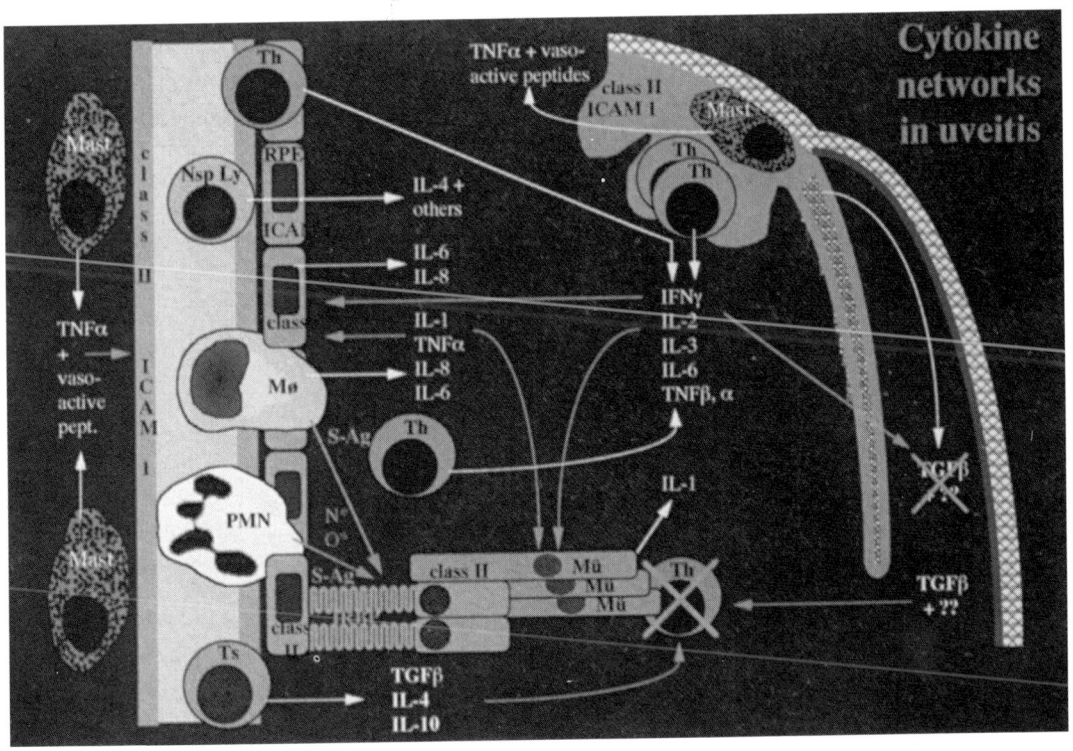


**Fig. 1-8.** Schematic representation of (1) numerous interactions within eye of immune system's cells and (2) cells resident in eye. (Courtesy Rachel Caspi, Ph.D.) (See Color Plate 1.)

identified in the immune system's repertoire in the eye. Although many exceptions and alternative mechanisms (sometimes contradictory) have been proposed or partially demonstrated, certain useful basic concepts can be of help to the observer. The initiation of a response leading to immune memory requires antigen to be presented to T cells. This classically is performed by macrophages bearing the same class II (HLA-DR) antigens as the T cells. Other cells, however, may also be equally competent in performing this task. Potential candidates in the eye include the vascular endothelium, retinal pigment epithelium, and Müller cells. Macrophages release factors such as IL-1 that are imperative for the activation of the T cell. IL-1 also may be necessary as a cell-membrane component for antigen presentation to occur.

The mechanism of antigen presentation is a most interesting question, still not fully understood. However, it appears that macrophages internalize antigen for processing, whereas nonimmune cells capable of performing such a task may perform the processing of antigen at the cell-surface membrane, with no internalization being necessary. Factors released by the T cell after activation, such as interferon, can also affect the antigen-presenting cell by stimulating class II antigen expression and thereby enhancing antigen presentation. The inducer T cell may then recruit other T cells capable of doing specific tasks or will itself become one of these "effector" cells.

The subsets of T cells, discussed earlier, cover a wide range of functions, from aiding B cells to produce antibody, to cell-mediated killing, to downregulation of the immune response (suppression). Two points are worth bearing in mind. The first is that T-cell recruitment is very much dependent on the release of factors (cytokines), which will help to recruit and activate other initially noncommitted T cells. This seems to be a basic underlying mechanism for T-cell functioning. The second point is the concept of T-cell circuitry, in which detailed schemes similar to chemical reactions are frequently hypothesized. Although this undoubtedly is an invaluable method by which the observer can begin to come to grips with this complex system, a counter theory that deserves to be mentioned is one that disclaims the existence of such circuits. This theory argues that a specific T cell may be pluripotential and that its functional role is determined not only by what antigens it is expressing on its cell surface but also by what the surrounding cells in the environment are expressing on their cell surface.

Other cells also have a major impact on this T-cell, B-cell macrophage axis. Mast-cell degranulation may help egress of immune cells into an organ, and the eosinophils, as well as neutrophils, will aid in killing and/or preparing pathogens for disposal by other parts of the immune system. T cells have a direct effect on mast-cell maturation in the bone marrow by the release of IL-3, whereas the T cell and other immune components have similar effects on other cells of the nonlymphoid series by the release of colony-stimulating factors.

### Classic immune hypersensitivity reactions

Although it is not rare for any inflammatory response to involve several arms of the immune repertoire, it frequently appears that one arm of the system predominates. Inflammatory reactions were originally classified into four types or "hypersensitivity reactions" by the British immunologists Philip Gell and Robin Coombs, with some recent additions.

**Type I.** This inflammatory reaction is mediated by antibodies, especially IgE. The binding of this antibody to mast cells or basophils results in the degranulation of these cells and the release of pharmacologically active products as already mentioned. An ocular example of this reaction is that of hay fever. Typically a large amount of edema without structural damage is noted. The role for this immune mechanism in intraocular inflammatory disease is still quite unclear. It is not inconceivable that mast cells could play an ancillary role in some cases, but hard evidence is still lacking.

**Type II.** This type of reaction is mediated by cytotoxic antibodies. This reaction is one that is thought to mediate hemolytic disorders, such as occurs in blood mismatch reactions and the scarring seen in ocular pemphigoid. It is clear that in ocular pemphigoid antibodies directed to the basement membrane of mucosal surfaces are present and may indeed be cytotoxic. However, T cells can be noted to be infiltrating into the lesion in this disease. Some have suggested including within this category those reactions termed *antibody-dependent cell-mediated cytotoxicity* (ADCC), thereby making this category one that has a mixed mechanism.

**Type III.** This reaction frequently is referred to as an immune complex–mediated inflammatory response. The binding of antibody to an antigen—either fixed in tissue or free-floating that then deposits as a complex—can initiate the complement cascade, which in turn attracts cells capable of causing tissue damage. An example is the Arthus reaction, seen some 4 hours after the injection of antigen into the skin of a sensitized person or animal having substantial levels of circulating antibody directed to the antigen being injected locally. This hypersensitivity reaction had been suggested as being one of the major immune mechanisms leading to intraocular inflammatory disease, such as Behçet's disease. However, more recent evidence suggests that its role in the uveitic process is more limited. Phacoanaphylaxis is a disorder that appears to be immune complex driven, at least in part.

**Type IV.** This category of immune response is for those mediated solely by T cells. It is therefore termed a *cell-mediated immune mechanism,* rather than humoral, as was the case for the other three types of hypersensitivity reactions. The positive skin test reaction noted 48 hours after a PPD test is placed in the skin is an example of a type IV hypersensitivity reaction. Granulomatous responses as seen in sarcoid are mediated by this mechanism as well, as is sympathetic ophthalmia. In all of these cases the role of the humoral arm of the immune system is thought not to play a significant role in the inflammatory reaction. Most recent evidence suggests, indeed, that T-cell dysregulation or T cell–controlled inflammatory responses are an extremely important, perhaps even preeminent, mechanism for intraocular inflammatory disease.

**Type V.** This reaction has been added to the original four. In this reaction an antibody can act as a stimulant to a target cell or organ. An example is long-acting thyroid stimulator (LATS) antibody. LATS is directed toward a portion of the hormone receptor in the thyroid and mimics the function of thyroid-stimulating hormone.

## SUGGESTED READINGS

Gallin JI, Goldstein IM, Snyderman R, editors: *Inflammation: basic principles and clinical correlates,* ed 2, New York, 1992, Raven Press.

Paul WE, editor: *Fundamental immunology,* ed 3, New York, 1993, Raven Press.

Roitt I, Brostoff J, Male D: *Immunology,* ed 3, St Louis, 1993, Mosby.

Detrick B, Hooks JJ: Cytokines in human immunology. In Leffell MS, Bias WB, Donnenberg DD, et al, editors: *CRC handbook of human immunology,* Boca Raton, Fla, 1995, CRC Press.

# CHAPTER 2

# Concepts of Disease Pathogenesis

The potential mechanisms by which tissue damage is mediated by the immune system pose a question that has been hotly debated for some time. The debates are particularly vociferous because most arguments are difficult to prove. Recently these potential mechanisms have opened some of their secrets to observers, and the arguments of a previous generation are no longer acceptable. With our increased understanding of immune mechanisms comes the realization of the network's complexity—that the system has many alternative choices and that there is an extraordinary intertwining of events that appears to be needed for the immune system to respond appropriately, as well as inappropriately. It still is conceptually valid to simplify these potential mechanisms, and the following pages attempt to do that—to provide the reader with concepts rather than numerous specifics. The understanding of these mechanisms is certainly an intellectually stimulating undertaking. However, this understanding has as well a clearly practical aspect. Therapeutic interventions will be increasingly specific, tailored to the problem at hand. Therefore, in the not too distant future, understanding mechanisms of ocular inflammatory disease will be invaluable in choosing the appropriate therapy for the patient.

## IMMUNE CHARACTERISTICS OF EYE

It seems reasonable to begin a chapter on immune mechanisms that may be responsible for intraocular inflammatory disease by reviewing the characteristics of the eye that may influence these responses. For years the eye was considered to be a "privileged" immune site. The implication of this term was that the immune system somehow ignored or was tolerant to the antigens in the eye. We think it appropriate to consider the eye as being immune-privileged, but in a different way than the original notion implied. Although the characteristics to be reviewed are not always unique to the eye, the combination of all these factors does elevate this organ to a special relationship with the immune system.

### Absence of lymphatic drainage

As with the brain, placenta, and testes, the eye has no normal lymphatic drainage. The environment in which antigen presentation occurs plays an important role in the type of immune response that the organism may mount. Experimentally, for example, antigen placed in an area with good lymphatic drainage will elicit an excellent immune response, with a measurable antibody response and cell-mediated immune response. However, the same antigen given intravenously may elicit a very different immune response, with the ultimate response being that of immune tolerance (or anergy). Therefore this anatomic phenomenon may have a profound effect on the types of immune responses that are elicited in the eye.

## Intraocular microenvironment

**Anterior chamber–associated immune deviation.** The immune response elicited by antigen placement into the anterior chamber has interested immunologists for some time. Allogeneic tissue implants (i.e., tissue from the same species but not an identical twin) in the anterior chamber were noted to survive longer than those placed in other orthotopic sites.[1] The placement of alloantigens into the anterior chamber of the eye has been noted to elicit a transient depression of cell-mediated immunity but an intact humoral response. This was initially called an $F_1$-lymphocyte–induced immune deviation.[2] A continued refinement and understanding of the phenomenon led to it being called the *anterior chamber–associated immune deviation* (ACAID).[3] The model has been further extended to include hapten-specific suppressor T-cell responses to syngeneic splenocytes that are coupled with azobenzenearsonate[4] (i.e., cell-bound antigens) and also has been obtained with soluble antigen alone,[5] such as histocompatibility and tumor antigens. In addition, the induction of ACAID can be enhanced by placing a cell line or tumor that is syngeneic to the major histocompatibility complex (MHC) of the host,[6] and the capacity of the immune system to enhance or suppress tumor growth can be successfully manipulated by use of this phenomenon. Good antibody responses and cytotoxic T cells directed against the intraocularly placed tumor (or antigen) develop. However, although cells that mediate delayed hypersensitivity reactions do not form, antigen-specific suppressor cells do.

ACAID can be induced in primates,[7] rats, and mice.[5,8] An antigen-specific ACAID will develop with the injection of interphotoreceptor retinoid-binding protein (IRBP) into the anterior chamber of rats or mice.[5,8] Of interest as well is the fact that the mice susceptible to IRBP-induced experimental autoimmune ureoretinitis (EAU) will not develop the disease if IRBP is injected into the eye before systemic immunization.[7]

Of prime import in ACAID is the presence of an intact ocular-splenic axis. The induction of suppressor T cells is enhanced when antigen processing bypasses the lymphatic drainage system normally present. There appears to be a unique processing of antigen in the dendritic cells of the eye. Cells then will carry the ACAID signal to the spleen for the activation of regulatory T cells. It has been reported that this signal in the blood was associated with F4/80+ macrophages, which populate the anterior uvea.[9] It appears that this signal is water soluble. Of interest is that in vitro exposure of antigen-presenting cells to aqueous humor—or transforming growth factor–β (TGF-β)—will confer ACAID-like properties on these cells.[10] Indeed, TGF-β appears to be playing one of the important roles in ACAID. Other investigators[11] have noted a soluble factor that could be transferred by serum alone. This apparent contradiction might reflect the different experimental methods that were used. It could, however, also reflect that several mechanisms may exist for the induction of ACAID. Indeed, the disruption of the normal ACAID mechanism with the addition of INF-γ into the eye, prostaglandins may replace TGF-β as the mediator of suppression.[12]

The role of ACAID in clinical situations still needs to be evaluated; however, it is not difficult to speculate as to its potential role in ocular tumor, as well as autoimmune and even infectious immune responses. This could be a mechanism by which nature attempts to limit unwanted inflammatory responses in the eye.[13]

**Resident ocular cells and immune system.** Although communication between resident organ cells and the immune system is not unique to the eye, the number of cells potentially capable of fulfilling this role in the eye is indeed remarkable. The list begins at the cornea with Langerhans cells, to cells in the ciliary body that can express Ia antigens on their surfaces, to the Müller cells, which are capable of profound effects on the immune response, to the retinal pigment epithelium, with characteristics very similar to those of macrophages. Finally, the vascular endothelium of the eye, as in other organs, may be of great import in regulating immune system activity.

Müller cells have been shown to have a profound affect on T cells.[14] Isolated pure cultures of rat Müller cells will downregulate the proliferative capabilities of S antigen–specific T cells capable of inducing experimental uveitis. Cell-to-cell contact is needed to see this phenomenon. It is interesting to note that when Müller cells are killed with a specific poison, the disease induced by S-antigen immunization in rats appears to be worse than in rats with "intact" retinal Müller cells in the retina.[15] Such experiments would suggest that Müller cells play a similar role as does ACAID—that is, part of the protective mechanisms in the eye that downregulate "nuisance" inflammatory responses in the eye.

A very different story seems to emerge with both corneal endothelial cells and the retinal pigment epithelium (RPE). Kawashima and Gregerson[16] reported that corneal endothelial cells block T-cell proliferation, but T-cell activation signals from an antigen-presenting cell were not blocked. This inhibition was not neutralized by the addition of neutralizing antibodies to TGF-β1 or TGF-β2.

As mentioned, the RPE has many characteristics of macrophages. These cells have the capacity to migrate and engulf particles. They have characteristics that strongly suggest a capacity to participate in the local immune response. The RPE has been shown to produce cytokines, perhaps the one of most note to date being interleukin-6 (IL-6),[17] a lymphokine capable of inducing intraocular inflammatory disease when injected into the eye. RPE cells, which express MHC class I antigens constitutively on their surface, can express class II antigens when activated[18] (see later discussion). Further, RPE cells in culture can act as antigen-presenting cells for S antigen–specific T cells.[19] Here then it would appear that we have an example of an ocular resident cell capable of augmenting (or initiating?) an immune response in the eye.

**Cytokines and eye.** A large number of cytokines, some produced locally by ocular resident cells, others made by cells of the immune system, have been implicated in the ocular immune response. In addition to cytokines, numerous neuropeptides and other factors have been cited as being involved in the ocular immune response. (See Fig. 1-8, which shows the complex nature of this response.) As a result of numerous experiments, cytokines can be termed "proinflammatory" or "immunosuppressive" in the intraocular milieu (see Box 2-1). Some cytokines have been noted to both stimulate and suppress the immune response, depending on the environment in which the cytokine is found. Instead of considering it contradictory, this phenomenon should be viewed as evidence of the complex immune response we are studying. IL-6 (produced locally), IL-2, and IFN-γ are perhaps the most important cytokines to be considered when an intraocular inflammatory response occurs.

**Box 2-1**
**Cytokines**

**PROINFLAMMATORY CYTOKINES**

| | |
|---|---|
| IL-1 | TNF |
| IL-6 | IL-2 |
| IL-3 | IL-8 |
| IFN-γ | IL-4 |

**ANTIINFLAMMATORY CYTOKINES**

| | |
|---|---|
| TGF-β | IL-4 (systemic) |
| IFN-γ | IL-10 |

The ocular immunosuppressive microenvironment appears to be rich in factors, as already noted; in addition to TGF-β,[20,21] which has been localized to trabecular cells,[22] α-melanocyte-stimulating hormone,[23] calcitonin gene-related peptide,[24] vasoactive intestinal peptide,[25] and IL-10 can be found. Other factors, such as hormones, may significantly affect the microenvironment. Sternberg and colleagues[26] have shown that rats not capable of mounting a major intrinsic cortisol response to trauma (or immunization with protein) are more prone to the development of autoimmune disorders. This observation is of further interest because the aqueous is deficient in cortisol-binding globulin; therefore this hormone could play a most important role in downregulating an immune response in the eye.[27]

**Oral tolerance.** It seems reasonable to speak about a novel approach at immunosuppression at this point because it is one dependent on the body's own immunosuppressive mechanisms. Oral tolerance is a long-recognized method to induce systemic tolerance. It was first described by Wells in 1911 who prevented anaphylaxis in guinea pigs by feeding them egg protein.[28] Chase[29] showed in 1946 that feeding the hapten dinitrofluorobenzene (DNFB) suppressed contact sensitivity. Information about positive mechanisms has been gained over the past few years.[30] Three possible immune mechanisms can be hypothesized: clonal deletion of autoaggressive cells, clonal anergy, and active suppression. Most information would suggest that active suppression is perhaps a predominant mechanism, but it is also clear that clonal anergy can be demonstrated under certain circumstances.[31,32] TGF-β appears to be the basic mediator of the active suppression seen after feeding. In studies using myelin basic protein, Miller and coworkers[33] showed that the epitopes of myelin basic protein that triggers TGF-β after feeding were distinct from the encephalitogenic epitopes.

Oral tolerance has been shown to markedly alter the expression of S-antigen–induced experimental autoimmune uveoretinitis (EAU).[34] Feeding S-antigen to Lewis rats before immunization with this antigen suppressed the expression of EAU. Feeding S-antigen even after immunization with S-antigen still was capable of suppressing EAU. Further, regulatory cells could be isolated from the spleen of fed animals. These are Th2 cells, cells that are capable of downregulating, as opposed to immune augmenting Th1 cells (see Chapter 1). An intact spleen appears to be important in the development of this phenomenon.[35] It is of interest to note that nasal administration of retinal antigens can also suppress EAU,[36] but in our hands it did not appear to be as effective as oral administration of antigen.

Because of these initial data and information being gathered from our collaborators working in the realm of other animal models and with patients having multiple sclerosis, we embarked on a pilot study in which we fed S-antigen to two patients with uveitis who were receiving immunosuppressive therapy for their disease. We hoped that we could induce immune tolerance and therefore stop or decrease their immunosuppressive therapy.[37] In one patient with pars planitis, oral prednisone was discontinued after the initiation of S-antigen feeding. The therapeutic response was so dramatic that S-antigen feeding was stopped. This resulted in a recurrence of his disease. Retreatment with prednisone and then subsequent feeding of S-antigen resulted in a similar positive therapeutic response (see Chapter 8). The two patients' responses have been so positive that a randomized double-masked study has begun.

### Uveitogenic antigens

The presence of uveitogenic antigens in the eye that are capable of inducing disease is an old concept, proposed as early as 1910 by Elschnig.[38] As we will see in some detail in the later section on autoimmunity, several antigens have been isolated that are capable of inducing ocular disease—in many respects similar to that seen in humans. This number of identifiable antigens capable of stimulating the immune system makes the eye unique, and it suggests that the old concept of autoimmunity may be an important factor in ocular disease.

### Choroidal circulation and anatomy

The choroid has a blood flow that is comparable only to that of the kidney. Therefore systemic influences can be assumed to rapidly affect this portion of the eye. Indeed, the relatively large blood flow and its anatomy would act as a sort of trap for many blood-borne problems, most notably fungal disorders. Therefore most fungal lesions begin as a choroiditis.[39] The choroid has the capacity to function as a repository for immunoreactive cells, in the extreme taking on the anatomic structure of a lymph node (lymphoid hyperplasia). Therefore this organ can be the center for profound immune responses, as is the case in many disorders to be discussed. The high concentration of mast cells in the choroid may be one mechanism by which immunoreactive cells in the choroid could spread to other parts of the eye. The mast cell's release of immunoreactive factors could help T-cell egress and ingress from this compartment.

### Retina

In addition to the uveitogenic antigens resident in its layers, the retina's being an "extension of the brain" makes it particularly prone to certain neurotropic organisms. Examples include *Toxoplasma gondii* and many viruses of the herpes family, which have a propensity for central nervous system tissue.

It is also important to remember that under normal circumstances the retinal vasculature has tight junctions, thus being impermeable to many molecules. Any perturbation, such as an inflammatory one, that alters this permeability can result in a profound change in retinal functioning. Further, it is interesting to speculate that because the retina maintains a high degree of oxidative metabolism, the potential for the generation of oxygen radicals may lead to autotoxicity.

## IMMUNOGENETICS

The capacity to respond to a specific immune stimulant is genetically determined. It has been noted that various mouse strains are variably susceptible to the same bacterial infection.[40] Another example of such a variable response is that seen against an allograft—that is, tissue taken from the same species but not from an identical twin or another animal of an inbred strain. The strength of the immune reaction against the allograft is in large part determined by antigens sitting on cell surface membranes that are the products of genes classified as being in the MHC. The MHC region is termed the *H-2 region* in mice and the histocompatibility lymphocyte antigen (HLA) region in human beings. Immune response (IR) genes were discovered by Benacerraf and colleagues[41] in their experiments evaluating the immune response of guinea pigs to amino acid polymers. Breeding and crossbreeding led to the realization that a genetic region was responsible for this responsiveness or nonresponsiveness.[42] McDevitt and Chinitz[43] showed that antibody responses in mice to synthetic polypeptides were indeed linked to the MHC region. The observation that one region appeared responsible for both transplantation and general immune responses evoked enormous interest and led to the realization of the import of this region. The HLA gene loci are located on chromosome 6 in human beings. Three major classes of antigens are controlled by these genes.

### Class I antigens

The class I antigens, which are proteins found on essentially all nucleated cells, are controlled by three loci in human beings, A, B, and C. The class I molecule has a molecular weight of about 45,000 daltons, is a glycoprotein, and is noncovalently linked to a beta$_2$-microglobulin (Fig. 2-1, *A*). The beta$_2$-microglobulin molecule is not encoded within the MHC region but rather on chromosome 15, and it is linked to the class I molecule at a later stage. A strong homology has been shown between moieties of the class I molecule and immunoglobulins, suggesting similar early evolutionary paths. Class I molecules are quite heterogeneous, and several cell surface membrane antigens controlled by each of the loci are defined. Complement-fixing cytotoxic antibodies can be raised against each variation, and these antigens are determined by serologic methods. The molecule will have an extracellular portion of the molecule, with the molecule extending through the membrane into the cytoplasm of the cell. Although the precise mechanisms are still unknown, it is known that the class I antigens participate in transplantation immunity by being the principal antigenic targets in allograft rejection. They also serve as recognition antigens for cytotoxic T cells when attacking virally infected cells.

### Class II and class III antigens

The class II antigens are produced by the HLA-D/DR locus. Identification of the HLA-D cell surface antigen products is determined by the mixed lymphocyte culture, whereas the DR is determined by use of serologic methods. There has been considerable debate as to whether the D/DR systems are the same. Some discrepancies in typing by means of the two methods have been noted in some nonwhite populations. At least 10 alleles have been identified in the DR system. The test is performed on B cells by means of a complement-dependent microcytotoxicity assay and use of sera from multiparous women. The HLA-D/DR loci are thought to be the equivalent of the IR gene region already discussed. Further, the cell surface molecule expression these loci control have been given the generic term *Ia antigens*. The class II molecule is different from that of the class I. Here it is made up of an alpha chain with a molecular weight of 35,000 daltons and a beta chain of about 28,000 daltons, which are noncovalently bound. No beta$_2$-microglobulin is present (Fig. 2-1, *B*).

The importance of the IR gene products cannot be overstated, because large components of the immune response are histocompatibility restricted, meaning that immune cooperation will occur only if both components share identical D/DR antigens. B- and T-cell cooperation and T-cell cooperation with macrophages are such examples. This means that macrophages from one individual cannot present antigen to T cells from another unless they express the same class II antigens. In the case of the eye, the appearance of DR (or Ia) antigens on the cell surface of resident ocular cells (not usually thought of as part of the immune system) may indicate the potential for their role as accessory immune cells. Forrester

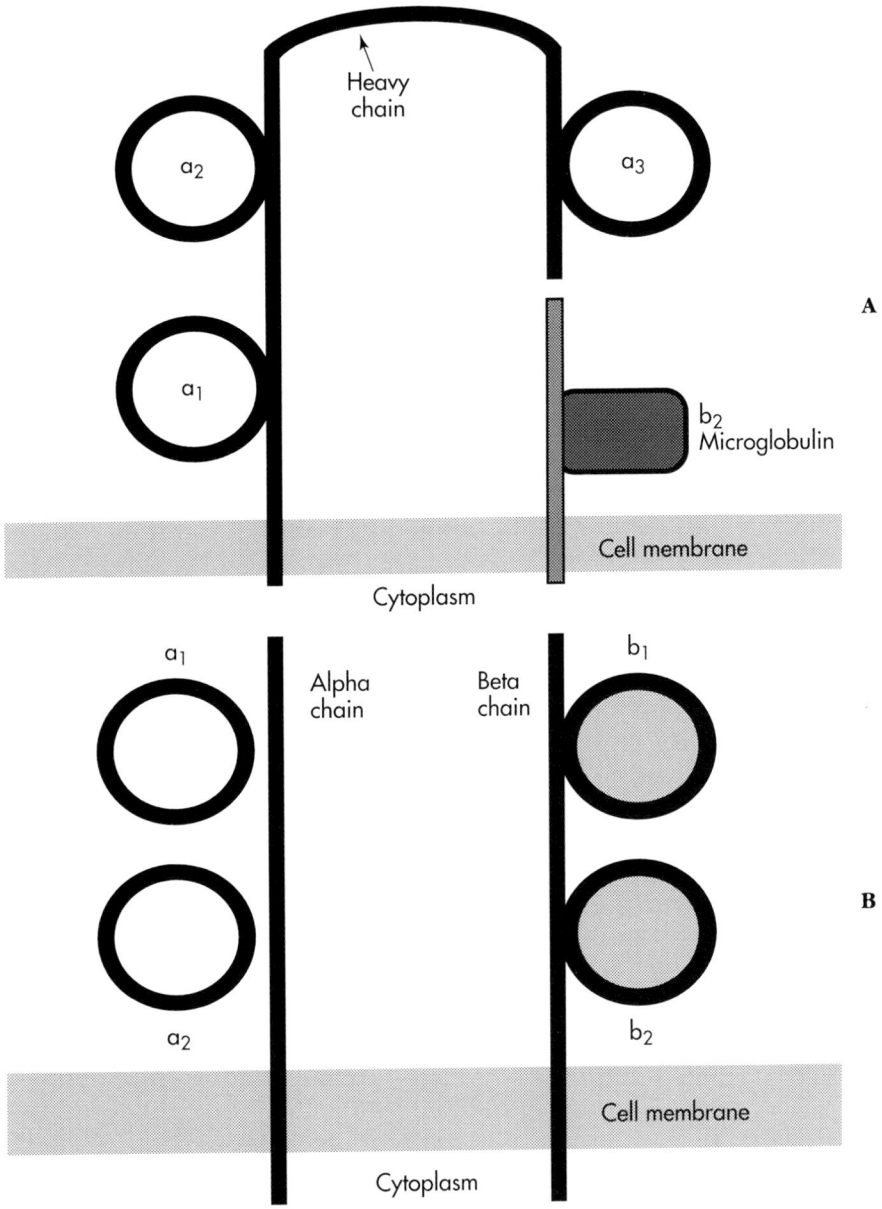


**Fig. 2-1. A,** Structure of class I antigen. **B,** Structure of class II antigen.

and colleagues[44] have found that the posterior uveal tract is richly populated with classic dendritic cells that constitutively express high levels of MHC II antigens. They further speculate about the important role in the interaction of resident ocular cells with the immune system and by extension their initiation of autoimmune responses in the posterior pole.

Class III antigens produced within the MHC region are components of the complement cascade. The control of the levels of C1, C2, and C4 may also be encoded in this region.

### Histocompatibility lymphocyte antigens

A logical adjunct to the recognition of the critical role the MHC region plays in the organism's immune response was the attempt to correlate certain disease processes with HLA antigens. Because there are four loci determining class I and II antigens, each human being has the capacity to bear a total of eight different alleles (four from each parent). Early on, testing could not reveal that number in many persons, either because they bear yet undetermined antigens or they are homozygote for a specific allele. Associations have been made with cer-

**Table 2-1.** Distribution of HLA haplotypes in patients with birdshot retinochoroidopathy and in control subjects

| HLA antigen | Phenotype frequency (%) | | Exact *p* | Relative risk |
|---|---|---|---|---|
| | Controls (*n* = 418) | Patients (*n* = 20) | | |
| **HLA-A** | | | | |
| 1 | 24.4 | 20.0 | 0.7935 | 0.78 |
| 2 | 52.6 | 35.0 | 0.1687 | 0.49 |
| 3 | 27.3 | 15.0 | 0.3044 | 0.47 |
| 9 | 17.9 | 10.0 | 0.5493 | 0.51 |
| 10 | 13.9 | 10.0 | 1.0000 | 0.69 |
| 11 | 13.6 | 5.0 | 0.4955 | 0.33 |
| 23 | 2.6 | 5.0 | 0.4335 | 1.95 |
| 24 | 14.6 | 5.0 | 0.3337 | 0.31 |
| 25 | 5.5 | 0.0 | 0.6147 | 0.00 |
| 26 | 8.1 | 10.0 | 0.6751 | 1.26 |
| 28 | 8.4 | 5.0 | 1.0000 | 0.58 |
| 29 | 7.4 | 80.0 | 0.0000* | 49.94 |
| 30 | 5.5 | 0.0 | 0.6147 | 0.00 |
| 31 | 4.3 | 0.0 | 1.0000 | 0.00 |
| 32 | 9.3 | 10.0 | 1.0000 | 1.08 |
| 33 | 1.4 | 0.0 | 1.0000 | 0.00 |
| 36 | 0.2 | 0.0 | 1.0000 | 0.00 |
| **HLA-B** | | | | |
| 5 | 13.6 | 5.0 | 0.4955 | 0.33 |
| 7 | 20.1 | 30.0 | 0.2676 | 1.70 |
| 8 | 14.4 | 20.0 | 0.5133 | 1.49 |
| 12 | 27.5 | 50.0 | 0.0409† | 2.64 |
| 13 | 4.8 | 0.0 | 0.6147 | 0.00 |
| 14 | 7.7 | 20.0 | 0.0719 | 3.02 |
| 15 | 13.6 | 0.0 | 0.0911 | 0.00 |
| 16 | 11.7 | 10.0 | 1.0000 | 0.84 |
| 17 | 10.5 | 10.0 | 1.0000 | 0.94 |
| 18 | 8.1 | 10.0 | 0.6751 | 1.26 |
| 21 | 9.3 | 10.0 | 1.0000 | 1.08 |
| 22 | 3.1 | 0.0 | 1.0000 | 0.00 |
| 27 | 8.9 | 0.0 | 3.978 | 0.00 |
| 35 | 19.4 | 15.0 | 0.7775 | 0.073 |
| 37 | 2.4 | 0.0 | 1.0000 | 0.00 |
| 38 | 7.4 | 5.0 | 1.0000 | 0.66 |
| 39 | 4.3 | 5.0 | 0.5964 | 1.17 |
| 40 | 12.0 | 10.0 | 1.0000 | 0.82 |
| 42 | 0.5 | 0.0 | 1.0000 | 0.00 |
| 44 | 25.4 | 45.0 | 0.6690 | 2.41 |
| 45 | 1.9 | 5.0 | 0.3460 | 2.70 |
| 47 | 0.7 | 0.0 | 1.0000 | 0.00 |
| 48 | 0.2 | 0.0 | 1.0000 | 0.00 |
| 49 | 5.7 | 5.0 | 1.0000 | 0.86 |
| 50 | 3.1 | 5.0 | 0.4855 | 1.64 |
| 51 | 6.0 | 5.0 | 1.0000 | 0.83 |
| 52 | 3.8 | 0.0 | 1.0000 | 0.00 |
| 53 | 3.4 | 0.0 | 1.0000 | 0.00 |
| 54 | 1.0 | 0.0 | 1.0000 | 0.00 |
| 55 | 0.7 | 0.0 | 1.0000 | 0.00 |
| **HLA-C** | | | | |
| 1 | 8.4 | 5.0 | 1.0000 | 0.58 |
| 2 | 9.1 | 10.0 | 0.7028 | 1.11 |
| 3 | 25.4 | 10.0 | 0.1819 | 0.33 |
| 4 | 20.6 | 15.0 | 0.7769 | 0.68 |
| 5 | 5.7 | 10.0 | 0.3358 | 1.82 |
| 6 | 5.5 | 5.0 | 1.0000 | 0.90 |

From Nussenblatt RB, Mittal KK, Ryan S et al: Birdshot retinochoroidopathy—an association with HLA-A29 and immune responsiveness to retinal S-antigen, *Am J Ophthalmol* 94:147-158, 1982. Used by permission.

*$P < .0001$.

†$P < .05$.

MEDICAL COLLEGE OF PENNSYLVANIA
AND HAHNEMANN UNIVERSITY
UNIVERSITY LIBRARY, CENTER CITY


tain diseases and HLA antigens. Brewerton and colleagues[45] were among the first to observe that an extremely high percentage of white patients with ankylosing spondylitis showed HLA-B27 positivity. The testing of other racial groups could not demonstrate as strong a correlation. Indeed, Khan and coworkers[46] demonstrated that HLA-B7 was associated with ankylosing spondylitis in African-Americans to a greater degree than was HLA-B27. One can infer from this and other studies that HLA associations may be different for various ethnic groups and perhaps that different genes initiate responses that lead ultimately to a common pathway that we identify as disease. HLA allele distributions can vary dramatically from one ethnic group to another.[47] Therefore testing for an HLA association in patients with a specific disease requires testing as well a large group of persons from the same gene pool who do not have the disease in question. This is done to determine the normal distribution of HLA antigens in that ethnic group. Only with this approach can a determination be made as to whether a specific HLA antigen is more prevalent in a disease entity.

An example of such an HLA distribution can be seen from our studies dealing with birdshot retinochoroidopathy (Table 2-1) (see Chapter 24). One can see from this table the distribution of alleles in both the white control and the white patient populations. Although not perhaps apparent initially, certain antigens may appear together more frequently than estimated by chance. This phenomenon is termed *linkage disequilibrium.* It indicates that certain HLA antigens appear consistently together more often than chance would allow. Such examples are HLA-A1, which is in known linkage disequilibrium with HLA-B8 and HLA-DR3; another would be HLA-A3 with HLA-B7 and HLA-DR2. In Table 2-1 it is HLA-A29 and HLA-B44. The percentage of patients bearing specific antigens can be seen, and the relative risk is calculated.

$$\text{Relative risk} = \frac{\text{Antigen-positive patients} \times \text{Antigen-negative control subjects}}{\text{Antigen-negative patients} \times \text{Antigen-positive control subjects}}$$

The relative risk is a most important indicator of the strength of the observation, because it indicates the increased risk for development of a given disease in persons carrying the antigen relative to those not carrying it. For birdshot retinochoroidopathy, it tells the observer that a white person who bears the HLA-A29 antigen has an almost 50 times greater potential risk for developing this disease. Relative risks that are 3 to 5 or below are usually of little practical help in determining risk. Some studies have used historic HLA data—that is, results obtained by others, at perhaps a different institution, with perhaps different anti-HLA sera. It is clear that use of such control subjects should be avoided if possible. Because of the great possible variation of HLA alleles in different groups, the use of control subjects of the same ethnic or racial group to that of the disease group is imperative.

Although mathematic programs exist to attempt to mix information gained from different ethnic or racial groups, the data obtained from these attempts are quite suspect. This basic rule poses real problems for those doing this type of research in countries with large numbers of citizens who are of mixed racial and ethnic parentage, such as in Brazil, where regional differences in terms of HLA distribution is great. Such problems also exist in India, where because of a strict caste system, groups never intermarried, thereby creating a large number of "mini-gene pools" in a society, which, to an outsider, may appear as homogeneous.

Ocular diseases have been evaluated extensively for their HLA associations (Table 2-2). Some of these associations have large relative risks associated with them. The reader should always scrutinize the findings carefully, bearing in mind the aforementioned principles.

Why should there be an HLA association with certain diseases? The simple answer is that it is unclear. The answer probably lies in multiple reasons. Some of the potential theories can be seen in Figure 2-2. The association may indeed reflect a specific immune response gene or one with which that gene is in linkage disequilibrium. Other concepts deal with HLA antigens and the exogenous environment. A provocative theory is one that was suggested by Botazzo and colleagues[48] some years ago. The reasoning behind this hypothesis is requirement of Ia antigens for antigen presentation and the initiation of the immune response. The inappropriate expression of Ia coupled with other lapses of immune surveillance could lead to disease. A report that would support this notion was recently reported by Taurog and

**Table 2-2.** Selected ocular diseases and their HLA associations

| Disease | Antigen | Relative risk |
|---|---|---|
| Acute anterior uvetis | HLA-B27(W)<br>HLA-B8,(AA) | 10<br>5 |
| Ankylosing spondylitis | HLA-B27(W)<br>HLA-B7 (AA) | 100 |
| Behçet's disease | HLA-B51(O)(?W) | 4-6 |
| Birdshot retinochoroidopathy | HLA-A29(W) | 49 |
| Ocular pemphigoid | HLA-B12(W) | 3-4 |
| Presumed ocular histoplasmosis | HLA-B7(W) | |
| Reiter's syndrome | HLA-B27(W) | 40 |
| Rheumatoid arthritis | HLA-DR4(W) | 11 |
| Sympathetic ophthalmia | HLA-A11(M) | 3.9 |
| Vogt-Koyanagi-Harada disease | MT-3(O) | 74.5 |

*AA,* African-American; *M,* mixed ethnic study; *O,* Oriental; *W,* white.

coworkers.[49] Taurog and group have produced rats transgenic for HLA-B27 and beta-2 microglobulin. They found that the B27 transgene was expressed in a copy number–dependent fashion, and inflammatory disease was dependent on the expression of B27 above a critical threshold. The implication of essentially all the theories is that the mechanisms are multifactorial and that exogenous and endogenous immune factors need to combine to produce disease. If not, disease expression would be far more common. A long series of experiments in mice with experimentally induced uveitis by Caspi and colleagues[50] supports this idea. From their observations, it is clear that the MHC plays a very important role in determining disease susceptibility. In mice certain permissive MHC types would include the H-$2^k$. However, the genetic background of the mice plays a very important role in determining the severity of the disease, so that a permissive MHC in a nonpermissive background will result in either very mild or no disease at all.

## IMMUNE COMPLEX–MEDIATED DISEASE

Type III hypersensitivity reactions were once thought to be the predominant mechanism of ocular inflammation. Immune complexes have a potentially important role in tissue destruction, but there may be an alternative role for immune complexes other than mediation of disease.

Immune complexes are formed by the association of an antibody with an autologous or exogenous antigen in the circulation, in the extravascular space, or on a cell surface. If the antibody molecule is of the IgM or IgG family, it has the capacity to bind to complement, therefore inducing tissue damage. The complexes often contain several immunoglobulin molecules and have a high molecular weight. One theory is that bivalent antigens are needed for the formation of immune complexes. Low levels of circulating immune complexes can be found in all normal persons. Immune complexes can function as an efficient way for the body to rid itself of unwanted tissue debris (or antigens), recognized more readily and removed more rapidly if bound to an antibody.

As mentioned, immune complexes can bind to tissue antigens, as in the kidney (an organ particularly prone to this type of immune-mediated damage) or to the vascular endothelium of many organs. With the fixing of complement, chemotactic factors could be released and neutrophils are attracted and activated. During this process they will release enzymes, which can degrade both proteins and collagen. This immune response will leave tissue damage, most frequently as areas of fibrinoid necrosis. In some models of immune complex–mediated disease of the lungs, tumor necrosis factor–α (TNF-α) appears to be an important cytokine that is a proinflammatory cytokine. This is mediated at least in part by the ability of TNF-α to upregulate the expression of adhesion molecules such as E-selectin and intercellular-adhesion molecule (ICAM)–1. The addition of IL-4 or IL-10, not only affects the production of TNF-α, but also reduces nitric oxide production, protecting animals from immune complex–mediated lung injury.[51]

Several disorders have been hypothesized as being mediated by the type III hypersensitivity reaction. Serum sickness seen after the administration of a foreign protein is one of the classic examples. At least part of the pathologic process noted in patients with systemic lupus erythematosus is thought to be mediated by this same mechanism, as is lens-induced endophthalmitis. Several infectious disorders are

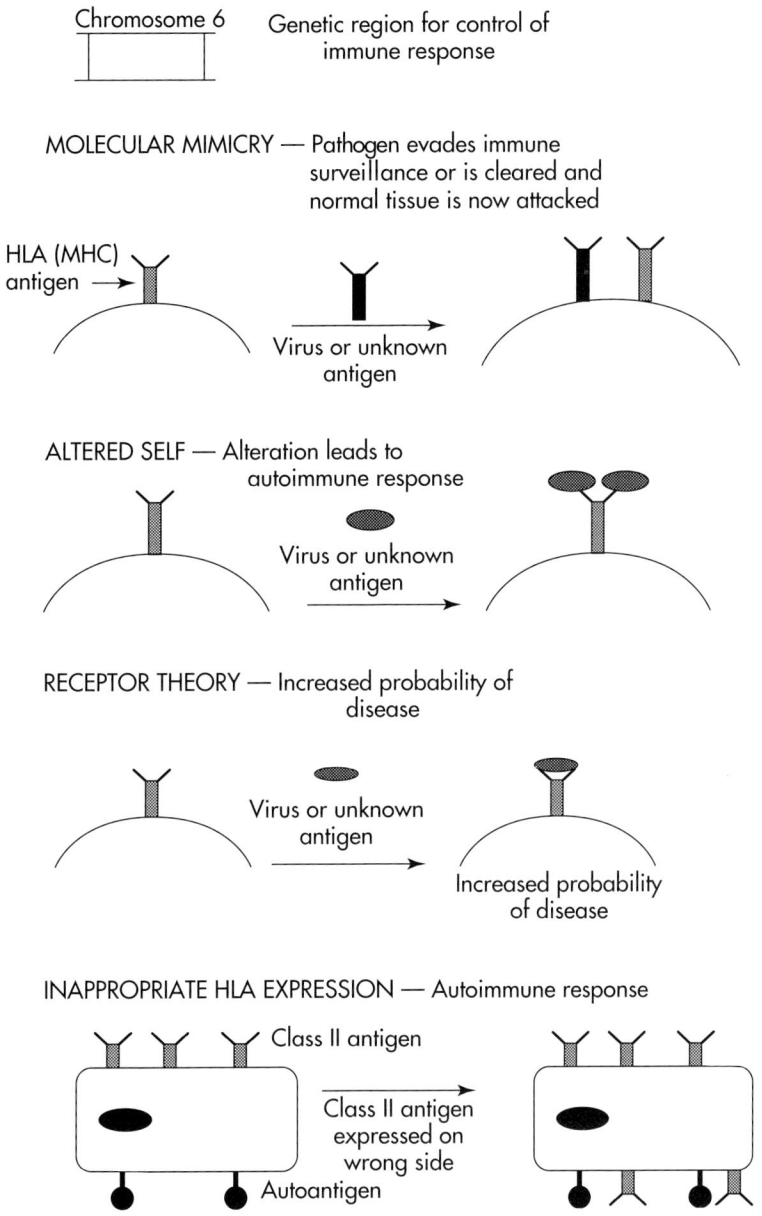


**Fig. 2-2.** Theoretic considerations that link HLA haplotypes to disease.

believed to have severe sequelae mediated by immune complexes as well. One such example is the severe renal disease seen after complexes form with soluble antigens of *Plasmodium falciparum.*

### Tissue damage in eye

The role of immune complex–mediated tissue damage in the eye still needs to be defined. Immune complexes can be demonstrated in the aqueous humour of patients with uveitis.[52,53] Circulating immune complexes have been reported in patients with Behçet's disease (see Chapter 25) and HLA-B27+ uveitis (see Chapter 19).[54,55] These findings, as well as others, have led some to speculate that immune complex–mediated tissue destruction could explain intraocular inflammatory disease and that recurrence of disease may be due to a repeated localization of immune complexes in the uveal tract.[56]

Experimentally one is able to induce inflammatory ocular disease by probable immune complex mediation. The placing of a foreign antigen (such as bovine serum albumin) into the eye, with a rechallenge some time later, will lead to an immune complex–mediated inflammatory response. Antigen antibody complexes in the aqueous can be demonstrated only during the time of active disease.[57] However, circulating immune complexes have not been shown to cause ocular inflammation.

Recent observations would not support the notion that immune complexes are playing a pivotal role in severe sight-threatening intermediate and posterior uveitis. In a review of iris specimens taken at the time of surgery from patients with uveitis, our laboratory has noted not plasma cells and evidence of immune complex–mediated disease (such as fibrinoid necrosis) but rather an influx of T cells.[58] Of particular note are the recent observations made concerning Behçet's disease, thought to be perhaps the most classic example of an "immune complex–mediated" uveitis. Anterior chamber paracentesis of well-established disease accompanied by hypopyon (see Chapter 25) reveals a large number of lymphocytes with a small number of neutrophils, the cell expected to predominate in an antigen-antibody reaction. An histologic review of a large number of Behçet's disease globes failed to demonstrate evidence of immune complex–mediated disease. Of particular note was the pronounced perivasculitis and not fibrinoid changes of the retinal vasculature.[59] The deposition of complement and once again the lack of fibrinoid changes in the aphthous ulcers of these patients have led others also to conclude that other immune mechanisms were at play.[60] A final note is the observation by our group that circulating immune complexes either remained the same or increased in patients with Behçet's disease whose condition was being therapeutically controlled with cyclosporine.[61]

The concept that the demonstration of immune complexes cannot be taken as prima facie evidence for an immune mechanism of destruction has begun to develop over the past few years. Kasp and colleagues[62] compared patients with retinal vasculitis who had circulating immune complexes and those who did not. They found that circulating immune complex formation seemed to protect against the more severe forms of retinal inflammatory disease. The possible explanation for this observation was that complexes seen in the

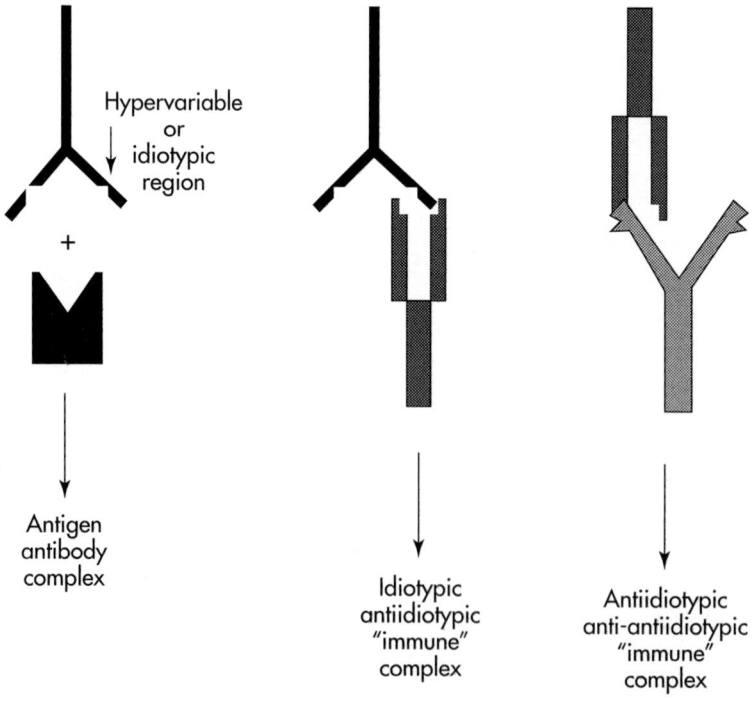


**Fig. 2-3.** Alternative theory to explain presence of immune complexes during uveitis. Immune complexes may be made up of two antibodies, and not antigen and antibody. Second antibody may be helping to "clear" first antibody, which could be detrimental. Thus presence of these immune complexes may be beneficial for organism.

group with the more favorable prognosis was made up of two antibodies, one harmful and the other produced by the body to neutralize the first. All assays for immune complexes rely on the detection of immunoglobulin aggregates.

It is important to remember that the hypervariable portion or idiotypic region of the immunoglobulin molecule, that part of the molecule directed against a specific antigen, can itself be an antigen for another immunoglobulin (the antiidiotypic antibody). This type of idiotypic-antiidiotypic complex is one that has been recognized to form in several situations and may be a common immune mechanism (Fig. 2-3). With the polyclonal response to a complex antigen, several idiotypic determinants may appear and be recognized as being foreign, thereby initiating a response against these idiotypes. These antiidiotypes as well could initiate an anti-antiidiotypic response, and so on. The import of these observations is that this cascade can affect the immune response. de Kozak and Mirshahi[63] have shown that preimmunization with a monoclonal antibody directed against an epitope of the retinal S-antigen will result in protection of animals from subsequent immunization with the retinal S-antigen. Another hypothesis is the induction of suppressor cells by antiidiotypic antibodies. This is the most probable explanation to a series of experiments by de Kozak and colleagues in which protection against EAU could be transferred with a lymph node preparation from antibody-immunized animals but not with the immunoglobulin fraction.[64] Another possibility is the blocking effect of the second antibody, effectively removing the first antibody from circulation and preventing its intended effect on the immune response.

An example of putative antibody mediated–ocular disease is that of cancer-related retinopathy. These patients produce antibodies that are believed to cross-react with their tumor and retinal elements, now thought to be the protein recoverin. The binding of the antibody to the retina will damage these elements and lead to poor vision.

## T-CELL RESPONSES AND AUTOIMMUNITY

On the basis of the present concepts of autoimmunity and their apparent relevance to the eye, it seems appropriate to discuss T-cell mechanisms here inasmuch as they appear to be inextricably intertwined. T-cell mechanisms are mediated not by the humoral route but rather through the direct contact of the T cell or through its release of lymphokines, thereby controlling the recruitment of other cells into the site of an immune response, with these cells ultimately being the effector cells. In addition, a major suppressive role, both specific and nonspecific, is played by T cells. Therefore dysregulation of this exquisite balance leading to autoimmunity would logically need to involve T cells.

Autoimmunity is an immune response directed against the host. This phenomenon is a common one and in the vast number of cases does not lead to obvious disease. It is when these initial autoimmune mechanisms lead to tissue damage that we denote it as autoimmune disease.[65] The mechanisms for autoimmune disease may vary considerably depending on the organ in question. Several mechanisms may lead ultimately to one final disease entity because of the relatively restricted way an organ is capable of responding to any immune response. Some general immune scenarios can be seen in Figs. 2-4 and 2-5. In Fig. 2-4, the drawings demonstrate concepts expressed by both Allison[66] and Weigle.[67] They both theorized that although sensitization may occur, the expression of disease would not occur as long as the effector T cell is rendered "tolerant" to the antigen in question. Such tolerance can occur if small amounts of the antigen are constantly circulating. This tolerant state is abrogated, however, if the effector T cell is now presented a new moiety of the antigen, this situation then leading to disease expression. Another hypothesis is that molecular mimicry is the initiating event (see earlier discussion of immunogenetics). The invading organism is quickly cleared, and the immune response is directed toward tissue components that are structurally similar. The final proposed mechanism in Fig. 2-4 would suggest that nonspecific polyclonal activation of the immune system, either by virus or immunostimulatory agents such as gram-negative bacterial cell wall components, will overwhelm the normal regulatory mechanisms and permit "forbidden clones" of cells to proliferate and cause tissue damage.

Fig. 2-5 attempts to combine two concepts that have gained some attention. The initial antigen presentation to the T cell may occur via Ia-bearing resident cells in the organ (see HLA discussion) as suggested by Bottazzo[48] or by a

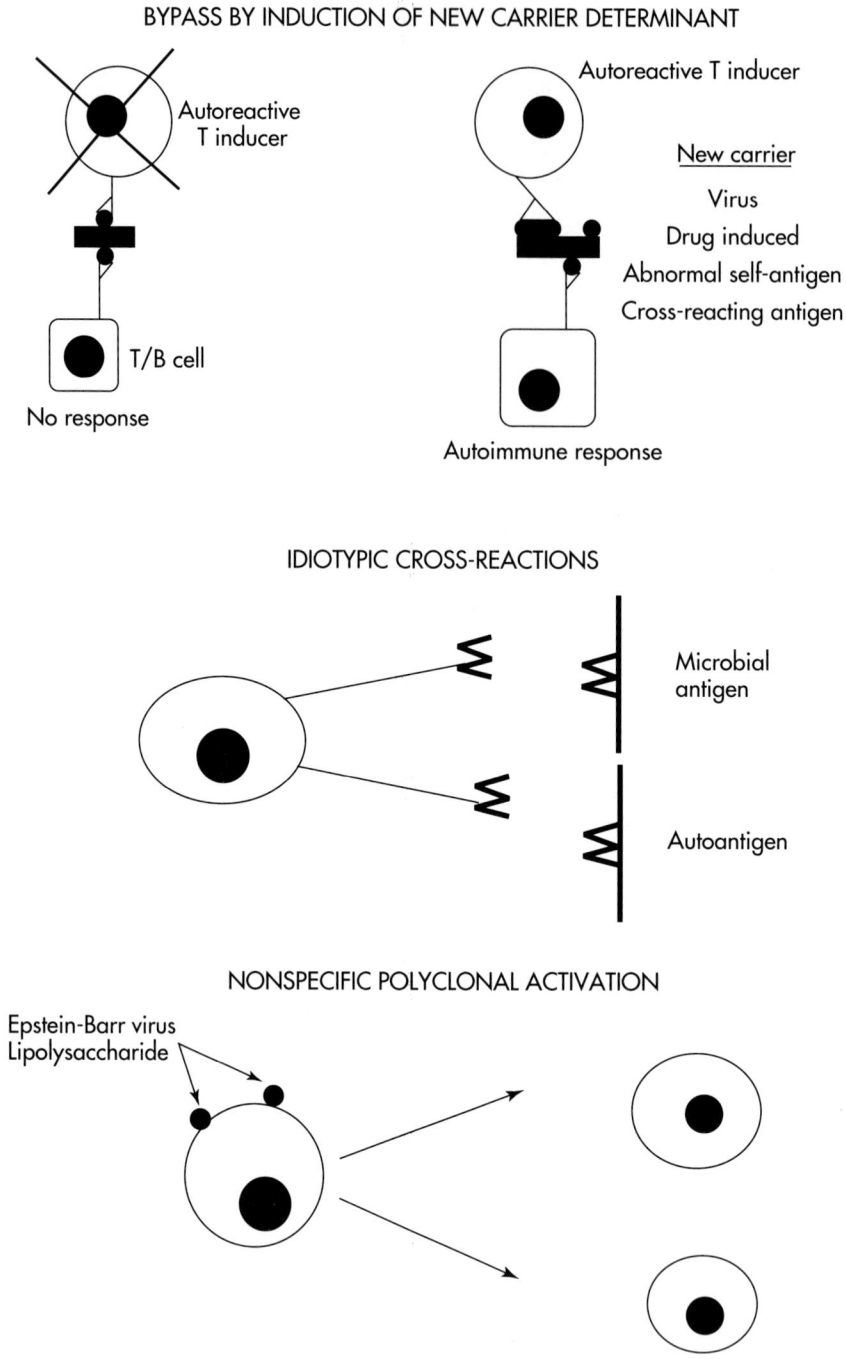


**Fig. 2-4.** Induction of autoimmunity I.

macrophage. This transfer of information will lead to sensitization but not to the expression of disease, because the presence of "surveillance" suppressor cells prevents this from occurring. The production of regulatory cells may be under the influence of a subset of the $CD4^+$ T cells that are identified with the 2H4 antibody (i.e., $CD4^+$ $2H4^+$ cells).

Fig. 2-5 shows two examples of dysregulation occurrence. In example A, either the number or the effectiveness of these suppressor cells has diminished dramatically, thereby permitting the clonal expansion of these sensitized T cells, the recruitment of other cells, and the clinical manifestation of disease. It has been proposed that antecedent viral infections, as well as other

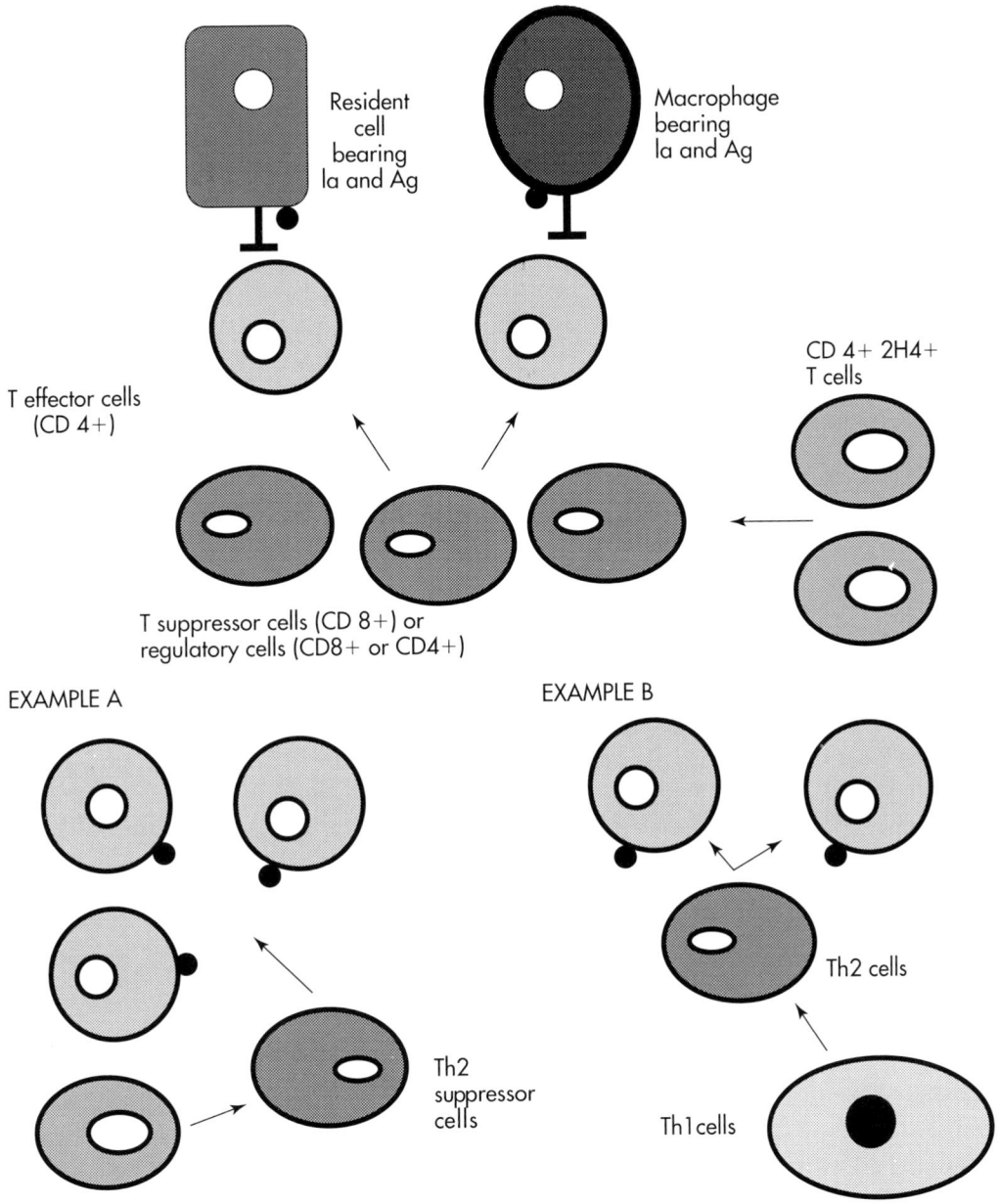


**Fig. 2-5.** Induction of autoimmunity II.

poorly understood endogenous regulating factors, could lead to such a problem. Such an alteration has been reported by Gibson and coworkers,[68] in which they demonstrated that the elimination of suppressor cells in mice led to the appearance and activation of "forbidden" B-cell clones, as well as the subsequent abrogation of the "self-tolerant" state maintained by these animals. An additional example is the recent observation that there is a selective loss in the $CD4^+$ $2H4^+$ subset of cells in patients with progressive multiple sclerosis.[69] Example B emphasizes the potential role of what was called a contrasuppressor cell and probably would be now called a Th1 cell. This mechanism, described initially by Gershon and colleagues,[70] has shown that suppression could be abrogated by a cell that directly downregulates the suppressor cells' functioning (see Green and Gershon[71] for a review of this mechanism). Kelly and Neilson[72] have demonstrated the counterbalancing effects of suppressor T cells ($T_s$) and contrasuppressor T cells ($T_{cs}$) in a model of autoimmune nephritis, so that if the $T_s$ predominates, tolerance is seen clinically, and if the $T_{cs}$ predominates, then disease expression occurs. Such an example is seen in Fig. 2-5.

### T-cell receptor

Much interest has centered around the antigen receptor expressed on the T-cell surface. The T-cell receptor (TCR) has a complex structure, made up of several chains controlled by different genes. It has been suggested that a specific subfamily, the beta chain of the TCR, was preferentially expressed on autoaggressive lymphocytes. In rats the Vβ8.2 subfamily epitope is expressed on a disproportionately large number of T cells capable of inducing EAU in naive animals.[73,74] Further work has refined this concept to a degree. It would appear that the Vβ8 family is expressed in these cells, but not necessarily exclusively. Egwuagu and coworkers[75] found that in rats the T cells invading the retina in S antigen–induced EAU express preferentially Vβ8.2, but IRBP-immunized animals had in their retinas at an early stage of EAU T cells bearing both the Vβ8.2 and Vβ8.3 phenotypes. Further, in mice, Rao and colleagues demonstrated a preferential usage of Vβ2, Vβ12, and Vβ15.[76] The implications of these findings have both basic scientific and practical clinical implications. If it were true that one subfamily of Vβ8 was always expressed on T cells that are autoaggressive (i.e., induce autoimmune disease), then one could use this as a marker to identify such cells in the body, and perhaps more important, these TCR peptide fragments could be used as a vaccinating agent to induce protection against all cells bearing this particular structure. Indeed, immunization (i.e., vaccination) with the Vβ8.2 fragments suppressed experimental autoimmune encephalomyelitis.[77] These results could not be reproduced in the experimental autoimmune uveitis model.[78] Human studies are underway to see if an overexpression of one epitope of the TCR is seen.

## OCULAR AUTOIMMUNITY

As mentioned previously, the concept that the eye harbors autoimmune-inducing or uveitogenic materials is one that has been suggested by many since the beginning of this century. It was Uhlenhuth's demonstration[79] of autoantibody production to the lens that pioneered this whole area of investigation. Several investigators used homogenates from the eye, which when injected into an animal, appeared capable of inducing an intraocular inflammatory response. Particular tribute must be paid to Drs. Waldon Wacker and colleagues[80] (Louisville, Ky.) and to Jean-Pierre Faure and coworkers[81] (Paris, France) for their zeal and scientific prowess in this area.

### Uveitogenic antigens of eye

**Retinal S-antigen (arrestin).** Wacker and colleagues reported the isolation, partial characterization, and immunologic properties of the retinal S-antigen (S-Ag) in 1977, with the French group soon after adding important new dimensions to this most important observation. The retinal S-Ag is one of the most potent of the uveitogenic antigens defined to date. This 48-kd intracellular protein is localized to the photoreceptor region of the retina and the pineal gland in some species (Fig. 2-6). Preparations from various species demonstrate high levels of cross-reactivity, reflecting the fact that the molecule appears to be highly conserved through evolution. The S-Ag has a molecular weight of about 50,000 daltons and contains a small amount of phospholipid. It is presently believed that S-Ag (or arrestin)[82] has the ability to mediate rhodopsin-catalyzed adenosine triphosphate (ATP) binding and to quench cyclic guanosine monophosphate (GMP) phosphodiesterase (PDE) activation. It will bind to photoactivated phosphorylated rhodopsin, preventing the transducin-mediated activation of PDE.[83]

The S-Ag will cause an immune-mediated, bilateral inflammatory response in the eye (EAU) when injected in microgram quantities at a site far from the globe (Fig. 2-7, *A* and *B*). The disease will begin as a retinitis in animals with angiotic retinae such as the monkey and rat,

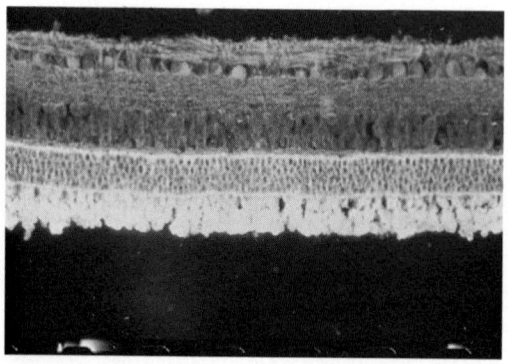

**Fig. 2-6.** Distribution of retinal S-antigen in photoreceptor region. (Courtesy Waldon Wacker, M.D.)

with more choroidal involvement in animals with pauangiotic retinae as in the guinea pig (Fig. 2-8, *A* to *C*). Several S-Ag-fragments have been shown to be pathogenic for Lewis rats.[84-87] Craft and colleagues[88] have demonstrated that the complementary DNA (cDNA) of the bovine S-Ag's antigenic site can be isolated and placed into a bacteriophage gene.

**Interphotoreceptor retinoid-binding protein.** A second uveitogenic retinal antigen more recently evaluated is that of the interphotoreceptor retinoid-binding protein (IRBP). This 140-kd molecule has been identified, purified, and characterized by Wiggert and Chader.[89] IRBP is believed to carry vitamin A derivatives between the photoreceptors and the RPE. It has four homologous domains.[90] Fox and colleagues[91] have demonstrated that IRBP, purified to homogeneity, has potent uveitogenic properties, with disease induction occurring at dosages as low as 0.3 μg per rat. The course of the disease in the IRBP-induced EAU is shorter than that seen with S-Ag, and the meninges surrounding the pineal glands of animals immunized with IRBP showed inflammatory disease whereas those receiving S-Ag did not have these changes. The disease induced in nonhuman primates with IRBP immunization shares similarities with that seen after S-Ag immunization, but it has less vitreous inflammation and seems somewhat more chronic[92] (Fig. 2-9). Several IRBP fragments have been reported as being pathogenic for Lewis rats.[93-95]

**Recoverin.** Recoverin, a 23-kd protein, is a member of the calcium-binding proteins, which localizes to the retina and the pineal. This antigen has been shown to be the target of antibodies in the cancer-associated retinopathy syndrome.[96] Immunization of rats with as low as 10 μg of recoverin induced both uveitis and pinealitis.[97] The disease appears to be similar to that seen with S-Ag. EAU can be transferred to naive animals by lymph node cells from recoverin-immunized animals.

**Bovine melanin protein.** Bovine melanin protein is derived from choroid-containing remnants of adherent retinal pigment epithelium. Broekhuyse and associates[98,99] reported that immunization was capable of inducing an autoimmune uveitis in rats. In the initial report, an anterior uveitis was the prominent aspect of the disease, with minimal choroidal involvement, and was therefore first called *experimental autoimmune anterior uveitis* (EAAU). However, Chan and coworkers[100] showed choroidal disease to be a more constant finding. Broekhuyse and Chan have thus proposed the term *experimental melanin protein–induced uveitis* to describe this disorder. Of interest was the finding that recurrent disease could be induced in this model with a footpad injection of lipopolysaccharide.

**Rhodopsin.** High concentrations of rhodopsin will induce an S-Ag–like EAU.[101,102] However, a dose of 100 to 250 μg of the antigen is usually used, but this causes severe ocular disease and pinealitis, whereas lower doses give a comcomitantly intermediate type of response. Opsin (rhodopsin's form in the light) seems to be less uveitogenic than rhodopsin.[103] Several fragments have been reported to be pathogenic in rat.[104]

**Phosducin.** Phosducin is a 33-kd retinal protein that is thought to play a role in the phototransduction of rods.[105] It does not appear to be as potent as some of the other antigens mentioned; at a dose of 50 μg injected

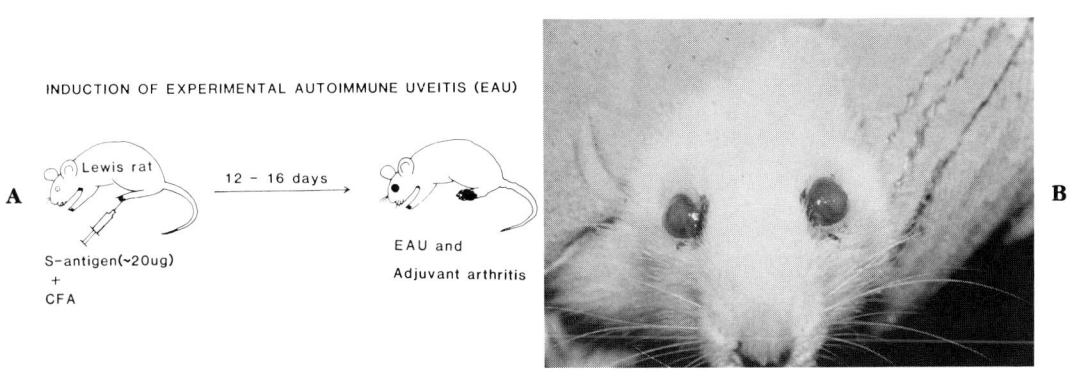


**Fig. 2-7. A,** Active immunization scheme for induction of EAU. **B,** Appearance of rat immunized 2 weeks before with high-dosage retinal S-antigen. Bilateral panuveitis is clinically apparent.

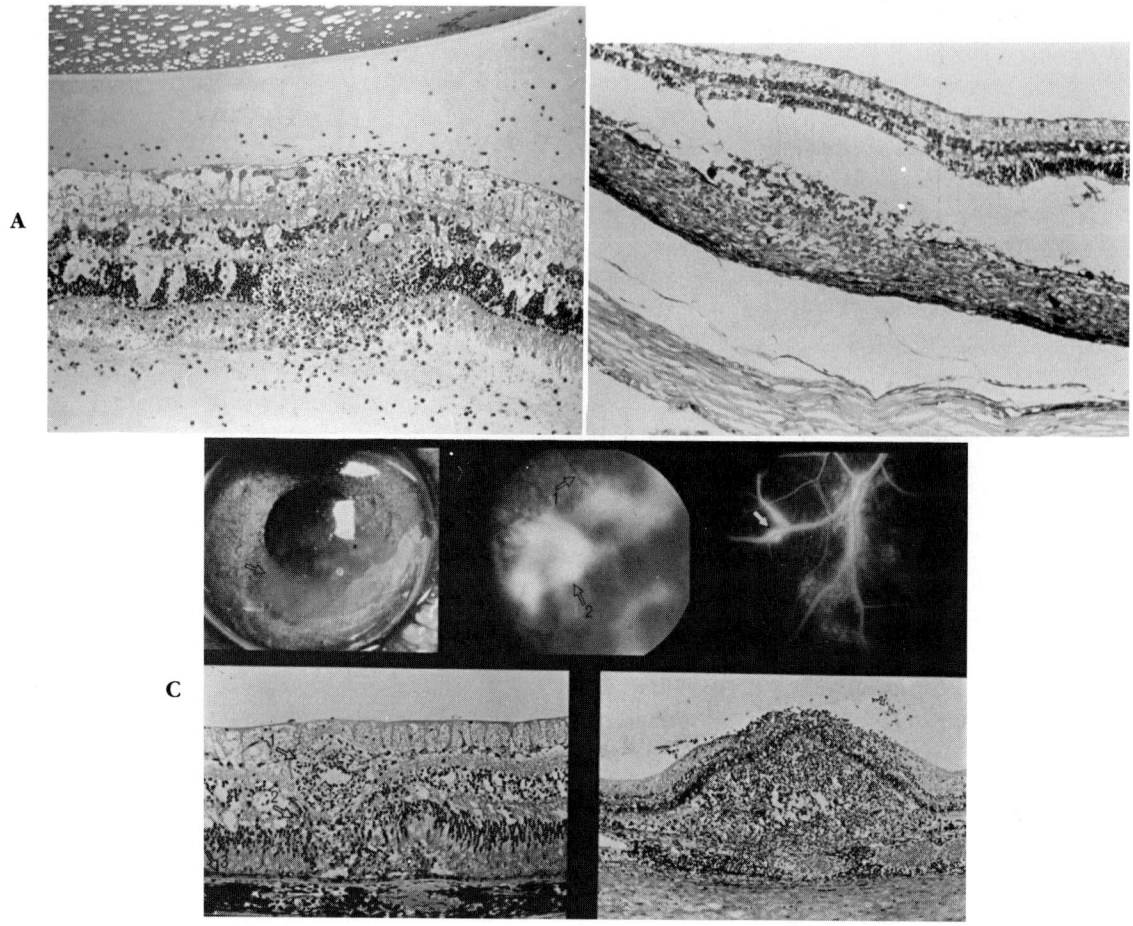


**Fig. 2-8. A,** Retinitis seen in Lewis rat after immunization with retinal S-antigen. Inflammatory disease has destroyed normal retinal architecture. Severe anterior segment inflammatory response occurs when higher dosages of antigen are used. **B,** S-antigen–induced inflammatory disease is more of a choroiditis when induced in a pauangiotic animal, such as guinea pig. **C,** S-antigen–induced EAU in monkey. Note anterior chamber changes. Posterior retinal lesions, with fluorescein angiography showing periphlebitis. Histologic focal destruction of photoreceptor region, with perivasculitis. *Lower right,* Massive subretinal inflammatory response pushing retina upward. (From *Arch Ophthalmol* 99:1090-1092. Copyright 1981, American Medical Association.)

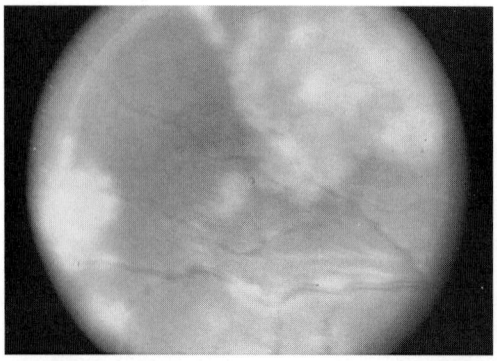

**Fig. 2-9.** Posterior segment disease in monkey immunized with IRBP. Note deep retinal lesions and sheathing of retinal vessels.

into a footpad, about 50% of the animals will develop disease. Patchy focal chorioretinal lesions with vitritis and retinal vascular involvement have been reported.[106]

**Immunology and histopathology.** The S-Ag– and IRBP-induced models and the antigens themselves have been the ones best investigated to date.[107] The study of these immune-mediated models for human intraocular inflammatory disease has yielded information invaluable for our understanding of the human condition. Perhaps the most important observation was the dominant role of the T cell in this disorder. This was first reported when Salinas-Carmona and colleagues[108] noted that active immunization of nude rats (animals

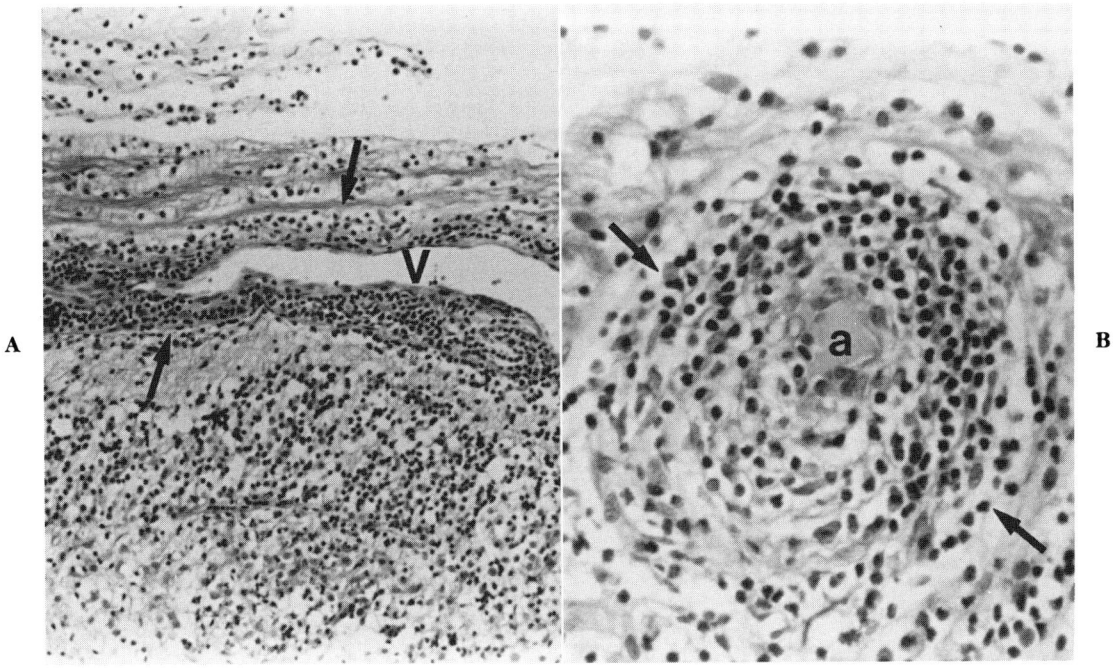


**Fig. 2-10.** Photomicrographs of rat eye with EAU. **A,** Vessel *(V)* in cross section demonstrating perivasculitis, with lymphocytes cuffing vessel along its route. **B,** Artery *(a)* with marked lymphocytic cuffing. (Courtesy Chi Chan, M.D.)

lacking an intact cell-mediated system) would not readily induce disease, whereas the heterozygote nude, having an intact T-cell circuitry, readily developed the disease. Further, transfer of splenic lymphocytes from S-Ag–immunized heterozygote animals to the nude rat (homozygote) did yield EAU. However, if the T-cell fraction was removed from this cell transfer, the disease did not occur.

Further support for the mandatory role of the T cell was the development of uveitogenic T-cell lines from Lewis rats.[109,110] These $Ia^{-0}$, IL-2 receptor$^{+}$ helper T cells will induce a disease that histologically is identical to that seen with active immunization.[111] The participation of other immune pathways in EAU has been examined. The transfer of hyperimmune serum containing anti–S-Ag antibodies to naive hosts will not induce disease. Immune complexes appear only in the reparative phase of the disease, suggesting that their appearance is one by which the immune system is downregulating the response or clearing the debris left from the primary immune reaction.[112] The addition of cobra venom, a potent method by which the complement system will be depleted and therefore an excellent way to test the role of immune complexes in the mediation of disease, did not prevent the development of the posterior pole disease, but it did dampen the anterior segment response.[113]

Mochizuki and coworkers[114] have noted that rat strain susceptibility to EAU induced with S-Ag was dramatically associated with the number of mast cells in the choroid, and de Kozak and colleagues[115] have impressively shown that mast cells in the choroid degranulate just before the influx of T cells into the eye, thus suggesting that these cells "open the door" into the eye for the T cells. This concept is especially provocative because Askenase and associates[116] have shown that mast-cell degranulation can be induced not only by IgE antibodies but also by T cells.

The changing patterns of cellular components and markers in the eye have given us a new understanding to this rapidly changing, finely orchestrated "ballet." Chan and colleagues[117] have shown that during the initial phase of S-Ag–induced EAU, helper T cells invade the eye, but later on it is the suppressor/cytotoxic T subset that predominates (Fig. 2-10). This pattern has been seen in human disease as well (see Chapter 22). The widespread expression of Ia antigens on several resident ocular cells is seen in EAU and in

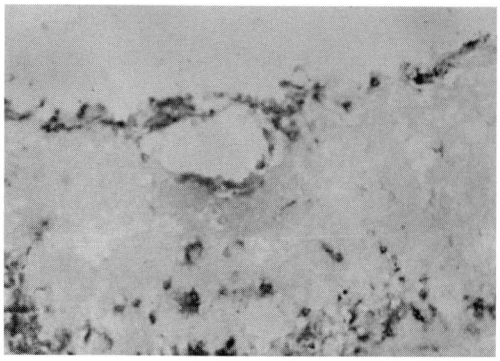

**Fig. 2-11.** Immunohistochemical staining showing expression of Ia molecules on retinal endothelium of rat that has EAU.

human uveitis, strengthening the observations seen in the animal model. It would also support the notion that these cells may be playing a role in the localized immune response (Fig. 2-11). The melanin protein–induced uveitis model has been noted to be characterized by a bilateral uveal infiltrate made up mostly of lymphocytes and monocytes, with most infiltrating T cells being $CD4^+$. MHC class II antigens were expressed intraocularly. This model is suggestive of both the IRBP and S-Ag models.[107]

**Endotoxin.** Another experimental model (but not autoimmune) is the injection into rats of the endotoxin lipopolysaccharide (LPS), a normal component of gram-negative bacterial cell walls, at a site far from the globe. This will induce a relatively fleeting anterior segment inflammatory response characterized mostly by an infiltration of polymorphonuclear cells[118] and cytokine release.[119] This model has potential relevance because patients with ankylosing spondylitis[120] and uveitis[121] have been reported to have a higher incidence of *Klebsiella* organisms in their stool or infection with another gram-negative bacteria during or shortly before the active portion of their disease than when their disease is quiet or as compared with control subjects. Although these observations have not been universally corroborated, the findings do bring into question the potential role these gram-negative organisms might play in immunomodulation. These antigens may activate complement without the participation of antibody. However, it is known that LPS can cause B cell clonal expansion, with a bypassing of the normal T-cell circuitry present to control such responses. The abundant B cell response could cause large amounts of antibody formation and possibly immune complex formation leading to an immune response. Either mechanism may be playing a role in the induction of anterior uveitis. One observation was the demonstration of homology of six consecutive amino acids between HLA-B27 and *Klebsiella pneumoniae* nitrogenase residues, with autoantibodies against this residue being found in HLA-$B27^+$ Reiter's syndrome and in patients with ankylosing spondylitis.[122]

**Importance of antigen studies.** This short synopsis concerning noninfectious ocular inflammatory animal models may convince the reader just how powerful a tool these models can be. The diseases induced have many features seen in the human situation, allowing us to dissect the ocular immune response and drawing attention to the potential role of ocular resident cells in the immune response. Many of the clinical and pathologic alterations seen in the animal models are seen also in human disease. These models (particularly the S-Ag model) have been excellent templates by which newer approaches to immunosuppression can be tested.[123-125]

Cyclosporine (CSA) was first evaluated for ocular autoimmune disease with the use of the S-Ag–induced model of experimental uveitis. Experiments clearly demonstrated the efficacy of this agent in preventing the expression of disease in rats even if therapy was begun 1 week after immunization, at a time when immunocompetent cells capable of inducing disease are present.[126,127] Further, lymphocytes from the animals protected from EAU by CSA therapy possessed immune memory to the antigen, giving positive in vitro proliferative responses to the S-Ag. Thus clonal deletion appears not to occur with CSA therapy, but rather a shift in the immune kinetic occurs, so that the immune repertoire still functions but not in a synchronized way. These initial observations led to the use of CSA in human disease. FK506 has been evaluated in a similar fashion and found to be quite effective in preventing EAU, as was rapamycin, as well as the induction of tolerance with oral administration of the retinal S-Ag (see Chapter 8).

The continued evaluation of immunomodulation in EAU will lead to a variety of new therapeutic approaches as this model is increasingly used as a template by which new

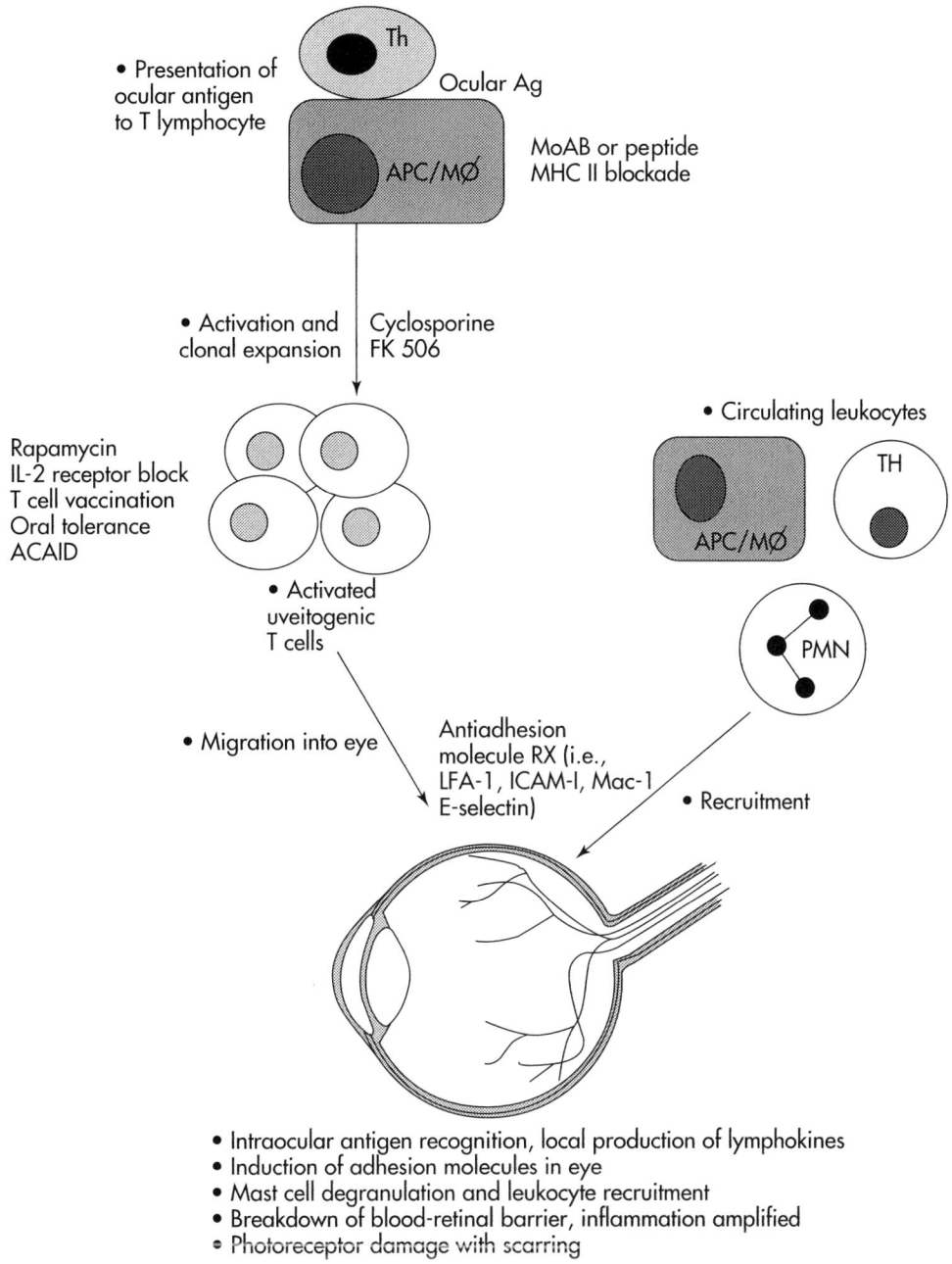


**Fig. 2-12.** Scheme showing induction of uveitis. Bullets (•) indicate what may be occurring based on evaluation of S-antigen uveitis model. Underlining indicates possible intervention strategies. (Modified from Caspi RR, Nussenblatt RB: Natural and therapeutic control of ocular autoimmunity: rodent and man. In Coutinho A, Kazatchkine MD, editors: *Autoimmunity: physiology and disease,* New York, 1994, Wiley-Liss.)

therapies are evaluated. Some of these strategies can be seen in Fig. 2-12. Here the reader can see that numerous points of the immune system can be delineated and appropriate strategies employed.

What is the potential role of the S-Ag or the other uveitogenic antigens found in the retina? Of course this still remains speculative. We have reported that patients with posterior and intermediate uveitis have exhibited in vitro cell-mediated proliferative responses to the S-Ag, not unlike those seen in the immunized animals.[128] It could be argued that these observations are epiphenomena and are not relevant to the disease process. It is difficult to accept this hypothesis in view of the devastat-

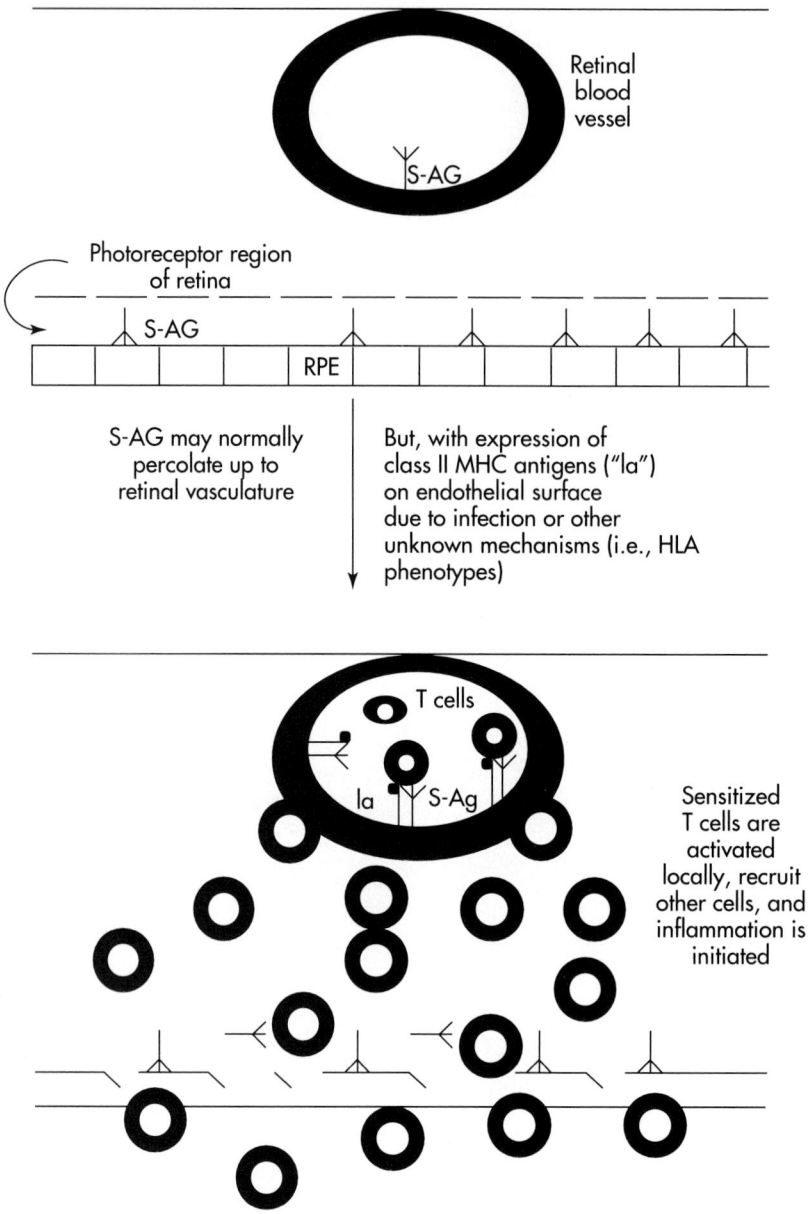


**Fig. 2-13.** Proposed scheme for role of S-antigen or other uveitogenic antigens in uveitis.

ing disease induced by these antigens. It is certainly possible that the initial event was not initiated by the S-Ag alone but that the release of S-Ag followed an infectious process, whether viral or even toxoplasmic. It is also clear that the events leading to an "autoimmune" uveitis are multifactorial. Such a scenario can be seen in Fig. 2-13, where the loss of surveillance suppressor cells by mechanisms already described combined with the abnormal expression of Ia on the vascular endothelium of the retina could lead to intraocular inflammatory disease.

## CELL-ADHESION MOLECULES

Cell-adhesion molecules (CAMs) are cell-surface glycoproteins important for the interaction of cells with other cells and for the interaction of cells with the extracellular matrix. CAMs play an integral role in the development of the inflammatory response. These adhesion molecules are especially important for directing leukocytes to areas of inflammation. The up-regulation of CAM expression on the vascular endothelium and surrounding area allows inflammatory cells to home to inflamed tis-

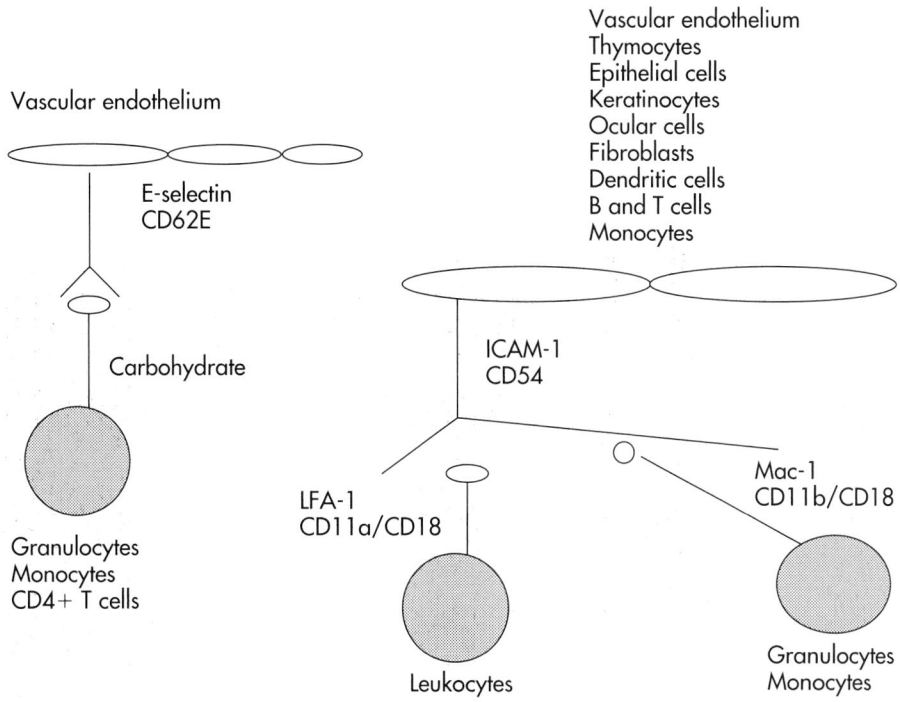


**Fig. 2-14.** Adhesion molecules and their in-organ resident cell and immune-cell interactions.

sues.[129,130] In addition, CAMs are involved in the interaction of lymphocytes and antigen-presenting cells, important for lymphocyte stimulation.

CAMs are divided into three structural groups: the selectins, the integrins, and the immunoglobulin gene superfamily. The CAMs discussed in this chapter and their counter-receptors are shown in Fig. 2-14. The selectins are a group of CAMs that appear to mediate the initial adhesion of inflammatory cells to the vascular endothelium, leading to a rolling of the cells along the vascular wall.[131] The integrins and members of the immunoglobulin supergene family, two other groups of CAMs, then interact to form a more firm adherence between the leukocytes and the vascular endothelium, leading to transendothelial migration of the cells into the inflamed tissue.[132]

E-selectin, also known as *endothelial leukocyte adhesion molecule*–1 (ELAM-1, CD62E), mediates the attachment of polymorphonuclear leukocytes to endothelial cells in vitro and appears to be important in the recruitment of neutrophils in a local endotoxin response in the skin.[133] We investigated the expression of E-selectin in eyes with endotoxin-induced uveitis (EIU), a useful animal model for the study of acute ocular inflammation,[134] which is characterized by iris hyperemia, miosis, increased aqueous humor protein, and inflammatory cell infiltration into the anterior uvea and anterior chamber.[135-138] Inflammatory cells first enter the eye 6 hours after endotoxin injection, and the resultant uveitis peaks within 24 hours. EIU is thought to result from mediators released by activated cells, including macrophages, but the exact mechanism causing inflammatory cell infiltration into the eye is not clearly defined. Recent data suggest that CAMs play an important role in the pathogenesis of this animal model of disease and that CAM expression is important for the recruitment of leukocytes into eyes with EIU.

ICAM-1 binds not only to Mac-1, but also to lymphocyte function-associated molecule–1 (LFA-1, CD11a/CD18), a second β2-integrin expressed on all leukocytes predominantly involved in lymphocyte trafficking. A number of groups have studied how ICAM-1 and LFA-1 affect the development of EIU. In eyes with EIU in C3H/HeN mice, ICAM-1 is first expressed on the ciliary body epithelium 6 hours after endotoxin injection and, later, on the vascular endothelium of the ciliary body and iris and on the corneal endothelium.[139] Elner and colleagues[140] demonstrated the expression of intercellular adhesion molecule–1 (ICAM-1,

CD54) on the corneal endothelium, and the expression of this cell adhesion molecule also appears important to the development of keratic precipitates. In experiments on Lewis rats, we have seen that EIU can be prevented by treating animals with anti–ICAM-1 or anti–LFA-1 antibody at the time of endotoxin injection,[141] even when administered 6 hours after endotoxin injection, when the eyes are already clinically inflamed. Rosenbaum and Boney[142] also showed that antibody to LFA-1 significantly reduced the cellular infiltrate associated with rabbit models of uveitis but that vascular permeability was less affected.

The secretion of cytokines, particularly by infiltrating T lymphocytes, appears to regulate adhesion-molecule expression. IFN-γ, IL-1, and tumor necrosis factor induce strong ICAM-1 expression at a transcriptional level, although the response to cytokines varies among cell types.[143-146] In vitro studies have shown that ICAM-1 expression on the cornea and retinal pigment epithelium is upregulated by cytokines such as IL-1.[147,148] It is clear that one of the major effects of cytokines in the pathogenesis of EIU involves the upregulation of adhesion molecule expression.

CAMs have also been shown to play a critical role in the pathogenesis of experimental autoimmune uveoretinitis (EAU). We first studied the expression of ICAM-1 and LFA-1 in B10.A mice with EAU.[149] ICAM-1 was first expressed on the vascular endothelium of the retina and ciliary body by 7 days after immunization, whereas infiltrating leukocytes expressing LFA-1 were not observed until 9 days after immunization, and clear histologic evidence of ocular inflammation did not occur until 11 days after immunization.

The effect of monoclonal antibodies against ICAM-1 and LFA-1 on the development of EAU has been examined. Ocular inflammation graded clinically at 14 and 21 days after immunization was significantly decreased in animals treated with anti–ICAM-1 ($p < 0.01$ at 14 and 21 days) or anti–LFA-1 antibody ($p < 0.01$ at 14 and 21 days). The inflammation graded histologically was also significantly decreased 21 days after immunization in animals treated with anti–ICAM-1 antibody ($p < 0.02$). Histologically graded inflammation was also decreased in animals treated with anti–LFA-1 antibody; however, the difference did not reach statistical significance ($p < 0.10$). These data suggest that anti–adhesion molecule antibodies could inhibit EAU either by interfering with immunization and antigen sensitization or by blocking leukocyte homing and migration into the eye. These data indicate that antibodies against ICAM-1 and LFA-1 inhibit EAU by interfering with both the induction and the effector phase of the disease. Adhesion molecules are also involved in the pathogenesis of lens-induced uveitis. Till and colleagues[150] showed that antibodies against adhesion molecules decreased ocular inflammation in lens-induced uveitis.

Recent studies in human beings have also shown that cell-adhesion molecules are important in the development of ocular inflammation. We have shown that ICAM-1 is expressed in the retina and choroid of human eyes with posterior uveitis.[151] In addition, we demonstrated increased expression of ICAM-1 in corneas with allograft rejection.[152] Based on animal data, clinical trials are underway to examine the use of anti–adhesion molecule antibodies to treat inflammatory disease in humans. A recent phase I clinical trial in 18 patients who received cadaver donor renal allografts showed that immunosuppression with anti–ICAM-1 antibody resulted in significantly less rejection.[153] These data show not only that CAMs are involved in the pathogenesis of inflammation but that drugs to block these adhesion molecules may provide effective therapy for inflammatory disease.

**Table 2-3.** Immune mechanisms at play in infectious disease

| Infectious agent | Mode of defense |
|---|---|
| Bacteria, virus | For neutralization, IgG with complement and neutrophils |
| Bacteria, virus | GI, respiratory infections: IgA, alternative complement pathway |
| Helminths | Intestinal IgE with mast cells |
| Pneumocci, encapsulated organisms | IgM, macrophages and complement |
| Mycobacteria, virus | Cytotoxic T cells and perforin |
| Mycobacteria, virus, syphilis, fungus | Macrophages and delayed type of hypersensitivity |

## IMMUNE RESPONSES TO INVADING VIRUSES AND PARASITES

The host's response to invading organisms is critical to its survival. Essentially all types of organisms can invade the eye, and responses of the immune system will vary (Table 2-3).

Viral infections are of course of great concern to the ophthalmologist, particularly to those with special interest in the anterior segment. However, the immune response to virus has taken on greater import for those involved with intraocular inflammatory disease because of both theoretic and practical considerations. Certain viruses have a particular propensity for retinal tissue, with herpes family infections, particularly cytomegalovirus, being of ever-increasing concern.

The invasion of a virus into the organism leads to the mobilization of several aspects of the immune response (Fig. 2-15). Antibody responses are abundant and may directly kill the virus. More frequently, however, cellular immune mechanisms appear to play a crucial role in eliminating the invading virus. T-cell responses against an invading virus have been well documented. The T-cell response is MHC-

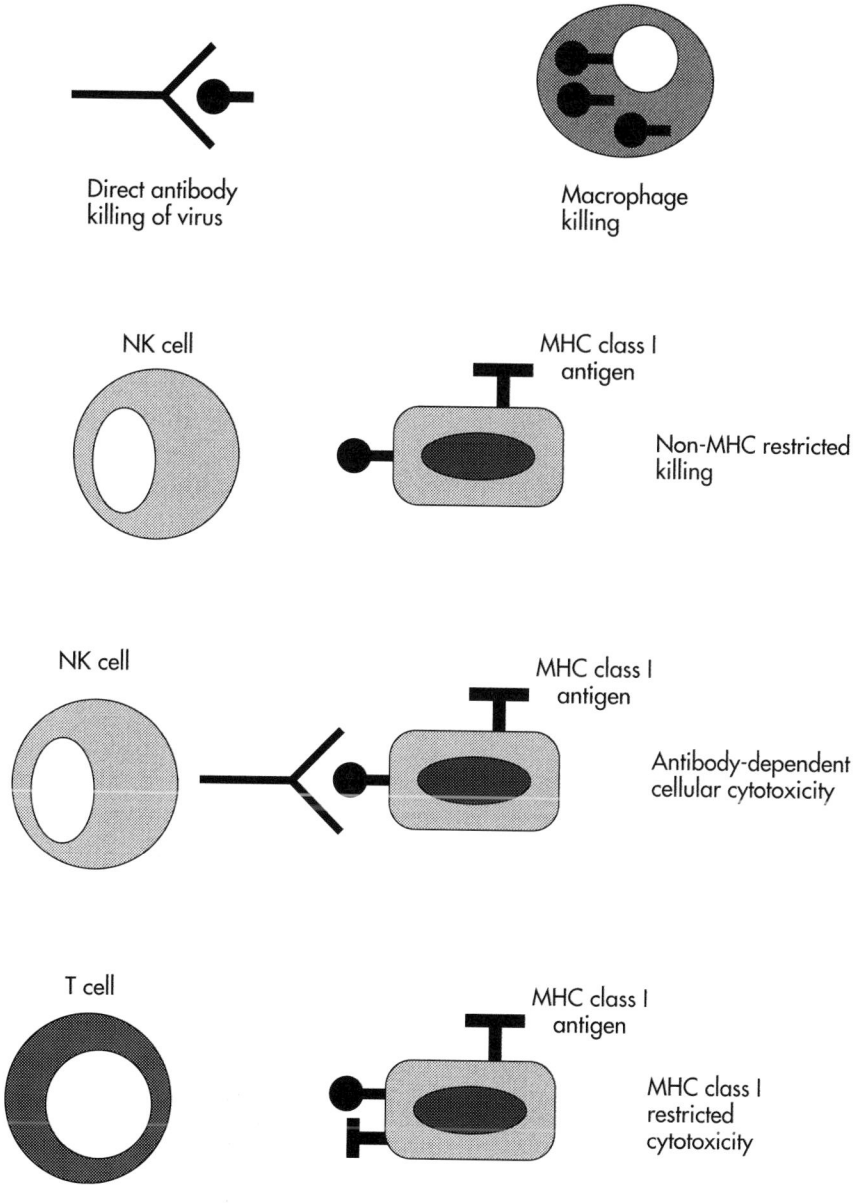


**Fig. 2-15.** Immune responses to viral invasion.

restricted. The T-cell is required to respond to a dual signal, that of the viral antigen and to class I antigens sitting on a target cell membrane. Natural killer cell (NK) activity is also seen to be directed against viral invasion. Found in the systemic circulation, these spontaneously cytotoxic cells, known as well as large granular lymphocytes, have probably a mixed lymphocyte and macrophage lineage. NK cell activity is not MHC-restricted, and virus infected cells seem to be particularly vulnerable to this cell's attack, but the mechanism of recognition still remains unclear. These cells are thought to participate in antibody-dependent cell-mediated cytotoxicity (ADCC), in which a specific antibody binds to the cell to enhance its destruction by cytotoxic cells. Macrophages also have important antiviral activity and will kill some engulfed virus particles. Others can be cleared if adequate macrophage activation occurs (see following discussion).

The immune system is rapidly activated to efficiently handle a viral infection in large part through the production of interferon. In response to a viral infection, both IFN-α and IFN-β are produced. Interferon's effect on a virally infected cell seems at least twofold: the production of a protein kinase, which inhibits viral protein synthesis, and the production of 2′5′–adenylate synthetase, which inhibits viral RNA synthesis. In addition to this direct effect on the virus, the IFNs, because of their immunomodulatory properties,[154] profoundly affect the immune response as well. The appearance of Ia on cell surface membranes could have an important effect on the rapidity of the immune response.

Because the immune response to the virus is in large part cell-mediated, any damage to this system could lead to grave consequences. This is the case with infection due to the human immunodeficiency virus (HIV, HTLV-III, LAV), the virus of the acquired immunodeficiency syndrome (AIDS). This RNA virus, which has a marked propensity for helper T cells, uses a reverse transcriptase to effectively incorporate its genetic library into that of the host cell. As the T cell becomes activated through antigen presentation by macrophages or other cells, the virus genome is also stimulated. The assembling and release of the HIV often lead to cell death. This virus then severely damages an important part of the immune system's mechanism for clearing such infections. This has secondary repercussions in the body's attempt to clear other virus infections, such as cytomegalovirus, which leads to a blinding retinitis in some patients with AIDS (see Chapter 26).

Parasitic infections of the eye include many types of organisms, from helminths to protozoa. The classically described response to parasitic infections is that of an eosinophilia. The release of the basic protein and other toxic products (see Chapter 1) from the eosinophil is thought to kill the organism. Certainly eosinophilia is characteristic for some forms of ocular parasitic infections, such as toxocariasis (see Chapter 16). However, for others, such as toxoplasmosis and onchocerciasis (see Chapters 14, 17), this appears not to be the case. T cells seem to predominate in the eye in the more chronic forms of these diseases, and deficient T-cell functioning can lead to serious consequences. An example of this is the systemic and ocular toxoplasmic infection seen in patients with AIDS, in patients immunosuppressed because of neoplasms, or in those iatrogenically suppressed for graft survival.

Parasitic invaders have an additional capacity to evade immune surveillance. Immunosuppressive factors appear to be elaborated by the parasite, leading to a downgrading of macrophage and T-cell activity around it. Certain parasites cloak themselves in nonantigenic proteins, thereby avoiding immune attack. The cyst of the *Toxoplasma gondii* found in the eye is such an example, with the wall incorporating antigens from the host. Other parasites vary their antigenic appearance frequently to avoid the T-cell and macrophage-directed responses.

## REFERENCES


1. Medawar PB: Immunity to homologous grafted skin. III. The fate of skin homografts transplanted to brain, to subcutaneous tissue and to the anterior chamber of the eye, *Br J Exp Pathol* 29:58-69, 1948.
2. Kaplan HJ, Streilein JW: Immune response to immunization via the anterior chamber of the eye. I. $F_1$-lymphocyte-induced immune deviation, *J Immunol* 118:809-814, 1977.
3. Streilein JW, Neiderkorn J: Induction of anterior chamber–associated immune deviation requires an intact, functional spleen, *J Exp Med* 153:1058-1067, 1981.
4. Wetzig RP, Foster CS, Greene MI: Ocular immune responses. I. Priming of A/J mice in the anterior chamber with azobenzenearsonate derivatized cells induces second-order–like suppressor T cells, *J Immunol* 128:1753-1757, 1982.
5. Mizuno K, Clark AF, Streilein JW: Anterior chamber associated immune deviation induced by soluble

antigens, *Invest Ophthalmol Vis Sci* 30:1112-1119, 1989.
6. Neiderkorn J, Streilein JW, Shadduck JA: Deviant immune responses to allogeneic tumors injected intracamerally and subcutaneously in mice, *Invest Ophthalmol Vis Sci* 20:355-363, 1981.
7. Eichorn M, Horneber M, Streilein JW et al: Anterior chamber associated immune deviation elicited via primate eyes, *Invest Ophthalmol Vis Sci* 34:2926-2930, 1993.
8. Hara Y, Caspi RR, Wiggert B et al: Suppression of experimental autoimmune uveitis in mice by induction of anterior chamber associated immune deviation with interphotoreceptor retinoid binding protein, *J Immunol* 148:1685-1692, 1992.
9. Wilbanks GA, Streilein JW: Studies on the induction of anterior chamber–associated immune deviation (ACAID). I. Evidence that an antigen-specific, ACAID-inducing, cell-associated signal exists in the peripheral blood, *J Immunol* 146:2610-2617, 1991.
10. Wilbanks GA, Mammolenti MM, Streilein JW: Studies on the induction of anterior chamber–associated immune deviation (ACAID). III. Induction of ACAID depends upon intraocular transforming growth factor–β, *Eur J Immunol* 22:165-173, 1992.
11. Ferguson TA, Hayashi JD, Kaplan HJ: The immune response and the eye. III. Anterior chamber–associated immune deviation can be adoptively transferred by serum, *J Immunol* 143:821-826, 1989.
12. Streilein JW, Wilbanks GA, Taylor A et al: Eye-derived cytokines and the immunosuppressive intraocular microenvironment: a review, *Curr Eye Res* 11 (suppl): 41-47, 1992.
13. Streilein JW: Immune privilege as the result of local tissue barriers and immunosuppressive microenvironments, *Curr Opinion Immunol* 5:428-432, 1993.
14. Caspi RR, Roberge FG, Nussenblatt RB: Organ-resident, nonlymphoid cells suppress proliferation of autoimmune T-helper lymphocytes, *Science* 237: 1029-1032, 1987.
15. Chan CC, Roberge FG, Ni M et al: Injury of Müller cells increases the incidence of experimental autoimmune uveoretinitis, *Clin Immunol Immunopathol* 59:201-207, 1991.
16. Kawashima H, Gregerson DS: Corneal endothelial cells block T cell proliferation, but not T cell activation or responsiveness to exogenous IL-2, *Curr Eye Res* 13:575-585, 1994.
17. Planck SR, Dang TT, Graves D et al: Retinal pigment epithelial cells secrete interleukin-6 in response to interleukin-1, *Invest Ophthalmol Vis Sci* 33:78-82, 1992.
18. Chan CC, Detrick B, Nussenblatt RB et al: HLA-DR antigens on retinal pigment epithelial cells from patients with uveitis, *Arch Ophthalmol* 104:725-729, 1986
19. Percopo CM, Hooks JJ, Shinohara T et al: Cytokine-mediated activation of a neuronal retinal resident cell provokes antigen presentation, *J Immunol* 145:4101-4107, 1990.
20. Granstein R, Stszewski R, Knisely T et al: Aqueous humor contains transforming growth factor–gb and a small (<3500 daltons) inhibitor of thymocyte proliferation, *J Immunol* 144:3021-3027, 1990.
21. Cousins SW, McCabe MM, Danielpour D et al: Identification of transforming growth factor-beta as an immunosuppressive factor in aqueous humor, *Invest Ophthalmol Vis Sci* 32:2201-2211, 1991.
22. Tripathi RC, Li J, Borisuth NSC et al: Trabecular cells of the eye express messenger RNA for transforming growth factor β1 and secrete this cytokine, *Invest Ophthalmol Vis Sci* 34:2562-2569, 1993.
23. Taylor AW, Streilein JW, Cousins SW: Identification of alpha–melanocyte stimulating hormone as a potential immunosuppressive factor in aqueous humor, *Curr Eye Res* 11:1199-1206, 1992.
24. Wahlestedt C, Beding B, Ekman R et al: Calcitonin gene-related peptide in the eye-release by sensory nerve stimulation and effects associated with neurogenic inflammation, *Regul Pept* 16:107-115, 1986.
25. Taylor AW, Streilein JW, Cousins SW: Vasoactive intestinal peptide (VIP) contributes to the immunosuppressive activity of normal aqueous humor, *J Immunol* 153:1080-1086, 1994.
26. Sternberg EM, Hill JM, Chrousos GP et al: Inflammatory mediator-induced hypothalamic-pituitary-adrenal axis activation is defective in streptococcal cell wall arthritis–susceptible Lewis rats, *Proc Natl Acad Sci USA* 86:2374-2378, 1989.
27. Knisely TL, Hosoi J, Nazareno R et al: The presence of biologically significant concentrations of glucocorticoids but little or no cortisol binding globulin within aqueous humor: relevance to immune privilege in the anterior chamber of the eye, *Invest Ophthalmol Vis Sci* 35:3711-3723, 1994.
28. Wells H: Studies on the chemistry of anaphylaxis. III. Experiments with isolated proteins, especially those of hen's eggs. *J Infect Dis* 9:147-151, 1911.
29. Chase MW: Inhibition of experimental drug allergy by prior feeding of the sensitizing agent, *Proc Soc Exp Biol Med* 61:257-259, 1946.
30. Weiner HL, Friedman A, Miller A et al: Oral tolerance: immunologic mechanisms and treatment of animal and human organ specific autoimmune diseases by oral administration of autoantigens, *Annu Rev Immunol* 12:809-834, 1994.
31. Friedman A, Weiner HL: Induction of anergy or active suppression following oral tolerance is determined by antigen dosage, *Proc Natl Acad Sci USA* 91:6688-6692, 1994.
32. Gregerson DS, Obritsch WF, Donoso LA: Oral tolerance in experimental autoimmune uveoretinitis. Distinct mechanisms of resistance are induced by low dose vs high dose feeding protocols, *J Immunol* 151:5751-5761, 1993.
33. Miller A, Al-Sabbagh A, Santos LMB et al: Epitopes of myelin basic protein that trigger TGF-β release after oral tolerization are distinct from encephalitogenic epitopes and mediate epitope-driven bystander suppression, *J Immunol* 151:7307-7315, 1993.
34. Nussenblatt RB, Caspi RR, Mahdi R et al: Inhibition of S-antigen induced experimental autoimmune uveoretinitis by oral induction of tolerance with S-antigen, *J Immunol* 144:1689-1695, 1990.
35. Suh EDW, Vistica B, Chan CC et al: Splenectomy abrogates the induction of oral tolerance in experimental autoimmune uveoretinitis, *Curr Eye Res* 12:833-839, 1993.

36. Dick AD, Cheng YF, McKinnon A et al: Nasal administration of retinal antigens suppresses the inflammatory response in experimental allergic uveoretinitis. A preliminary report of intranasal induction of tolerance with retinal antigens, *Br J Ophthalmol* 77:171-175, 1993.
37. Nussenblatt RB, de Smet MD, Weiner HL et al: The treatment of the ocular complications of Behęt's disease with oral tolerization. In *Sixth International Conference on Behçet's disease,* Amsterdam, 1993, Elsevier Press.
38. Elschnig A: Studien zur sympathischen ophthalmis. Die antigene wirkung des augenpigmentes, *Albrecht von Graefes Arch Ophthalmol* 76:509-546, 1910.
39. Cogan DG: Immunosuppression and eye disease (first Vail lecture), *Am J Ophthalmol* 83:777-788, 1977.
40. Shutze H, Gorer PA, Finlayson MH: The resistance of four mouse lines to bacterial infections, *J Hyg* 36:37-49, 1936.
41. Benacerraf B, Green I, Paul WE: The immune response of guinea pigs to hapten-poly-L-lysine conjugates as an example of the genetic control of the recognition of antigenicity, *Cold Spring Harbor Symp Quant Biol* 32:569-575, 1967.
42. Bluestein HG, Green I, Benacerraf B: Specific immune response genes of the guinea pig. II. Relationship between the poly-L-lysine gene and the genes controlling immune responsiveness to copolymers of L-glutamic acid and L-tyrosine in random bred Hartley guinea pigs, *J Exp Med* 134:471-481, 1971.
43. McDevitt HO, Chinitz A: Genetic control of the antibody response: relationship between immune response and histocompatibility (H-2) type, *Science* 163:1207-1208, 1969.
44. Forrester JV, McMenamin PG, Holthouse I et al: Localization and characterization of major histocompatibility complex class II–positive cells in the posterior segment of the eye: implications for induction of autoimmune uveoretinitis, *Invest Ophthalmol Vis Sci* 35:64-77, 1994.
45. Brewerton DA, Hart FD, Nicholls A et al: Ankylosing spondylitis and HL-A27, *Lancet* 1:904, 1973.
46. Khan MA, Kushner I, Braun WE et al: HLA-B7 and ankylosing spondylitis in American blacks, *N Engl J Med* 297:513, 1977.
47. Terasaki P: *Histocompatibility testing 1980,* Los Angeles, 1980, UCLA Tissue Typing Laboratory.
48. Bottazzo GF, Pujol-Borrell R, Hanafusa T et al: Role of aberrant HLA-DR expression and antigen presentation in induction of endocrine autoimmunity, *Lancet* 2:1115-1119, 1983.
49. Taurog JD, Maika SD, Simmons WA et al: Susceptibility to inflammatory disease in HLA-B27 transgenic rat lines correlates with the level of B27 expression, *J Immunol* 150:4168-4178, 1993.
50. Caspi RR, Grubbs BG, Chan CC et al: Genetic control of susceptibility to experimental autoimmune uveoretinitis in the mouse model: concomitant regulation by MHC and non-MHC genes. *J Immunol* 148:2384-2389, 1992.
51. Mulligan MS, Jones ML, Vaporciyan AA et al: Protective effects of IL-4 and IL-10 against immune complex–induced lung injury, *J Immunol* 151:5666-5674, 1993.
52. Dernouchamps JP, Vaerman JP, Michiels J et al: Immune complexes in the aqueous humor and serum, *Am J Ophthalmol* 84:24-31, 1977.
53. Char DH, Stein P, Masi R et al: Immune complexes in uveitis, *Am J Ophthalmol* 87:678-681, 1979.
54. Lehner T, Almedida JD, Levinsky RJ: Damaged membrane fragments and immune complexes in the blood of patients with Behçet's syndrome, *Clin Exp Immunol* 34:206-212, 1978.
55. Vinje O, Miller P, Mellbye J: Immunological variables and acute phase reactants in patients with ankylosing spondylitis (Bechterew's syndrome) and their relatives, *Clin Rheumatol* 3:501-513, 1984.
56. O'Connor GR: Factors related to the initiation and recurrences of uveitis, (Fortieth Edward Jackson memorial lecture), *Am J Ophthalmol* 96:577-599, 1983.
57. Howes EL Jr, Char DH, Christenson M: Aqueous immune complexes in immunogenic uveitis, *Invest Ophthalmol Vis Sci* 23:715-718, 1982.
58. Stevens G Jr, Chan CC, Wetzig RP et al: Iris lymphocytic infiltration in patients with clinically queiscent uveitis, *Am J Ophthalmol* 104:508-515, 1987.
59. Cogan DG: Personal communication, 1987.
60. Poulter LW, Lehner T, Duke O: Immunohistochemical investigations of recurrent oral ulcers and Behçet's disease. In Lehner T, Barnes CG, editors: *Recent advances in Behçet's disease,* London, 1986, Royal Society of Medicine Services.
61. Nussenblatt RB, Palestine AG, Chan CC et al: Effectiveness of cyclosporine therapy for Behçet's disease, *Arthritis Rheum* 26:671-679, 1985.
62. Kasp E, Graham E, Stanford MR et al: A point prevalence study of 150 patients with idiopathic retinal vasculitis. II. Clinical relevance of antiretinal autoimmunity and circulating immune complexes, *Br J Ophthalmol* 73:722-730, 1989.
63. de Kozak Y, Mirshahi M: Experimental autoimmune uveoretinitis: idiotypic regulation and disease suppression, *Int Ophthalmol* 14:43-56, 1990.
64. de Kozak Y, Mirshahi M, Boucheix C et al: Modulation of experimental autoimmune uveoretinitis by adoptive transfer of cells from rats immunized with anti–S antigen monoclonal antibody, *Reg Immunol* 2:311-320, 1989.
65. Rose NR, Bona C: Defining criteria for autoimmune diseases (Wetebsky's postulates revisited), *Immunol Today* 14:426-430, 1993.
66. Allison A: Unresponsiveness to self antigens, *Lancet* 2:1401-1403, 1971.
67. Weigle WO: Recent observations and concepts in immunological unresponsiveness and autoimmunity, *Clin Exp Immunol* 9:437-447, 1971.
68. Gibson J, Basten A, Walker KZ et al: A role of suppressor T cells in induction of self-tolerance, *Proc Natl Acad Sci USA* 82:5150-5154, 1985.
69. Morimoto C, Hafler DA, Weiner HL et al: Selective loss of the suppressor-inducer T-cell subset in progressive multiple sclerosis, *N Engl J Med* 316:67-72, 1987.
70. Gershon RK, Eardley DD, Durum S et al: Contrasuppression. A novel immunoregulatory activity, *J Exp Med* 153:1533-1546, 1981.
71. Green DR, Gershon RK: Contrasuppression. The second law of thymodynamics, revisited, *Adv Cancer Res* 42:277-335, 1984.
72. Kelly CJ, Neilson EG: Contrasuppression in autoimmunity. Abnormal contrasuppression facilitates expression of nephritogenic effector T cells and interstitial nephritis in kdkd mice, *J Exp Med* 165:107-123, 1987.

73. Egwuagu CE, Chow C, Béraud E et al: T cell receptor beta-chain usage in experimental autoimmune uveoretinitis, *J Autoimmunol* 4:315-324, 1991.
74. Gregerson DS, Fling SP, Merryman CF et al: Conserved T cell receptor V gene usage by uveitogenic T cells, *Clin Immunol Immunopathol* 58:154-161, 1991.
75. Egwuagu CE, Mahdi RM, Nussenblatt RB et al: Evidence for selective accumulation of Vβ8+ T lymphocytes in experimental autoimmune uveoretinitis induced with two different retinal antigens, *J Immunol* 151:1627-1636, 1993.
76. Rao NA, Naida YM, Bell R et al: Usage of T cell receptor β-chain variable gene is highly restricted at the site of inflammation in murine autoimmune uveitis, *J Immunol* 150:5716-5721, 1993.
77. Vandenbark AA, Hashim G, Offner H: Immunization with a synthetic T-cell receptor V-region peptide protects against experimental autoimmune encephalomyelitis, *Nature* 341:541-544, 1989.
78. Kawano Y, Sasamoto Y, Kotake S et al: Trials of vaccination against experimental autoimmune uveoretinitis with a T-cell receptor peptide, *Curr Eye Res* 10:789-795, 1991.
79. Uhlenhuth PT: Zur lehre von der unterscheidung verschiedener eiweissarten mit hilfe spezifischer sera. In *Festschrift zum 60 Geburstag von Robert Koch,* Jena, Germany, 1903, Fischer.
80. Wacker WB, Donoso LA, Kalsow CM et al: Experimental allergic uveitis. Isolation, characterization, and localization of a soluble uveitopathogenic antigen from bovine retina, *J Immunol* 119:1949-1958, 1977.
81. Faure JP: Autoimmunity and the retina, *Curr Top Eye Res* 2:215-302, 1980.
82. Pfister C, Dorey C, Vadot R et al: Identité de la protéine dite "48k" qui interagit avec la rhodopsine illuminée dans les batonnets retiniens et de l'"antigène S retinien" inducteur de l'uvéo-rétinite autoimmune expérimentale, *C R Acad Sci Paris* 299:261-265, 1984.
83. Pfister C, Chabre M, Plouet J et al: Retinal S antigen identified as the 48k protein regulating light-dependent phosphodiesterase in rods, *Science* 228: 891-893, 1986.
84. Donoso LA, Merryman CF, Shinohara T et al: S-antigen. Identification of the MAbA9-C6 monoclonal antibody binding site and the uveitopathogenic sites, *Curr Eye Res* 5:995-1004, 1986.
85. de Smet MD, Bitar G, Roberge FG et al: Human S-antigen: presence of multiple immunogenic and immunopathogenic sites in the Lewis rat, *J Autoimmun* 6:587-599, 1993.
86. Gregerson DS, Merryman CF, Obritsch WF et al: Identification of a potent new pathogenic site in human retinal S-antigen which induces experimental autoimmune uveoretinitis in LEW rats, *Cell Immunol* 128:209-219, 1990.
87. Merryman CF, Donoso LA, Zhang XM et al: Characterization of a new, potent, immunopathogenic epitope in S-antigen that elicits T cells expressing V beta 8 and V alpha 2–like genes, *J Immunol* 146:75-80, 1991.
88. Craft C, Stein P, Klein DC et al: Isolation of cDNA clones for S-antigen, *Invest Ophthalmol Vis Sci* 26(suppl):28, 1985.
89. Wiggert B, Chader GJ: Monkey interphotoreceptor retinoid-binding protein (IRBP): isolation, characterization, and synthesis. In Bridges CD, Adler AJ, editors: *The interphotoreceptor matrix in health and disease,* New York, 1985, Alan R. Liss.
90. Borst DE, Redmond TM, Elser JE et al: Interphotoreceptor retinoid-binding protein. Gene characterization, protein repeat structure, and its evolution, *J Biol Chem* 264:1115-1123, 1989.
91. Fox GM, Kuwabara T, Wiggert B et al: Experimental autoimmune uveoretinitis (EAU) induced by retinal interphotoreceptor retinoid-binding protein (IRBP): differences between EAU induced by IRBP and by S-Antigen, *Clin Immunol Immunopathol* 43:256-264, 1987.
92. Hirose S, Kuwabara T, Nussenblatt RB et al: Uveitis induced in primates by interphotoreceptor retinoid-binding protein, *Arch Ophthalmol* 104:1698-1702, 1986.
93. Donoso LA, Merryman CF, Sery T et al: Human interstitial retinoid binding protein. A potent uveitopathogenic agent for the induction of experimental autoimmune uveitis, *J Immunol* 143:79-83, 1989.
94. Kotake S, Redmond TM, Wiggert B et al: Unusual immunologic properties of the uveitogenic interphotoreceptor retinoid-binding protein-derived peptide R23, *Invest Ophthalmol Vis Sci* 146:2995-3001, 1991.
95. Sanui H, Redmond TM, Kotake S et al: Identification of an immunodominant and highly immunopathogenic determinant in the retinal interphotoreceptor retinoid-binding protein (IRBP), *J Exp Med* 169:1947-1960, 1989.
96. Thirkill CE, Tait RC, Tyler NK et al: The cancer-associated retinopathy antigen is a recoverin-like protein, *Invest Ophthalmol Vis Sci* 33:2768-2772, 1992.
97. Gery I, Chanaud NP III, Anglade E: Recoverin is highly uveitogenic in Lewis rats, *Invest Ophthalmol Vis Sci* 35:3342-3345, 1994.
98. Broekhuyse RM, Kuhlmann ED, Winkens HJ et al: Experimental autoimmune anterior uveitis (EAAU), a new form of experimental uveitis. I. Induction by a detergent-insoluble, intrinsic protein fraction of the retina pigment epithelium, *Exp Eye Res* 52:465-474, 1991.
99. Broekhuyse RM, Kuhlmann ED, Winkens HJ: Experimental autoimmune anterior uveitis (EAAU). II. Dose-dependent induction and adoptive transfer using a melanin-bound antigen of the retinal pigment epithelium, *Exp Eye Res* 55:401-411, 1992.
100. Chan CC, Hikita N, Dastgheib K et al: Experimental melanin-protein–induced uveitis in the Lewis rat. Immunopathologic processes, *Ophthalmology* 101: 1275-1280, 1994.
101. Schalken JJ, Winkens HJ, Van Vugt AHM et al: Rhodopsin-induced experimental autoimmune uveoretinitis: dose-dependent clinicopathological features, *Exp Eye Res* 47:135-145, 1988.
102. Schalken JJ, Winkens HJ, Van Vugt AHM et al: Rhodopsin induced experimental autoimmune uveoretinitis in monkeys, *Br J Ophthalmol* 73:168-172, 1989.
103. McMenamin PG, Broekhuyse RM, Forrester JV: Ultrastructural pathology of experimental autoimmune uveitis: a review, *Micron* 24:521-546, 1993.
104. Adamus G, Schmied JL, Hargrave PA et al: Induction of experimental autoimmune uveitis with rhodopsin synthetic peptides in Lewis rats, *Curr Eye Res* 11:657-667, 1992.

105. Lee RH, Fowler A, McGinnis JF et al: Amino acid and cDNA sequence of bovine phosducin, a soluble phosphoprotein from photoreceptor cells, *J Biol Chem* 265:15867-15873, 1990.
106. Dua HS, Lee RH, Lolley RN et al: Induction of experimental autoimmune uveitis by the retinal photoreceptor cell protein, phosducin, *Curr Eye Res* 11:107-111, 1992.
107. Caspi RR: Experimental autoimmune uveoretinitis—rat and mouse. In Cohen I, Miller A, editors: *Autoimmune disease models: a guidebook,* San Diego, 1994, Academic Press.
108. Salinas-Carmona MC, Nussenblatt RB, Gery I: Experimental autoimmune uveitis in the athymic nude rat, *Eur J Immunol* 25:481-484, 1982.
109. Rozenszajn LA, Muellenberg-Coulombre C, Gery I, et al: Induction of experimental autoimmune uveoretinitis (EAU) in rats by T cell lines, *Immunology* 57:559-565, 1986.
110. Nussenblatt RB, Palestine AG, El-Saied M et al: Long-term antigen specific and non-specific T-cell lines and clones in uveitis, *Curr Eye Res* 3:299-305, 1984.
111. Caspi RR, Roberge FG, McAllister CG et al: T cell lines mediating experimental autoimmune uveoretinitis (EAU) in the rat, *J Immunol* 136:928-933, 1986.
112. Sakai J: Immune complexes in experimental autoimmune uveoretinitis, *Nippon Ganka Gakkai Zasshi* 87:1288-1299, 1983.
113. Marak GE Jr, Wacker WB, Rao NA et al: Effects of complement depletion on experimental allergic uveitis, *Ophthalmic Res* 11:97-107, 1979.
114. Mochizuki M, Kuwabara T, Chan C et al: An association between susceptibility to experimental autoimmune uveitis and choroidal mast cell numbers, *J Immunol* 133:1699-1701, 1984.
115. de Kozak Y, Sainte-Laudy J, Benveniste J et al: Evidence for immediate hypersensitivity phenomena in experimental autoimmune uveoretinitis, *Eur J Immunol* 11:612-617, 1981.
116. Askenase PW, Rosenstein RW, Ptak W: T-cells produce an antigen-binding factor with in vivo activity analogous to IgE antibody, *J Exp Med* 157:862-873, 1983.
117. Chan CC, Mochizuki M, Palestine AG et al: Kinetics of T-lymphocyte subsets in the eyes of Lewis rats with experimental autoimmune uveitis, *Cell Immunol* 96:430-434, 1985.
118. Rosenbaum JT, McDewitt HO, Guss RB et al: Endotoxin-induced uveitis in rats as a model for human disease, *Nature* 286:611, 1980.
119. De Vos AF, Hoekzema R, Kijlstra A: Cytokines and uveitis, a review, *Curr Eye Res* 11:581-597, 1992.
120. Ebringer RW, Cowdell DR, Cowling P: Sequential studies in ankylosing spondylitis, *Ann Rheum Dis* 37:146-151, 1978.
121. Saari KM: Acute anterior uveitis. In Saari KM, editor: *Uveitis update,* Amsterdam, 1984, Excerpta Medica.
122. Schwimmbeck PL, Yu DTY, Oldstone MBA: Autoantibodies to HLA B27 in the sera of HLA B27 patients with ankylosing spondylitis and Reiter's syndrome, *J Exp Med* 166:173-181, 1987.
123. Gery I, Mochizuki M, Nussenblatt RB: Retinal specific antigens and immunopathogenic processes they provoke. In Osborne N, Chader J, editors: *Progress in retinal research,* vol 5, Oxford, 1986, Pergamon Press.
124. Nussenblatt RB: Experimental autoimmune uveitis: mechanisms of disease and clinical therapeutic indications (Proctor lecture), *Invest Ophthalmol Vis Sci* 32:3131-3141, 1991.
125. Caspi RR, Nussenblatt RB: Natural and therapeutic control of ocular autoimmunity: rodent and man, *Autoimmunity: physiology and disease,* New York, 1994, Wiley-Liss.
126. Nussenblatt RB, Rodrigues MM, Wacker WB et al: Cyclosporin A. Inhibition of experimental autoimmune uveitis in Lewis rats, *J Clin Invest* 67:1228-1231, 1981.
127. Nussenblatt RB, Rodrigues MM, Salinas-Carmona MC et al: Modulation of experimental autoimmune uveitis with cyclosporin A, *Arch Ophthalmol* 100:1146-1149, 1982.
128. Nussenblatt RB, Gery I, Ballintine EJ et al: Cellular immune responsiveness of uveitis patients to retinal S-antigen, *Am J Ophthalmol* 89:173-179, 1980.
129. Bevilacqua MP, Stengelin S, Gimbrone MAJ et al: Endothelial leukocyte adhesion molecule–1: an inducible receptor for neutrophils related to complement regulatory proteins and lectins, *Science* 243:1160-1164, 1989.
130. Luscinskas FW, Brock AF, Arnaout MA Jr: Endothelial-leukocyte adhesion molecule-1–dependent and leukocyte (CD11/CD18)-dependent mechanisms contribute to polymorphonuclear leukocyte adhesion to cytokine-activated human vascular endothelium, *J Immunol* 142: 2257-2263, 1989.
131. Mulligan MS, Varani J, Dame MK et al: Role of endothelial-leukocyte adhesion molecule 1 (ELAM-1) in neutrophil-mediated lung injury in rats, *J Clin Invest* 88:1396-1406, 1991.
132. Springer TA: Traffic signals for lymphocyte recirculation and leukocyte emigration: the multistep paradigm, *Cell* 76:301-314, 1994.
133. Munro JM, Pober JS, Cotran RS: Recruitment of neutrophils in the local endotoxin response: association with de novo endothelial expression of endothelial leukocyte adhesion molecule–1, *Lab Invest* 64: 295-299, 1991.
134. Whitcup SM, Wakefield D, Li Q et al: Endothelial leukocyte adhesion molecule–1 in endotoxin-induced uveitis, *Invest Ophthalmol Vis Sci* 33:2626-2630, 1992.
135. Ayo C: A toxic ocular action. New property of Shwartzman toxins, *J Immunol* 46:113-132, 1943.
136. Rosenbaum JT, McDevitt HO, Guss RB et al: Endotoxin-induced uveitis in rats as a model for human disease, *Nature* 286:611-613, 1980.
137. Forrester JV, Worgul BV, Merriam GR Jr: Endotoxin-induced uveitis in the rat, *Albrecht von Graefes Arch Klin Ophthalmol* 213:221-233, 1980.
138. Kogiso M, Tanouchi Y, Mimora Y et al: Endotoxin-induced uveitis in mice. I. Induction of uveitis and role of T lymphocytes, *Jpn J Ophthalmol* 36:281-290, 1992.
139. Whitcup SM, DeBarge LR, Rosen H et al: Monoclonal antibody against CD11b/CD18 inhibits endotoxin-induced uveitis, *Invest Ophthalmol Vis Sci* 34:673-681, 1993.
140. Elner VM, Elner SG, Pavilack MA et al: Intercellular adhesion molecule–1 in human corneal endothelium: modulation and function, *Am J Pathol* 138:525-536, 1991.

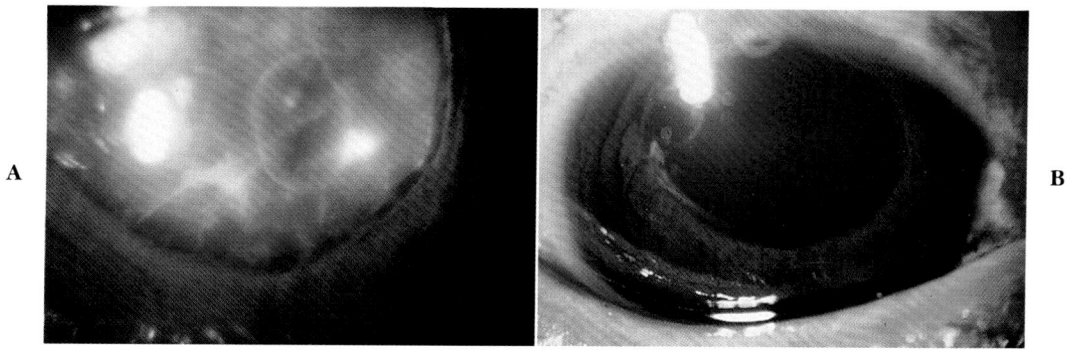


**Plate 8. A,** Uveitic eye after extracapsular cataract extraction (ECCE) (phacoemulsification) and intraocular lens (IOL) placement. Postoperative inflammatory response was severe, with development of fibrin in anterior chamber. **B,** Clinical improvement occurred 24 hours after injection with tissue plasminogen activator (TPA). (Courtesy Rubens Belfort, Jr., M.D., Sao Paulo, Brazil.)

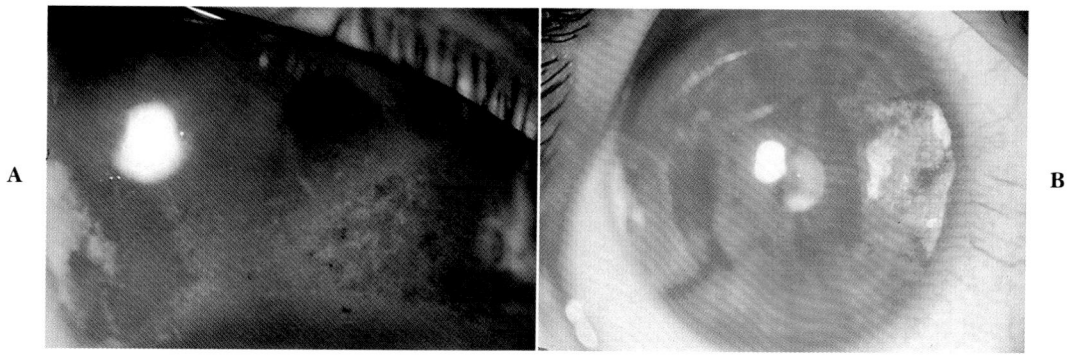


**Plate 9. A,** Band keratopathy in 6-year-old boy with bilateral uveitis. **B,** Same eye 2 days after excimer laser surgery performed with use of topical anesthesia. (Courtesy Rubens Belfort, Jr., M.D., Sao Paulo, Brazil.)

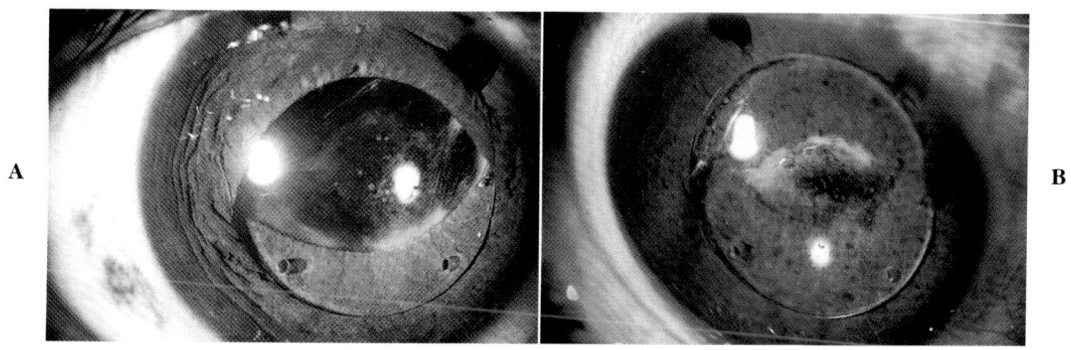


**Plate 10.** Uveitic eye that underwent cataract surgery and posterior chamber IOL placement. **A,** Inferior portion of lens has migrated anterior to lens plane. **B,** Whole lens is now forward. This "iris capture" occurred without marked inflammatory disease. (Courtesy Rubens Belfort, Jr., M.D., Sao Paulo, Brazil.)

A

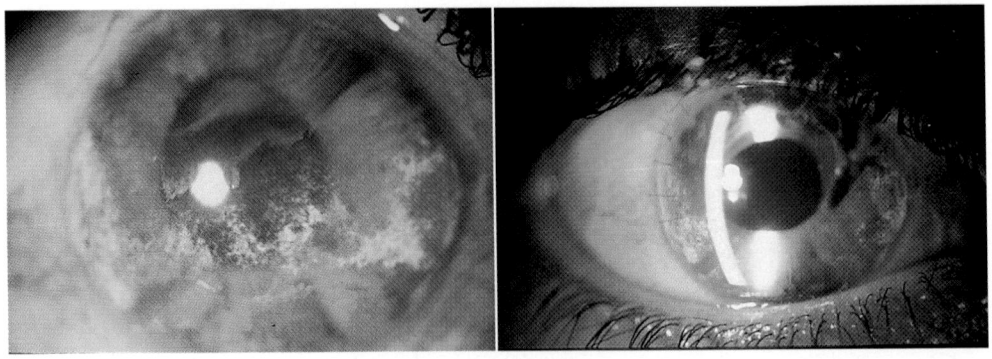

B

**Plate 11.** When his disease was quiescent, an 11-year-old boy with anterior uveitis underwent cataract extraction and IOL placement. **A,** After multiple YAG capsulotomies and EDTA treatments, a persistent anterior chamber reaction required topical steroid therapy. **B,** After IOL removal and normalization of intraocular pressure, inflammation was absent, steroid therapy had been discontinued, and visual acuity was 20/100. (Courtesy Rubens Belfort, Jr., M.D., Sao Paulo, Brazil.)

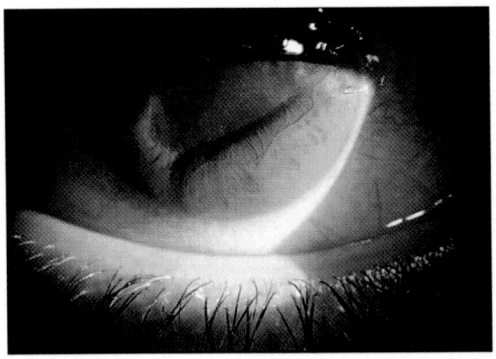

**Plate 12.** Slit-lamp photograph of patient with uveitis and pupillary block glaucoma. Iris bombé, due to broad iris-lens synechiae, localized from 3 to 6 o'clock position.

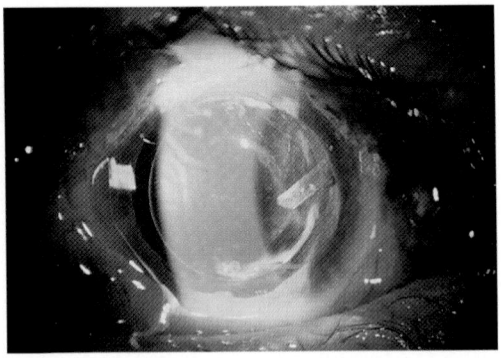

**Plate 13.** Uveitic eye with secondary glaucoma that could not be controlled with maximum medication or trabeculectomy surgery. Tube from single-plate Molteno implant can be seen in anterior chamber at 2 o'clock position.

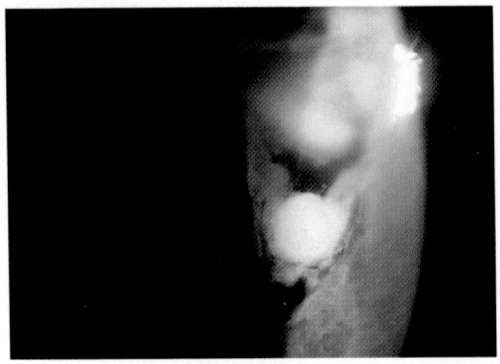

**Plate 14.** YAG laser membrane discission in patient with dense post–cataract surgery pupillary membrane.

141. Whitcup SM, Hikita N, Shirao M et al: Effect of monoclonal antibodies against ICAM-1 (CD54) an LFA-1 alpha (CD11a) in the prevention and treatment of endotoxin-induced uveitis (EIU), *Invest Ophthalmol Vis Sci* 34 (suppl):1143, 1993.
142. Rosenbaum JT, Boney RS: Efficacy of antibodies to adhesion molecules, CD11a or CD18, in rabbit models of uveitis, *Curr Eye Res* 12:827-831, 1993.
143. Springer TA: Adhesion receptors of the immune system, *Nature* 346:425-434, 1990.
144. Springer TA, Dustin ML, Kishimoto TK et al: The lymphocyte function-associated LFA-1, CD2, and LFA-3 molecules: cell adhesion receptors of the immune system, *Annu Rev Immunol* 5:223-252, 1987.
145. Dustin ML, Springer TA: Lymphocyte function-associated antigen–1 (LFA-1) interaction with intercellular adhesion molecule (ICAM-1) is one of at least three mechanisms for lymphocyte adhesion to cultured endothelial cells, *J Cell Biol* 107:321-331, 1988.
146. Norris DA: Cytokine modulation of adhesion molecules in the regulation of immunologic cytotoxicity of epidermal targets, *J Invest Dermatol* 95:11S-120S, 1990.
147. Kaminska GM, Niederkorn JY, McCulley JP: Intercellular adhesion molecule–1 (ICAM-1) expression in normal and inflamed human cornea: induction by recombinant interferon gamma and interleukin-1, *Ophthalmol Vis Sci* 32 (suppl):677, 1991.
148. Liversidge J, Sewell HF, Forrester JV: Interactions between lymphocytes and cells of the blood-retina barrier: mechanisms of T lymphocyte adhesion to human retinal capillary endothelial cells and retinal pigment epithelial cells in vitro, *Immunology* 71:390-396, 1990.
149. Whitcup SM, DeBarge LR, Caspi RR et al: Monoclonal antibodies against ICAM-1 (CD54) and LFA-1 (CD11a/CD18) inhibit experimental autoimmune uveitis, *Clin Immunol Immunopathol* 67:143-150, 1993.
150. Till GO, Mulligan MS, Lee S et al: Adhesion molecules in experimental phacoanaphylactic endophthalmitis, *Invest Ophthalmol Vis Sci* 33 (suppl):795, 1992.
151. Whitcup SM, Chan CC, Li Q et al: Expression of cell adhesion molecules in posterior uveitis, *Arch Ophthalmol* 110:662-666, 1992.
152. Whitcup SM, Nussenblatt RB, Price FW et al: Expression of cell adhesion molecules in corneal graft failure, *Cornea* 12:475-480, 1993.
153. Haug CE, Colvin RB, Delmonico FL et al: A phase I trial of immunosuppression with anti-ICAM–1 (CD54) mAb in renal allograft recipients, *Transplantation* 55:766-773, 1993.
154. Hooks JJ, Detrick B:Immunoregulatory functions of interferon. In Torrence P, editor: *Biological response modifiers,* San Diego, 1985, Academic Press.

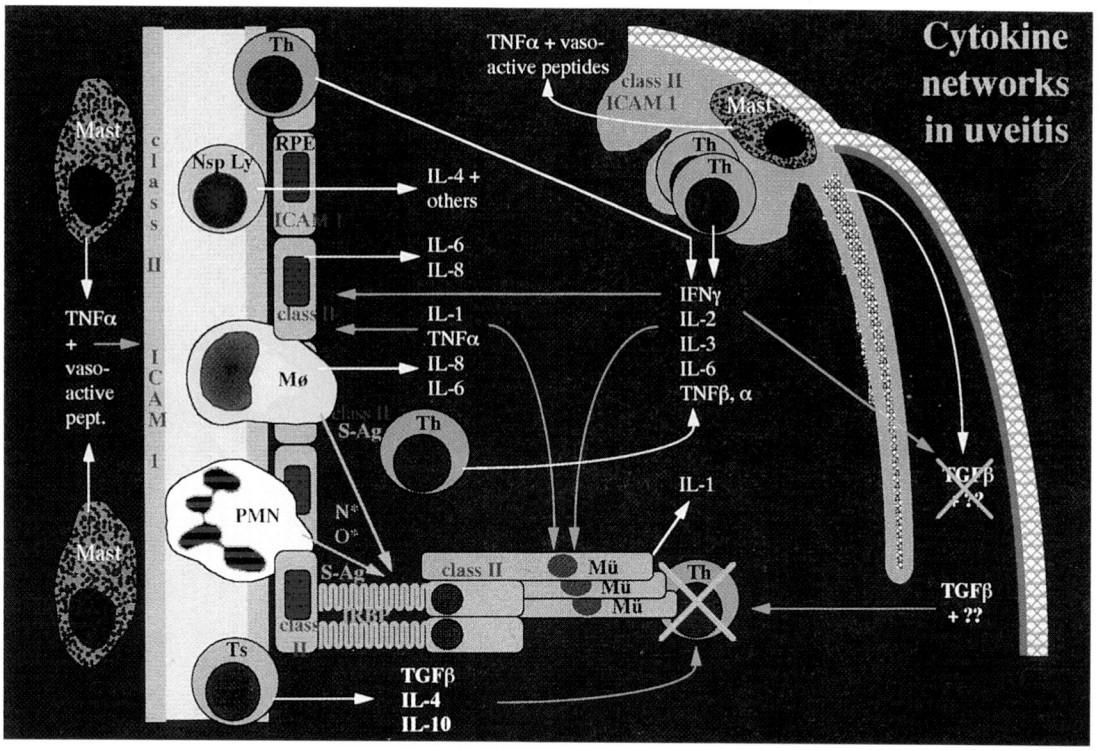


**Plate 1.** Schematic representation of (1) numerous interactions within eye of immune system's cells and (2) cells resident in eye. (Courtesy Rachel Caspi, Ph.D.)

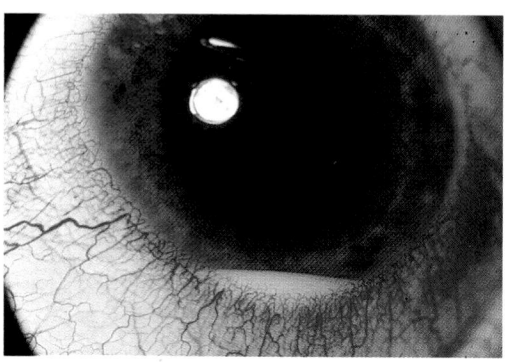

**Plate 2.** Hypopyon in patient with Behçet's disease.

**Plate 3.** Grading of vitreous haze. (From Nussenblatt RB, Palestine AG, Chan CC et al: Standardization of vitreal inflammatory activity in intermediate and posterior uveitis, *Ophthalmology* 92:467-471, 1985.)

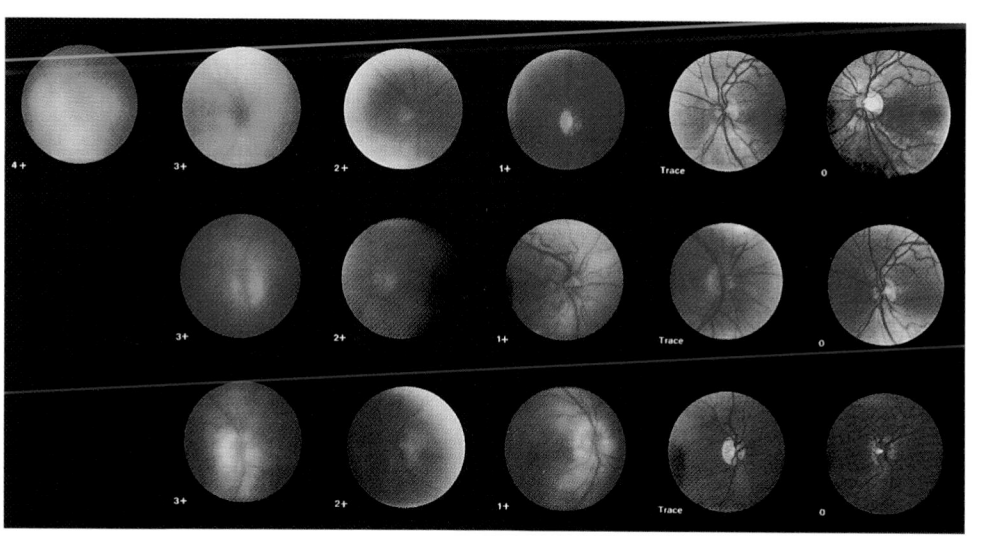

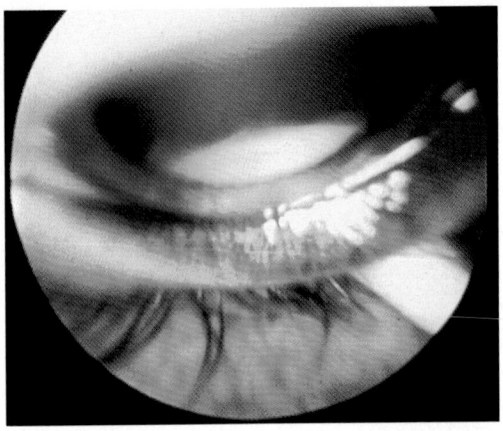

**Plate 4.** Exudate on pars plana (snowbank) in patient with pars planitis. (Courtesy Ronald Smith, M.D.)

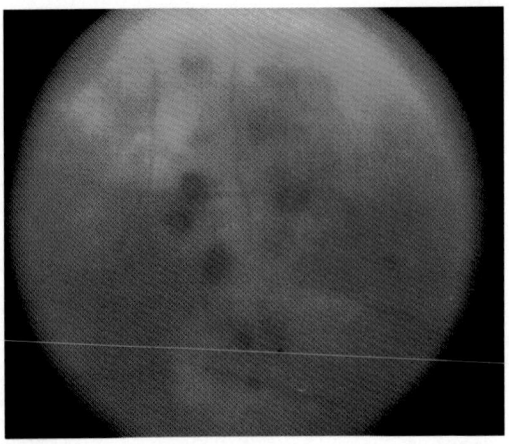

**Plate 5.** Fundus photograph showing yellow-colored subretinal infiltrates, retinal hemorrhage, and retinal edema in eye with 20/125 visual acuity and moderate vitritis.

A

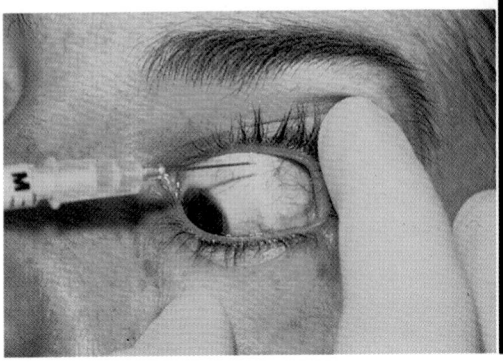

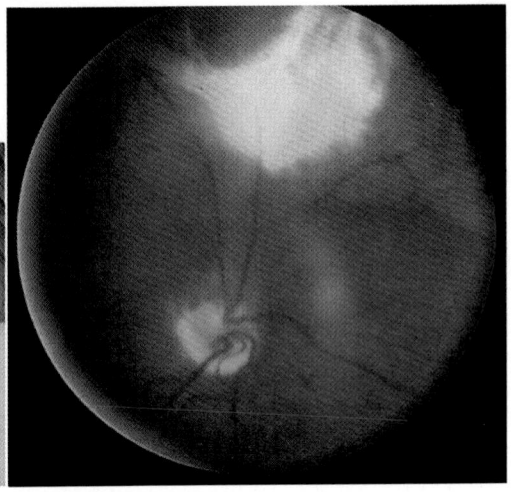

B

**Plate 6. A,** Temporal approach to giving periocular injection. **B,** Although possibility is markedly decreased if precautions are taken, perforation of globe can occur, as seen here.

A

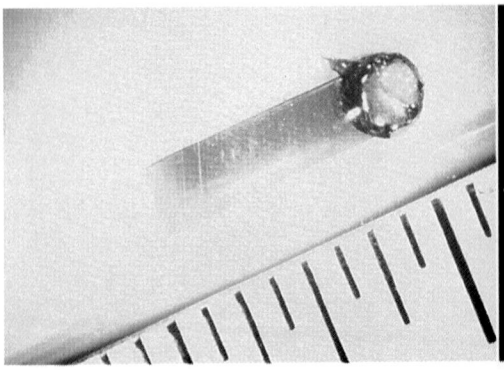

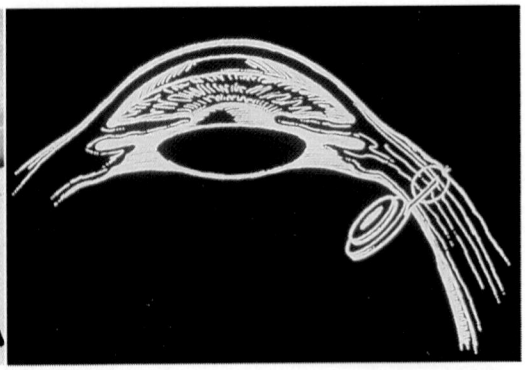

B

**Plate 7. A,** Intraocular device used for delivery of ganciclovir. **B,** Position in vitreous after suturing into sclera at pars plana level. (Courtesy Chiron Corp.)

A

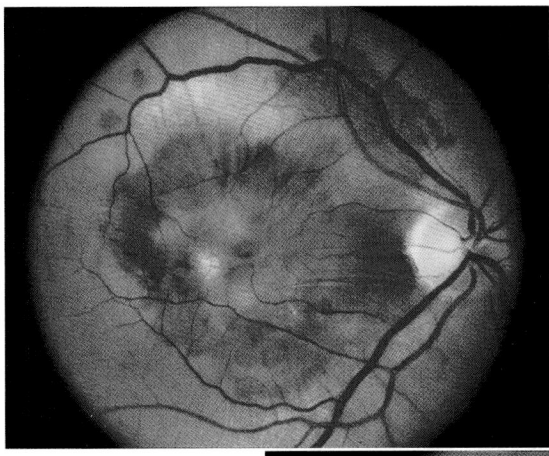

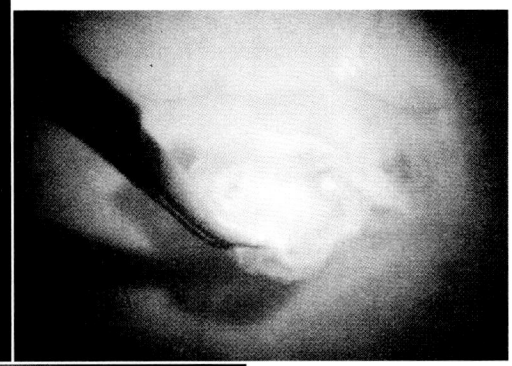

B

C

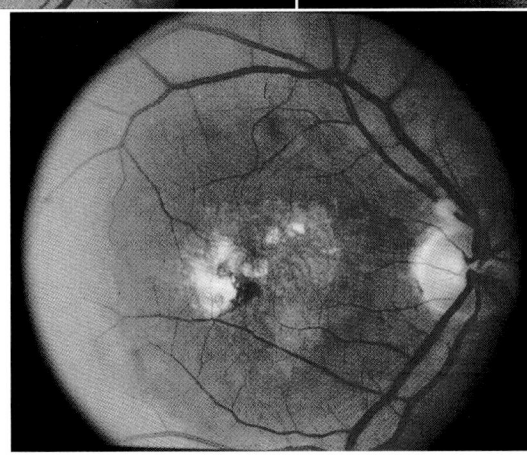

**Plate 15. A,** Subretinal neovascular lesion in macular region. **B,** Removal of lesion with special subretinal forceps. **C,** Fundus as it appears after surgery. (Courtesy Antonio Capone Jr., M.D., and Daniel Martin, M.D., Emory University, Atlanta, Ga.)

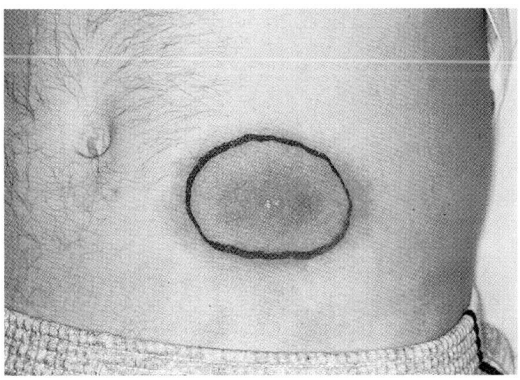

**Plate 16.** Erythema migrans, rash characteristic of Lyme disease, is seen on abdomen of patient. Rash is usually oval or annular with expanding borders. Black circle was drawn to outline border of rash 24 hours before time of this photograph. Note that borders of rash have expanded substantially since previous day.

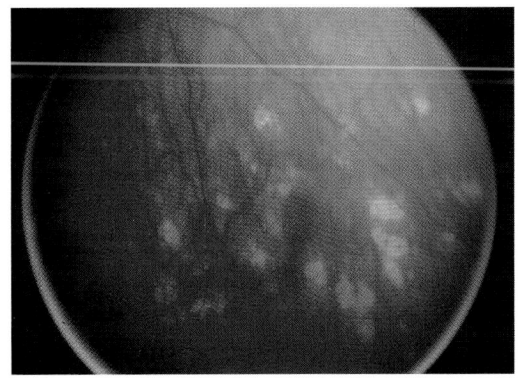

**Plate 17.** Well-circumscribed lesions in periphery of choroid in patient with brucellosis. (Courtesy Narsing A. Rao, M.D.)

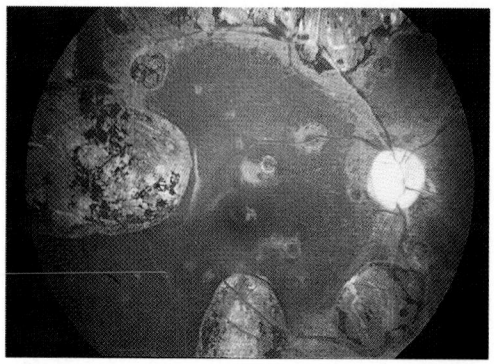

**Plate 18.** Chorioretinal lesions in young patient with chronic granulomatous disease. Macular involvement resulted in decreased visual acuity.

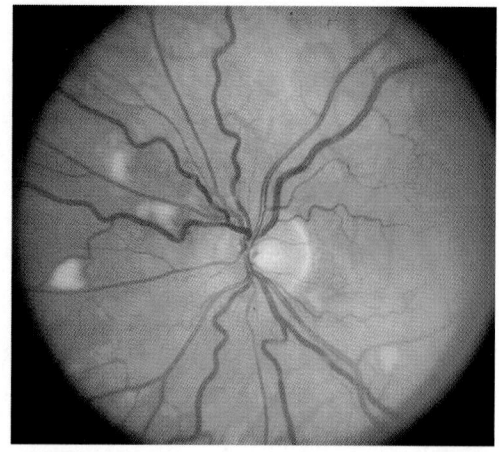

**Plate 19.** Multiple nerve fiber layer infarcts (cotton-wool spots) in patient with AIDS.

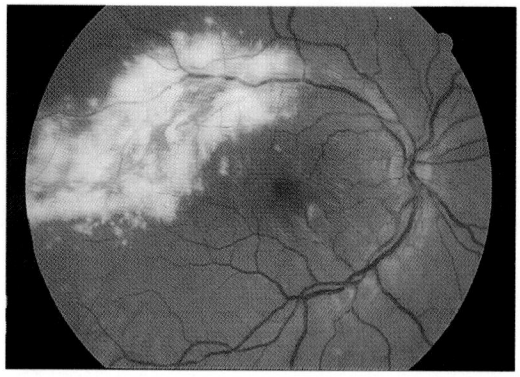

**Plate 20.** Cytomegalovirus retinitis in vascular distribution characterized by fluffy-white retinal infiltration and small area of retinal hemorrhage.

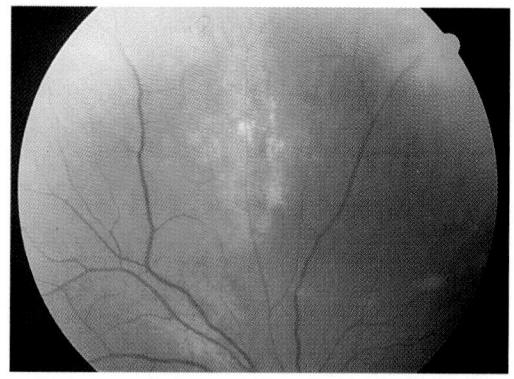

**Plate 21.** Cytomegalovirus retinitis may also have granular appearance with mottling of retinal pigment epithelium and little associated retinal hemorrhage.

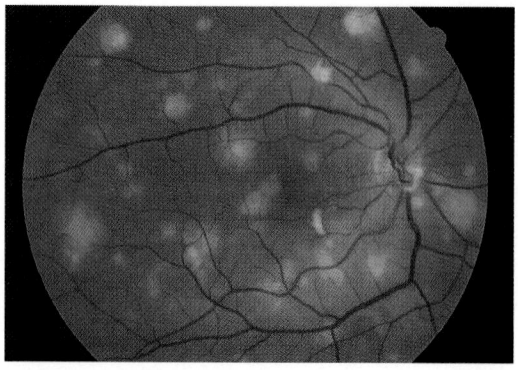

**Plate 22.** Fundus photograph of patient with AIDS and *Pneumocystis carinii* pneumonia shows multiple yellow deep choroidal lesions. Histopathologic examination revealed not only *P. carinii* cysts but also cytomegalovirus (see Plate 23) and *Mycobacterium avium–intracellulare* (see Plate 24). (From *Retina* 12:331-335, 1992.)

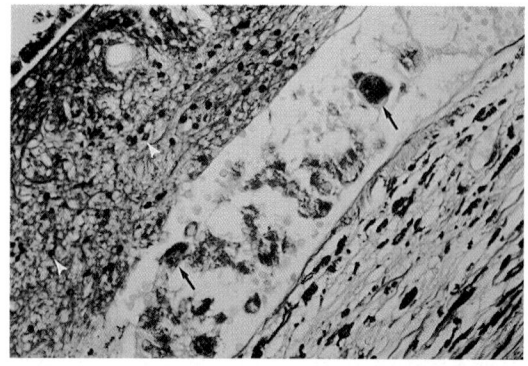

**Plate 23.** Photomicrograph of choroidal lesion of right eye shows numerous *Pneumocystis carinii* cysts *(white arrowheads)* and cytomegalovirus cells in choroidal blood vessel *(arrows)*. (Gomori's methenimine-silver stain; ×400.) (From *Retina* 12:331-335, 1992.)

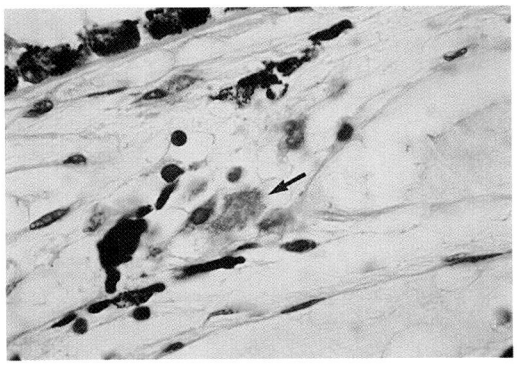

**Plate 24.** Photomicrograph of choroid adjacent to area infiltrated with *Pneumocystis carinii* shows cluster of acid-fast bacilli *(arrow)*. (Ziehl-Neelsen stain; ×100.) (From *Retina* 12:331-335, 1992.)

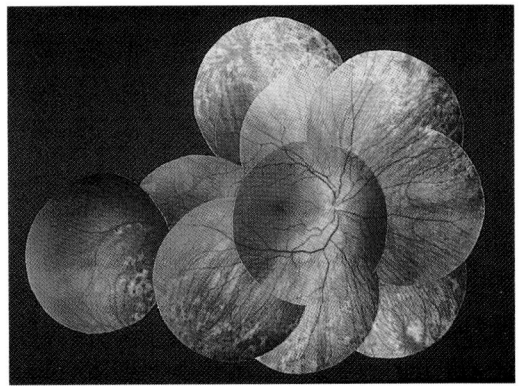

**Plate 25.** Photographic montage of patient with didanosine-related retinal lesions. Atrophic areas of retinal pigment epithelium hypopigmentation and hyperpigmentation are seen in midperiphery of fundus.

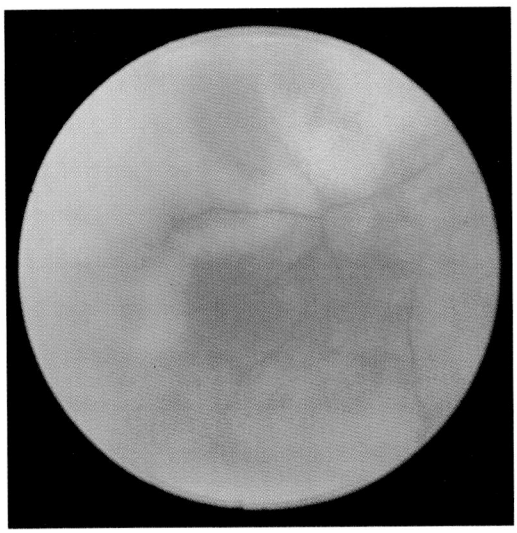

**Plate 26.** Acute retinal necrosis with dense white retinal infiltrate in retinal periphery.

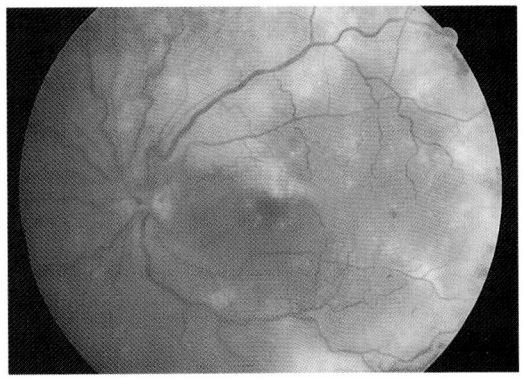

**Plate 27.** Diffuse retinitis involving posterior pole in patient with progressive outer retinal necrosis. Retinitis appears to involve outer retina with little evidence of retinal vasculitis. (Courtesy Christopher Walton, M.D., National Eye Institute, Bethesda, Md.)

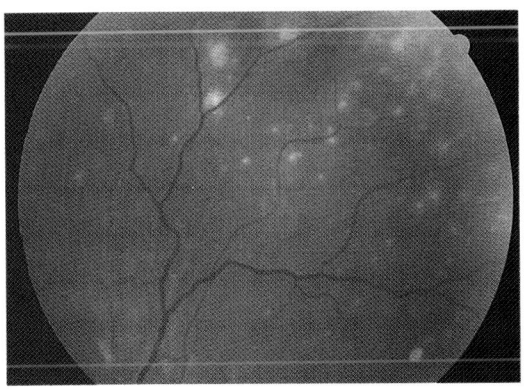

**Plate 28.** Multifocal punctate lesions involving outer retina early in course of progressive outer retinal necrosis. These lesions quickly spread and coalesced despite therapy. (Courtesy Christopher Walton, M.D., National Eye Institute, Bethesda, Md.)

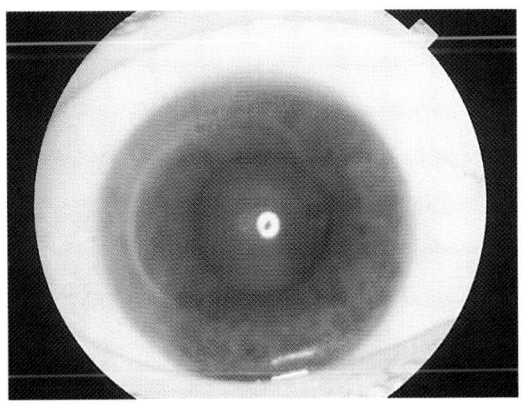

**Plate 29.** Twelve-year-old girl with herpes simplex virus keratitis complicated by anterior uveitis, disciform stromal keratitis, and formation of Wesseley immune ring. (Courtesy Roger George, M.D.)

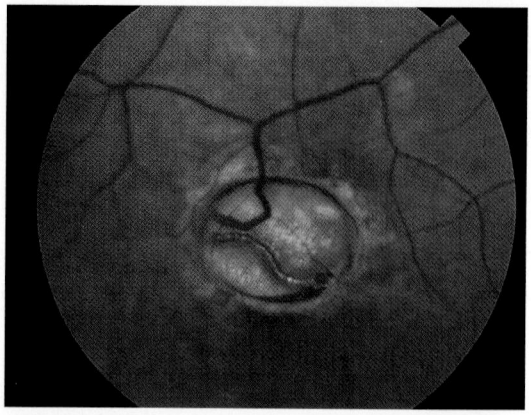

**Plate 30.** Fundus photograph of eye with congenital toxoplasmosis, with retinochoroidal shunt. (Courtesy J. Melamed, M.D., Porto Alegre, Brazil.)

A

B

C

D

E

**Plate 31.** Fundus photographs and angiograms of 30-year-old patient who reported metamorphopsia for several weeks in left eye. Visual acuity was 20/40, with 20/20 vision in right eye. **A** shows raised macular lesion. Angiogram **(B)** shows hyperfluorescence compatible with subfoveal neovascularization. Vision in left eye decreased to 20/100 at 3 months and was 20/80 at 6 months. However, pigmented ring around lesion **(C)** was noted. By 24 months, vision had returned to 20/20, with atrophic lesion in macula present **(D),** with staining but not leakage noted on angiogram **(E).** (Courtesy Peter A. Campochiaro, M.D.)

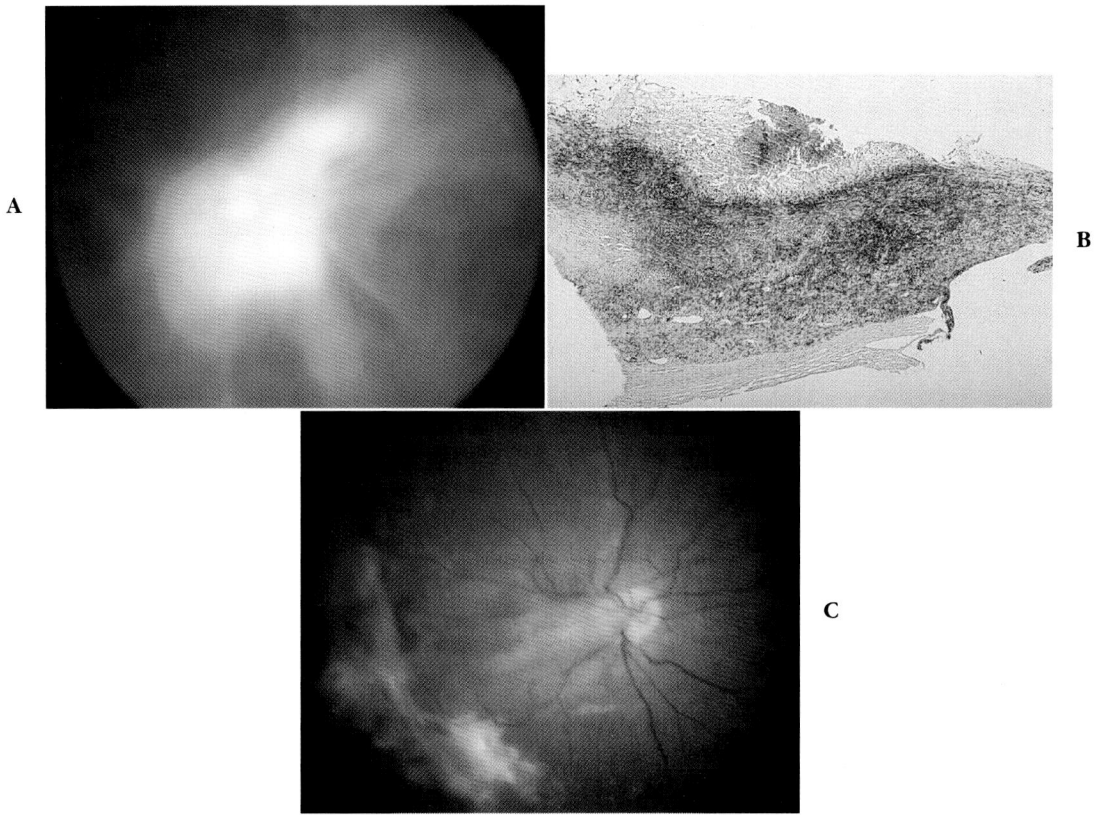


**Plate 32. A,** Posterior traction detachment caused by large granuloma. After pars plana vitrectomy, lesion was removed in toto through retinotomy site. **B,** Histologic findings of lesion were characteristic of toxocariasis lesion. Result of ELISA for *Toxocara canis* found vitreous sample markedly positive. **C,** Posterior pole after surgery. Vision improved from hand motion to 15/200. (Courtesy Prof. M. Gonvers, Lausanne, Switzerland.)

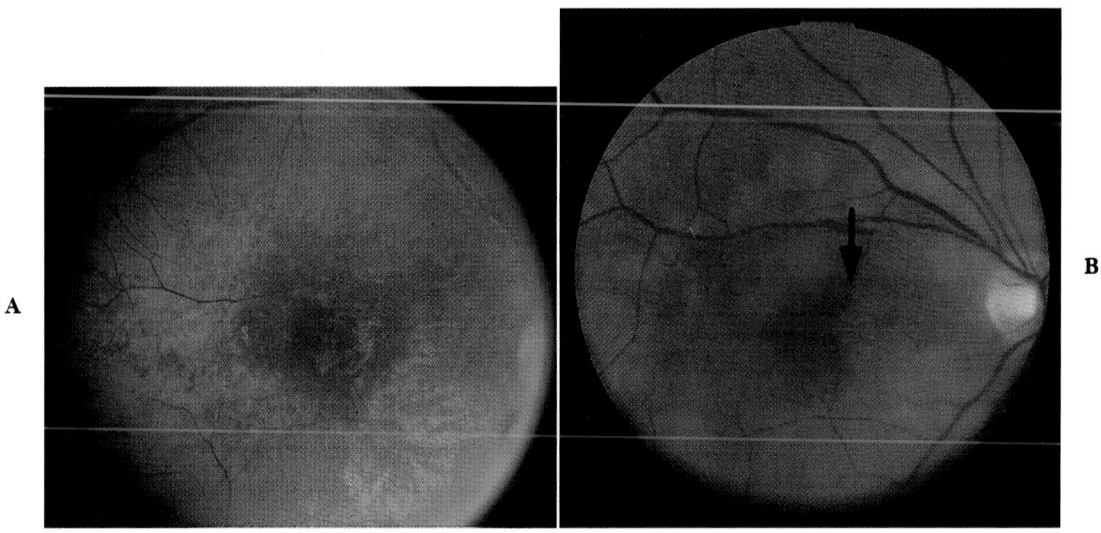


**Plate 33.** Fundus photographs of worms causing diffuse unilateral subacute neuroretinitis from, **A,** southern part of United States and, **B,** northern part of United States. (Courtesy J. Donald Gass, M.D.)

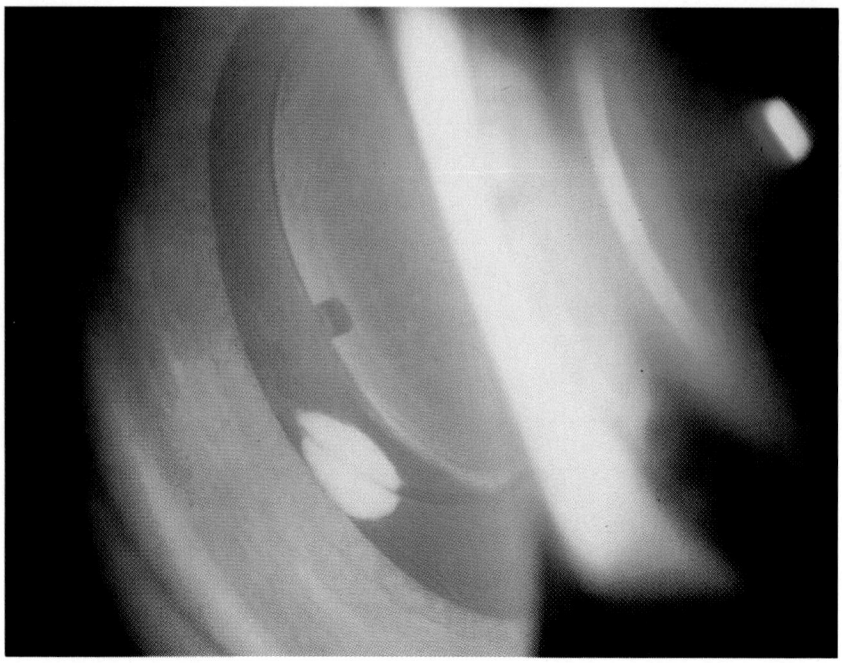

**Plate 34.** Infiltrate on lens haptic in patient with late-onset postoperative endophthalmitis caused by *Propionibacterium acnes*. (Courtesy Robert Martin, M.D.)

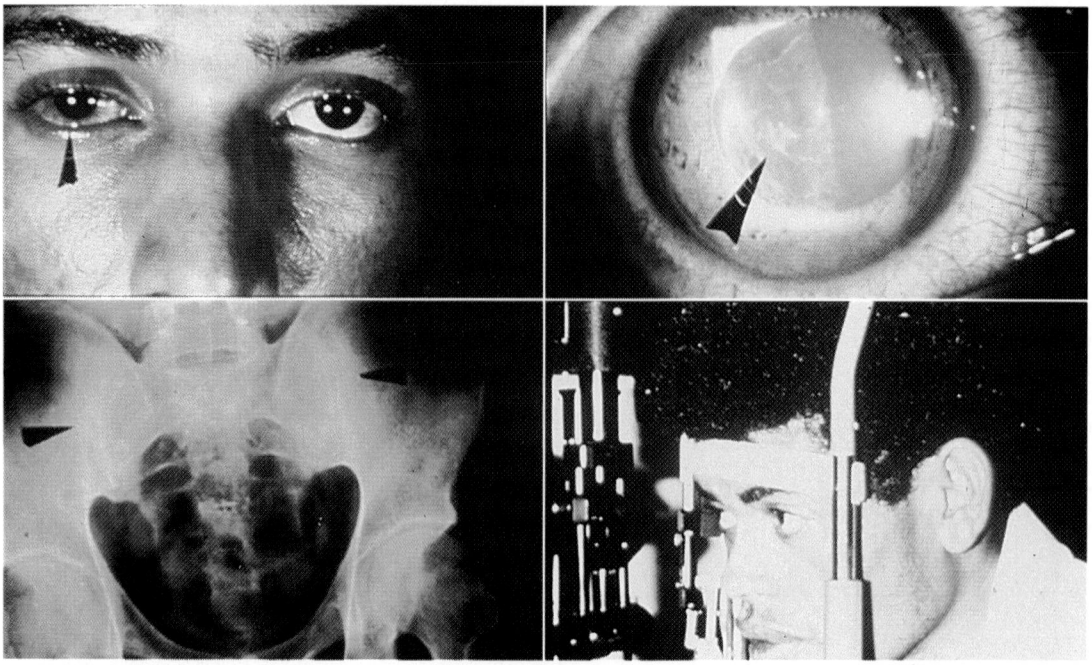


**Plate 35. A,** Unilateral redness caused by iritis associated with ankylosing spondylitis. **B,** Fibrin clot in anterior chamber in iritis associated with ankylosing spondylitis. **C,** X-ray film of sacroiliac joints demonstrating increased radiodensity caused by ankylosing spondylitis. **D,** Flexed neck caused by ankylosis of cervical spine in ankylosing spondylitis. (Courtesy Fernando Oréfice, M.D., and Rubens Belfort, Jr., M.D.)

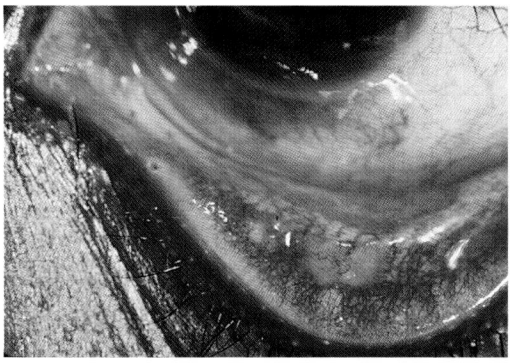

**Plate 36.** Biopsy proven conjunctival granulomas in patient with sarcoidosis.

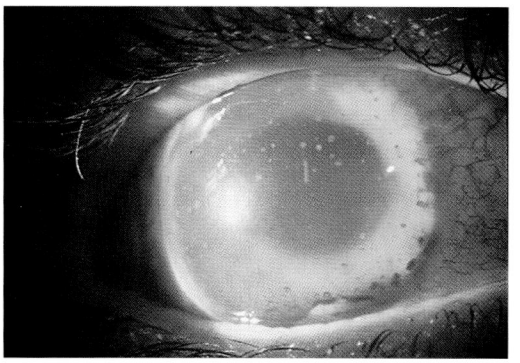

**Plate 37.** Large granulomatous mutton-fat keratic precipitates in patient with chronic uveitis and sarcoidosis.

A

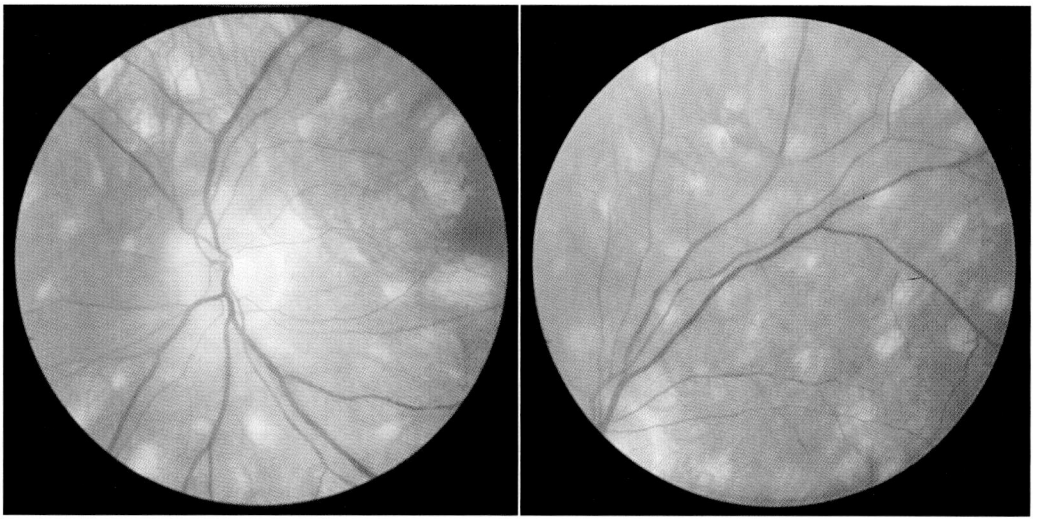

B

**Plate 38.** Multiple cream-colored lesions, circular or oval, deep to retina, are seen in birdshot retinopathy. They tend to be clustered in posterior pole **(A)** out to midperiphery **(B).**

A

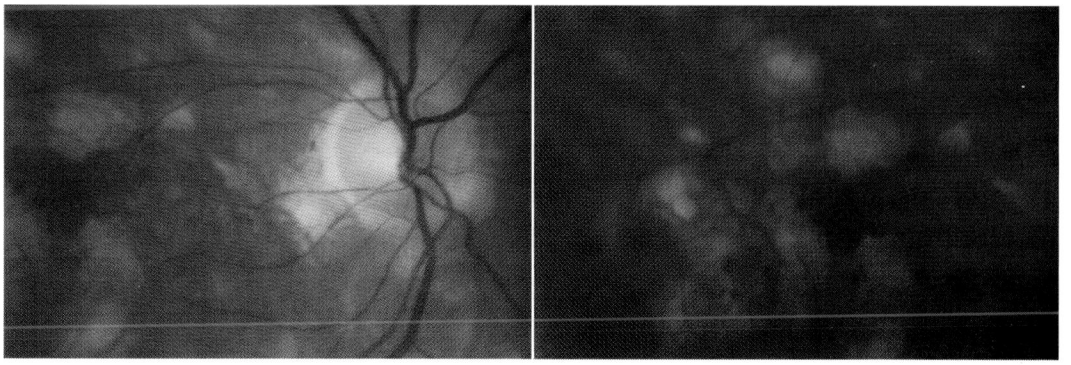

B

**Plate 39. A** and **B,** High-magnification fundus photographs of lesions in long-standing disease. There is loss of retinal pigment epithelium in some areas, and choroidal vessels are apparent.

A

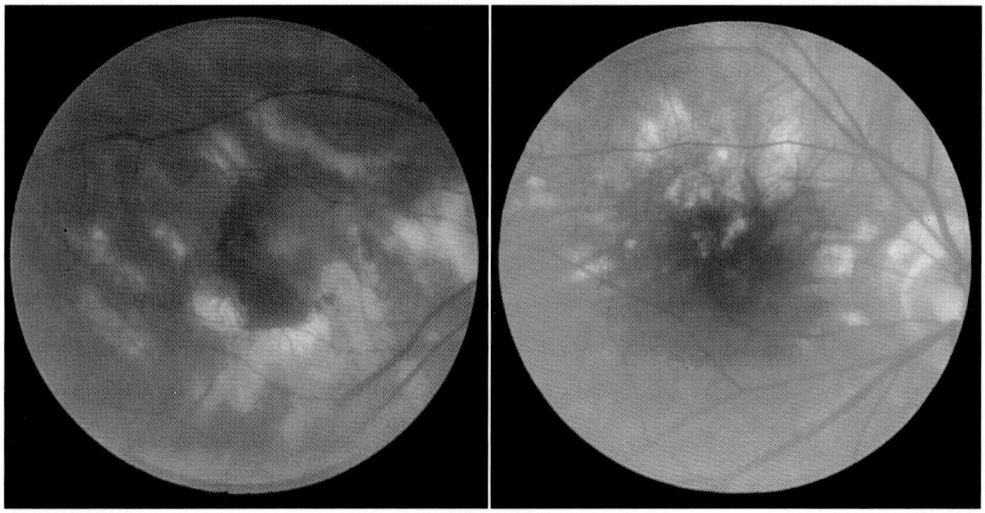

B

**Plate 40.** Patient with birdshot lesions strewn throughout posterior pole of both eyes. **A,** Right eye has subfoveal net that has bled and raised macula. **B,** Left eye has lesion in macula.

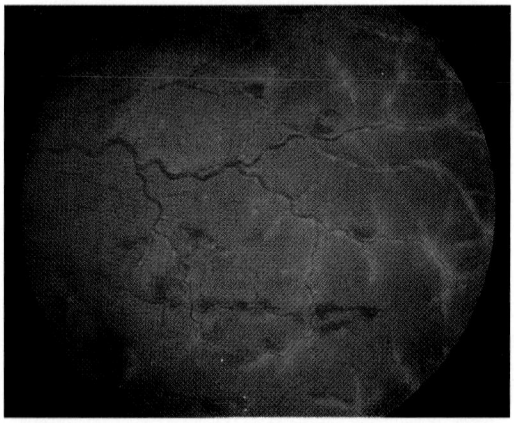

**Plate 41.** Fundus of young boy with idiopathic frosted-branch angiitis. Yannuzzi has suggested that angiitis is seen in children whereas periphlebitis generally is noted in young adults. (Courtesy L.A. Yannuzzi, M.D.)

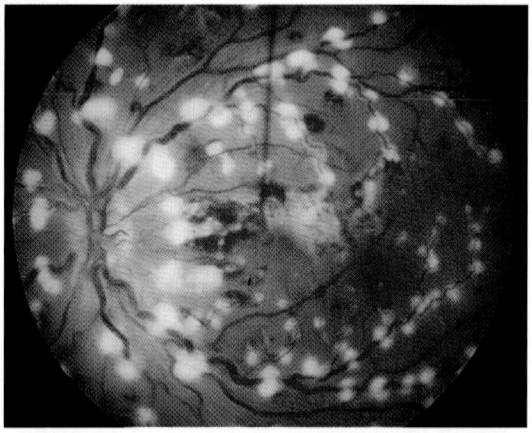

**Plate 42.** Fundus of young woman with difficult-to-control systemic lupus erythematosus. Extensive nerve fiber infarcts and hemorrhage create dramatic picture, with maintenance of good visual acuity. Retinopathy cleared after disease was controlled.

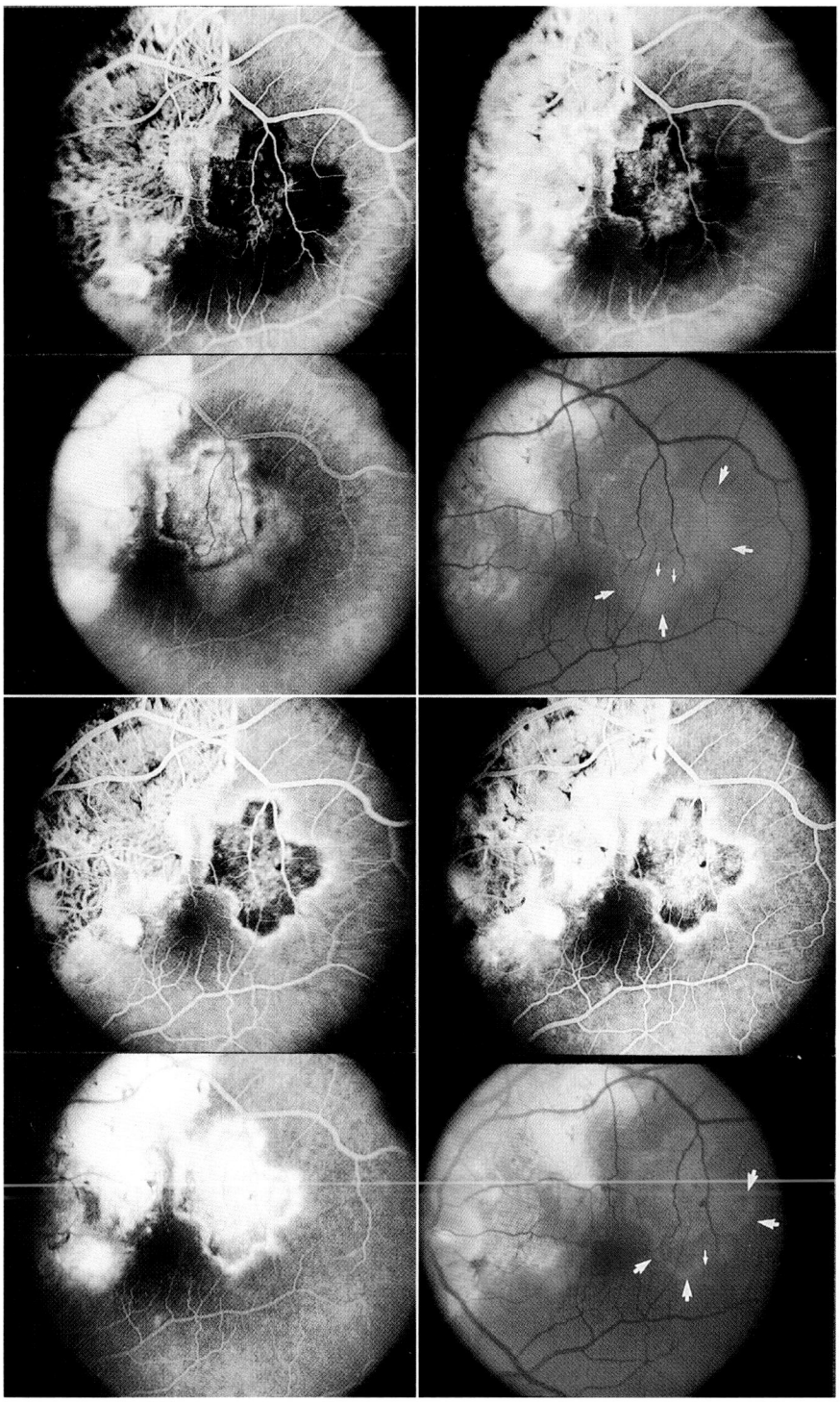

A

B

**Plate 43. A,** Fluorescein angiogram and fundus photograph of patient with serpiginous choroiditis, complaints of slightly decreased visual acuity, and metamorphopsia in left eye. Early blocked fluorescence and late leakage are seen at borders of active lesions. Late frame also shows late leakage compatible with serous detachment of adjacent retina *(arrows).* **B,** Fluorescein angiogram and fundus photograph of same patient 9 days after pulse intravenous methylprednisolone. Patient had noted decreased metamorphopsia. Early blocked fluorescence is no longer seen at border of lesion, and serous retinal detachment has resolved *(arrows).* (From *Ophthalmology* 98:952, 1991.)

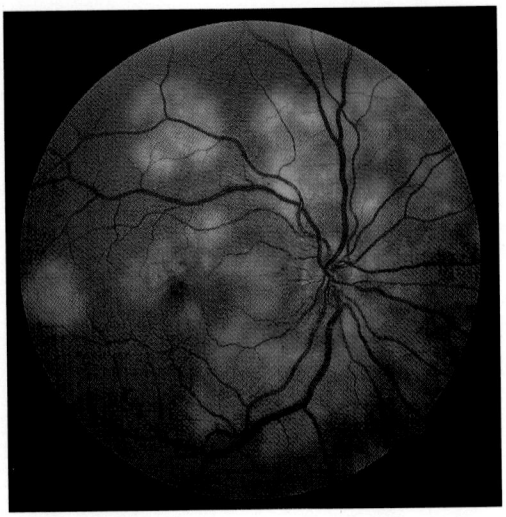

**Plate 44.** Early lesions of acute posterior multifocal placoid pigment epitheliopathy.

A

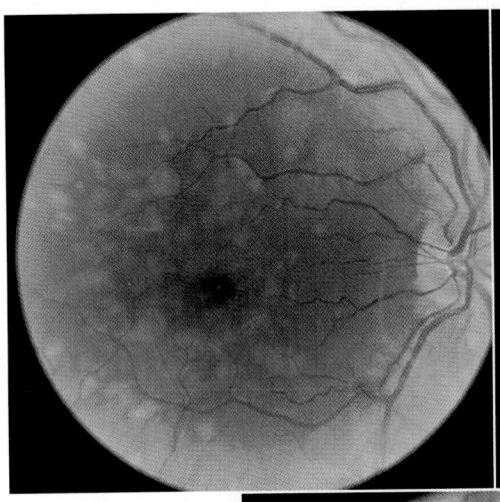

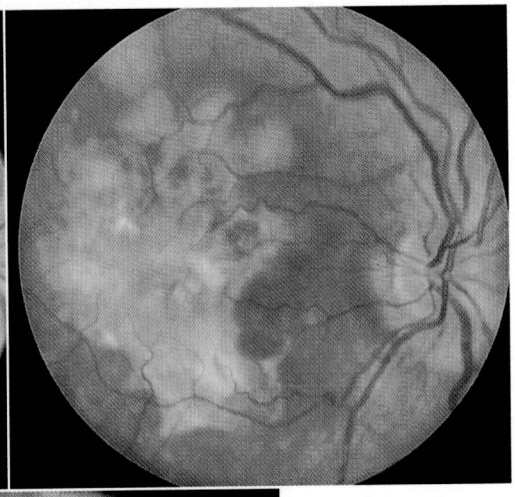

B

C

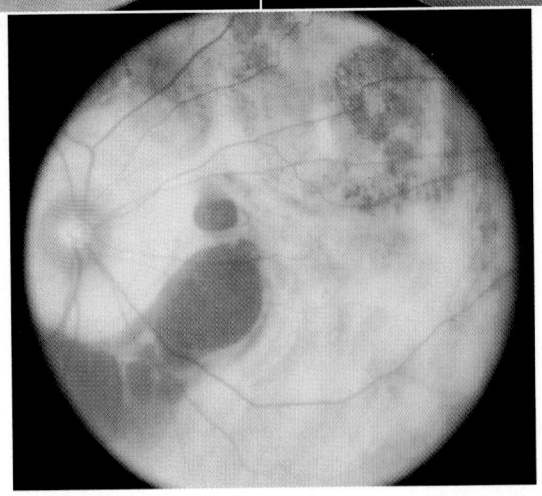

**Plate 45. A,** Early changes of subretinal fibrosis syndrome and uveitis. With time these changes coalesced to form picture seen in **B. C,** Extensive subretinal fibrosis involving disc and then extending into macula region.

A

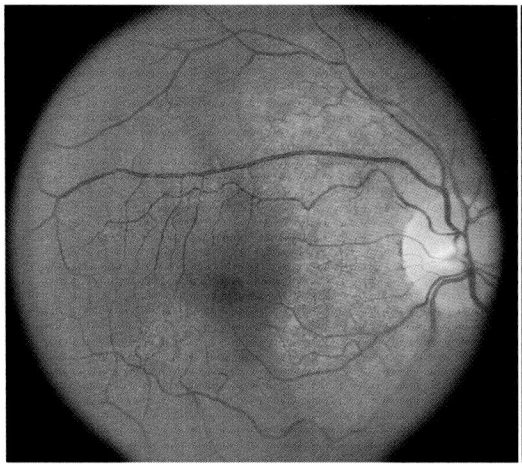

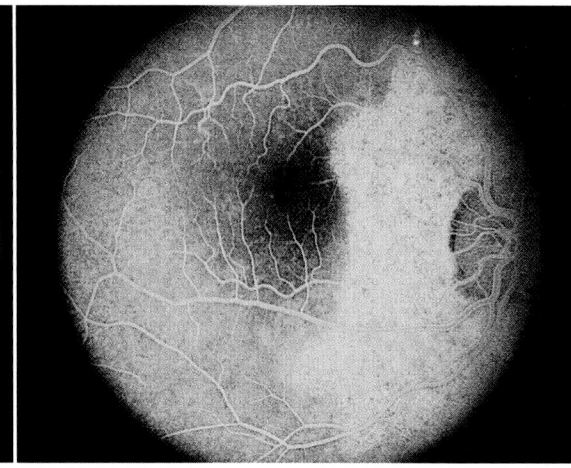

B

**Plate 46. A,** Fundus photograph. **B,** Fluorescein angiogram of patient with acute zonal occult outer retinopathy.

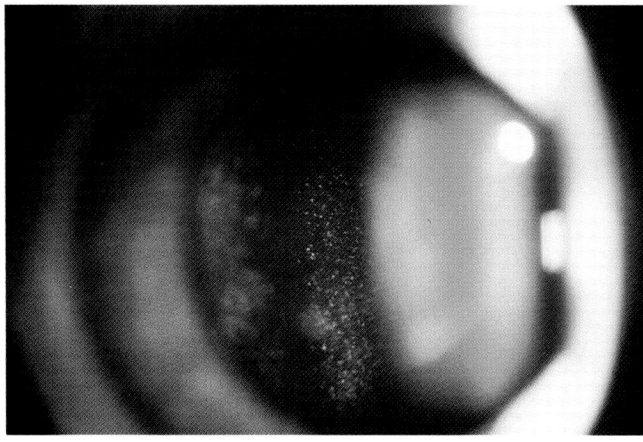

**Plate 47.** Slit-lamp biomicroscopy examination revealing sheets of vitreous cells characteristic of intraocular lymphoma.

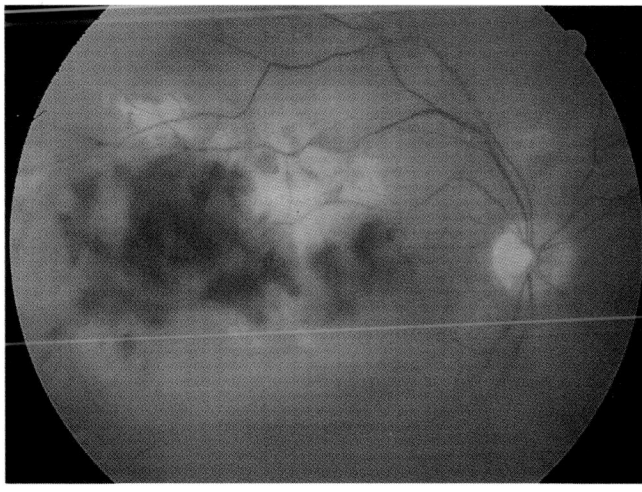

**Plate 48.** Fundus photograph of patient with intraocular lymphoma showing retinal infiltrates and hemorrhage mimicking cytomegalovirus retinitis. Findings resolved with therapy for lymphoma.

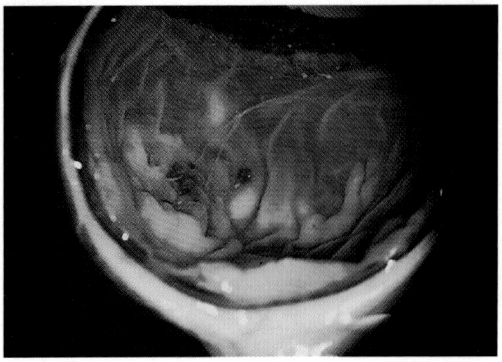

**Plate 49.** Enucleation specimen of patient with intraocular lymphoma shows multiple white areas of retinal and subretinal tumor infiltration with adjacent areas of retinal hemorrhage.

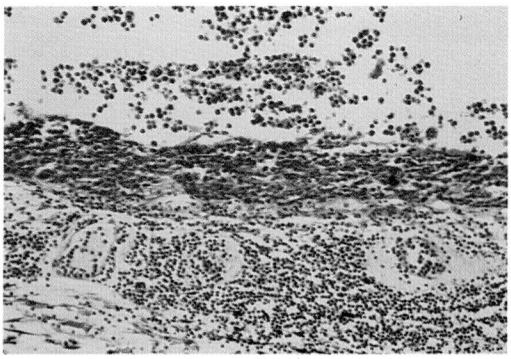

**Plate 50.** Photomicrograph of enucleated globe shown in Plate 49 reveals tumor infiltration between Bruch's membrane and retinal pigment epithelium. Reactive lymphocytes and some tumor cells are seen in overlying vitreous (hematoxylin and eosin; original magnification ×200.).

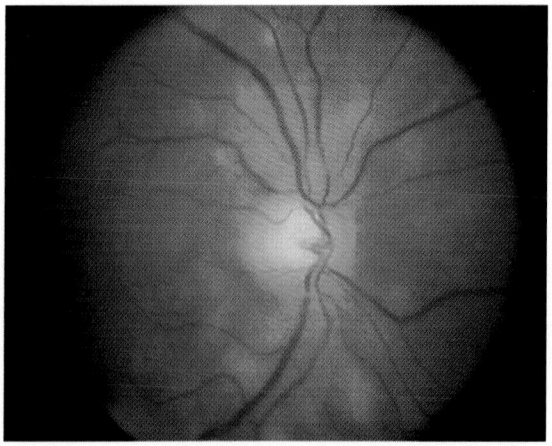

**Plate 51.** Multiple yellow choroidal infiltrates in patient with lymphoid hyperplasia of uvea.

# PART 2

# DIAGNOSIS

# CHAPTER 3

# History Taking in the Patient With Uveitis

The word *diagnosis* comes from the Greek word meaning to distinguish and discern. Diagnosis encompasses both data collection and analysis of the compiled clinical information. The facts used in diagnosis come from a detailed medical history and a thorough physical examination. In the case of patients with uveitis, one must look beyond the eye for important diagnostic clues because the rheumatologic, infectious, and oncologic diseases that cause uveitis are often easier to diagnose after a careful medical history has been taken and a detailed physical examination has been performed. The ophthalmologist who does not examine the skin or joints of the patient with uveitis will miss the opportunity to correctly diagnose many cases of uveitis. Observing the course of the disease as well as the response to therapy can also provide additional insights to the correct causes of the disease.

A careful and detailed medical history is one of the keys to correctly diagnosing the patient with uveitis. It has been estimated that over 90% of diagnoses can be made on the basis of the medical history alone. It is important not only to obtain a series of medical facts but also to form an impression about the overall course of the disease and the impact that the disease is having on the patient's quality of life. Are there defined disease episodes or is the condition truly chronic? Is inflammation accompanied by pain and redness or by floaters and visual loss? In chronic disease, the level of visual disability and discomfort that is tolerable for one patient is intolerable for another, and it is important to understand the patient's perspective before recommending therapy. In addition, some aspects of the disease can be modified by therapy, but others cannot. By determining what is really bothering the patient, the physician can attempt to focus therapy on the most troublesome aspect of the disease. For example, some patients are most concerned about recurrent episodes of inflammation and the need for taking medications on a frequent basis. Others are more concerned about the distortion of vision that may result, even if it is mild, and do not mind taking frequent medications if slight visual improvement may result. Most importantly, the perception of visual loss differs greatly among patients. Only by fully understanding the patient and his/her relationship with the disease can the physician best counsel the patient to put the disorder into proper perspective.

Floaters and decreased vision are the two most common complaints of patients with inflammation of the vitreous, retina, and choroid. Most patients describe floaters as multiple small- or medium-sized spots that move as their eye moves. Other patients complain of blurred or decreased vision. In fact, when acuity is severely diminished, patients may be unable to visualize the floaters, and these patients may only complain of floaters as vision starts to improve after therapy. A change in the pattern of floaters or visual impairment often signals a change in the underlying ocular disease such as an increase in inflammation, the development of vitreous hemorrhage, or the condensation of the vitreous into a more organized opaque tissue. A careful history can also differentiate causes of brief visual impairment, such as vascular emboli, shifting subretinal fluid, or neurologic diseases such as migraine, from visual disability caused by ocular inflammatory disease.

A detailed family history, social history, and sexual history are frequently omitted from the ophthalmic evaluation but are integral to the evaluation of the patient with uveitis. Patients should complete a uveitis questionnaire before the examination; our questionnaire was developed in conjunction with Dr. C. Steven Foster at the Massachusetts Eye and Ear Infirmary (see following Appendix). The questionnaire is then reviewed with the patient during the medical history when additional questions can be asked. The survey helps to guarantee that a core of medical information is gathered on all patients and that important medical questions are not neglected.

Although uveitis rarely occurs within families, many uveitidies such as ankylosing spondylitis and birdshot retinochoroidopathy have strong HLA associations that suggest an important inherited component. In addition, a patient's social situation can influence not only the type and severity of the diseases he/she acquires but also the physician's ability to effectively treat the condition. Social problems can impede a patient's compliance with medical or surgical therapy. Furthermore, patients who are not able to take medication reliably or to comply with frequent laboratory monitoring of hematologic and renal status are not good candidates for immunosuppressive therapy that can impair the immune system.

# APPENDIX

# Sample Uveitis Questionnaire

**FAMILY HISTORY**

These questions refer to your parents, grandparents, children, grandchildren, brothers, sisters, aunts, and uncles.

Has anyone in *your family* had:

Cancer ..... Yes No
Diabetes ..... Yes No
Allergies ..... Yes No
Arthritis or rheumatism ..... Yes No
Syphilis ..... Yes No
Tuberculosis ..... Yes No
Sickle cell disease or trait ..... Yes No
Lyme disease ..... Yes No

Has anyone in *your family* had medical problems of the:

Eyes ..... Yes No
Skin ..... Yes No
Kidneys ..... Yes No
Lungs ..... Yes No
Stomach or bowel ..... Yes No
Nervous system or brain ..... Yes No

**SOCIAL HISTORY**

Age (years) _____ Current job _____

Have you lived outside of the U.S. ..... Yes No
If yes, where? _____
Have you ever owned a dog? ..... Yes No
Have you ever owned a cat? ..... Yes No
Have you ever eaten raw meat or uncooked sausage? ..... Yes No
Have you ever been exposed to sick animals? ..... Yes No

Do you drink untreated stream, well, or lake water? ..... Yes No
Do you smoke cigarettes? ..... Yes No
How many alcoholic drinks do you have each day? _____
Have you ever used intravenous drugs? ..... Yes No
Have you ever taken birth control pills? ..... Yes No
Have you ever had a bisexual or homosexual relationship? ..... Yes No

**PERSONAL MEDICAL HISTORY**

Are you allergic to any medications? ..... Yes No
If yes, which medications? _____

Please list the *medicines* you are currently taking including nonprescription drugs such as aspirin, ibuprofen, antihistamines, etc.

_____
_____
_____
_____

**MEDICAL HISTORY**

Please list all *eye* operations you have had (including laser surgery) and the dates of the surgeries.

_____
_____
_____
_____
_____
_____
_____
_____
_____

Please list all *other* operations you have had and the dates of the surgeries.

_____
_____
_____
_____
_____
_____
_____
_____

Have *you* ever had any of the following illnesses?

Cancer ..... Yes No
Diabetes ..... Yes No
Hepatitis ..... Yes No
High blood pressure ..... Yes No
Anemia (low blood counts) ..... Yes No
Pneumonia or pleurisy ..... Yes No
Tuberculosis ..... Yes No
Herpes (cold sores) ..... Yes No
Chicken pox ..... Yes No
Shingles (zoster) ..... Yes No

German measles (rubella) ..... Yes No
Measles (rubeola) ..... Yes No
Mumps ..... Yes No
Chlamydia or trachoma ..... Yes No
Syphilis ..... Yes No
Any other sexually transmitted disease ..... Yes No
Leprosy ..... Yes No

Have *you* ever had any of the following illnesses?

Leptospirosis ..... Yes No
Lyme disease ..... Yes No
Histoplasmosis ..... Yes No
Candidiasis or moniliasis ..... Yes No
Coccidioidomycosis ..... Yes No
Sporotrichosis ..... Yes No
Cryptococcal infection ..... Yes No
Toxoplasmosis ..... Yes No
Amoeba infection ..... Yes No
Giardiasis ..... Yes No
Toxocariasis ..... Yes No
Cysticercosis ..... Yes No
Trichinosis ..... Yes No
Whipple's disease ..... Yes No
AIDS ..... Yes No
Hay fever ..... Yes No
Allergies ..... Yes No
Vasculitis ..... Yes No
Arthritis ..... Yes No
Rheumatoid arthritis ..... Yes No
Lupus (systemic lupus erythematosus) ..... Yes No
Scleroderma ..... Yes No
Reiter's syndrome ..... Yes No
Colitis ..... Yes No
Crohn's disease ..... Yes No
Ulcerative colitis ..... Yes No
Behçet's disease ..... Yes No
Sarcoidosis ..... Yes No
Ankylosing spondylitis ..... Yes No
Erythema nodosum ..... Yes No
Temporal arteritis ..... Yes No
Multiple sclerosis ..... Yes No
Serpiginous choroidopathy ..... Yes No
Fuchs' heterochromic iridocyclitis ..... Yes No
Vogt-Koyanagi-Harada syndrome ..... Yes No

Have *you* ever had any of the following symptoms?

***General health***

Chills ..... Yes No
Fevers (persistent or recurrent) ..... Yes No
Night sweats ..... Yes No
Fatigue (tire easily) ..... Yes No
Poor appetite ..... Yes No

Unexplained weight loss ..... Yes No
Do you feel sick? ..... Yes No

***Neurologic***

Frequent or severe headaches ..... Yes No
Fainting ..... Yes No
Numbness or tingling in your body ..... Yes No
Paralysis or weakness in parts of your body ..... Yes No
Seizures or convulsions ..... Yes No
Psychiatric conditions ..... Yes No

Have *you* ever had any of the following symptoms?

***Ears***

Hard of hearing or deafness ..... Yes No
Ringing or noises in your ears ..... Yes No
Frequent or severe ear infections ..... Yes No
Painful or swollen ear lobes ..... Yes No

***Nose and throat***

Sores in your nose or mouth ..... Yes No
Severe or recurrent nosebleeds ..... Yes No
Frequent sneezing ..... Yes No
Sinus trouble ..... Yes No
Persistent hoarseness ..... Yes No
Tooth or gum infections ..... Yes No

***Skin***

Rashes ..... Yes No
Skin sores ..... Yes No
Sunburn easily (photosensitivity) ..... Yes No
White patches of skin or hair (vitiligo or poliosis) ..... Yes No
Loss of hair ..... Yes No
Tick or severe insect bites ..... Yes No
Painfully cold fingers ..... Yes No
Severe itching ..... Yes No

***Respiratory***

Severe or frequent colds ..... Yes No
Constant coughing ..... Yes No
Coughing up blood ..... Yes No
Recent flu or viral infection ..... Yes No
Wheezing or asthma attacks ..... Yes No
Difficulty in breathing ..... Yes No

***Cardiovascular***

Chest pain ..... Yes No
Shortness of breath ..... Yes No
Swelling of your legs ..... Yes No

***Blood***

Frequent or easy bruising ..... Yes No
Frequent or easy bleeding ..... Yes No
Have you received blood transfusions? ..... Yes No

***Gastrointestinal***

Trouble swallowing ..... Yes No
Diarrhea ..... Yes No

Bloody stools.....Yes No
Stomach ulcers.....Yes No
Jaundice or yellow skin.....Yes No

***Bones and joints***

Stiff joints.....Yes No
Painful or swollen joints.....Yes No
Stiff lower back.....Yes No
Back pain while sleeping or on awakening.....Yes No
Muscle aches.....Yes No

Have *you* ever had any of the following symptoms?

***Genitourinary***

Kidney problems.....Yes No
Bladder trouble.....Yes No
Blood in your urine.....Yes No
Urinary discharge.....Yes No
Genital sores or ulcers.....Yes No
Prostatitis.....Yes No
Testicular pain.....Yes No
Are you pregnant?.....Yes No
Do you plan to become pregnant in the near future?.....Yes No

# CHAPTER 4

# Examination of the Patient With Uveitis

The ocular examination of patients with uveitis is important not only to the appropriate diagnosis of the disease but also to determine the appropriate therapy. The examination will provide information that enables the examiner to generate a differential diagnosis and will allow the patient's subjective complaints to be placed into the framework of objective clinical findings. In addition, the baseline examination becomes an important yardstick against which treatment success or failure will be measured. Because many inflammatory diseases are chronic and require potentially toxic therapy, the physician must assess whether a patient is benefiting from treatment. A thorough review of the patient's record provides critical information for planning new therapeutic approaches and guards against repeating therapies that were unsatisfactory in the past. Because a patient's medical record is important in assessing response to therapy, it is extremely important to accurately record the presence or absence of important physical findings in a reproducible and standardized manner. Because many of the ophthalmic findings in inflammatory disease, such as vitreous cells and haze, can be evaluated only by subjective means, the examiner should strive for internal consistency in grading the severity of the observations and to standardize these observations whenever possible. However, when standard grading scales are available in the literature, the examiner must also attempt to use the same grading criteria as other ophthalmologists in order to compare the patient's examination with reports of other similar patients.

## VISUAL ACUITY

Several factors can lead to decreased visual acuity in patients with uveitis or retinitis. A combination of corneal, anterior chamber, lenticular, and vitreal haze may overlie a disturbance in retinal function caused by retinal edema, retinal necrosis, or retinal scarring. In addition, optic nerve function may be compromised after inflammation or glaucoma. It is important for the clinician to determine the cause of diminished vision because the therapeutic approach will differ according to the cause. For example, it would be inappropriate to increase a patient's dose of prednisone to treat worsening vision that is due to a progressive posterior subcapsular cataract. Whatever type of visual acuity measurement is used, it must be performed under the same lighting conditions each time; otherwise, the fluctuations induced by the testing environment will mask changes in vision caused by worsening disease or response to therapy. A best-corrected visual acuity measurement should be obtained, either by refraction or at the very least, with the use of a pin hole. Near-vision measurement is also helpful because we have observed that the improvement in near vision often precedes an improvement in distance vision by several weeks in patients with chronic macular edema.

The most common method to measure visual acuity uses the Snellen eye chart. Like all eye charts, the Snellen chart tests a patient's ability to resolve high contrast letters and is satisfactory if the patient's vision is good. Unfortunately, the chart does not have enough sensitivity for patients with poor vision. There are no lines between 20/100 and 20/200 or between 20/200 and 20/400. In addition, there are too few letters on the lines above 20/100. Although an improvement in visual acuity from 20/200 to 20/125 may not be significant to the patient, the ability to measure this improvement is an important indicator that the current therapeutic approach is working. Because many patients with macular edema have a visual acuity of less than 20/80, initial improvement might be missed with a standard Snellen chart.

For these reasons, we have used the ETDRS chart developed by Ferris and colleagues for the evaluation of patients in the Early Treatment for Diabetic Retinopathy Study (Fig. 4-1).[1] This chart has five letters per line starting with the 20/200 line, and every three lines represents a doubling of the visual angle. Therefore improving from 20/40 to 20/20 represents the same level of improvement in visual function as 20/80 to 20/40. If patients cannot read the 20/200 line while sitting 4 meters from the chart, they are moved to 1 meter from the chart and the acuities are recorded as 5 over the appropriate denominator, that is, 5/200. Because each line has 5 letters, the acuity can be expressed as the total number of letters read. The 1 and 4 meter scales can be made continuous by adding 30 letters to the number read at 4 meters. The scale of visual acuity is then linear and continuous from 5/200 (5 letters) to 20/12.5 (95 letters).

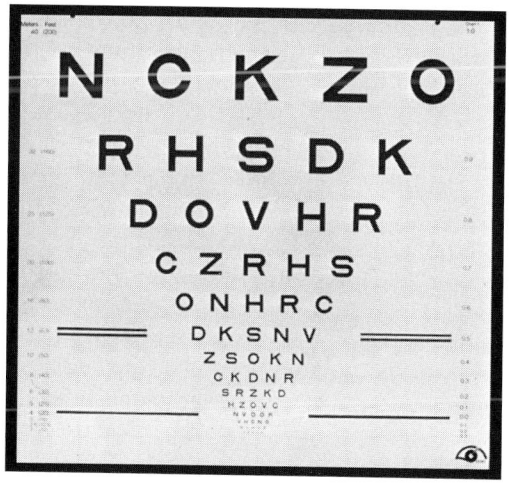


**Fig. 4-1.** Visual acuity chart from Early Treatment of Diabetic Retinopathy Study (ETDRS). (Courtesy Frederick Ferris, M.D.)

## EXTERNAL EXAMINATION

As stated earlier, a detailed examination of the skin can provide useful diagnostic clues for the astute clinician. Not only should the skin of the lids be closely examined, but the entire skin should be evaluated for presence of rashes, nodules, or vitiligo. Eyelid lesions may hold the key to diagnosis. We have diagnosed sarcoidosis on the basis of the presence of lid granulomas and of lesions on the extremities and chest, and we have diagnosed Kaposi's sarcoma based on characteristic vascular lesions on the upper eyelid.

## PUPILS AND EXTRAOCULAR MUSCLES

Evaluation of the pupils is frequently difficult in the patient with uveitis because of synechiae or chronic cycloplegic therapy. The inflamed pupil, even without synechiae, may not move well as a result of iris atrophy. When examination is possible, the status of the optic nerve can be assessed with the standard swinging flashlight test to detect an afferent pupillary defect.

Extraocular muscle involvement in intraocular inflammatory disease is unusual. Esotropia or exotropia resulting from long-standing visual loss as a result of cataract, retinal, or optic nerve disease may develop. The finding of a new vertical tropia or internuclear ophthalmoplegia should alert the physician to underlying diseases of the central nervous system that may be associated with causes of uveitis such as multiple sclerosis, sarcoidosis, or non-Hodgkin's lymphoma.

## INTRAOCULAR PRESSURE MEASUREMENT

Either elevated intraocular pressure or hypotony can occur as a result of intraocular inflammation. Goldmann applanation tonometry is usually sufficient to measure the intraocular pressure in patients with uveitis;

however, fluorescein should not be instilled until the slit-lamp examination and ophthalmoscopy are completed because fluorescein enters the eye and prevents an accurate assessment of the amount of flare in the anterior chamber. In addition, fluorescein may obscure the view of the posterior segment if the pupil is small and may persist in the eye for more than 24 hours, especially in eyes with hypotonia and decreased aqueous flow. Therefore applanation tonometry should either be done with anesthetic without fluorescein, done with a pneumotonometer, or performed at the end of the examination.

## SLIT-LAMP BIOMICROSCOPY

### Conjunctiva

Conjunctival injection is a common sign of acute anterior inflammation but is rare in chronic posterior segment disease. Usually conjunctival injection is uniform in the perilimbal region and represents ciliary body inflammation. The conjunctival injection of uveitis can be differentiated from conjunctivitis by the lack of involvement of the fornix and palpebral conjunctiva. Scleritis and episcleritis may occur in conjunction with some types of intraocular inflammation. Injected deep scleral vessels, a purple scleral hue, and severe pain distinguish true scleritis from more superficial inflammation. Scleritis associated with uveitis is often nodular and confined to a section of the globe, whereas ciliary body injection tends to involve the globe more diffusely. Some confusion may arise when a patient with intraocular inflammation develops an allergic reaction to topical medication. The eye becomes more painful and red during treatment, and this may be misinterpreted as worsening disease and failure of the treatment. However, patients with a superimposed allergic reaction often develop itching, dermatitis, and significant conjunctival injection that involves the palpebral conjunctiva.

### Cornea

**Keratic precipitates.** Keratic precipitates (KP) are the most common corneal finding in uveitis (Fig. 4-2). They are small aggregates of inflammatory cells that accumulate on the endothelial surface of the cornea. The presence of these deposits on the endothelium of the cornea can provide useful diagnostic information and indicates the current level of inflammatory activity. Also, in an eye without active anterior segment inflammation manifested by cells and flare, the presence of KP tells the practitioner that the eye was previously inflamed.

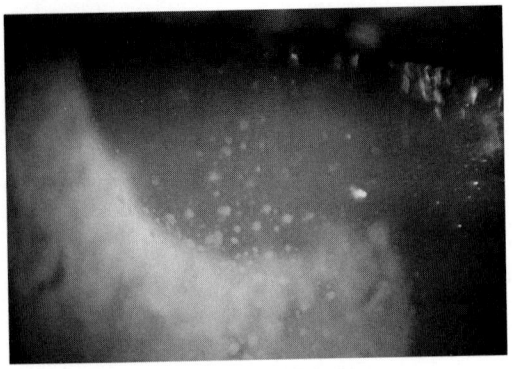

**Fig. 4-2.** Granulomatous keratic precipitates present in patient with sarcoidosis.

KP usually accumulates on the lower half of the cornea, often in a base-down triangle configuration; however, in some disorders, such as Fuchs' iridocyclitis, KP may be present superiorly. The precipitates vary in size from flecks the size of cornea guttata to 1 mm in diameter. Because cornea guttata may be present in patients with uveitis, very fine small KP can be distinguished by an inferior corneal location and slightly elongated shape. KP can be easily seen with the slit lamp and direct or retroillumination. The small aggregates have been conventionally referred to as "nongranulomatous," whereas the larger, more greasy-appearing ones have been termed "mutton-fat" or "granulomatous" (Fig. 4-2). These terms may be misleading because they imply a pathologic correlation that is rarely known. There is no objective way of defining granulomatous versus nongranulomatous KP. The extreme cases are clear, but one may see both types coexisting in one patient at the same time or see variations during the course of the disease or therapy. In general, the larger granulomatous aggregates are composed of macrophages and giant cells and occur in chronic inflammation, whereas the smaller nongranulomatous ones occur in acute inflammation and are more likely to be composed of neutrophils and lymphocytes. Nevertheless, there are a number of diseases typically associated with granulomatous KP (see Box 5-3), and the presence of these precipitates can help in developing a differential diagnosis. In most inflammatory reactions, the neutrophil is the first cell present, and the transformed macro-

**Table 4-1.** Grading of anterior chamber cells

| Schlaegel* | | Hogan† | | Authors' approach† | |
|---|---|---|---|---|---|
| Grade | Cells | Grade | Cells | Grade | Cells |
| — | — | 0 | 0 | 0 | 0 |
| ½ | Rare (normal) | Rare cells | 1-2 | | |
| — | — | Occasional Cells | 3-7 | | |
| — | — | — | — | Trace‡ | 1-5 |
| 1 | Occasional cell | 1+ | 7-10 | 1+‡ | 6-15 |
| 1½ | 2-7 | 1-2+ | 10-15 | — | — |
| 2 | 8-15 | 2+ | 15-20 | 2+ | 16-25 |
| 2½ | 16-30 | — | — | — | — |
| 3 | Too many to count | 3+ | 20-50 | 3+ | 26-50 |
| 3½ | Too many to count | — | — | — | — |
| 4 | Most ever seen | 4+ | >50 | 4+ | >50 |

Data from Schlaegel TF Jr: *Essentials of uveitis,* Boston, 1967, Little, Brown, p 7; Hogan MJ et al: *Am J Opthalmol* 47:155-170, 1959.

*Using a wide beam with a narrow slit.

†Using a 1 × 1 mm slit.

‡For grades of trace and 1 + the exact number of cells is recorded parentheses, that is, 1+ (11).

phages (epithelioid cells) and lymphocytes accumulate as the inflammation becomes more chronic. KP therefore mimics the course of the inflammation in the tissue. For example, patients with documented pulmonary sarcoidosis may have acute anterior inflammatory episodes with small nongranulomatous KP. If the inflammatory disease becomes chronic, the KP aggregates may become larger and more granulomatous. After the resolution of active inflammation, the KP aggregates may disappear completely or become smaller, translucent, or pigmented. KP may also be washed away during intraocular surgery.

**Other corneal findings.** Other corneal findings can provide clues to the correct diagnosis. For example, corneal dendrites may be seen with uveitis as a result of herpes simplex virus infection. Interstitial keratitis may be associated with syphilis or Cogan's syndrome; the clinician should examine the cornea carefully because the presence of stromal ghost vessels extending more than several millimeters from the limbus may easily be overlooked. Finally, we have seen several patients with corneal grafts who were referred with conditions diagnosed as idiopathic uveitis. In a number of these cases, the uveitis was actually caused by early allograft rejection.

### Anterior chamber

The anterior chamber is easily examined with the slit lamp for signs of ocular inflammation. Because inflammatory cells do not arise in the aqueous, the presence of cells or increased protein (flare) in the anterior chamber is evidence of spillover from the inflamed iris or ciliary body. Not infrequently, a patient with recurrent iritis will come to the ophthalmologist complaining of pain, but because of a lack of cells or flare on examination, the patient will be told that there is no uveitis and that no therapy is needed. To the practitioner's dismay, the patient returns the next day with a full-blown iritis. The explanation for this is that the inflammation begins in the iris and ciliary body, and only when sufficient inflammatory cells accumulate within these tissues do the cells begin to enter the aqueous and become visible to the clinician. Therefore anterior chamber inflammation is a convenient but somewhat indirect measure of the inflammatory reaction in the iris and ciliary body.

Anterior chamber cells are primarily lymphocytes in most episodes of anterior uveitis, but a significant number of neutrophils may be present early in the course of disease. Anterior chamber cells are best seen by directing the slit-lamp beam obliquely across the eye and focusing posterior to the cornea. There is considerable variation among physicians on the grading of the number of cells. Because the cells represent an index of activity but not a direct measure of the active inflammation, we do not believe that the grading system must discriminate between small increments of disease. Table 4-1 summarizes the system proposed by Hogan and colleagues,[2] the system proposed by Schlaegel that uses a wide beam with a narrow slit,[3] and our preferred system that uses a 1 × 1 mm slit beam. The smaller slit allows some resolution for more severe inflammation and less resolution at the milder end of the spectrum. We are most interested in quantifying anterior chamber cells during the early stages of acute inflammation when a change in cellularity may signal an early response to therapy and when a lack of response might dictate a change in therapy. The problem with most classification systems is that it is impossible for clinicians to remember how many cells are associated with a trace grade of trace, occasional, or rare cells. Therefore we have modified our grading system; for grades of trace cells (1 to 5) and 1+ cells (6 to 15 cells), we will put the exact number of cells counted in parentheses after the grade, for example, 1+ (11) or trace (3). In many chronically inflamed eyes, it may be impossible to eliminate every last cell, and these rare cells may not require treatment. Nevertheless, persistence of more than a rare cell may place the patient at increased risk for inflammatory complications and worsen the prognosis after cataract extraction.

It is also our experience that the size of the individual cells in the anterior chamber will decrease as the inflammation begins to resolve. This may occur before the number actually decreases. A change from large activated lymphocytes to smaller cells may account for this clinical observation. It is important to differentiate inflammatory cells from other types of cells in the anterior chamber. Red blood cells, iris pigment cells, and malignant cells may be mistaken for inflammatory cells. The differentiation is especially difficult if a lymphoid malignancy is present; monoclonal antibody staining of cells obtained by paracentesis may be critical in identifying the type of cell.

Increased protein content in the anterior chamber is a manifestation of a breakdown of the blood-ocular barrier. When the slit beam is obliquely aimed across the anterior chamber, the ability to visualize the path of the beam is termed *flare.* There are approximately 7 g of protein/100 ml of blood, but only 11 mg of protein/100 ml of aqueous. A faint amount of flare is normal if a bright light is used. The amount of light scattering is proportional to the concentration of protein in a solution, and hence more flare indicates increased protein in the anterior chamber fluid. Flare can be clinically graded on a 0 to 4+ scale (Table 4-2). We have reserved the 4+ grade for leakage of protein so extensive that a fibrin clot is present.

**Table 4-2.** Grading of anterior chamber flare

| Grade | Schlaegel[3] | Hogan et al.[2] |
|---|---|---|
| 0 | Complete absence | |
| ½ | Faint (normal) | – |
| 1 | Very slight (normal) | Very slight |
| 1½ | Mild | – |
| 2 | Mild to moderate | Moderate (iris and lens clear) |
| 3 | Moderate | Marked flare (iris and lens hazy) |
| 4 | Severe | Intense (fibrin, plastic aqueous) |

Data from Schlaegel TF Jr: *Essentials of uveitis*, Boston, 1967, Little, Brown, p7; Hogan MJ et al: *Am J Ophthalmol* 47:155-170, 1959.

In addition to the subjective grading of flare, it is possible to more accurately measure the degree of light scattering and quantify the amount of protein. A technique described by Herman and colleagues[4] uses the principle that fluorescein in the anterior chamber will bind to albumin and the amount of bound fluorescein will alter the polarization of fluorescein as measured by fluorophotometry. This method is able to quantify alterations in blood-ocular barrier leakage of albumin. A newer technique of objectively assessing aqueous flare measures the scattering of a laser beam projected across the anterior chamber. This laser flare meter is more fully described in Chapter 6.

There is some disagreement as to whether the presence of flare by itself, without cells or other signs of active inflammation, should be treated. In our opinion, without objective quantification of a change in the leakage across the blood ocular barrier, chronic flare alone is not a sign of active inflammation. Damaged blood vessels may be leaky for a long time after the active inflammation has resolved. Continued treatment with drugs such as corticosteroids probably does little to alter the repair of these vessels in the absence of active inflammation. There is no evidence that small amounts of increased protein in the anterior chamber are detrimental to the eye, and there appears to be no reason for continued therapy in this situation. Specifically, children with juvenile rheumatoid arthritis with flare but no cells should not be treated with topical corti-

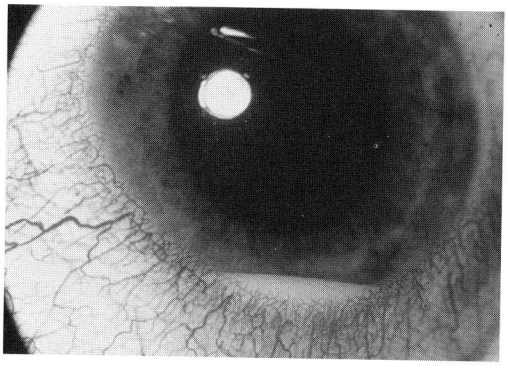

**Fig. 4-3.** Hypopyon in patient with Behçet's disease.(See Color Plate 2.)

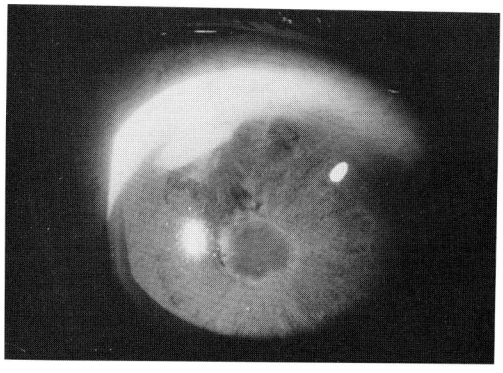

**Fig. 4-4.** Posterior synechiae and closure of iridectomy.

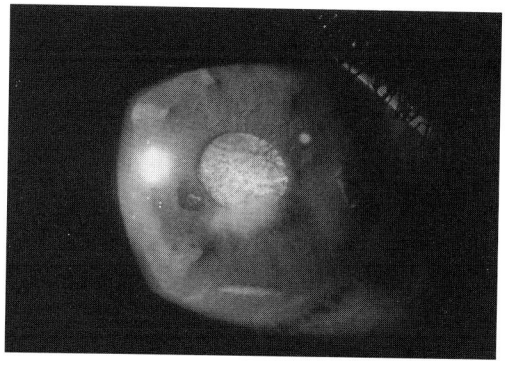

**Fig. 4-5.** Anterior synechia in patient with sarcoidosis demonstrating iris-cornea adhesions.

costeroids. Therefore flare should be considered a marker of inflammation but not a pathognomonic finding of active inflammation.

A hypopyon (Fig. 4-3) is a collection of leukocytes that settles in the lower angle of the anterior chamber. The cause of a hypopyon is unclear and is not solely related to the number of cells in the anterior chamber. It is also related to the presence of sufficient fibrin to cause the cells to clump and settle. Hypopyon is a dramatic but short-lived finding in ocular inflammation that has been associated with Behçet's disease, endophthalmitis, and rifabutin toxicity in patients with AIDS. A hypopyon may also occur sporadically in severe acute inflammation associated with many other types of uveitis.

## Iris

Inflammation is often accompanied by the release of mediators that promote fibrin deposition, clotting, and fibroblast proliferation that are the probable cause of synechia. Synechiae are adhesions between the iris and the lens capsule (posterior synechiae) (Fig. 4-4) or the iris and the cornea near the anterior chamber angle (peripheral anterior synechiae, PAS). The former are responsible for the development of pupillary block glaucoma, and the latter contribute to the development of obstruction of aqueous outflow. In general, the presence of synechia indicates that the inflammation has been chronic or recurrent; however, these adhesions may occasionally develop within a few days in patients with severe inflammation. Although most peripheral anterior synechiae can be seen only by gonioscopy, some patients will develop more profound anterior adhesions (Fig. 4-5). Most posterior synechiae are located at the pupillary border, but patients with severe chronic inflammation can develop adhesions of the entire posterior iris surface to the anterior lens capsule. A fibrovascular membrane may develop in patients with long-standing and recurrent inflammation in whom the pupil size has been reduced to a few millimeters by posterior synechia (Fig. 4-6). This membrane may be translucent and adherent to the surface of the lens and not apparent until cataract removal is attempted.

Iris nodules are accumulations of inflammatory cells in the iris or on its surface. The Koeppe nodule develops on the pupillary border, whereas the Busacca's nodules occur on the iris surface (Fig. 4-7). Iris nodules tend to be found in diseases that have been termed granulomatous and are more specific for these conditions than granulomatous KP.

## Anterior chamber angle

Because glaucoma is a frequent (and often the most severe) complication of uveitis, a thor-

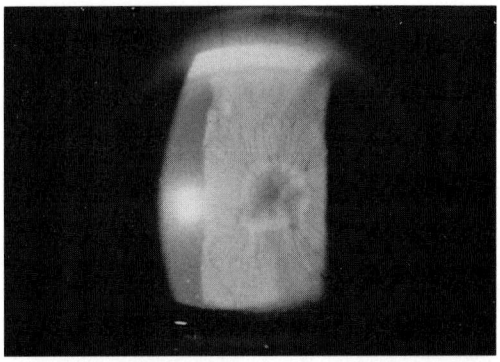

**Fig. 4-6.** Posterior synechia with fibrin membrane and totally occluded pupil.

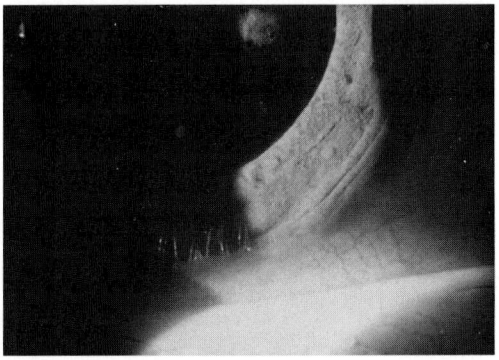

**Fig. 4-7.** Busacca's nodules of iris in patient with Vogt-Koyanagi-Harada syndrome.

ough examination of the anterior chamber angle is indicated. The finding of neovascularization may indicate a need for panretinal photocoagulation. In addition, in patients with a uniocular uveitis, examination of the angle may reveal an occult foreign body or ciliary body malignancy.

### Lens

Many patients with uveitis develop cataracts because of underlying inflammation and the use of corticosteroids to treat the disease. Posterior subcapsular opacities are commonly seen early, but the advanced cataract in uveitis is frequently a complicated cataract with nuclear, cortical, and capsular opacities. It is important to determine how much of a uveitis patient's diminished vision is a result of a progressive cataract because the therapy for cataract is surgical extraction and not increased immunosuppressive therapy. Again, evaluation of the contribution of lens opacity to decreased vision is discussed in greater depth in Chapter 6 on diagnostic testing.

**Table 4-3.** Grading of vitreous cells with use of Hruby lens

| Cells in retroilluminated field | Description | Grade |
|---|---|---|
| 0-1 | Clear | 0 |
| 2-20 | Few opacities | Trace |
| 21-50 | Scattered opacities | 1 |
| 51-100 | Moderate opacities | 2 |
| 101-250 | Many opacities | 3 |
| >251 | Dense opacities | 4 |

## VITREOUS

Inflammation in the vitreous, as in the anterior chamber, is characterized by increased cells and protein. The vitreous is rarely the source of the inflammatory cells, which instead arise from the choroid, retina, and ciliary body. However, in certain infections, the focus of the inflammation may be in the vitreous. Both vitreal cells and vitreal haze are more difficult to quantify than aqueous cell and flare. The vitreous is larger, and cells or haze may be localized to only a part of the vitreous. Therefore the quantification may depend on how the eye was examined. For example, the anterior-posterior location of small numbers of cells in a relatively clear vitreous can be determined with the use of the slit lamp, but in the severely inflamed eye, the mid and posterior vitreous may be obscured by anterior vitreal cells and haze. Small pupil size, corneal opacity, and cataract will also make the grading process more difficult.

The grading of vitreous cells described by Kimura and colleagues[5] uses the Hruby lens to view the cells in retroillumination. The cells appear as black dots, and it may be difficult to differentiate vitreal debris from active inflammatory cells in some eyes. Debris is often pigmented and forms clumps that are larger than individual cells. We grade overall vitreous cells and opacities in a manner similar to the scale devised by Kimura and colleagues (Table 4-3). We then note whether the major accumulation of cells is immediately behind the lens, in the anterior or posterior vitreous, or adjacent to a retinal lesion. Location of the cells is a function of both the ocular disease and its severity. The location of the cells is important in classifying the inflammation, but we have noted, for example, that patients with pars planitis who usually have cells in the anterior

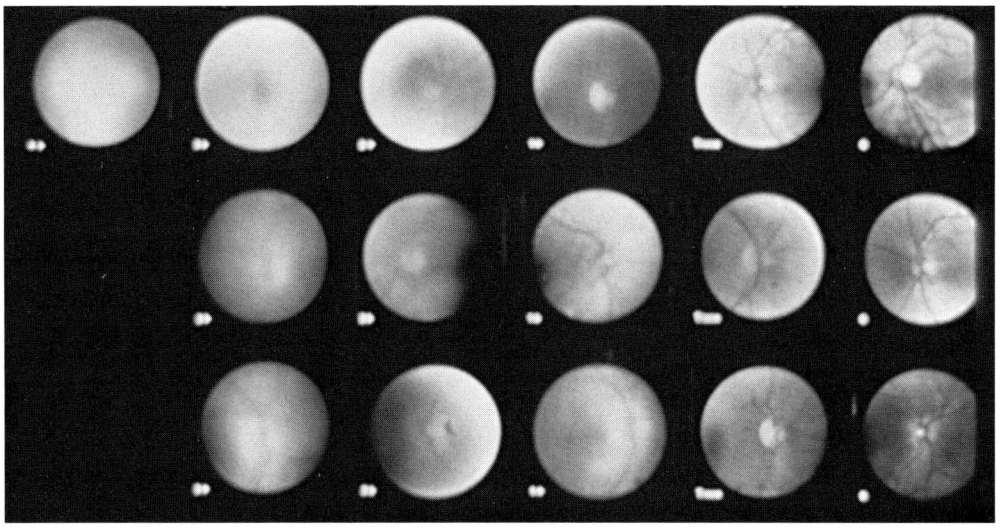

**Fig. 4-8.** Grading of vitreous haze. (From Nussenblatt RB, Palestine AG, Chan CC et al: Standardization of vitreal inflammatory activity in intermediate and posterior uveitis, *Ophthalmology* 92:467-471, 1985.) (See Color Plate 3.)

vitreous will develop many cells in the posterior vitreous if the inflammation is more severe. In many diseases, but especially in sarcoidosis and pars planitis, vitreous cells tend to aggregate into clumps called "snowballs." These snowballs settle in the inferior periphery near the retinal surface and are seen best with the indirect ophthalmoscope.

It is our strong opinion that vitreous haze is a better indicator of active inflammation than vitreous cells are because it combines the optical effect of cellular infiltration and protein leakage. We have developed a grading scale based on the view of the optic disc and posterior retina with the use of the indirect ophthalmoscope and a 20 diopter lens (Fig. 4-8).[6] It is important to mentally correct for lens opacities, anterior segment inflammation, and corneal disease; however, the use of the indirect ophthalmoscope prevents mild media opacities from interfering with the grading. The use of photographic standards makes this system more reproducible than other subjective grading systems. In practice it is useful to have the standard color photographs in the examining room. One can then examine the patient's eye and look at the grading chart to select the standard that best matches the degree of haze.

Vitreous strands, membranes, and areas of vitreoretinal traction are not uncommon in intermediate and posterior uveitis. They are best seen with the indirect ophthalmoscope but may be studied in detail with a contact lens or a +90 diopter lens at the slit lamp. There is frequently a posterior vitreous detachment in patients with long-standing vitreous inflammation as the fibrin in the vitreous contracts and pulls the posterior vitreous face forward. Recently, investigators have suggested that vitreous traction that causes an incomplete posterior vitreous detachment may be associated with the development of cystoid macular edema.[7]

## RETINA AND CHOROID

Examination of the retina in inflammatory disease is best done with a combination of the indirect ophthalmoscope, the Hruby lens, the +90 diopter lens, and a mirrored contact lens. Because of coexisting vitreous inflammation, each of these has advantages and disadvantages. The indirect ophthalmoscope is ideal for defining the extent and height of retinal and choroidal lesions; it penetrates vitreous haze and other media opacities better than any other instrument. It is not good for defining the relative depth of a lesion within the retina or determining the presence of macular edema. The Hruby lens is somewhat better at penetrating haze than the +90 diopter or +78 diopter lens and is better for assessing macular edema. If the media is reasonably clear, the +90 diopter or +78 diopter lens, which provides an inverted view of the fundus, is ideal for viewing vascular abnormalities, intraretinal lesions, and

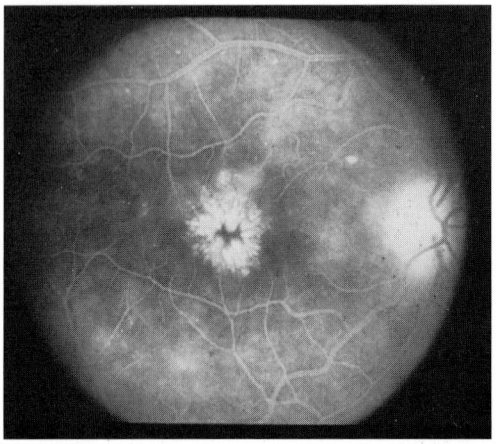

**Fig. 4-9.** Fluorescein angiogram demonstrating cystoid macular edema caused by pars planitis.

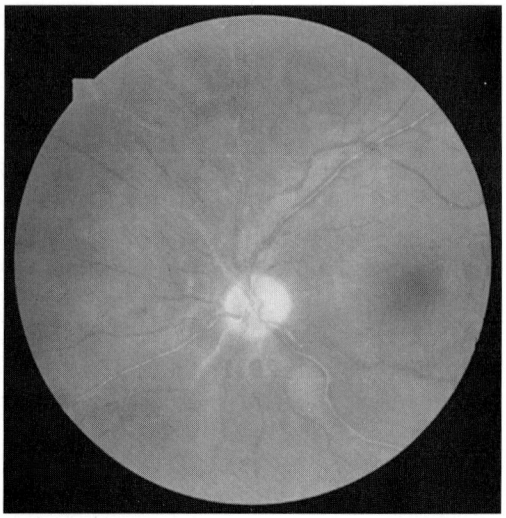

**Fig. 4-10.** Retinal vascular sheathing in patient with idiopathic retinal vasculitis.

vitreoretinal traction in the posterior retina. The midperiphery of the retina also can be seen with this lens, but the mirrored contact lens is more useful for the detailed examination of peripheral chorioretinal lesions.

Cystoid macular edema is a common retinal finding in patients with uveitis (Fig. 4-9). Although fluorescein angiography can more objectively document the presence of macular edema, clinical examination with the Hruby lens is easier, is cost-effective, and can be performed on each visit. In addition, examination with the Hruby lens allows the examiner to determine the extent of macular thickening associated with the edema. In the absence of vitreous haze, cystoid macular edema is easily seen. However, macular edema may be obscured by overlying vitreous haze and is best observed by viewing the macula with the light directed slightly to one side of the fovea. Cystoid macular edema may then be visualized by indirect illumination and will "light up" in contrast to the surrounding retina. This technique also decreases light scattering from the vitreous. The surface of a cyst can sometimes be visualized as a subtle surface elevation, distinguishing it from a true macular hole. If the pupil is small, the viewing aperture will be reduced, and only a faint glimpse of the macular cysts will be seen by this method. Macular holes and lamellar holes as well as retinal pigment epithelial clumping are also commonly observed, and it is possible to see cloudy white areas of retinal edema without a classic cystoid pattern.

Retinal vascular alterations are also a common finding in patients with intermediate or posterior uveitis. Vascular sheathing of the arteries or veins, usually caused by infiltration of inflammatory cells around the vessels, is easily seen in the posterior pole (Fig. 4-10). Peripheral vascular sheathing is more subtle and may be missed if it is not specifically sought. Sheathing is often accompanied by vessel narrowing and sometimes by vascular obliteration. Peripheral vascular narrowing and obliteration is best evaluated with the indirect ophthalmoscope; it manifests as an absence of small peripheral vessels. Acute vascular occlusion is accompanied by retinal edema, but old areas of vascular loss show only atrophic retina and retinal pigment epithelial stippling.

Retinal hemorrhages and cotton-wool spots frequently accompany retinal vasculitis. These are presumably related to the retinal ischemia produced by the inflammation. In addition, cellular retinal infiltrates can be observed in certain types of retinitis. These appear as white areas similar to cotton wool spots but may be located deep within the retina as compared with the superficial location of cotton wool spots. In addition, active retinal infiltrates frequently have fuzzy edges, overlying vitreal cells, and surrounding retinal edema. Hard retinal exudates are relatively uncommon in inflammatory disease. It is possible that the retinal vessels do not leak large lipid-containing proteins from the plasma. When hard exudates are observed, they frequently occur between an area of retinal ischemia and an area of essentially normal retina. The presence of a subretinal neovascular membrane should be suspected if hard exudates, retinal edema, hemorrhage, or gray-white elevated lesions are seen.

Careful examination with the Hruby, +90 diopter, or contact lens is crucial in distinguishing a lesion that involves the neurosensory retina from lesions at the level of the retinal pigment epithelium or choroid. Examination of the edge of the lesion is often helpful in determining its depth and its cause. At times it may still be difficult to know the location of an infiltrate without the aid of a fluorescein angiogram. Many lesions will have associated subretinal fluid or be covered by increased cellularity in the vitreous, and this should be documented.

In addition to subretinal fluid, the subretinal space can be infiltrated with glial and retinal pigment epithelial cells that have proliferated as a consequence of the inflammation. These appear as plaques and bands of yellow-white tissue, which for lack of a more specific term are often referred to as subretinal fibrosis. The inflammatory process stimulates the growth of fibroblasts and the metaplasia of the retinal pigment epithelium and possibly Müller cells. The bands of this tissue, combined with epiretinal and vitreoretinal bands, produce retinal traction and distortion.

Choroidal lesions, with or without retinal involvement, are common in posterior inflammatory disease. When inflammatory lesions are deep and isolated to the choroid, they often appear as grayish-yellow elevated masses (Fig. 4-11). They are best seen with the indirect ophthalmoscope but may be missed as they can be subtle in both elevation and pigmentary change. One or more choroidal nodules may be present and can vary in size from 50 μm to 500 μm in diameter. Atrophic chorioretinal lesions with surrounding hyperpigmentation are a striking sign of inflammatory disease in the uveitis patient. However, these lesions do not represent areas of active inflammation, and although they are the most prominent clinical feature of some diseases, they represent old inactive disease. Only active inflammation, not residual scarring, can be treated by drugs that modulate the immune response. Thus therapy is not indicated in patients with multiple chorioretinal scars without infiltrative lesions of the retina or choroid or active vitritis.

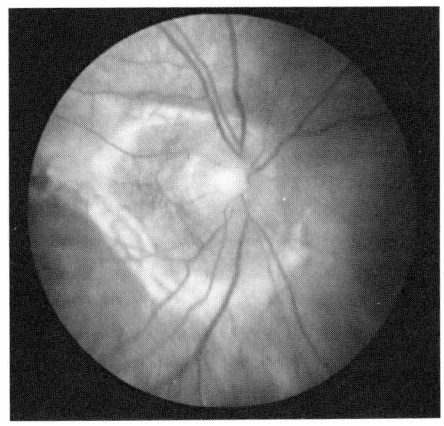

**Fig. 4-11.** Large choroidal granuloma around optic disc in patient with sarcoidosis.

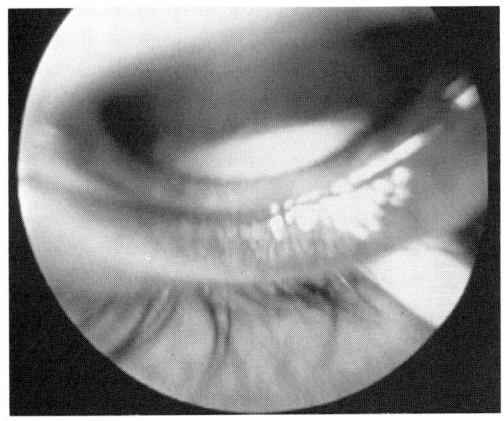

**Fig. 4-12.** Exudate on pars plana (snowbank) in patient with pars planitis. (Courtesy Ronald Smith, M.D.) (See Color Plate 4.)

Examination of the retinal periphery and pars plana is an important part of the ocular examination of patients with uveitis. Pars plana snowbanking is the accumulation of a white fibroglial mass over the pars plana and adjacent retina (see Chapter 20). It is usually restricted to the inferior pars plana but may extend superiorly. Scleral depression is usually required to see the pars plana exudate, but in some cases the inflammatory mass may be large enough to be seen with the indirect ophthalmoscope without a lens (Fig. 4-12). Peripheral vitreous infiltrates lying on the retinal surface should not be interpreted as snowbanking. Peripheral neovascularization may be present within the snowbank, increasing the risk of vitreous hemorrhage. If the pars plana exudate is sparse and located only along the ora serrata, it may be difficult to identify unless immediate comparison is made with the ora serrata in other locations within the eye.

## OPTIC NERVE

Uveitis may affect the optic nerve in several ways. Disc hyperemia, papillitis, or papilledema may be seen. Disc hyperemia may persist even in an eye with little other clinically active inflammation elsewhere. The optic disc may develop neovascularization, glaucomatous damage, or optic atrophy in the presence of ocular inflammation. In determining the cause of vision loss in eyes with uveitis, optic nerve disease is frequently overlooked. Not only can the optic nerve be damaged by the intraocular inflammation, but inflammatory diseases such as sarcoidosis may directly involve the nerve. In addition, patients with intermediate uveitis have a higher incidence of associated multiple sclerosis. Examination of the optic disc with the Hruby lens or +90 diopter lens, serial disc photographs, and electrophysiologic testing are often helpful in evaluating the uveitis patient with visual loss.

## REFERENCES

1. Ferris FL III, Kassoff A, Bresnick GH, et al: New visual acuity charts for clinical research, *Am J Ophthalmol* 94:91-96, 1982.
2. Hogan MJ, Kimura SJ, Thygeson P: Signs and symptoms of uveitis. I. Anterior uveitis, *Am J Ophthalmol* 47:155-170, 1959.
3. Schlaegel TF Jr: *Essentials of uveitis,* Boston, 1967, Little, Brown, p 7.
4. Herman DC, McLaren JW, Brubaker RF: A method of determining concentration of albumin in the living eye, *Invest Ophthalmol Vis Sci* 29:133-137, 1988.
5. Kimura SJ, Thygeson P, Hogan MJ: Signs and symptoms of uveitis. II. Classification of the posterior manifestations of uveitis, *Am J Ophthalmol* 47:171-176, 1959.
6. Nussenblatt RB, Palestine AG, Chan CC, et al: Standardization of vitreal inflammatory activity in intermediate and posterior uveitis, *Ophthalmology* 92:467-471, 1985.
7. Hikichi T, Trempe CL: Role of the vitreous in the prognosis of peripheral uveitis, *Am J Ophthalmol* 116:401-405, 1993.

# CHAPTER 5

# Development of a Differential Diagnosis

The correct diagnosis of uveitis is often challenging not only for the general ophthalmologist but also for the uveitis specialist. Patients present with a plethora of ocular findings as well as associated systemic symptoms and signs. Ocular inflammation may be the initial presentation of an underlying systemic disease that if undiagnosed and untreated may lead to significant morbidity and even death. For example, we have seen a number of patients with intraocular lymphoma whose conditions are misdiagnosed and inappropriately treated as a case of idiopathic uveitis. Even in cases of uveitis without an underlying systemic disease, misdiagnosis can lead to inappropriate therapy. A patient with fungal endophthalmitis who is thought to have sarcoidosis may be treated with corticosteroids, leading to an exacerbation of the infection, when appropriate antifungal therapy could be curative. In this chapter we review our diagnostic approach to patients with uveitis and present two cases to illustrate our approach.

The first step in developing a differential diagnosis for patients with inflammatory eye disease is to classify the uveitis in as detailed a fashion as possible. We do this by systematically asking the eight questions listed in Box 5-1. We then generate a list of possible diagnoses by combining the data obtained from the answers to these eight questions. Some of the information is obtained from the history such as the age and demographics of the patient and associated systemic symptoms. Other data, such as the type and anatomic location of the inflammation, are obtained from the ocular examination. Again, the need for information about systemic and neurologic signs necessitates a careful physical and neurologic examination of the uveitis patient by the ophthalmologist or by a consulting internist, internal medicine subspecialist, neurologist, or general medical practitioner.

Once the uveitis has been classified, a preliminary differential diagnosis should be generated. The answers to each of the questions in Box 5-1 will generate a list of possible diagnoses. The diagnoses that appear most frequently on these lists are then the most likely cause of the disorder. Ancillary examinations including laboratory tests or specialized examinations such as radiography, electrophysiology, or surgery such as a diagnostic vitrectomy can then be obtained to discern among the most likely diagnoses. In the following chapter on diagnostic testing, we show that the "shotgun approach" of ordering every diagnostic test available will mislead the clinician into making the wrong diagnosis.

## CLASSIFYING UVEITIS

### 1. Is the disease acute or chronic?

Acute cases of uveitis usually have a sudden onset and last up to 6 weeks. A list of the most common causes of acute uveitis are listed in

**Box 5-1**
**Classification of uveitis**

1. Is the disease acute or chronic?
2. Is the inflammation granulomatous or nongranulomatous?
3. Is the disease unilateral or bilateral?
4. Where is the inflammation located in the eye?
5. What are the demographics of the patient?
6. What associated symptoms does the patient have?
7. What associated signs are present on physical examination?
8. How did the disease respond to previous therapy?

**Box 5-2**
**Causes of acute and chronic uveitis**

**ACUTE UVEITIS**

Most cases of anterior uveitis: idiopathic, ankylosing spondylitis, Reiter's syndrome, Fuchs' heterochromic iridocyclitis
Vogt-Koyanagi-Harada syndrome
Toxoplasmosis
White-dot syndromes: acute posterior multifocal placoid pigment epitheliopathy and multiple evanescent white-dot syndrome
Acute retinal necrosis
Postsurgical bacterial infection
Trauma

**CHRONIC UVEITIS**

Juvenile rheumatoid arthritis
Birdshot choroidopathy
Serpiginous choroidopathy
Tuberculous uveitis
Postsurgical uveitis (*Propionibacterium acnes,* fungal)
Intraocular lymphoma
Sympathetic ophthalmia
Multifocal choroiditis
Sarcoidosis
Intermediate uveitis/pars planitis

Box 5-2. Most cases of anterior uveitis such as HLA-B27–associated iritis and idiopathic anterior uveitis fall into this category. Other diseases that typically cause acute uveitis include Vogt-Koyanagi-Harada disease, postsurgical bacterial infection, toxoplasmosis, many of the "white-dot syndromes" such as acute posterior multifocal placoid pigment epitheliopathy and multiple evanescent white-dot syndrome, and traumatic iritis. Although many diseases can cause an acute uveitis, these are the conditions to consider first in the differential diagnosis of an acute uveitis. Chronic forms of uveitis have an insidious onset and typically last longer than 6 weeks. Again, although many diseases can cause a uveitis that persists longer than 6 weeks, the uveitides that are characteristically chronic are listed in Box 5-2. Knowing if the uveitis is acute or chronic is never sufficient to make a diagnosis, but it may aid in the diagnostic process.

### 2. Is the inflammation granulomatous or nongranulomatous?

The ocular examination offers the unique opportunity to determine the type of infiltrating inflammatory cells involved in the disease process without taking a biopsy sample for histologic analysis. In cases of anterior uveitis, inflammatory cells attach to the corneal endothelium in conglomerates called keratic precipitates (KP). The appearance of KP has been used to classify the inflammatory process as granulomatous or nongranulomatous. The more common nongranulomatous type of KP is characterized by fine white-colored collections of lymphocytes, plasma cells, and pigment. These precipitates can form in any disease and cause an anterior uveitis; the finding of nongranulomatous KP does not help tremendously in the formulation of a differential diagnosis other than to alert the clinician that anterior inflammatory disease has occurred in the eye. Granulomatous keratic precipitates are large greasy-appearing collections of lymphocytes, plasma cells, and giant cells (see Fig. 4-2). The finding of granulomatous KP, also called "mutton-fat" KP, on the slit-lamp examination can be a useful diagnostic clue. Patients with granulomatous KP usually have a history of a chronic disease with an insidious onset and frequently have posterior segment disease in addition to their anterior segment inflammation. Other ocular findings suggestive of granulomatous inflammation are iris nodules and choroidal granulomas. Importantly, the finding of granulomatous inflammation in the eye suggests a unique set of diagnostic possibilities that are listed in Box 5-3.

**Box 5-3**
**Causes of granulomatous inflammation in eye**

Sarcoidosis
Sympathetic ophthalmia
Uveitis associated with multiple sclerosis
Lens-induced uveitis
Intraocular foreign body
Vogt-Koyanagi-Harada syndrome
Syphilis
Tuberculosis
Other infectious agents

**Box 5-4**
**Causes of unilateral uveitis**

Sarcoidosis
Postsurgical uveitis
Intraocular foreign body
Parasitic disease
Acute retinal necrosis
Behçet's disease

### 3. Is the disease unilateral or bilateral?

Although one eye may be affected first, most causes of uveitis involve both eyes within the first several months. Therefore the history that the disease is unilateral can help in diagnosing the condition. Diseases that frequently involve a single eye, even after months or years of the disorder, are listed in Box 5-4. Parasitic disease typically involves one eye, although some of the diseases, such as toxoplasmosis, occur bilaterally. Uveitis after ocular surgery or an intraocular foreign body are almost exclusively unilateral diseases. The one disease that most ophthalmologists think of as a bilateral disease but that we see involving a single eye in a number of patients is sarcoidosis. Similarly, we have seen a number of cases of Behçet's disease that involved a single eye, especially in patients of Asian descent.

### 4. Where is the inflammation located in the eye?

It is important to determine the anatomic position of the inflammation within the eye. Table 5-1 delineates two similar methods for the anatomic classification of intraocular inflammatory disease. We tend to base our anatomic classification on the scheme proposed by the International Uveitis Study Group.[1] In addition to classifying patients as having anterior, intermediate, posterior, or panuveitis, we note if there is a predominant involvement of the cornea (keratouveitis), sclera (sclerouveitis), or retinal vasculature (retinal vasculitis) because these findings point to specific causes.

Anterior uveitis describes a disease predominantly limited to the anterior segment of the eye. Other terms used in the literature for anterior uveitis are iritis, iridocyclitis, and anterior cyclitis. The inflammation is characterized by conjunctival hyperemia, anterior chamber cell and flare, KP, and iris abnormalities including posterior synechiae and peripheral anterior synechiae. A mild cellular inflammatory response in the anterior vitreous is often seen. The common causes of anterior uveitis are listed in Box 5-5.

Intermediate uveitis is the anatomic diagnosis that causes the most confusion among ophthalmologists. However, the proper classification of a uveitis as intermediate uveitis is very important because an underlying cause for

**Table 5-1.** Anatomic classification of uveitis

| IUSG* | Tessler† |
|---|---|
| – | Sclerouveitis |
| – | Keratouveitis |
| Anterior uveitis | Anterior uveitis |
| Iritis | Iritis |
| Anterior cyclitis | Iridocyclitis |
| Iridocyclitis | |
| Intermediate uveitis | Intermediate uveitis |
| (formerly known as pars planitis) | Cyclitis |
| Posterior cyclitis | Vitritis |
| Hyalitis | Pars planitis |
| Basal retinochoroiditis | |
| Posterior uveitis | Posterior uveitis |
| Focal, multifocal, or diffuse choroiditis, chorioretinitis, retinochoroiditis, or neurouveitis | Retinitis<br>Choroiditis |
| Panuveitis | – |

*From Bloch-Michel E, Nussenblatt RB: International Uveitis Study Group recommendations for the evaluation of intraocular inflammatory disease, *Am J Ophthalmol* 103: 234-235, 1987.

†From Tessler HH: Classification and symptoms and signs of uveitis. In Duane TD, Jaeger EA, editors: *Clinical ophthalmology*, vol 4, Philadelphia, 1987, JB Lippincott; Chapter 32, pp 1-10.

**Box 5-5**
**Causes of anterior uveitis**

Idiopathic
Ankylosing spondylitis
Reiter's syndrome
Inflammatory bowel disease
Psoriatic arthritis
Behçet's disease
HLA-B27–associated disease
Juvenile rheumatoid arthritis
Fuchs' heterochromic iridocyclitis
Sarcoidosis
Syphilis
Glaucomatocyclitic crisis
Masquerade syndromes

**Box 5-6**
**Causes of intermediate uveitis**

Sarcoidosis
Inflammatory bowel disease
Multiple sclerosis
Lyme disease
Pars planitis*

*Not an etiologic diagnosis, but patients with intermediate uveitis of the par planitis subtype tend to have worse prognosis.

the disease can often be determined. Intermediate uveitis is characterized by inflammation that primarily affects the vitreous and peripheral retina. Aggregates of inflammatory cells are frequently seen in the inferior vitreous and have been termed *vitreous snowballs.* Similarly, the accumulation of inflammatory cells and debris along the pars plana and ora serrata that have been called *snowbanks.* A mild anterior uveitis often coexists, and cystoid macular edema is a frequent finding. The conditions associated with intermediate uveitis are listed in Box 5-6.

Disease limited to the posterior segment of the eye, particularly the retina and choroid are termed *posterior uveitis.* A large number of diseases cause posterior uveitis, so to further subdivide the disorders we classify posterior uveitis as predominantly a retinitis or choroiditis and as a focal or multifocal disease. A list of the disorders that cause focal and multifocal retinitis and choroiditis are listed in Box 5-7. The term *panuveitis* is reserved for diseases that involve all segments of the eye, typically with a severe sight-reducing inflammatory response. The common causes of panuveitis are listed in Box 5-8.

**Box 5-7**
**Causes of posterior uveitis**

**FOCAL RETINITIS**

Toxoplasmosis
Onchocerciasis
Cysticercosis
Masquerade syndromes

**MULTIFOCAL RETINITIS**

Syphilis
Herpes simplex virus
Cytomegalovirus
Sarcoidosis
Masquerade syndromes
Candidiasis
Meningococcus

**FOCAL CHOROIDITIS**

Toxocariasis
Tuberculosis
Nocardiosis
Masquerade syndromes

**MULTIFOCAL CHOROIDITIS**

Histoplasmosis
Sympathetic ophthalmia
Vogt-Kayanagi-Harada syndrome
Sarcoidosis
Serpiginous choroidopathy
Birdshot choroidopathy
Masquerade syndromes (metastatic tumor)

**Box 5-8**
**Causes of panuveitis**

Syphilis
Sarcoidosis
Vogt-Koyanagi-Harada syndrome
Infectious endophthalmitis
Behçet's disease

Severe scleritis in association with uveitis is most frequently seen in patients with underlying connective tissue diseases such as rheumatoid arthritis and ankylosing spondylitis. Inflammatory bowel disease such as Crohn's disease and ulcerative colitis also cause sclerouveitis. Finally, severe retinal vasculitis is associated with a subset of diseases that cause uveitis. Like scleritis, retinal vasculitis is often associated with underlying connective tissue disease. A full list of the disorders that cause retinal vasculitis can be found in Chapter 26.

### 5. What are the demographics of the patient?

Demographic considerations can lead the ophthalmologist to suspect certain types of uveitis, although there are always patients who present outside of the usual age, sex, race, ethnic heritage, and residence parameters for any particular disease. The age of the patient can be particularly useful in developing a differential diagnosis because certain causes of uveitis are more common among patients of specific age groups. A list of age considerations in patients with uveitis is found in Table 5-2. One must be careful, however, not to rigidly apply these guidelines to patients. For example, although intraocular lymphoma is typically found in patients over the age of 65 years, we have seen patients with this disease in their 30s. Nevertheless, these guidelines are clearly useful, especially in diagnosing uveitis in children. Other demographic considerations in patients with uveitis are listed in Table 5-3.

### 6. What associated symptoms does the patient have?

Specific symptoms, both those relating to the eye and those suggesting systemic disease, should lead the clinician to suspect certain types of uveitis. We find that carefully defining a patient's symptoms is the most important step to determine the correct diagnosis. Many of the symptoms that suggest specific diagnoses are listed in Table 5-4. However, the enthusiasm to classify the patient within a diagnostic category may tempt the clinician to stretch the symptoms to fit a particular disease. For example, a patient who noted mild knee pain after playing basketball for the first time in 2 years should not be classified as having a chronic arthritis consistent with rheumatoid arthritis. Similarly, ringing in the ears after a 4-hour rock concert does not qualify as tinnitus suggestive of Vogt-Koyanagi-Harada syndrome. Similarly, the clinician must also be careful not to suggest symptoms to the patient. Avoid asking questions like, "You must have had some joint pain with this, haven't you?"

**Table 5-2.** Age considerations in patients with uveitis

| Age (yr) | Diagnostic considerations |
|---|---|
| <5 | Juvenile rheumatoid arthritis<br>Toxocariasis<br>Postviral neuroretinitis<br>(Retinoblastoma)<br>(Juvenile xanthogranuloma)<br>Leukemia |
| 5-15 | Juvenile rheumatoid arthritis<br>Pars planitis<br>Toxocariasis<br>Postviral neuroretinitis<br>Sarcoidosis<br>Leukemia |
| 16-25 | Pars planitis<br>Ankylosing spondylitis<br>Idiopathic anterior uveitis<br>Toxoplasmosis<br>Sarcoidosis<br>Acute retinal necrosis |
| 25-45 | Ankylosing spondylitis<br>Idiopathic anterior uveitis<br>Fuchs' heterochromic iridocyclitis<br>Idiopathic intermediate uveitis<br>Toxoplasmosis<br>Behçet's disease<br>Idiopathic retinal vasculitis<br>Sarcoidosis<br>White-dot syndromes<br>Vogt-Koyanagi-Harada syndrome<br>AIDS, syphilis<br>Serpiginous choroidopathy |
| 45-65 | Birdshot retinochoroiditis<br>Idiopathic anterior uveitis<br>Idiopathic intermediate uveitis<br>Idiopathic retinal vasculitis<br>Behçet's disease<br>Serpiginous choroidopathy<br>Acute retinal necrosis |
| >65 | Idiopathic anterior uveitis<br>Idiopathic intermediate uveitis<br>Idiopathic retinal vasculitis<br>Serpiginous choroidopathy<br>(Masquerade syndromes) |

NOTE: Parentheses indicate noninflammatory diseases.

### 7. What associated signs are present on physical examination?

If it is rare to find ophthalmologists taking a detailed medical history in the office, it is almost unheard of for a detailed physical examination to be performed. Unless you are prepared to do a thorough physical examination, it is probably more practical to refer patients to their primary care physician for this part of the evaluation. Nevertheless, it is fruitful

**Table 5-3.** Demographic considerations in uveitis

| Factor | Disease risks |
|---|---|
| Female | Pauciarticular juvenile rheumatoid arthritis, chronic anterior uveitis |
| Male | Ankylosing spondylitis, sympathetic ophthalmia |
| American black | Sarcoidosis |
| Native American | Vogt-Koyanagi-Harada syndrome |
| Midwestern American | Presumed ocular histoplasmosis |
| Japanese* | Vogt-Koyanagi-Harada syndrome<br>Behçet's syndrome |
| Mediterranean ancestry | Behçet's syndrome |
| Central American | Cysticercosis, onchocerciasis |
| South American | Cysticercosis |
| West African | Onchocerciasis |
| Intravenous drug user | Fungal endophthalmitis, AIDS |
| Promiscuous heterosexual or homosexual | AIDS, syphilis |
| Frequent hiking in wooded areas | Lyme disease |

*Not in Americans of Japanese extraction.

**Table 5-4.** Systemic signs and symptoms in uveitis

| Symptom or sign | Possible associated conditions |
|---|---|
| Headaches | Sarcoidosis, Vogt-Koyanagi-Harada syndrome |
| Neurosensory deafness | Vogt-Koyanagi-Harada syndrome, sarcoidosis |
| Cerebrospinal fluid pleocytosis | Vogt-Koyanagi-Harada syndrome, sarcoidosis, acute posterior multifocal placoid pigment epitheliopathy, Behçet's syndrome |
| Paresthesia, weakness | Intermediate uveitis associated with multiple sclerosis, Behçet's syndrome, steroid myopathy |
| Psychosis | Vogt-Koyanagi-Harada syndrome, sarcoidosis, Behçet's disease, steroid psychosis, systemic lupus erythematosus |
| Vitiligo, poliosis | Vogt-Koyanagi-Harada syndrome |
| Erythema nodosum | Behçet's syndrome, sarcoidosis |
| Skin nodules | Sarcoidosis, onchocerciasis |
| Alopecia | Vogt-Koyanagi-Harada syndrome |
| Skin rash | Behçet's syndrome, sarcoidosis, viral exanthem, syphilis, herpes zoster, psoriatic arthritis, Lyme disease |
| Oral ulcers | Behçet's syndrome, inflammatory bowel disease |
| Genital ulcers | Behçet's syndrome, Reiter's syndrome, sexually transmitted diseases |
| Salivary or lacrimal gland swelling | Sarcoidosis, lymphoma |
| Lymphoid organ enlargement | Sarcoidosis, AIDS |
| Diarrhea | Whipple's disease, inflammatory bowel disease |
| Cough, shortness of breath | Sarcoidosis, tuberculosis, malignancy |
| Sinusitis | Wegener's granulomatosis |
| Systemic vasculitis | Behçet's syndrome, sarcoidosis, relapsing polychondritis |
| Arthritis | Behçet's syndrome, Reiter's syndrome, sarcoidosis, juvenile rheumatoid arthritis, rheumatoid arthritis, Lyme disease, inflammatory bowel disease, Wegener's granulomatosus, systemic lupus erythematosus, other connective tissue diseases |
| Sacroileitis | Ankylosing spondylitis, Reiter's syndrome, inflammatory bowel disease |
| Chemotherapy or other immunosuppression | Cytomegalovirus retinitis, *Candida* retinitis, other opportunistic organisms |

for the ophthalmologist to examine a few things before making the referral. We have found that examination of the skin can be extremely rewarding in diagnosing uveitis. We have discovered sarcoid granulomas, rashes consistent with Lyme disease and syphilis, and Kaposi's sarcoma. A brief examination of the joints for signs of inflammation is also useful, and a screening neurologic examination is warranted, especially in patients who may have intraocular lymphoma, sarcoidosis, or Behçet's disease. Table 5-4 lists the systemic

**Table 5-5.** Common causes of anterior and posterior uveitis

| Diagnosis | Perkins et al.* (%) | Henderly et al.† (%) |
|---|---|---|
| **ANTERIOR UVEITIS** | | |
| Idiopathic anterior uveitis | 32.7 | 12.1 |
| HLA-B27–associated anterior uveitis | – | 3.0 |
| Juvenile rheumatoid arthritis | 5.1 | 2.8 |
| Fuchs' heterochromic iridocyclitis | 6.3 | 1.8 |
| Ankylosing spondylitis | 5.7 | 1.5 |
| Reiter's syndrome | 5.2 | 1.0 |
| Inflammatory bowel disease | 2.9 | 0.3 |
| Syphilis | 1.2 | 0.8 |
| Intraocular lens-related anterior uveitis | | 1.0 |
| **POSTERIOR UVEITIS** | | |
| Toxoplasmic retinochoroiditis | 9.2 | 7.0 |
| Idiopathic retinal vasculitis | 4.6 | 6.8 |
| Idiopathic posterior uveitis | 6.9 | 3.7 |
| Ocular histoplasmosis | – | 3.5 |
| Toxocariasis | 2.9 | 2.6 |
| Serpiginous choroidopathy | – | 2.0 |
| Acute posterior multifocal placoid pigment epitheliopathy | – | 1.8 |
| Acute retinal necrosis | – | 1.3 |
| Birdshot choroidopathy | – | 1.2 |
| Intraocular lymphoma | 1.1 | 1.2 |

*Data from Perkins ES, Folk J: Uveitis in London and Iowa, *Ophthalmologica* 36:189, 1984.
†Data from Henderly DE, Genstler AJ, Smith RE, et al: Changing patterns of uveitis, *Am J Ophthalmol* 103:131-136, 1987.

signs associated with specific uveitic conditions.

### 8. How did the patient respond to previous therapy?

The course of the disease, in particular the response to therapy, can provide useful information in determining the cause. Is the disease responsive to antiinflammatory therapy? Does the disease require continued corticosteroid therapy? If so, how much corticosteroid is needed? Is the disease resistant to corticosteroid therapy? These questions can help the clinician come to the correct diagnosis. In general, infectious diseases may initially improve with antiinflammatory therapy but later worsen. Postsurgical endophthalmitis caused by *Propionibacterium acnes* typically improves temporarily with topical or systemic corticosteroids but then recurs. Temporary and partial response to therapy also suggests that the ocular inflammation may be associated with a chronic systemic disease such as sarcoidosis or a malignancy-like lymphoma. A long history of intermittent response to therapy tends to be more suggestive of a chronic noninfectious and nonmalignant disease because both infection or malignancy often declare themselves after several years.

Of course the old adage, "when you hear hoofbeats, think of horses and not zebras," also applies to the evaluation of the uveitis patient. Common diseases are frequently the cause of uveitis even in the difficult cases to diagnose. Table 5-5 lists the most common causes of anterior and posterior uveitis from two published surveys of uveitis patients.

Once the above questions are answered, lists of possible diagnoses are generated. By determining the diagnoses that appear most frequently, a final list of the most likely conditions responsible for the patient's uveitis is generated. The clinician can then order diagnostic studies to discern among the most likely disorders. The following cases will help to illustrate the process of developing a differential diagnosis in the patient with uveitis.

#### Case 5-1

A 42-year-old white woman presented with a 10-year history of bilateral uveitis treated intermittently with topical and systemic corticosteroids and a chief complaint of blurred vi-

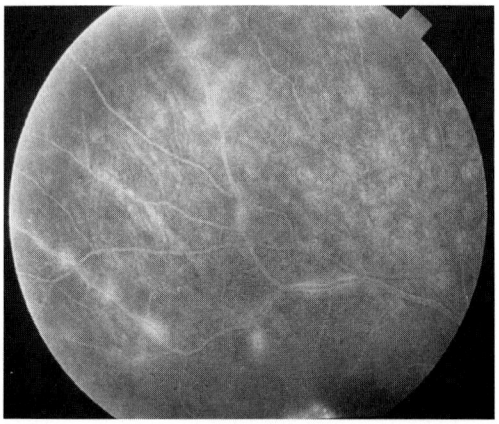

**Fig. 5-1.** Late phase of fluorescein angiogram showing staining of blood vessel walls and leakage of dye from peripheral retinal vasculature.

sion that was worse in the left eye. A detailed medical history was significant for sinusitis and depression. On examination, her visual acuity was 20/50 in the right eye and 20/100 in the left eye. Slit-lamp biomicroscopy showed mutton-fat KP in the left eye. There were trace vitreous cells and haze in the right eye and 2+ vitreous cells and haze in the left eye. There were peripheral retinal vasculitis and cystoid macular edema in both eyes (Fig. 5-1). Physical examination revealed no rash, joint findings, or other abnormalities. Neurologic examination was normal.

Just by reading the above case history, most clinicians find it difficult to derive an erudite differential diagnosis. But by classifying the uveitis with the eight questions previously outlined, lists of possible diagnoses can be generated. By comparing these lists, the most likely diagnoses can then be identified. Ques-

**Box 5-9**
**Lists of diagnoses generated for Case 5-1**

Chronic, granulomatous, bilateral, intermediate uveitis in a middle-aged white woman with intermittent response to topical and systemic corticosteroids

**CHRONIC UVEITIS**

Juvenile rheumatoid arthritis
Birdshot choroidopathy
Serpiginous choroidopathy
Tuberculous uveitis
Postsurgical uveitis (*Propionibacterium acnes,* fungal)
Intraocular lymphoma
Sympathetic ophthalmia
Multifocal choroiditis
Sarcoidosis
Intermediate uveitis/pars planitis

**INTERMEDIATE UVEITIS**

Sarcoidosis
Inflammatory bowel disease
Multiple sclerosis
Lyme disease
Pars planitis

**GRANULOMATOUS INFLAMMATION IN EYE**

Sarcoidosis
Sympathetic ophthalmia
Uveitis associated with multiple sclerosis
Lens-induced uveitis
Intraocular foreign body
Vogt-Koyanagi-Harada syndrome
Syphilis
Tuberculosis
Other infectious agents

**AGE 25-45 YR**

Ankylosing spondylitis
Idiopathic anterior uveitis
Fuchs' heterochromic iridocyclitis
Intermediate uveitis
Toxoplasmosis
Behçet's disease
Idiopathic retinal vasculitis
Sarcoidosis
White-dot syndromes
Vogt-Koyanagi-Harada syndrome
AIDS
Syphilis
Serpiginous choroidopathy

**ASSOCIATED SYMPTOMS AND SIGNS**

Sinusitis–Wegener's disease

tion 1 asks whether the disease is acute or chronic. Because the patient has a 10-year history of disease, the uveitis is clearly chronic, and this is associated with the diseases listed in Box 5-2. The patient has mutton-fat KP suggesting that the uveitis is granulomatous, and this suggests the list of diagnoses shown in Box 5-3. The disease is bilateral, which does not point to a specific set of diseases; however, with prominent vitritis and peripheral retinal vasculitis, the anatomic classification of an intermediate uveitis does suggest a specific set of possible diseases to the clinician (Box 5-6). The patient is white and in the 24- to 45-year-old range suggesting the diagnoses shown in Table 5-2. As seen in Table 5-4, a complaint of sinusitis suggests a possible diagnosis of Wegener's granulomatosis, but the patient had no specific findings on physical examination.

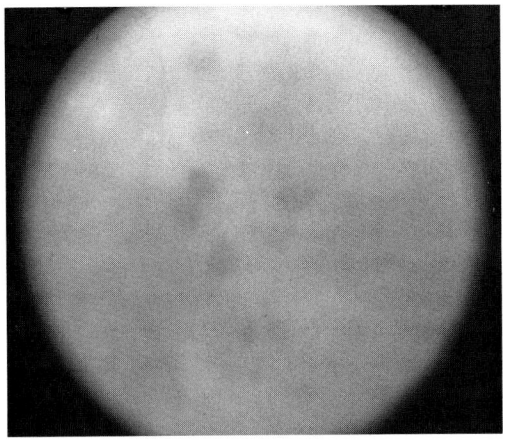

**Fig. 5-2.** Fundus photograph showing yellow-colored subretinal infiltrates, retinal hemorrhage, and retinal edema in eye with 20/125 visual acuity and moderate vitritis. (See Color Plate 5.)

In summary, the uveitis can be classified as a chronic, granulomatous, bilateral, intermediate uveitis in a middle-aged white woman with intermittent response to topical and systemic corticosteroids. The group of lists containing possible diagnoses for this patient are shown in Box 5-9. If you compare these lists, the most frequently mentioned disorders include sarcoidosis, other causes of intermediate uveitis such as multiple sclerosis and inflammatory bowel

**Box 5-10**
**Lists of diagnoses generated for Case 5-2**

Chronic, nongranulomatous, bilateral, multifocal retinitis in an elderly white woman

**CHRONIC UVEITIS**

Juvenile rheumatoid arthritis
Birdshot choroidopathy
Serpiginous choroidopathy
Tuberculous uveitis
Postsurgical uveitis (*Propionibacterium acnes*, fungal)
Intraocular lymphoma
Sympathetic ophthalmia
Multifocal choroiditis
Sarcoidosis
Intermediate uveitis/pars planitis

**GRANULOMATOUS INFLAMMATION IN EYE**

Sarcoidosis
Sympathetic ophthalmia
Uveitis associated with multiple sclerosis
Lens-induced uveitis
Intraocular foreign body
Vogt-Koyanagi-Harada syndrome
Syphilis
Tuberculosis
Other infectious agents

**MULTIFOCAL RETINITIS**

Syphilis
Herpes simplex virus
Cytomegalovirus
Sarcoidosis
Masquerade syndromes
*Candida*
Meningococcus

**AGE >65 YR**

Idiopathic anterior uveitis
Idiopathic intermediate uveitis
Idiopathic retinal vasculitis
Serpiginous choroidopathy
Masquerade syndromes
Sarcoidosis

**DEMOGRAPHIC CONSIDERATIONS**

Patient lives in an endemic area for Lyme disease

disease, and other chronic disorders such as Behçet's disease and Wegener's granulomatosis. Diagnostic tests were then ordered to discern between the most likely disorders. Results of a diagnostic evaluation for sarcoidosis and Wegener's granulomatosis including a chest x-ray, serum angiotensin-converting enzyme level, antineutrophil cytoplasmic antibody test, and computed tomography scan of the sinuses were normal. However, a magnetic resonance imaging scan of the brain revealed lesions consistent with a diagnosis of multiple sclerosis. The patient later developed an episode of lower extremity weakness followed by a second episode of paresthesia that extended to the level of the umbilicus diagnostic of this disease.

**Case 5-2**

A 73-year-old white woman presented with blurred vision in both eyes during the previous year. The patient first noted floaters in the left eye 1 year earlier but did not see an ophthalmologist until 3 months before, when she was found to have a slight decrease in visual acuity in the left eye and bilateral mild vitritis. Over the next 3 months her vision decreased in both eyes, and she was referred to the National Eye Institute. She had a history of type II diabetes mellitus controlled with oral hypoglycemic agents and of rheumatic fever as a child. She also complained of weight loss and unsteady gate. She lived in a wooded area in Glen Falls, N.Y.

On examination, visual acuity was 20/50 in the right eye and 20/125 in the left eye. Anterior segment examination was normal, but there were 2+ vitreous cells and 1+ vitreous haze in both eyes. Funduscopic examination revealed punctate yellow-colored subretinal infiltrates in both eyes and retinal hemorrhage and edema in the left eye (Fig. 5-2). Physical examination revealed ataxia.

Again, this patient presents difficulty in diagnosis, but with the approach detailed in case 5-1 a differential diagnosis can be readily developed. The disease is chronic, and the inflammation is nongranulomatous. It is a bilateral disease and is classified as a multifocal retinitis. Therefore the patient is classified as having a chronic, nongranulomatous, bilateral, multifocal retinitis. She is an elderly white woman, and the history of living in a wooded area suggests a demographic susceptibility to develop Lyme disease. Her symptoms of weight loss suggests the possibility of an underlying malignancy, malnutrition, or possible gastrointestinal disease, and the unsteady gait alerts the clinician to the possibility of neurologic disease. The list of diagnoses generated by this classification are shown in Box 5-10. As you can see, the most frequently listed diagnoses include sarcoidosis, infectious diseases, and the masquerade syndromes, most notably intraocular lymphoma.

Our first concern was that the patient had an underlying malignancy. Systemic evaluation was unrewarding, and a vitrectomy showed no malignant cells. However, two serum angiotensin-converting enzyme levels were elevated at 81 and 101 U/L (normal range: 8-52 U/L), and a bronchoscopy confirmed the diagnosis of sarcoidosis.

We hope that this chapter will provide the clinician with a pragmatic approach to generating a differential diagnosis. This then allows the ophthalmologist to order the appropriate tests to discern among the most likely possibilities. As you will see in Chapter 6, the alternative shotgun approach of indiscriminately ordering every diagnostic test in the book may be both expensive and misleading.

## REFERENCE

1. Bloch-Michel E, Nussenblatt RB: International Uveitis Study Group recommendations for the evaluation of intraocular inflammatory disease, *Am J Ophthalmol* 103:234-235, 1987.

# CHAPTER 6

# Diagnostic Testing

What diagnostic tests should you order in the evaluation of the patient with uveitis? This is one of the most difficult questions we are asked. It is clear, however, that a nonselective approach to testing is costly, inefficient, and provides information that is often irrelevant or, worse, may lead one far astray from the truth. It is important to understand how to interpret diagnostic data as this information will help the clinician to order the appropriate tests.

Why does the clinician order diagnostic tests? Usually diagnostic tests are ordered to aid in making the correct diagnosis. Unfortunately many clinicians are overly influenced when a positive or negative diagnostic test comes back from the laboratory. A clinical example will serve to illustrate this point. A 34-year-old African-American woman from San Antonio, Tex., presents with an intermediate uveitis in both eyes for the past 7 months. There is no history of rash, arthritis, or fever, but the patient does complain of wheezing and shortness of breath on exertion. The ophthalmologist orders a battery of diagnostic tests including a serologic test for Lyme disease that has a positive result. Of course, the ophthalmologist is ecstatic in diagnosing the patient and treats her with a 2-week course of ceftriaxone. There are only three problems with this scenario. The patient probably does not have Lyme disease, did not need the expensive 2-week course of intravenous antibiotics, and more likely has sarcoidosis that is not being treated!

Before one can appropriately interpret what the results of a diagnostic test mean, three pieces of information are needed. First, one needs to know the sensitivity of the diagnostic test (Fig. 6-1). The sensitivity of a test is calculated by dividing the number of patients who actually have the disease and who on testing have a positive result by the total number of patients with the disease who are tested. Another name given to the patients with a disease who have a positive test result is true positives; they have a positive test and actually have the disease. Patients who have the disease but who have a negative test result are called false negatives. Many of the commonly used serologic tests for Lyme disease have a sensitivity of 90%. What does that mean? It means that if 100 patients with Lyme disease were tested, 90 would have a positive result (true positives), but 10 would have a negative result (false negatives).

The second piece of information you need to have to interpret a diagnostic test result is the specificity (Fig. 6-1). The specificity of a diagnostic test is calculated by dividing the number of patients who do not have the disease in question and who have had an appropriately negative result by the total number of people without the disease who are tested. People who do not have the disease and who have a negative test result are called true negatives. Similarly, people who do not have the disease but who have a positive test result anyway are called false positives. In the case of the serologic test for Lyme disease, the specificity is also 90%. This means that if 100 patients without Lyme disease take this test, 90 will have an appropriately negative result, but 10 will have a misleading positive result!

## PRETEST LIKELIHOOD OF DISEASE

The critical piece of information needed for test interpretation is one that is completely

| | Disease present | Disease absent | |
|---|---|---|---|
| Test + | True positives<br>a | False positives<br>b | |
| Test − | False negatives<br>c | True negatives<br>d | |

**Fig. 6-1.** Sensitivity and specificity of diagnostic tests. Sensitivity = a/a + b. Specificity = d/b + d.

ignored by many doctors. This piece of information is called the pretest likelihood of the disease and is defined as the chance that the patient has a particular disease before the diagnostic test is ordered. The pretest likelihood can be based on a number of factors such as the patient's history and physical examination and the incidence of a particular disease in that area. This is the figure that most depends on the clinician's prowess and ability; the more accurate the physician's calculation of the pretest likelihood of disease, the more accurate the subsequent interpretation of the test result will be.

What is the pretest likelihood of Lyme disease in the case of the 34-year-old woman from San Antonio with intermediate uveitis who has no other symptoms and signs of Lyme disease and who does not live in an endemic area for the disease? The prevalence of Lyme disease in that area is probably less than 1 per 1000, and with no other evidence of the disease the pretest likelihood of the disease would probably be less than this. But let's be generous and say that the pretest likelihood of this patient having Lyme disease is 1 in 1000 or 0.1%. How do we interpret her positive test result for Lyme disease?

The likelihood that the diagnosis of Lyme disease is correct in this patient can be calculated because we now have the sensitivity of the test (90%), the specificity of the test (90%), and the pretest likelihood of the disease (0.1%). This calculation of what is called the posttest likelihood of disease is carried out with the use of a formula derived by the mathematician Bayes and is called Bayes' theorem. The standard form of Bayes' theorem states the following:

$$\text{Posttest probability} = \frac{\text{Pretest probability} \times \text{sensitivity}}{(\text{Pretest probability} \times \text{sensitivity}) + (1 - \text{pretest probability})(1 - \text{specificity})}.$$

Bayes' theorem has been understood for two centuries but has only been applied to clinical reasoning over the past 30 years.[1–5] Although formulas may appear daunting to some clinicians, computer programs and nomograms have been developed to help the clinician interpret the data.[6,7] So what is the likelihood that our patient has Lyme disease given her positive laboratory test? With Bayes' theorem the chance that she has Lyme disease is still only 0.9%, or a chance of 9 out of 1000! Although this represents an almost 10-fold increase in likelihood compared with the pretest likelihood, because there was a very small chance that she had Lyme disease before the test, she still probably does not have the disease. Knowing that the posttest likelihood of the patient having Lyme dis-ease is less than 1%, the clinician probably would not opt to treat the patient with antibiotics.

Diagnostic tests are also not as useful if there is a very strong likelihood that a patient has the disease before the test is ordered. If this same patient came from Lyme, Conn., had a history of a tick bite followed by an erythematous, round rash, and now presented with an intermediate uveitis and arthritis, even without testing she would probably have over a 99% chance of having the disease. Even if her Lyme serologic test result was negative, after applying Bayes' theorem the patient would still have about a 99% chance of having the disease!

Diagnostic tests are most helpful when the pretest likelihood of the disease is about 50%. In the case of our patient with intermediate uveitis, if after our initial assessment we thought that her chance of having Lyme disease was 50%, a positive serologic test result would increase the posttest likelihood of the disease to 90%. So in this case, we start with a 50:50 chance of Lyme disease but end up with Lyme disease being far and away the most likely diagnosis.

So now that you have the knowledge to analyze data, it should be easy to interpret your patients' test data, right? Unfortunately, it is not that easy. It is difficult to obtain the sensitivities and specificities for many of the common diagnostic tests we order. Many laboratories are considering providing a nomogram listing the

**Table 6-1.** Laboratory tests in uveitis

| Tests | Conditions/comments |
|---|---|
| Angiotensin-converting enzyme | Sarcoidosis; may be elevated in children without sarcoidosis |
| Antiphospholipid Ab (lupus anticoagulant and anticardiolipin Ab) | Thrombosis, CNS disease, and spontaneous abortions in patients with systemic lupus erythematosus |
| Antinuclear antibody | Systemic lupus erythematosus and other rheumatic diseases |
| Antifungal Ab | Fungal disease |
| Antineutrophil cytosplasmic Ab (ANCA) | Wegener's granulomatosis (cANCA)<br>Polyarteritis nodosa (pANCA) |
| Antinuclear antibody (ANA) | Systemic lupus erythematosus and other rheumatic diseases |
| Antitoxoplasma Ab | Toxoplasmosis |
| Antiviral Ab | Viral infection |
| Calcium | Sarcoidosis |
| Chlamydia complement-fixation test | Chlamydia |
| Cultures | Bacterial, fungal, mycobacterial, and viral diseases |
| Erythrocyte sedimentation rate | Underlying systemic diseases (i.e., rheumatic disease, malignancy) |
| Complete blood cell count | Underlying systemic disease |
| HIV ELISA | HIV |
| HTLV-1 | HTLV-1 infection |
| HLA typing | (Specific HLA types associated with specific diseases) |
| Immune complexes | Rarely useful |
| Liver function tests | Sarcoidosis, hepatitis |
| Lumbar puncture for cell count | APMPPE, VKH, infection, malignancy |
| Lumbar puncture for CSF VDRL | Syphilis |
| Lumbar puncture for culture and Gram stain | Infection |
| Lumbar puncture for cytology | CNS lymphoma |
| Lyme serology | Lyme disease (be aware of false positives) |
| Rheumatoid factor (RF) | Rheumatoid arthritis; girls with JRA and uveitis often RF (−) but ANA (+) |
| Stool for ova and parasites | Parasitic disease |
| T-cell subsets | (Low CD4 count predisposes patient for opportunistic infections) |
| Thyroid function tests | Increased incidence of thyroid disease in uveitis patients |
| Urinalysis | (Blood suggests rheumatic disease) |
| VDRL/FTA-ABS | Syphilis |

*APMPPE,* Acute posterior multifocal placoid pigment epitheliopathy; *CSF,* cerebral spinal fluid; *CNS,* central nervous system; *HIV,* human immunodeficiency virus; *HTLV,* human T-cell leukemia/lymphoma virus; *JRA,* juvenile rheumatoid arthritis; *VKH,* Vogt-Koyanagi-Harada.

posttest likelihood of the disease for differing pretest likelihood as they already know the current sensitivity and specificity for that test. But how do we know what the sensitivity or specificity of a chest x-ray is for the diagnosis of sarcoidosis or of a diagnostic vitrectomy for intraocular lymphoma? These figures are difficult to obtain and may vary tremendously from institution to institution. More and more, however, articles are being published on the sensitivity and specificity of diagnostic procedures and tests. In addition, the clinician can do the calculations on the basis of hypothetical numbers. For example, one might ask that given a 95% sensitivity and a 95% specificity for a test in a patient who I think has a 10% chance of having the disease, what is the posttest likelihood of the disease? It is surprising how much such calculations can help you to decide on a diagnostic or therapeutic approach to complicated patients. Rosenbaum and Wernick[3] have written a recent review on how to apply Bayes' theorem to the evaluation of patients with uveitis, and this article should be useful to many clinicians.

## DIAGNOSTIC TESTS FOR UVEITIS

After your initial differential diagnosis is generated, diagnostic tests should be ordered to help discern among the most likely disorders. Remember that diagnostic tests will have the most utility in confirming or rejecting diagnoses that start with about a 50% chance of being correct. Table 6-1 and Box 6-1 list the

**Box 6-1**
**Other diagnostic tests in uveitis**

**IMAGING TESTS**

CT scan of head
CT scan of sinuses
Gallium scan
Hand x-ray
MRI of head
Sacroiliac x-ray

**SKIN TESTING**

Allergy testing
Anergy testing
Behcetin
Histoplasmin
Kveim
Pathergy
PPD

**ANCILLARY OPHTHALMIC TESTING**

Color vision testing
Electroretinogram
Electrooculogram
Fluorescein angiography
Laser interferometry
Laser flare reading
Manifest refraction
Ultrasound
Visual evoked potentials
Visual field testing

**BIOPSY SPECIMENS**

Conjunctiva
Lacrimal gland
Aqueous humor
Vitreous
Choroid and retina
Skin

common diagnostic tests useful for the evaluation of patients with uveitis. In addition to helping the clinician make the correct diagnosis, diagnostic tests are ordered in two other clinical settings. The first of these involves ordering tests to help the practitioner exclude the diagnosis of tumor and infection, because these disorders require specific therapy and would be exacerbated by antiinflammatory treatment. The second is to determine why a patient's vision has decreased and whether this change is reversible. In complicated uveitic eyes, the reasons for poor vision may be multifactorial, and the clinician needs as much information as possible.

The number of diagnostic tests available to the ophthalmologist have increased tremendously over the last decade. Many tests are expensive yet yield little useful information; others are critical for the appropriate management of patients. These tests can be arbitrarily grouped into laboratory tests, imaging techniques, skin testing, surgical specimens, and ancillary ophthalmic tests. Many of the tests listed in Tables 6-1 and Box 6-1 are more thoroughly discussed in later chapters on specific diseases; however, several points for each group of diagnostic tests deserve comment here.

### Laboratory tests

Laboratory tests usually are the first diagnostic tests that most physicians order. Although we have emphasized that laboratory tests should not be routinely used to screen uveitis patients for disease and that tests should be ordered only to discern among likely diagnoses, there is one exception. Practically all patients with uveitis should be tested for syphilis. There are a number of factors that support the use of laboratory tests to screen for syphilis in most patients with uveitis. Syphilis remains a common cause of uveitis and is easily treatable. Untreated patients with ocular syphilis often have devastating visual outcomes. Importantly, the fluorescent treponemal antibody absorption (FTA-ABS) test for syphilis is both extremely sensitive and specific. For patients with late syphilis, the stage of disease associated with uveitis, the sensitivity and specificity of the FTA-ABS test are both 99%. With this combination of a treatable, common disease, poor outcome in untreated patients, and a highly sensitive and specific diagnostic test with little risk and moderate cost, screening becomes useful. It is important to note, however, that other laboratory tests for syphilis are not as good for screening patients for late syphilis (see Chapter 10). The VDRL, for example, has a sensitivity of only 70% for late syphilis. Therefore the clinician should insist on an FTA-ABS in evaluating the uveitis patient. Also, the incidence of syphilis in patients with AIDS is also increasing.[8,9] As a result, all uveitis patients with syphilis should also be tested for HIV infection and vice versa.

A number of tests are used for research purposes but are commercially available. Many practitioners order these tests but do not know what to do with the results when they come back. Standardization of many of these tests is subpar, and many of these tests are better left unordered. One example is testing for circulating immune complexes. Circulating immune complexes were first thought to be the mechanism underlying the destruction of the eye in various forms of uveitis. Tests for circulating immune complexes were ordered, and if present they were attributed to be the cause of the disease. It is no longer clear that immune complexes are the cause of many cases of uveitis. Circulating immune complexes are found in many persons, and the evidence to date would suggest that their presence in ocular inflammatory disease may be protective rather than destructive (see Chapter 2).

One new diagnostic test that is being commonly used in the evaluation of patients with uveitis and retinal vasculitis is the antineutrophil cytoplasmic antibody test (ANCA). The test has been very helpful in diagnosing and following patients with Wegener's granulomatosis, a systemic vasculitis characterized by a necrotizing granulomatous vasculitis of the upper and lower respiratory tracts, a focal necrotizing glomerulonephritis, and systemic small vessel vasculitis involving a number of organ systems. Ocular involvement including uveitis, scleritis, and retinal vasculitis occurs in about 16% of patients.[10-12] Young[13] described 98 patients with uveitis tested for the presence of ANCA by an indirect immunofluorescence method and found a positive ANCA in patients with chronic uveitis with various causes. A cytoplasmic pattern of staining (cANCA) is felt to be more specific for Wegener's granulomatosis than a peripheral pattern (pANCA). Soukasian and colleagues[14] reported that ANCA test results were positive in seven patients with scleritis caused by Wegener's granulomatosis but negative in 54 patients with other ocular inflammatory diseases; this suggests that the test is both sensitive and specific. High specificity of the cANCA for Wegener's granulomatosis in patients with ocular inflammatory disease has been reported by other investigators as well.[15]

### Image analysis

Although newer techniques provide the practitioner with high resolution images, simple radiographic techniques, such as skull x-rays to evaluate patients with suspected congenital toxoplasmosis for calcifications, should not be overlooked. Chest x-rays should be obtained in patients suspected of having sarcoidosis or tuberculosis. A computed tomography (CT) scan or magnetic resonance imaging (MRI) scan of the brain is indicated for patients with possible intraocular lymphoma (see Chapter 29). In contrast, sinus x-rays are frequently ordered as part of the evaluation of patients with uveitis; however, it is not clear that this test is helpful on a routine basis. Patients with a history of sinus disease and uveitis may have an underlying systemic vasculitis such as Wegener's granulomatosis, but in these patients, an ANCA, otoloaryngology consult, and possibly a CT scan of the sinuses may be more appropriate and useful than sinus radiographs.

### Skin testing

Skin testing is often neglected by the practitioner, but these simple tests can give the observer a large amount of information. The purified protein derivative (PPD) and histoplasmin skin tests are easily placed and give important clinical data. The PPD is an important test in the evaluation of the uveitis patient with a history suggesting tuberculosis. In addition, patients should be tested with a PPD before they are placed on immunosuppressive therapy, because if the PPD is positive, these patients will require antituberculous therapy before immunosuppressive therapy is begun. Patients with a history of possible tuberculosis or a positive reaction to a tuberculosis skin test should be tested with a lower strength PPD, such as a 1 test unit dose, instead of the usual 5 test unit dose. If these test results are negative, then the higher test dose can be given. The histoplasmin skin test is useful in evaluating patients with presumed ocular histoplasmosis syndrome; however, the test may activate an old, inactive histoplasmosis lesion and should be avoided in patients with macular lesions.

Skin testing can also be used to document anergy. Patients with sarcoidosis are typically anergic and should have depressed responses to skin testing with control antigens such as tetanus. Systemic corticosteroid administration sometimes reverses anergy in these patients, whereas cyclosporine may prevent type IV hypersensitivity reactions in the skin and yield a negative result to the skin test. In the past, the Kveim test was a commonly performed test for sarcoidosis but was very dependent on the batch of Kveim that was used. Currently, Kveim antigen cannot be obtained, and the test is no longer used. The Behcetin skin test is also infrequently performed. In this test, patients with suspected Behçet's disease are stuck with a sterile needle, and the skin is observed or biopsied for evidence of a Type IV reaction. The hypothesis is that patients with Behçet's disease will display a positive delayed hypersensitivity response to the needle stick (pathergy). Although the test is rarely performed, a history of skin reactions to phlebotomy draws or after intravenous line placements may suggest pathergy and the diagnosis of Behçet's disease.

Allergy testing was at one time a very important component to the evaluation of the uveitis patient. The relevance of atopy or a specific allergy to uveitis is not clear. Hard evidence showing that type I hypersensitivity reactions are a major, underlying force in intraocular inflammatory disease is lacking; only anecdotal information suggests perhaps a secondary role.[16] As a result, we only occasionally obtain allergy testing in our patients.

### Tissue samples

The diagnosis of many forms of uveitis are based on the history and the typical appearance of the ocular disease. Nevertheless, the definitive diagnosis of many cases of uveitis requires histologic confirmation. No oncologist or radiation therapist would agree to treat a patient with presumed intraocular lymphoma without a tissue diagnosis. Similarly, the definitive diagnosis of sarcoidosis also requires histologic confirmation. In many other cases, analysis of ocular fluid or tissue can provide a wealth of information to the clinician. The information is, however, only as good as the ability to evaluate the specimen. It is imperative that the tissue is processed expeditiously by a person experienced in a variety of histologic and immunologic techniques including immunohistochemical staining.

**Box 6-2**
**Analysis of aqueous humor for antibody**

A = Inverse titer of specific IgG in aqueous
B = Total IgG in aqueous
X = Inverse titer of specific IgG in serum
Y = Total IgG in serum
If (A/B)/(X/Y) > 1, then there is local antibody production within the eye, suggesting intraocular infection

EXAMPLE:
Aqueous titer to toxoplasmosis = 1:200; aqueous IgG = 0.1 g/dl
Serum titer to toxoplasmosis = 1:400; serum IgG = 3 g/dl
*Therefore:* A/B = 60, suggesting uveitis is due to toxoplasmosis

The evaluation of intraocular fluid is of great potential value. An area in which the analysis of intraocular fluids has aided the clinician in diagnosis is toxoplasmosis. Problems arise when atypical lesions are noted in a patient with low levels of circulating antitoxoplasma antibody. Desmonts[17] proposed that local production (that is, intraocular) of specific antitoxoplasmosis antibody strongly suggests an active ocular lesion as a result of toxoplasmosis. To demonstrate local production of antibody, the specific antibody in the eye is measured relative to the total amount of globulin in the eye. This led Desmonts to calculate the antibody coefficient (C). The formula for determining this value is:

$$C = \text{Antibody titer}\,\frac{\text{Aqueous humor}}{\text{Serum}} \times \text{Immunoglobulin}\,\frac{\text{Serum}}{\text{Aqueous humor}}$$

Ideally, the antibody coefficient should be 1.0. A coefficient from 2 to 7 is compatible with local production of specific antibody, but a coefficient above 8 is considered highly suggestive of local production. An example of the use of this formula is presented in Box 6-2.

Similar evaluations have been performed to look for local antibody production to virus. Timsit and colleagues[18] detected herpes simplex virus (HSV) antibodies in the aqueous of half of clinically confirmed herpes keratouveitis cases. Kaplan and colleagues[19] found antibodies against either HSV or vesicular stomatitis virus in the aqueous of 4 of 20 patients with idiopathic uveitis. Samples may, however, become contaminated with peripheral serum. Further, local production of specific antibody may be related to a polyclonal B-cell activation totally unrelated to the virus in question. Clearly, these methods require further refinement, and only with continued attempts at such refinement can this technique help in the diagnosis of intraocular inflammatory disease. Although this approach is not generally used in the United States, it is commonly used by many specialists in Europe.[20]

Intraocular inflammation as a result of autoimmune disease may look similar to the inflammation after infection. In patients with a history of postsurgical uveitis, a diagnostic vitrectomy and anterior chamber tap are often warranted. Recently, a number of slow-growing bacteria have been identified as causes of chronic insidious postsurgical uveitis. One of these organisms, *Propionibacterium acnes,* is described in detail in the chapter on postsurgical uveitis (see Chapter 18) and the chapter on masquerade syndromes (see Chapter 29).

Many clinicians routinely biopsy the conjunctiva and lacrimal gland in the search for histologic evidence of sarcoidosis. Most studies, however, report disappointing results with random "blind biopsies."[21] We suggest only biopsing the conjunctiva if a specific lesion is noted and biopsing the lacrimal glands only if they are clinically enlarged or show increased uptake on a gallium scan. We have, however, found that biopsy of skin lesions can be extremely helpful to the clinician. We have made the diagnosis of sarcoidosis in numerous patients on the basis of a noncaseating granuloma found on skin biopsy.

Finally, we have performed chorioretinal biopsy in patients with severe posterior uveitis that had caused severe visual loss in one eye and threatened the other eye despite therapy. This technique is more fully described in the chapter on the role of surgery in the diagnosis and treatment of uveitis (see Chapter 9).

### Ancillary ophthalmic tests

Electrophysiologic testing can help to determine the cause of visual loss in some patients with uveitis, but in general electrophysiologic testing rarely leads to a specific diagnosis. Both the electroretinogram and electrooculogram can be altered in many of the inflammatory disorders of the retina and choroid. Because of the general lack of specificity, the electroretinogram will only tell the observer if significant widespread damage has occurred, and to date we are not aware of changes noted on the electroretinogram or on the electrooculogram that are specific for entities within the broad category of posterior uveitis. Feurst and colleagues[22] reported that the electroretinograms of patients with birdshot retinochoroidopathy show a loss of blue cone responses in the dark adapted state (see Chapter 24). We have noted a loss of blue cone responses not only in birdshot retinochoroidopathy but also in other posterior uveitis entities. This may reflect a general effect of the immune response on the retina's electrophysiologic responsiveness.

Early in our therapeutic studies, we wanted to know whether we could predict who among the uveitis patients might improve with immunosuppressive therapy. We had noted that there was a discrepancy between the visual acuity obtained with the standard Snellen and later Early Treatment Diabetic Retinopathy Study (ETDRS) eye chart and the laser interferometer. The visual acuity obtained with the laser interferometer is often better than that measured with eye charts. We hypothesized that these differences might be caused by potentially reversible macular changes as a result of the ongoing inflammatory disease. In a prospective study of 26 patients treated with cyclosporine for endogenous intermediate and posterior uveitis, we noted improvement in 86% of patients in whom the laser interferometer predicted a three line or better improvement in vision as compared with the standard measurement of visual acuity (Fig. 6-2). In contrast, only 52% of the patients in whom the laser interferometry showed less than a three line improvement later improved with cyclosporine therapy. There was a moderate correlation between the predicted number of lines of improvement with the laser interferometer and the number of lines actually improved with therapy ($R = 0.59$, $p < 0.001$). We therefore perform a laser interferometry visual acuity determination on all uveitis patients with poor vision. If the laser interferometry acuity is better than the visual acuity measured on an ETDRS chart, we expect to see an improvement in visual acuity

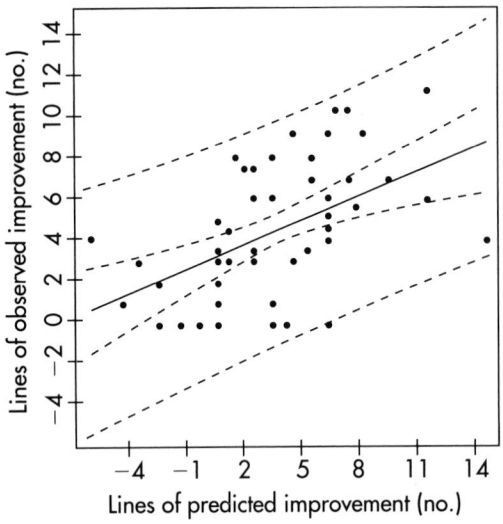


**Fig. 6-2.** Linear regression plot of number of lines of predicted improvement using laser interferometer (slope = 0.40, intercept = 2.96) and observed improvement after cyclosporine therapy ($R$ = 0.53). Outer dotted lines represent 95% confidence limits. (From Palestine AG, Alter GJ, Chan CC et al: Laser interferometry and visual prognosis in uveitis, *Ophthalmology* 92:1567-1569, 1985.)

with therapy even in patients with cystoid macular edema.

**Fluorescein angiography.** Fluorescein angiography is an invaluable aid in evaluating the numerous changes in uveitic eyes. The alterations seen are variable and frequently require the observer to evaluate the angiogram for some time before a satisfactory interpretation is made. Some of the more frequently noted ocular changes that are highlighted with fluorescein angiography are listed in Box 6-3. Corresponding stereo photographs may be helpful in establishing the level at which the pathology in the eye is occurring.

Macular edema is one of the major causes of decreased vision in many types of intraocular inflammatory disease. The cause for the decreased vision is not absolutely known. We assume, logically, that it is due to a swelling of the retinal layers, which disrupts the intimate association of the retinal elements that results in crisp vision or distorts the alignment of the photoreceptors. However, we certainly know that patients with angiographic evidence of mild or moderate macular edema can have good visual acuity. Further, we have been most struck that patients can have an improvement of vision after therapeutic intervention, yet the fluorescein angiogram shows no change in the leakage of fluorescein. Because late leakage seen on angiography is not strongly correlated with a drop in vision, we explored other possible alterations that might be evaluated with fluorescein angiography. We hypothesized that retinal thickening and not the leakage of fluorescein into the retina was one of the major causes of the decrease in vision. We measured the amount of retinal thickening with the use of standard angiographic photos taken early in the angiogram (Fig. 6-3).[23] We noted a strong correlation between retinal thickening and the visual acuity of these eyes (Figs. 6-4 and 6-5). The amount of leakage of dye in the late phase of the angiogram did not, however, correlate well with visual acuity.

**Box 6-3**
**Major fluorescein angiographic findings in uveitis**

- Cystoid macular edema
- Subretinal neovascular membranes
- Disc leakage
- Late staining of retinal vessels
- Neovascularization of retinal vessels
- Retinal vascular capillary dropout and reorganization
- Retinal pigment epithelium perturbations

In reading the angiogram, it is important to look at the early frames to best visualize the microvasculature surrounding the fovea. To best enhance the stereo effect, we have found it useful to use a "map reader." If one wishes to compare sequential fluorescein angiograms, the photos must taken with the Allan separator always set at the same value. Differences in the separator settings can induce an artificial increase or decrease in the height of lesions noted when viewing the photos with the stereo viewer.

Many inflammatory eye diseases are thought to be associated with abnormalities in the choroidal blood flow. Unfortunately, the excitation and fluorescence of fluorescein dye are absorbed and scattered by the retinal pigment. In addition, fluorescein dye rapidly leaks from the fenestrated vessels of the choriocapillaris leading to a diffuse background choroidal fluorescence. Both of these factors combine to obscure a detailed analysis of the choroidal blood flow with fluorescein angiography.

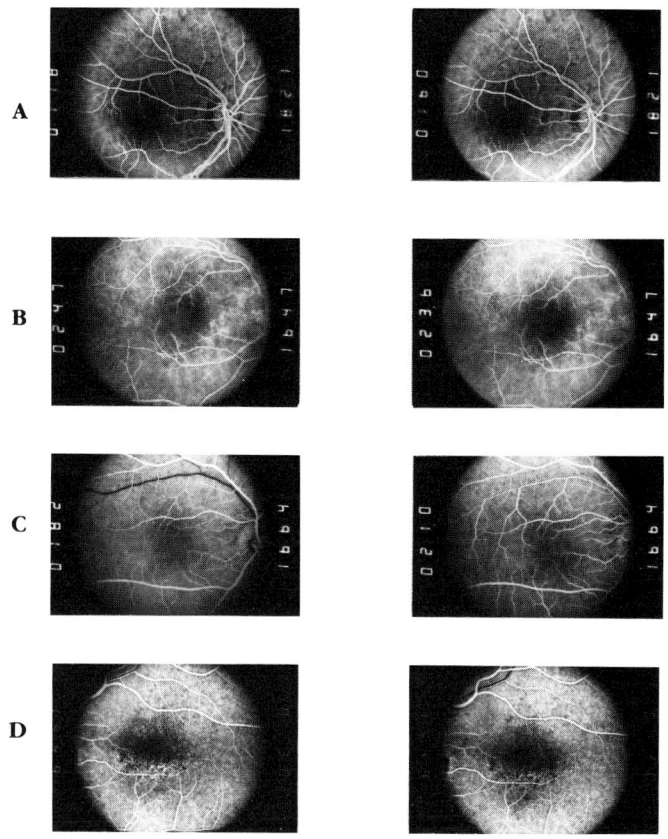


**Fig. 6-3.** Standard stereoscopic fluorescein angiographic photographs showing varying degrees of macular thickening. **A,** "Normal." **B-D,** In order of increasing macular thickening. Strong light source should be placed under photographs, and macular thickening can be best evaluated using "map reader" (Air Photo Supply, model PS-2 stereo viewer), which will yield maximum stereopsis. (From Nussenblatt RB, Kaufman SC, Palestine AG et al: Macular thickening and visual acuity, *Ophthalmology* 94:1134-1139, 1987.)

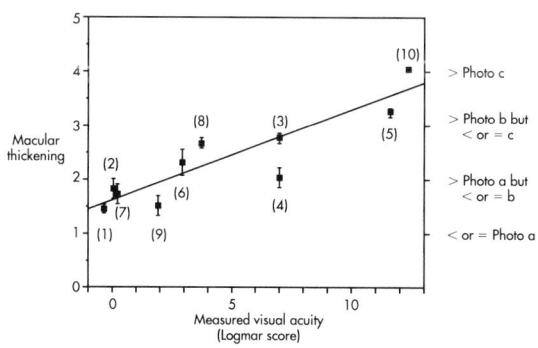


**Fig. 6-4.** Mean (± 1 standard error) of 13 gradings of macular thickening for eyes with cystoid macular edema (11 because of uveitis, 2 because of diabetes). Simple linear regression showed significant relationship between mean thickening and actual visual acuity. (From Nussenblatt RB, Kaufman SC, Palestine AG et al: Macular thickening and visual acuity, *Ophthalmology* 94:1134-1139, 1987.)

**Indocyanine green.** Indocyanine green (ICG) is a water-soluble tricarbocyanine dye that was first used to measure cardiac output.[24] Unlike fluorescein, ICG is almost completely bound to plasma proteins and does not leak from normal retinal or choroidal vessels. Importantly, the pigment of the retinal pigment epithelium and neurosensory retina does not significantly block the choroidal fluorescence when ICG dye is illuminated with infrared light. ICG fluorescence is also more easily detected through hemorrhage. As a result, ICG angiography, which is recorded on either infrared photography or video angiography, is a useful tool for demonstrating abnormalities of choroidal blood flow including choroidal neovascular membranes.[25–28]

ICG angiography has now been used to study patients with a number of uveitic conditions. In patients with serpiginous choroiditis, ICG angiography has demonstrated blockage of cho-

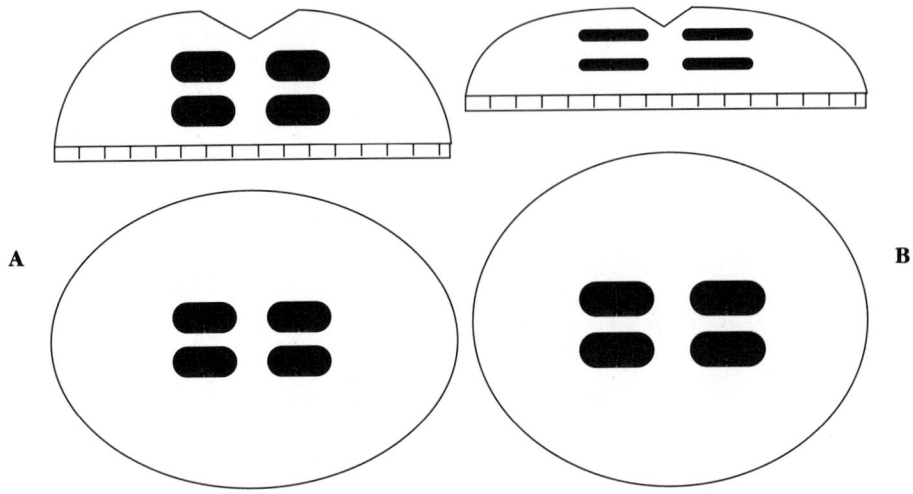


**Fig. 6-5.** Proposed scheme as to why fluorescein leakage may appear to be same but macular thickening may have decreased, resulting in improvement in visual acuity. **A,** During acute episode of uveitis, cystic spaces are filled with fluid, and macula is thickened. **B,** With therapy, there is decrease in macular thickening, but amount of leakage will appear to be same if angiogram is reviewed in standard fashion. (From Nussenblatt RB, Kaufman SC, Palestine AG et al: Macular thickening and visual acuity, *Ophthalmology* 94:1134-1139, 1987.)

roidal fluorescence in active areas of lesions with return of the normal choroidal fluorescence as the inflammation subsided.[29] In addition, the chorioretinal lesions associated with birdshot choroiditis are often difficult to observe clinically or to document with fluorescein angiography. However, Krupsky and colleagues[30] showed that ICG angiography was superior to fluorescein angiography in demonstrating these lesions that appeared as hypofluorescent areas suggesting loss of the choriocapillaris. A number of researchers are using ICG angiography to study patients with both active and quiescent chorioretinal lesions in patients with uveitis, and it is hoped this technique will provide new insight into the pathophysiology of the number of uveitic disorders.

### Neurologic tests

The eye is a part of the brain, and many forms of uveitis have associated central nervous system involvement. As the eye can be a window to the brain and provide insight into neurologic disease, evaluation of the brain and cerebrospinal fluid can give important clues to the underlying cause of ocular inflammatory disease. For example, lumbar puncture is useful in evaluating patients with possible Vogt-Koyanagi-Harada syndrome or intraocular lymphoma.

## NEW DIAGNOSTIC TESTS

Since its initial description by Saiki and colleagues,[31] the polymerase chain reaction (PCR) has become one of the most commonly used techniques in biomedical research. PCR provides a simple way to amplify a specific fragment of DNA, and this technique has proved useful for the study of genetic diseases and the detection of infectious agents. Pertinent to the field of uveitis, PCR has also been used to detect viruses, bacteria, and parasites in the eye.

To start the PCR four components are combined: (1) target DNA, (2) primers (short strands of DNA that tag the section of target DNA to be copied, (3) polymerase (the enzyme that catalyzes gene replication), and (4) nucleotides. PCR is based on the consecutive repetition of three reactions. First, the target DNA is denatured by heating the test tube to 95°C. Second, primers are annealed to a targeted strip of DNA as the temperature of the test tube is decreased. Finally, polymerase then triggers the synthesis of a new DNA molecule between the primers in the third step of the PCR. These three steps of the reaction are then repeated consecutively during 30 to 40 cycles and controlled by the raising and lowering of the temperature of the test tube.

At the end of the PCR, the amount of target DNA is increased by one million–to one billion–

fold. However, the extreme sensitivity of the technique requires very strict laboratory procedures to prevent the carry-over of positive substrate between samples that could lead to false-positive results. The PCR can be used to detect DNA fragments in many types of specimens including cells, body fluids, and paraffin-embedded sections. The PCR is currently being used to identify the DNA of infectious agents in the eye, because as we have seen, the interpretation of serologic tests is often misleading. Before PCR can be carried out, the sequence of the target DNA (specific for the organisms in question) must be known, and the appropriate primers then synthesized. Viral DNA has been identified by PCR in eyes with a number of disorders including acute retinal necrosis.[32] We currently use PCR in our laboratory to diagnose ocular toxoplasmosis.[33,34]

Presently, PCR is still a research tool. Because of its exquisite sensitivity, the chances of false-positive results are significant. In addition, a small piece of DNA found in the eye of a patient may represent a remnant from an infection that occurred long ago and may be totally unrelated to the patient's current illness. Nevertheless, the use of PCR will continue to proliferate in the ophthalmic literature and will probably be available clinically in the near future to detect infectious agents in ocular specimens.

### Rapid tests for herpes simplex and herpes zoster

Currently, biopsy specimens, including cells obtained from anterior chamber taps, are tested for herpes virus with the use of a direct fluorescent antibody test after 48 hours and 5 days of growth. Enzyme-linked immunosorbent assay tests, which gives almost immediate diagnostic information, are being developed and may be available clinically in the next year or two. However, problems with sensitivity and specificity may arise and need to be thoroughly investigated before these tests are routinely used in clinical practice.

### Laser cell/flare meter

Although standardized schemes for assessing anterior chamber cells and flare have been published in the literature, grading differs tremendously between clinicians and even varies by the same grader over time. A laser device has been developed to assess flare in the anterior chamber of the eye and should standardize the grading of anterior chamber inflammation; this is extremely useful in determining the response to therapy.[35,36] Furthermore, it is difficult to detect the induced flare caused by small amounts of protein in the aqueous humor resulting from early breakdown of the blood-aqueous barrier. After cataract surgery, for example, it would be nice to predict which eyes were at risk to develop uveitis and cystoid macular edema. The laser cell/flare meter is more sensitive than the eye in detecting flare and may be useful in predicting which eyes are at risk for developing worsening inflammatory disease and might be used to identify eyes requiring more aggressive antiinflammatory therapy.

### REFERENCES


1. Griner PF, Mayewski RJ, Mushlin Al et al: Selection and interpretation of diagnostic tests and procedures: principles and applications, *Ann Intern Med* 94:553-600, 1981.
2. Rembold CM, Watson D: Posttest probability calculation by weights: a simple form of Bayes' theorem, *Ann Intern Med* 108:115-120, 1988.
3. Rosenbaum JT, Wernick R: The utility of routine screening of patients with uveitis for systemic lupus erythematosus or tuberculosis, *Arch Ophthalmol* 108: 1291-1293, 1990.
4. Warner HR, Toronto AF, Veasey LG et al: A mathematical approach to medical diagnosis: application to congential heart disease, *JAMA* 177:177-183, 1961.
5. Warner HR, Toronto AF, Veasy LG: Experience with Bayes' theorem for computer diagnosis of congenital heart disease, *Ann N Y Acad Sci* 115:558-567, 1964.
6. Fagan TJ: Nomogram for Bayes' theorem. *N Engl J Med* 293:257, 1975.
7. Gorry GA, Barnett GO: Sequential diagnosis by computer, *JAMA* 205:849-854, 1968.
8. Passo MS, Rosenbaum JT: Ocular syphilis in patients with human immunodeficiency virus infection, *Am J Ophthalmol* 106:1-6, 1988.
9. Tramont EC: Syphilis in the AIDS era, *N Engl J Med* 316:1600-1601, 1987.
10. Fauci AS, Haynes BF, Katz P et al.: Wegener's granulomatosis: prospective clinical and therapeutic experience with 85 patients for 21 years, *Ann Intern Med* 98:76-85, 1983.
11. Nolle B, Specks U, Ludemann J et al.: Anticytoplasmic autoantibodies: their immunodiagnostic value in Wegener's granulomatosis, 111:28-40, 1989.
12. Cohen-Tervaert MD, van der Woude FJ, Fauci AS et al: Association between active Wegener's granulomatosis and anticytoplasmic antibodies, *Arch Intern Med* 149:2461-2465, 1989.
13. Young DW: The antineutrophil antibody in uveitis, *Br J Ophthalmol* 75:208-211, 1991.
14. Soukasian SH, Foster CS, Niles JL et al: Diagnostic value of anti-neutrophil cytoplasmic antibodies in scleritis associated with Wegener's granulomatosis, *Ophthalmology* 99:125-132, 1992.

15. Nolle B, Coners H, Guncker G: ANCA in ocular inflammatory disorders, *Adv Exp Med Biol* 336:305-307, 1993.
16. Bloch-Michel E, Timsit JC: Uveitis with allergy to candidin, *Ophthalmologica* 191:102-106, 1985.
17. Desmonts G: Definitive serological diagnosis to ocular toxoplasmosis, *Arch Ophthalmol* 76:839-853, 1966.
18. Timsit JC, Fortier B, Pontet F et al.: Value of the immunoenzyme method (ELISA) in determining serum and aqueous humor antiherpes immunoglobulin levels (apropos of 155 cases), *J Fr Ophtalmol* 5:669-674, 1982.
19. Kaplan HJ, Lee FK, Waldrep JC et al: Viral antibodies in the aqueous humor in idiopathic uveitis. In Saari KM, editor, *Uveitis Update,* Excerpta Medica, 1984:437-442.
20. Kijlstra A, Breebaart AC, Baarsma GS et al: Aqueous chamber taps in toxoplasmic chorioretinitis, *Doc Ophthalmol* 64:53-58, 1986.
21. Weinreb RN, Tessler H: Laboratory diagnosis of ophthalmic sarcoidosis, *Surv Ophthalmol* 28:653-664, 1984.
22. Feurst DJ, Tessler HH, Fishman GA et al: Birdshot retinochoroidopathy, *Arch Ophthalmol* 102:214-219, 1984.
23. Nussenblatt RB, Kaufman SC, Palestine AG et al.: Macular thickening and visual acuity, *Ophthalmology* 94:1134-1139, 1987.
24. Fox IJ, Wood EH: Indocyanine green: physical and physiologic properties, *Proc Mayo Clin* 35:732-744, 1960.
25. Kogure K, David NJ, Yamanouchi U et al: Infrared absorption angiography of the fundus circulation, *Arch Ophthalmol* 83:209-214, 1970.
26. Flower RW, Hocheimer BF: A clinical technique and apparatus for simultaneous angiography of the separate retinal and choroidal circulations, *Invest Ophthalmol* 12:248-261, 1973.
27. Flower RW, Hochheimer BF: Indocyanine green dye fluorescence and infrared absorption choroidal angiography performed simultaneously with fluorescein angiography, *Johns Hopkins Med J* 138:33-42, 1976.
28. Destro M, Puliafito CA: Indocyanine green videoangiography of choroidal neovascularizations, *Ophthalmology* 96:846-853, 1989.
29. Bischoff P: Bedeutung der infrarotangiographie für die differentialdiagnostik der aderhauttumoren, *Klin Mbl Augenheilk* 186:187-193, 1985.
30. Krupsky S, Friedman E, Foster CS et al: Indocyanine green angiography in choroidal diseases, *Invest Ophthalmol Vis Sci* 33(Suppl):723, 1992.
31. Saiki RK, Gelfand DH, Stoffel S et al.: Primer-directed enzymatic amplification of DNA with a thermostable DNA polymerase, *Science* 239:487-491, 1988.
32. Forster DJ, Dugel PU, Frangieh GT et al: Rapidly progressive outer retinal necrosis in the acquired immunodeficiency syndrome, *Am J Ophthalmol* 110: 341-348, 1990.
33. Chan CC, Palestine AG, Li Q, Nussenblatt RB: Diagnosis of ocular toxoplasmosis by the use of immunocytology and the polymerase chain reaction, *Am J Ophthalmol* 117:803-805, 1994.
34. Brezin AP, Egwuagu CE, Burnier M Jr et al: Identification of *Toxoplasma gondii* in paraffin-embedded sections by the polymerase chain reaction, *Am J Ophthalmol* 110:599-604, 1990.
35. Shah SM, Spalton DJ, Taylor JC: Correlations between laser flare measurements and anterior chamber protein concentrations, *Invest Ophthalmol Vis Sci* 33:2878-2884, 1992.
36. Guex-Crosier Y, Pittet N, Herbort CP: Evaluation of laser flare-cell photometry in the appraisal and management of intraocular inflammation in uveitis, *Ophthalmology* 101:728-735, 1994.

# CHAPTER 7

# Evaluation of the Uveitis Literature

The practice of medicine is based on applying what we have learned from our teachers during medical school, residency training, and fellowship in addition to the knowledge gained by reading books and articles. It is our hope, for example, that the book you are reading will assist you in the care of patients with uveitis. However, all medical literature, including our book, must be read critically. Much of the information that appears to be irrefutable scientific dogma, is actually based on inconclusive data derived from a handful of patients. Because the recommendations are in print and stated by seemingly reputable authorities, they are often followed blindly. It is frequently useful to scrutinize the original references on which various therapeutic approaches are based; what you find may surprise you.

When reading the medical literature it is important to determine the experimental methods used in the study. Sometimes this information can be discerned from the title of the article; at other times the methods section must be read. Occasionally the study method is not stated in the paper. If this is the case, the article is probably not worth reading. Many of the clinical studies in the literature are retrospective, meaning that the data were collected from previous patient visits. Retrospective studies can provide valuable information, but they are usually limited by the quality and thoroughness of the patient records. Patient's symptoms and clinical findings are often not recorded although present. For example, when there is no comment in a patient's record about vitreous haze, does this mean that vitreous haze was absent or that it may have been present but not recorded in the note? Fortunately, most ophthalmic notes contain a core of data including visual acuity, intraocular pressure, anterior segment examination, and retinal examination. Nevertheless, prospective studies, when specific data are collected during patient visits, are less prone to these errors.

There are four basic clinical studies: case series, case-control studies, cohort studies, and randomized clinical trials.[1] The case report or case series is probably the weakest method of deriving clinical data. Case series are usually retrospective reviews that list the clinical findings of patients with a specific disease. The case series can illustrate the variety of clinical manifestations of diseases and provide information about diagnosis, management, and prognosis. However, in addition to the problem of missing data from patient records, the reader should be aware of other pitfalls that may jeopardize the value of the report. First, the disease or condition may not be adequately defined. If patients with sympathetic ophthalmia are inadvertently included in a series of patients with Vogt-Koyanagi-Harada syndrome, the findings and conclusions may be altered. Second, the patient population reported may be dissimilar from the clinician's practice. Frequently uveitis specialists see more severe cases because these are the patients referred to their practice. Therefore a uveitis specialist may report that the visual prognosis for a given disease, such as sarcoidosis, is poor. If this is based on a series of patients composed of referrals with end-stage disease, the report may be biased. Be especially wary of retrospective reviews that make global dogmatic statements on the basis of a few patients. Finally, case series have no control group for comparison. If a report states that depression was found in 35% of patients with uveitis, it is not clear that this represents a causal relationship. Visual loss and not uveitis may be the cause of depression. It would be important to know how many patients with other ocular diseases that cause visual loss (a control group) have depression. For example, the same percentage of patients with visual loss from retinal degenerations may also be depressed.

The case-control study is a second type of clinical study in which the investigator compares a group of patients with a given condition to a control group without the condition. The records of both groups are then compared to see whether certain factors were more likely to occur in one group than in the other. The classic example of a case-control study would examine patients with lung cancer and a group without the disease and then determine their smoking history. It is then possible to determine an odds ratio that determines the relative risk for a given condition like lung cancer given a specific factor like smoking. Case-control studies, although more powerful than the case series, are prone to bias. Many case-control studies rely on a retrospective review of patients' records to determine the differences in a number of clinical parameters between cases and controls. Additional bias arises from the method of choosing the cases and controls. Despite the potential bias, case-control studies are becoming more common in the literature because they are easy to carry out, especially with the computerization of clinical records. In addition, they are often the only feasible method available to study rare disorders.

A cohort study identifies two groups or cohorts of patients; for example, one cohort that receives a certain treatment and one cohort that does not receive the treatment. The groups are then followed prospectively for the development of a specific outcome. However, because the treatments are not assigned randomly, it is possible that the two groups differ in important parameters. For example, if you followed two groups of patients with glaucoma, one treated with medications and one treated surgically, you may falsely conclude that surgical therapy is inferior for treating glaucoma because these patients had a worse visual outcome. However, it may be that the patients treated medically had more mild cases of disease and better initial visual acuity than patients who received surgical therapy.

The randomized clinical trial provides the most powerful evidence about the value of a new therapy or diagnostic approach. Because patients enrolled into the study are randomly assigned into a specific group, if the numbers of patients in the study are large enough the groups are usually equivalent clinically. From an ethical standpoint, randomized clinical trials should compare treatments when the investigator in unsure which therapy is better. There are a number of factors that should be included in a well-designed and well-conducted randomized trial.[2] The investigators should have performed previous studies in the area and include people with appropriate training in the conduct and analysis of the study. The primary outcome of the study should be clearly stated, even if multiple outcomes are examined. The procedure for enrolling patients into the trial should be clearly delineated and include the inclusion and exclusion criteria. In addition, the therapy should be clearly stated, and the control group should be clinically appropriate. For example, if one were designing a trial to study the benefits of phacoemulsification as a technique for cataract surgery, it would be clinically inappropriate to compare this technique to intracapsular cataract extraction because extracapsular cataract surgery is the more frequently performed procedure.

It is extremely important that the paper include a discussion of sample size calculation. Sample size is based not only on the event rate expected in the two groups, but also on the level of protection against type I and type II error. A type I error occurs when the study falsely concludes that the therapies tested are different when in fact they are the same. A type II error occurs when the study falsely concludes that there is no difference between the therapies when in fact a difference exists. Many randomized clinical trials in the literature are underpowered. What this means is that the potential for a type II error is high, sometimes 30% or higher. In these studies a conclusion that there was no statistically significant difference between the two groups is meaningless. There could in fact be a big difference between the two groups, but not enough patients were tested to show the difference. An example of an underpowered study is as follows. If we wanted to test the hypothesis that the two sides of a quarter are different, we could flip the coin a number of times and record the results. If you flipped the coin three times (similar to enrolling three patients) and got heads each time, you might falsely conclude that the two sides were the same. The chance that you would reach this wrong conclusion would, however, diminish as you increased the number of times you flipped the coin! You would then have more power to show a difference between the two sides of the coin and thus have more protection against a type II error. Remember studies can never definitively prove that two treatments are the same.

The data in randomized trials should be appropriately collected, and patients should have a reasonably high level of adherence to protocol procedures with little missed data or loss to follow-up. Observers should be masked to the treatments that patients receive. Statistical methods should be appropriate for the data, and the tables and figures easily read. Finally, it is important that the authors' conclusions are supported by the data and do not exceed the evidence.

## CLINICAL TRIALS IN UVEITIS

Unfortunately, most of the uveitis literature is comprised of case series and case reports. As stated above, these studies can provide useful information but are highly prone to bias and lack a control population to compare the findings. Despite their superior strength as a clinical design, few case-control studies or cohort studies of uveitis patients have been conducted. Even rarer are randomized controlled clinical trials of therapies for patients with uveitis. Part of the explanation for the small number of randomized trials of uveitis patients stems from difficulties that arise when studying patients with this disorder. Many forms of uveitis are rare; therefore, it is difficult to recruit enough patients to fulfill the sample size requirements. It is important that the observers are masked to the therapy, which may be difficult if surgical treatment is compared with medications. Patients with uveitis often have underlying systemic diseases making it difficult for patients to follow a predetermined therapeutic protocol because their other diseases often require systemic therapy.

Nevertheless, randomized clinical trials can be conducted in patients with uveitis. In these trials it is important to collect data in a standardized fashion. We record visual acuity according to a standard protocol with the use of ETDRS charts.[3] Inflammatory activity is similarly recorded with standardized methods, such as grading scales for vitreous haze or laser interferometry for anterior chamber haze.[4]

The National Eye Institute conducted a recent randomized, double-masked study of cyclosporine compared with prednisolone for the treatment of endogenous uveitis.[5] In this trial, 28 patients were treated with cyclosporine and 28 patients with prednisolone. Although no statistically significant difference was found between the primary outcomes of visual acuity or vitreous haze of patients in the two groups, because of the small numbers it would be wrong to conclude that the two therapies were the same. The authors were careful not to state that the study proved that the two therapies were equivalent and instead suggested that because similar outcomes were achieved, cyclosporine could be considered as an alternative to corticosteroid therapy.

## REFERENCES

1. Sackett DL, Haynes RB, Tugwell P: *Clinical epidemiology: a basic science for clinical medicine,* Boston, 1985:224-229, Little, Brown.
2. Meinert CL, Tonascia S: Clinical trials design, conduct, and analysis, New York, 1986:274-275, Oxford University Press.
3. Ferris FL III, Kassoff A, Bresnick GH et al: New visual acuity charts for clinical research, *Am J Ophthalmol* 94:91-96, 1982.
4. Nussenblatt RB, Palestine AG, Chan CC et al: Standardization of vitreal inflammatory activity in intermediate and posterior uveitis, *Ophthalmology* 92:467-471, 1985.
5. Nussenblatt RB, Palestine AG, Chan CC et al: Randomized, double-masked study of cyclosporine compared to prednisolone in the treatment of endogenous uveitis, *Am J Ophthalmol* 112:138-146, 1991.

# PART 3

# Medical Therapy and Surgical Intervention

# CHAPTER 8

# Philosophy, Goals, and Approaches to Medical Therapy

This chapter represents in some ways the very heart of the treating physician's role. How do you choose the best therapeutic agent for your patient? This decision is often tension provoking because patients requiring the types of therapy under discussion usually have bilateral sight-threatening disease, are afraid, and are depending on the physician to choose a therapeutic intervention that will quickly restore their vision. Oftentimes the task is fraught with many difficulties, which must be explained to the patient. It is truly a partnership. The more the patient knows about the physician's goals and concerns, the more they can help. It is fair to say that enormous gains have occurred in recent years in our understanding how to use many of the drugs under discussion. Further, pharmacology is an area that is burgeoning with real hope for the future[1]; indeed, other yet-untapped sources may also bring new immunosuppressive drugs to the growing armamentarium.[2] For the moment, there may not be any one ideal drug, but the treating physician's choices provide some latitude. However, each of these agents is a powerful medication that must be evaluated with care and respect.

## GOALS AND PHILOSOPHY

In the treatment of uveitis the decision to intervene with any therapeutic agent should be based on both a thorough clinical evaluation and philosophic guidelines. In general, the approach to therapy should take into account at least the following considerations.

### Pain, photophobia, and discomfort

Symptom relief is an important goal for several reasons. The first and foremost is of course the ethical imperative of the physician. However, practical considerations should not be overlooked. Pain relief helps in the establishment of a good patient-physician relationship, which is of primary importance in what is frequently a long therapeutic course with ups and downs. A second practical reason is that once relief is obtained the patient is able to cooperate more readily. The ability to examine the patient's ocular condition in greater detail and to obtain more reliable testing results, particularly visual acuity, is of immeasurable help to the physician.

### Degree and location of inflammatory disease

The type and frequency of administration of any therapeutic choice depend on the physician's evaluation of how "serious" the inflammatory disease is and what ocular structures are being affected. For instance, if the sequela of an intraocular inflammation is limited only to posterior synechiae, then the use of topical mydiratics and corticosteroids may be a reasonable approach to therapy. However, disease that is more posteriorly located would need to be approached by means of quite different strategies. If alternative therapies are available, the physician needs to decide which one to start initially. In addition, if vital structures, such as the macula, are involved, more aggressive immunosuppressive therapy may need to be employed, even though the potential for side effects may be greater.

### Evaluation of visual acuity and prospect of reversibility

Alteration in the patient's visual acuity is, in most cases of inflammatory disease involving the intermediate and posterior portion of the globe, the reason for a therapeutic intervention. It is, as well, the major reason that the patient consults the physician—in the hope that therapy will positively affect the condition. It is therefore imperative that the physician attempt to define as clearly as possible why the vision has decreased. On this decision will hinge the therapeutic approach. Has the vision decreased because of recently developed macular edema or because the patient's cataract progressed as a result of recurrent bouts of anterior uveitis? Or have both occurred? Does the patient need a cataract extraction only? Is this surgery needed to better follow the effects of long-term immunosuppressive therapy? The physician must constantly question his or her decisions, seeking to confirm the original hypothesis, since in as much as these patients frequently have multifactorial reasons for vision changes. The use of various tests in the clinic can help in this evaluation (see Chapter 6), but the ultimate decision still rests on the treating physician.

Before embarking on any therapy that has a significant risk for the patient, the physician must weigh this inherent risk with any benefit. It is therefore necessary to decide if any or all of the visual alteration is due to irreversible changes. Is there a macular hole so that the vision may never be better than 20/200, or should surgery be considered? Have subretinal neovascularization and resultant scarring left little hope for good vision in spite of a possible surgical procedure? It is wrong to begin therapy if no reasonable hope for visual improvement exists. In addition, when does one commence therapy? Although the answer is highly variable, it is always based on the physician's belief that the therapeutic intervention's side effects are outweighed by the potential good. It is the physician's duty to desist from inappropriate therapy as much as it is to institute beneficial treatment. Pressures on the physician for action are generally present that make him or her more readily accepting of therapeutic intervention. Why not try? Many times this is acceptable, but patients need to know if they are facing unfavorable odds, which makes their input in deciding if treatment should be given even more important.

### Follow-up procedures and standardization of observations

It is imperative that a reasonable time be allotted to evaluate whether a specific therapy is effective. We have found that up to 3 months is a reasonable period in which to evaluate whether an acute problem will improve. One should remember that ocular changes due to uveitis may resolve slowly, and the observer must use sometimes-subtle changes in the ocular examination to determine whether to continue therapy. The patient should adhere to a regular follow-up schedule and should know whom to contact if an emergency arises. At the start of systemic immunosuppressive therapy, patients should be examined at least weekly. These initial weekly examinations can later be replaced by visits every 2 weeks, with the patient eventually returning monthly for the initial half year. The physician needs to preset the definition of a therapeutic "success" and adhere to these criteria. Just as it is unwise to stop or alter therapy too soon, it is not reasonable to continue therapy if the minimal criteria for success are not met. These criteria may include an increase of vision, a decrease in the amount of vitreous haze, a decrease in the number of cells in the anterior chamber, or a decrease in the photophobia the patient is having.

The criteria that determine successful treatment presuppose that tests are performed in a standard manner and that test results reflect a change in the ocular status rather than the fact that a different person performed the test. Standardization of observations is critical to the successful evaluation of these patients' condition. We have taken great pains to standardize our visual acuity assessment and the evaluation of ocular inflammation.

### One eye or two

We generally avoid the use of systemic drugs in patients who have unilateral chronic uveitis and no underlying systemic disease. In our experience it is the rare case indeed in which unilateral disease is justification for long-term therapy. In the case of the patient with sight remaining in only one eye, a value judgment needs to be made concerning whether local therapy should be used before systemic therapy is employed.

### General health and age of patient

The very basic considerations of patient health and age must play a role in deciding what sort of therapy to utilize. We thoroughly evaluate all patients and examine therapeutic alternatives before starting systemic therapy, especially in children. The secondary effects of systemic immunosuppressive agents, such as steroids, can have major and lifelong effects on a growing child. A diagnosis of diabetes may be a relative contraindication for systemic corticosteroid therapy, whereas uncontrolled hypertension or renal disease may make cyclosporine a poor therapeutic choice. The physician must be always aware that most of these therapies have significant systemic and local effects.

### Patient's reliability, preferences, and understanding

The patient has come for expert advice concerning what frequently is a sight-threatening disorder that in many cases is irreversible. Time should be spent with the patient, who deserves an explanation of ocular (and systemic) findings, the seriousness of these findings, what type of therapy is warranted, and what the possible positive effects and adverse effects may be. We have found that the fully informed patient provides invaluable aid to the treating physician. Obtaining informed written consent may be a requirement under certain circumstances, such as with experimental therapies. Patients with uveitis usually require long-term care, and early on, the more the patient understands medical concerns, uncertainties, and possible therapeutic alternatives, the easier is the treating physician's task.

## NONSURGICAL THERAPEUTIC OPTIONS

### Corticosteroids

The corticosteroid family of medications has been the mainstay of therapy for ocular inflammatory disease since its introduction by Gordon in the early 1950s.[3] Its use in ophthalmology began soon after its introduction into the medical armamentarium.[4] The synthetic compounds usually used by the physician are variations of the compounds normally found in the body, and they profoundly affect many aspects of the organism's physiology. The synthetic preparations available to the physician were developed because of their particularly effective mediation of one aspect of these hormones' effects: immunosuppression. The treating physician should be totally at ease with the various therapeutic strategies available.

MODE OF ACTION. In humans, corticosteroids are not considered to be cytotoxic agents. Human immune cells are not susceptible to lysis by corticosteroid administration, even at higher dosages usually employed, unlike some of the agents to be covered in this chapter. Mice, rats, and rabbits are considered to be corticosteroid-sensitive animals, with their lymphocytes showing a marked tendency toward lysis after the administration of corticosteroids. Therefore extrapolation from animal experiments must take place only after careful evaluation.

The mechanism of entry into the cell by steroids has been evaluated by means of several systems. The underlying point for all the steroid hormones is the need for cellular receptors (Fig. 8-1). The steroid is met at the cell surface by the appropriate receptor and then complexes with it in the cytoplasm of the cell. This complex then migrates to the nucleus, where it exerts its effect on DNA transcription, leading to changes in RNA production. These RNA alterations result in changes in protein production and cell function. In steroid-sensitive animals, such as the rat, those cells with steroid receptors will be lysed. However, in humans, this is not the case, and in vivo and in vitro testing is therefore needed to fully evaluate the effect of hormone on the system in question.

The effects of steroids on the immune system are both local and systemic. Essentially all cellular components are affected. On the systemic level, a profound change is seen particularly with neutrophils and lymphocytes (Figs. 8-2 and 8-3). For lymphocytes, Clamen[5] and Fauci[6] have shown that a large number of the lymphocytes in the intravascular space continuously recirculate with the extravascular lymphocyte pool in such organs as the bone marrow, spleen, and lymph nodes. The addition of steroids induces a change in the recirculation pattern, with a large number of T cells, particularly the helper T subset, sequestered out of the intravascular circulation. This phenomenon results in a break in the

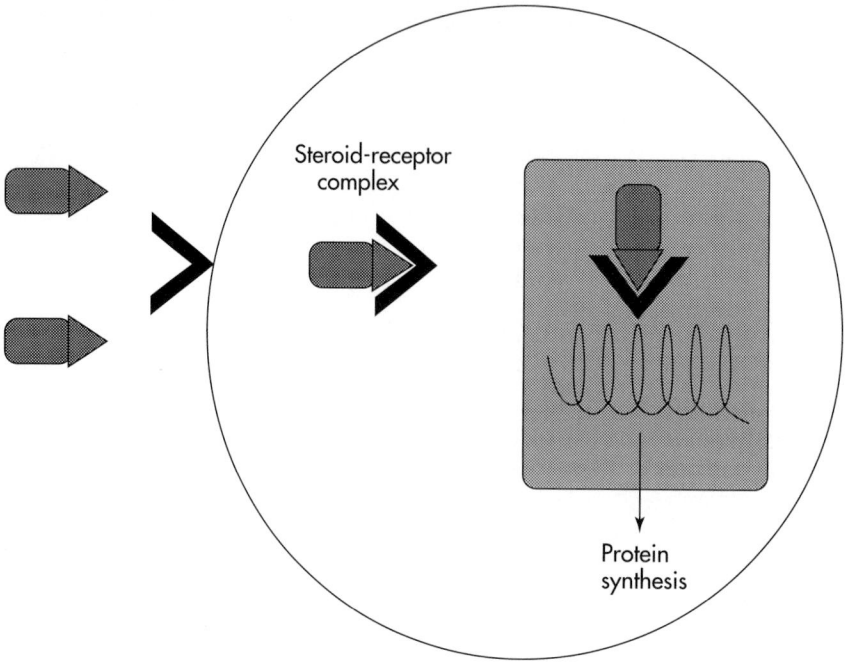


**Fig. 8-1.** Scheme showing entry of steroid molecule into cell via receptor.

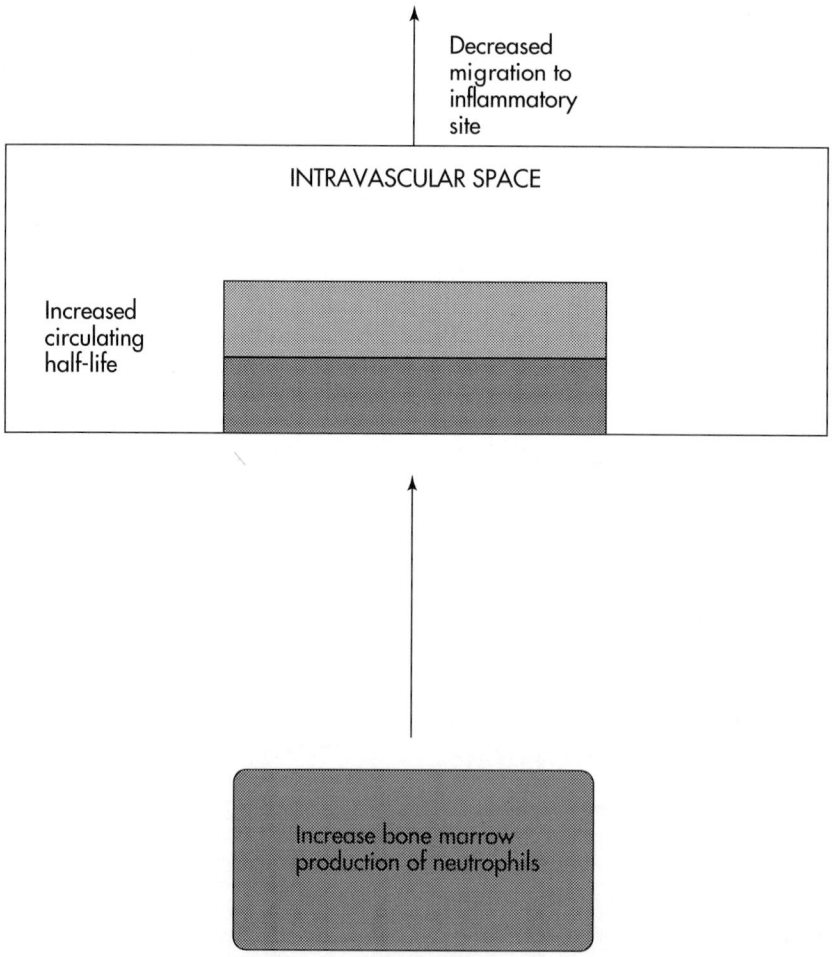


**Fig. 8-2.** Effect of corticosteroids on neutrophils.

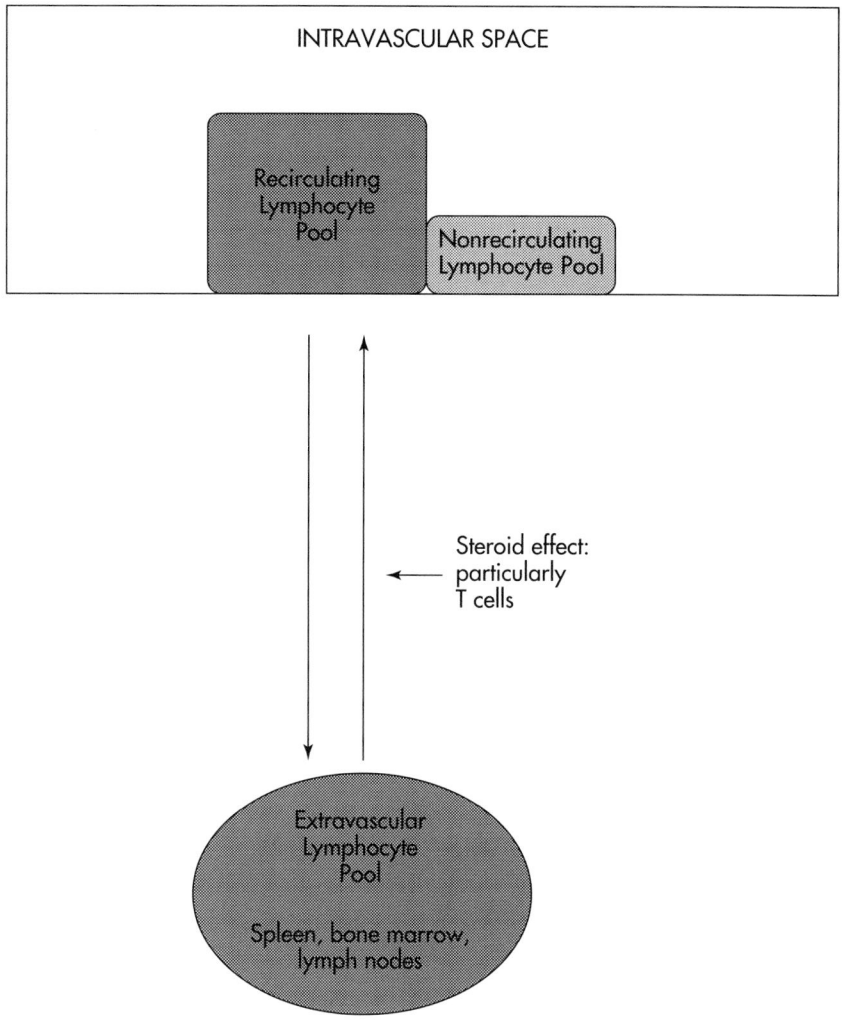


**Fig. 8-3.** Effect of corticosteroids on lymphocytes.

recruitment of immunoreactive cells to the site of the inflammatory reaction. The effect on neutrophils appears to be quite striking as well. Steroid therapy induces a larger number of neutrophils to be produced by the bone marrow. In addition to this increased production, the circulating half-life of these cells on reaching the intravascular space is prolonged. Concomitant with these effects is an impeding of neutrophil migration from this space to the site of inflammation. Decreases in the number of circulating monocytes, eosinophils, and basophils have also been observed.

Although the changes in the immune system are profound, it is important to remember that they are temporary. Fauci[6] has demonstrated that T-cell subsets return to essentially the presteroid ingestion state after about 24 hours. This observation is most important in developing a strategy for the treatment of an acutely active inflammatory condition, whether in the eye or elsewhere.

Profound effects on cell function have been noted with the addition of steroid. The effects on the various immune cell populations include a decrease in bactericidal activity, a decrease in delayed hypersensitivity reactions, a decrease in lymphokine production, and changes in immediate hypersensitivity reactions. In addition, steroid administration has a profound effect on local resident cells in an organ, particularly the vascular endothelium. A decrease of the leakage of fluid during an inflammatory episode from the capillary endothelium results with steroid administration, thus decreasing tissue swelling. Further, during an inflammatory response, there is a decrease

**Table 8-1.** Relative potencies of corticosteroids

| Preparation | Systemic equivalent (mg) | Antiinflammatory potency |
|---|---|---|
| Hydrocortisone | 20 | 1.0 |
| Cortisone | 25 | 0.8 |
| Prednisolone | 5 | 4.0 |
| Prednisone | 5 | 4.0 |
| Dexamethasone | 0.75 | 26 |
| Methylprednisolone | 4 | 5 |
| Triamcinolone | 4 | 5 |
| Betamethasone | 0.6 | 33 |

in the amount of intracellular fluid taken in by cells, thereby decreasing cell swelling and avoiding the resultant decrease in function and ultimate lysis. The effect of steroids on lysosome membranes, thought at one time to be an important stabilizing factor, now remains unclear.

PREPARATIONS, DOSAGE SCHEDULES, AND COMPLICATIONS. Many steroid preparations are now available. It should be remembered that the corticosteroid preparations have varying potencies; therefore, sometimes quite different concentrations of each drug need to be used (Table 8-1 and Fig. 8-4).

The topical application of corticosteroids is an excellent way to treat certain uveitides. Our own preference has been the use of prednisolone formulations for severe intraocular inflammatory disease. The basis for this choice is not scientific but merely the result of usage, convenience, and therefore a feeling of knowing what to expect with this formulation. Although studies do show differences of corneal penetration between phosphate and acetate preparations of steroids, we have not noted a major difference in efficacy between the two preparations when dealing with an active inflammation. When the diagnosis is made, it is imperative initially to treat the uveitis aggressively. We frequently ask the patient to take his or her drops every hour while awake. One can even consider asking patients to begin their topical therapy by taking a drop every 15 minutes for the first hour, as a sort of loading dose. Our opinion is that frequently "failures" of this therapy are due to infrequent dosaging schedules. Further, the longer and more chronic the disease, the more difficult it often is to bring under control. Once a dosaging schedule has

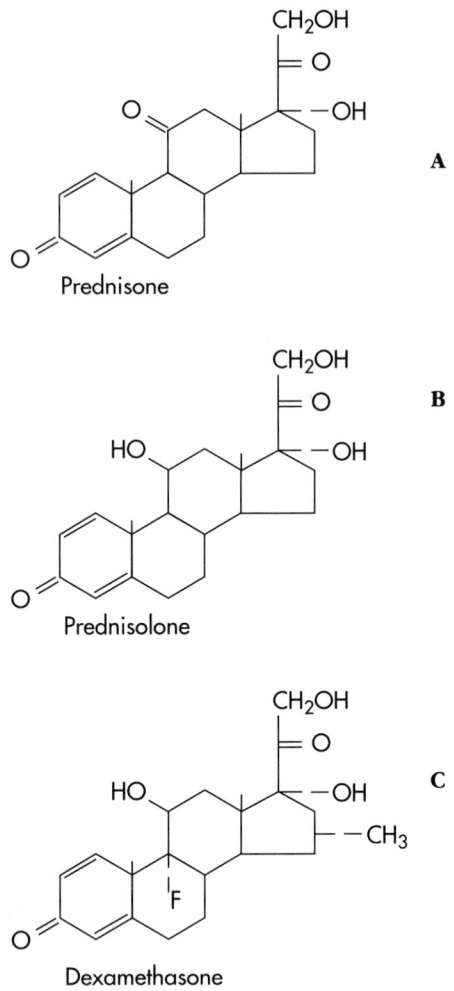


**Fig. 8-4.** Structures of more commonly used corticosteroids.

been found to be effective, as evidenced by a decrease in the flare and cell in the eye, we then see the patient often (every 2-3 days to once a week) and begin a very slow tapering of the drops. A tapering schedule is special to each patient, but persons who have had numerous attacks may need to take one or two drops a day for weeks or even months.

A second option is to inject the corticosteroid periocularly. This method, which permits a relatively high concentration of material to be given rapidly, is an effective way to treat particularly severe inflammatory conditions. There is the general choice between long-acting preparations (in a depot vehicle) and shorter-acting soluble preparations. These injections can be given every 1 to 2 weeks for short periods. In addition to severe anterior segment disease in general, this is a useful

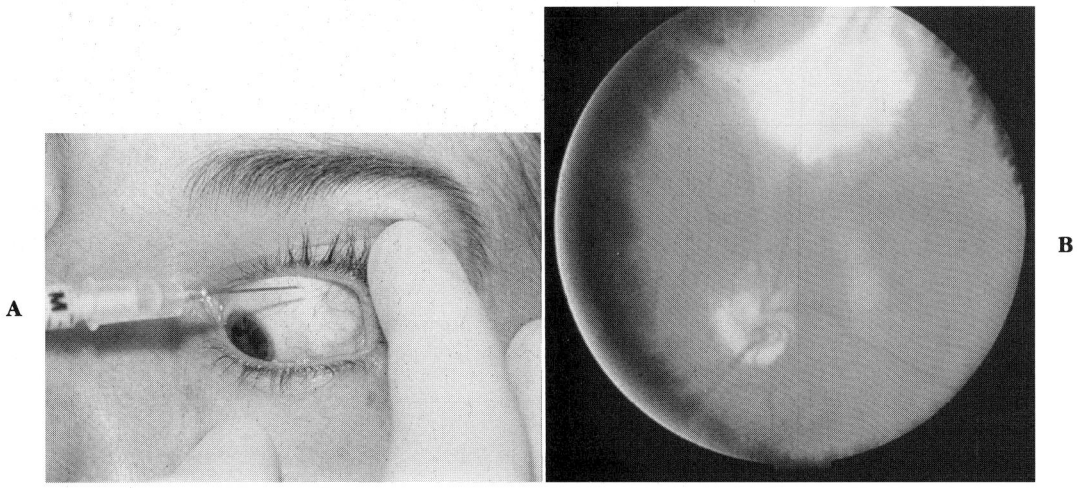


**Fig. 8-5. A,** Temporal approach to giving periocular injection. **B,** Although possibility is markedly decreased if precautions are taken, perforation of globe can occur, as seen here. (See Color Plate 6.)

approach in cases of unilateral disease, at time of surgery on an uveitic eye, and in cases in which the systemic effects of steroids are to be avoided. We have found this an effective way to treat cystoid macular edema, even in children, although the procedure may require that young children receive general anesthesia.

Several approaches to periocular injections have been suggested, and it probably is best to use the approach with which one feels the most comfortable. The approach from the superotemporal aspect of the globe, as described by Schlaegel,[7] is an approach that deserves to be reviewed by both the seasoned ophthalmologist and those beginning in the field. This approach is thought to decrease the possibility of ocular penetration and to truly place the medication under Tenon's capsule and in the region of the macula. Freeman and coworkers[8] have demonstrated that the temporal approach is efficient in placing the injected steroid close to the macula. Our own approach has been to modify the Schlaegel technique. Rarely do we need to systemically premedicate an adult. Topical anesthetics are liberally used, and the area where the injection is to be performed (invariably the superotemporal aspect of the globe) is further anesthesized with a cotton swab soaked in topical anesthetic (either 4% lidocaine or cocaine). By means of the temporal approach and the precautions recommended by Nozik,[8a] the corticosteroid is injected, either at the pars plana/peripheral retina or more posteriorly. If there are no contraindications, we generally inject triamcinolone (Kenalog), 40 mg in 1 ml, because this preparation appears to cause less fibrosis. Some practitioners have suggested mixing the steroid preparation with a local anesthetic. We generally do not do this because the increased volume needed increases the pain of the procedure. An alternate approach is to inject the steroid preparation directly through the lower lid (using a 25-gauge needle) while the patient looks upward. After the injection, for the patient's comfort, we patch the eye and give a mild analgesic. If the procedure is performed on an outpatient basis, the person will be observed for some time (30-90 minutes) to be sure there are no untoward problems. We use this technique over a 4- to 10-week interval, giving a series of two to four injections before declaring this method ineffective (Fig. 8-5).

SECONDARY EFFECTS. The topical application of steroid induces a rise in intraocular pressure in a significant number of persons. This should be monitored closely. It has been our experience that some patients with uveitis are extremely sensitive to steroid, with dramatic increases in intraocular pressure noted even when topical steroids are administered on a very modest schedule. The reactivation of corneal herpes simplex infection can occur with topical steroid therapy. This is even of greater import in those patients undergoing corneal grafts, inasmuch as a large proportion of these persons are undergoing this procedure because of corneal herpes.

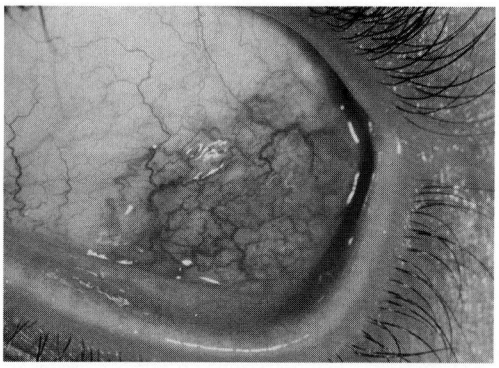

**Fig. 8-6.** Allergic response in conjunctiva after periocular injection of steroid. Patient underwent skin testing and was found to have profound allergic response to vehicle.

The periocular injection of steroid has secondary effects unique to the procedure as well. (1) Although periocular steroid injections are an effective therapy for childhood uveitis, they may require general anesthesia, with the potential side effects inherent with this. (2) Possible penetration of the globe with the needle should be a constant concern to the ophthalmologist. It is hoped that the placing of the needle temporally will reduce this possibility considerably. (3) Continued periocular injections can induce orbital problems, such as proptosis of the globe and fibrosis of the extraocular muscles. (4) Severe, intractable glaucoma can occur after periocular injections. This can become particularly problematic when a depot injection has been used. In such cases the surgical removal of the depot may need to be performed, which is sometimes a major undertaking. (5) Reactions to the vehicle in which the steroid injection has been placed can also occur (Fig. 8-6). (6) In cases of scleritis and ocular toxoplasmosis, periocular injections can be problematic. In the former the injections could potentially inhibit new collagen growth to a point that perforation of the globe may occur. In the case of toxoplasmosis, the acutely high intraocular steroid dose may effectively prevent the body's normal antitoxoplasma mechanisms, thereby causing an exacerbation of the ocular disease.

Systemic corticosteroids remain the initial drug of choice for most patients with severe bilateral endogenous sight-threatening uveitis. The striking exception to this rule is patients with Behçet's disease (see Chapter 25). When initiating systemic steroid therapy, one should keep in mind several considerations. It is imperative that the treating physician (to the best of his or her ability) rules out the possibility of infection or malignant disease as a cause for the intraocular inflammation. Uppermost is the clinical impression, based on the ocular examination, that there is an inflammatory response that requires systemic therapy. It is important to set standards by which the practitioner will decide that the therapy is successful or not. A detailed explanation should be given the patient before embarking on therapy. The subject matter should include length of therapy, goals, and side effects.

We generally find it advisable to begin therapy with prednisone 1 to 1.5 mg/kg/day (Table 8-2). The relatively high dose and daily therapy appear to increase the efficacy of this approach, which takes into account the known effects of corticosteroids in human beings, already described. The high dosages of corticosteroids should be maintained until one sees a clinical effect, but it is clear that the treating physician must set a reasonable time limit to decide whether this form of therapy is truly worthwhile. If the determination is made that the corticosteroids are having a beneficial effect, then a slow reduction of the therapeutic dose needs to be established. A too-rapid reduction can lead to a recurrence. The slow-tapering plan permits the treating physician to see if the reduction will cause a reactivation, which frequently manifests as a mild ocular inflammation and perhaps a minimal decrease in visual acuity. Some patients may need only a periodic short course of systemic steroids, whereas others require long-term maintenance. Antacids or other antiulcer medications and calcium supplements can be given to patients, particularly those receiving long-term therapy. We routinely give ranitidine, 150 mg once or twice a day, to all our patients receiving oral prednisone for any length of time.

Alternate-day therapy is certainly a logical goal to aim for since side effects of such administration are much less than with daily dosing. Fauci[9] has suggested that one way to attain this is to double the daily maintenance dosage and then slowly reduce the alternate-day dosage by 5 mg until zero is reached. In our experience those patients with severe inflammatory disease or persistent macular edema

**Table 8-2.** Common immunosuppressive agents used systemically to control intraocular inflammatory disease

| Agent | Usual dosage* |
|---|---|
| Prednisone | Oral: 1-2 mg/kg/day |
| Methylprednisolone | IV pulse: 1 g over 1-2 hr |
| Antimetabolites | |
| Methotrexate | Oral: 7.5-15 mg weekly; can be given intramuscularly |
| Azathioprine | Oral: 50-150 mg daily, 1-1.5 mg/kg, but up to 2.5 mg/kg/day per body weight |
| Alkylating agents | |
| Cyclophosphamide | Oral: 50-100 mg daily, up to 2.5 mg/kg/day per body weight<br>IV pulse: 750 mg/m$^2$ (adjusted to kidney function and WBC count) |
| Chlorambucil | Oral: 0.1-0.2 mg/kg/day |
| Cyclosporine | Oral: up to 5 mg/kg/day, usually given with prednisone, 10-20 mg/day |
| FK506 | Oral: 0.10-0.15 mg/kg/day per body weight |

*It is important to note that the dosages should ultimately be determined by a treating physician with experience using these medications on the basis of the medical state of the patient in question. Further, not all of these medications (or the route of therapy indicated) have been approved by various governmental agencies (i.e., U.S. Food and Drug Administration) for use in patients with uveitis. Therefore the physician needs to inquire about their specific use.

often do not do well on alternate-day therapy, but it still remains a logical goal. It is important to stress the method outlined by Fauci because it has been our experience in ophthalmology that the plan is rarely followed. If a patient is taking prednisone 20 mg/day and the decision has been made to attempt an alternate-day approach, then the treating physician needs to double the daily amount of prednisone from 20 to 40 mg/day and then begin a slow taper every other day.

How long does one treat? What is a reasonable long-term dosage? These are not easy questions to answer. Each patient's requirements, capacities, and willingness are very different. We believe that a reasonable daily adult maintenance dosage is from 15 to 20 mg of prednisone. This of course varies from patient to patient. For many cases of severe inflammatory disease, we commonly see patients undertreated, with treatment lasting only for 3 to 4 weeks followed by a rapid taper. Unfortunately this wishful thinking will not work in many patients. We will not consider lowering the steroid dosage below this level unless the ocular disease appears quiescent for an extended period, usually about 3 months. In some diseases, such as sympathetic ophthalmia (see Chapter 14), we have elected to treat at maintenance dosages for at least a year, fearing a recurrence if therapy were stopped earlier.

The potential side effects of corticosteroids should be familiar to those giving the medication. Some of the more common secondary problems are seen in Box 8-1. Other adverse reactions noted have included nonketotic hyperosmolar coma in young nondiabetic patients receiving systemic corticosteroids for a short time period[10] and central serous retinopathy.[11]

Intravenously administered "pulse" corticosteroid therapy can also be employed. We have used this approach in cases in which there is a severe bilateral process that needs to be treated as rapidly as possible, intravenously administering 1 g methlyprednisolone repeated each day for 3 days. Patients are hospitalized and examined by an internist before the administration of this therapy. It is not yet clear that this method indeed renders better results than does giving a high dosage of oral prednisone, such as 80 mg/day.

A constant question that must be asked is whether the desired effect warrants the potential or real side effects. No easy answer can be given, and a dialog between the patient and the physician is the only way such a question can be decided.

Although corticosteroids remain the mainstay of therapy for uveitis, some patients are resistant to steroids. Some, particularly those who receive long-term steroid therapy, develop unacceptable side effects at the dosages that need to be given to control the disease. In those patients immunosuppressive agents are added as steroid-sparing agents so that lower steroid doses can be used. Steroids combined with cytotoxic agents or cyclosporine are reasonable

**Box 8-1**
**Secondary effects of corticosteroid therapy**

**FLUIDS, ELECTROLYTES**
Sodium retention, potassium loss
Fluid retention
Hypokalemic alkalosis
Hyperosmolar coma

**MUSCULOSKELETAL**
Muscle weakness
Steroid myopathy
Osteoporosis
Aseptic necrosis of femoral and humeral heads
Tendon rupture

**GASTROINTESTINAL**
Nausea
Increased appetite
Peptic ulcer
Perforation of small and large bowel
Pancreatitis

**DERMATOLOGIC**
Poor wound healing
Easy bruisability
Increased sweating

**NEUROLOGIC**
Convulsions
Headaches
Hyperexcitability
Moodiness
Psychosis

**ENDOCRINE**
Menstrual irregularities
Cushingoid state
Suppression of growth in children
Hirsutism
Suppression of adrenocortical pituitary axis
Diabetes

**OPHTHALMIC**
Cataracts
Glaucoma
Central serous retinopathy
Activation of herpes (topical)

**OTHER**
Weight gain
Thromboembolism

and sometimes effective regimens and are discussed next.

## Cytotoxic agents

It is curious to note that cytotoxic agents have their roots in instruments of destruction, namely chemical warfare. Although synthesized earlier, it was the use of mustard gas during World War I, with the resultant lymphopenia and lymphoid aplasia, that led to this family of agents being evaluated for therapeutic purposes. On a practical basis, two major categories of cytotoxic agents are used today in the treatment of ocular inflammatory disease: alkylating agents, such as chlorambucil and cyclophosphamide (Fig. 8-7), and the antimetabolites, such as azathioprine and methotrexate (Fig. 8-8). They have been used by physicians for several decades, but their true efficacy still remains unclear for many ocular disorders; however, more information has recently been gained in their use for other putative autoimmune diseases. The physician treating severe sight-threatening disease should be aware of these agents and how they may fit into the general scheme of nonsurgical therapy for uveitis. Although, when viewed as a group, serious side effects are apparent, the role they play as steroid-sparing or replacing agents cannot be denied.[12,13]

### Alkylating agents

MODE OF ACTION. The alkylating agents have the property to undergo reactions that result in the formation of covalent links (alkylation) of neutrophilic substances. In interacting with DNA strands, alkylating agents are thought to interact with the 7-nitrogen guanine (Fig. 8-9).[14] This cross-linking of DNA would result in the inability of the cell's DNA to properly separate during division, ultimately leading to the death of the cell.

Nitrogen mustards are unstable compounds, and alterations in the structure were invariably tried to increase stability. An aromatic modification of mustard gas is chlorambucil (see Fig. 8-7), yielding it stable enough to be given by

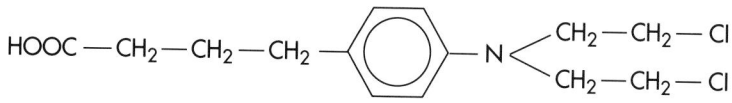


Chlorambucil

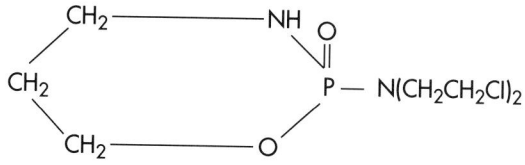


Cyclophosphamide

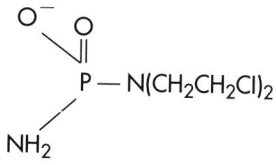


Phosphoramide mustard

**Fig. 8-7.** Structure and active moiety of two most used alkylating agents.

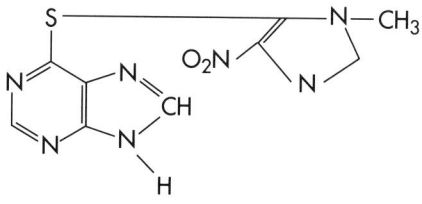


Azathioprine

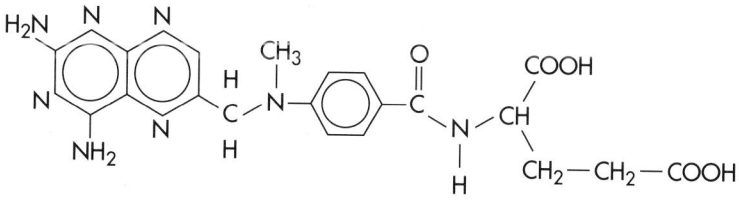


Methotrexate

**Fig. 8-8.** Structures of two antimetabolites.

mouth. Cyclophosphamide is yet another modification, with a cyclic phosphamide group added. For cyclophosphamide to become an active agent, it must be metabolized in the liver's microsomal system. It is theorized that phosphoramide mustard (see Fig. 8-7) is the most active of the metabolites.

The effect of alkylating agents on the immune system is rather profound. Higher doses are thought to more acutely affect B-cell function than T-cell function, but long-term lower dosages may have an equal or even

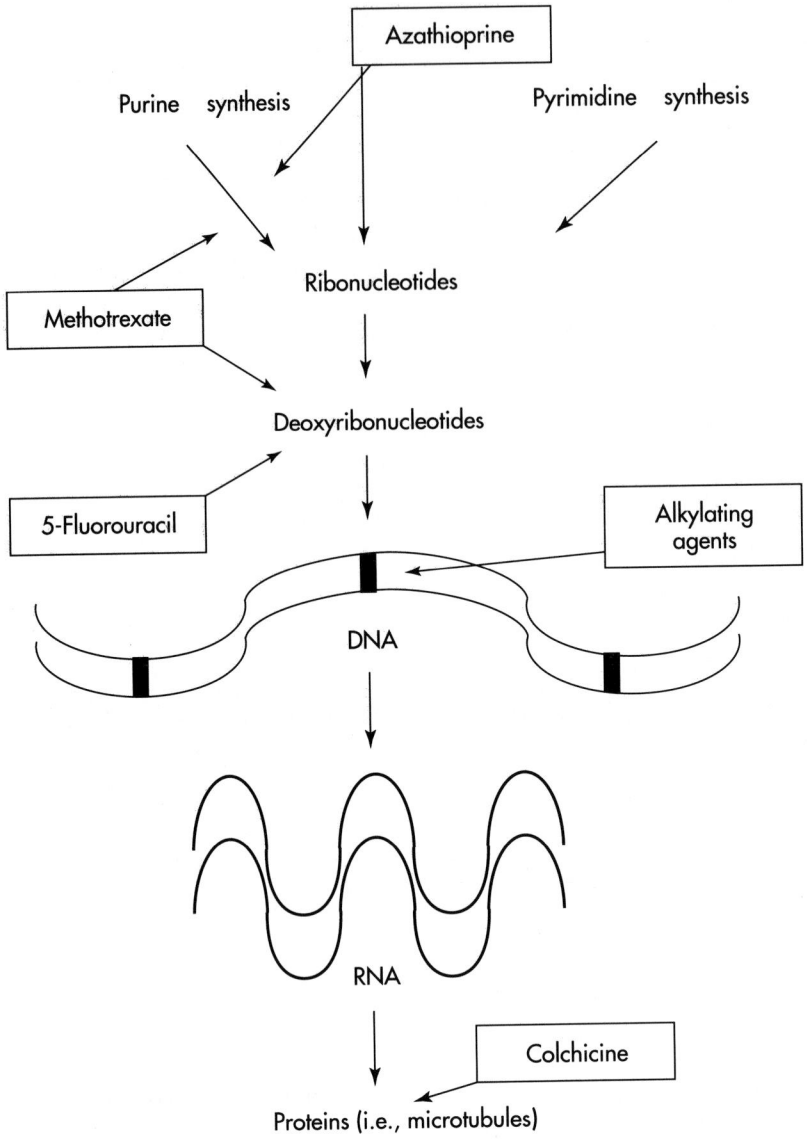


**Fig. 8-9.** Site of action of several cytotoxic agents.

greater effect on T-cell function. Paradoxically, alkylating agent administration to animals can result in the loss of suppressor cells, something certainly not advisable for patients with a poorly controlled immunoregulatory system. The alkylating agents are thought to be more potent in inducing a response as compared with the antimetabolites. However, with greater efficacy comes more potential for adverse secondary effects. These agents are thought to mediate ocular inflammatory disease through the killing of clones of cells that are effecting the damage in the eye. This may be occurring at some central location (e.g., lymph node, bone marrow) or at the end organ itself. The response is not specific and will theoretically affect any actively dividing cell.

INDICATIONS AND DOSAGES. Buckley and Gills[15] reported the efficacy of cyclosphosphamide therapy in the treatment of intermediate uveitis. In addition, alkylating agents have been frequently used in the treatment of Behçet's disease.[16] The recommendations of the International Uveitis Study Group for the use of cytotoxic agents were decided upon in the early 1980s. Although somewhat dated, the basic concepts of the group's recommendations still seem to hold true. Behçet's disease was one absolute recommendation, because corticosteroid therapy was not thought to adequately control the retinal/retinal vascular disease frequently observed in these patients. In general, alkylating agents are indicated for severe bilateral sight-threatening endogenous uveitis. Again, it cannot be overly stressed that the treating physician must be confident that the disease being treated does not have an infectious component. Further, the physician should consider therapy only if there is vision to save. It should not be considered in end-stage disease just to be sure "everything was tried." The potential side effects of these agents necessitate a good reason for their administration. The patient must be well informed of the physician's intentions and expectations, as well as any side effects. It is probably reasonable that the patient sign a consent form. In addition, an internist should examine the patient to be sure that there is no systemic contraindication for therapy and to help in the dosing and follow-up. Although this therapeutic approach is used in generalized life-threatening autoimmune diseases in children, we have not used it in pregnant women or children with uveitis, because of the concern of the potential long-term side effects of these drugs. If it is used in younger persons, the physician should discuss the side effects in depth. One important consideration is the possibility that the medication may induce azoospermia, and banking of sperm before the initiation of therapy might be considered. Harvesting ova, although performed less frequently, might also be considered.

For cyclophosphamide, adult patients can start at about 2 mg/kg/day by mouth, with the usual starting dose for a rapid effect being between 150 to 200 mg/day (see Table 8-2). The drug should be taken on an empty stomach because the drug can be activated in the gastrointestinal tract if taken with food. The white blood cell count with differential must be monitored constantly, beginning with a baseline value. One may begin to see a drop in the white blood cell count within a few days to a week. Once this occurs, the dosage may be decreased by 25 to 50 mg, with the object being a white blood cell count that stabilizes at no lower than 3000/mm$^3$. Neutrophils should not fall below a total count of 1500 to 2000/mm$^3$. Nevertheless, the dosage used should be based predominantly on the therapeutic effect of the drug on ocular inflammation.

Pulse cyclophosphamide (see Table 8-2) has been used widely in the treatment of systemic collagen vascular disease, such as the renal disease associated with systemic lupus erythematosus. This approach to therapy is thought to carry fewer risks than everyday oral therapy. Hoffman and associates[17] found that intermittent cyclosphosphamide therapy combined with steroid therapy yielded a long-term failure rate of 79% in patients with Wegener's granulomatosis. We as well have not found this approach to be particularly effective; breakthroughs of disease activity tend to occur between therapeutic courses. Rosenbaum[18] reported that in 11 patients with uveitis treated with pulse cyclophosphamide, 5 benefited but only 2 had a sustained improvement without the use of additional immunosuppressive therapy. Rosenbaum concluded that most patients with uveitis do not experience a prolonged benefit from this therapeutic approach. Systemic steroids can be administered along with the alkylating agent. This permits one to use lower dosages of both and therefore avoid some of the side effects of both.

Godfrey and colleagues[19] have used chlorambucil to treat several disorders, including Behçet's disease and sympathetic ophthalmia. Therapy with this medication can be administered on an outpatient basis. The total dose is usually between 6 to 12 mg/day. We generally give a lower initial dose (2 mg) to be sure that there are no idiosyncratic responses, and then increase the dose. As with cyclophosphamide, the white blood cell count and differential must be constantly monitored.

A somewhat different approach was discussed by Tessler and Jennings,[20] who reported the use of high-dose short-term chlorambucil in the treatment of Behçet's disease and sympathetic ophthalmia. These authors believe that they induced remission in all patients, using an average total dose of 2.2 g over 23 weeks for the patients with Behçet's disease and a total dose of 0.9 g over 11 weeks for the patients with sympathetic ophthalmia.

SECONDARY EFFECTS. A wide range of side effects has been reported with alkylating agents.[21] For these particular agents, the leukopenia is an integral part of the effect of these agents, yielding immunosuppression. Thrombocytopenia and anemia also occur. Increased incidence of infection, particularly viral, is another great concern. Interstitial fibrosis of the lungs, testicular atrophy, and hemorrhagic cystitis are associated with cyclophosphamide therapy, the latter being a relative indication for discontinuation of the drug. Renal toxicity has been attributed to the metabolites of alkylating agents,[22] and visual disturbances have been reported with high doses of cyclophosphamide.[23] Teratogenicity is a major concern, and cyclophosphamide is excreted in breast milk.

Perhaps the most disquieting adverse effects seen with these agents are those that may occur after long-term therapy. The first is the potential for secondary malignancy.[21] Secondary urinary bladder cancer seems to occur in patients who have hemorrhagic cystitis. Of course the underlying disorder being treated may also predispose some patients to the development of these disorders, particularly the myeloproliferative and lymphoproliferative neoplasms. A second troublesome observation is the finding of chromosomal damage with extended cyclophosphamide therapy.[24] In Hoffman and colleagues' review of 158 patients with Wegener's granulomatosis,[25] a series of disturbing complications ascribed to cyclophosphamide therapy were reported: 73 patients had 140 serious infections that required hospitalization and intravenous antibiotic therapy, 43% had cystitis, 2.8% had bladder cancer, and 2% had myelodysplasia. Of the women treated 57% stopped having their menses for 1 year, with testing supporting the diagnosis of ovarian failure. There was a calculated 24-fold increase in malignant conditions and a calculated 33-fold increase in bladder cancer, occurring 7 months to 10 years after the medication was stopped.

It should be added that during the past few years alkylating agent therapy, because of the aforementioned complications, has been less and less used by internists for the treatment of putative autoimmune diseases. However, the anecdotal evidence certainly suggests a positive therapeutic effect in curtailing severe intraocular inflammatory disease. For life-threatening systemic vasculitis or some cases of sight-threatening retinal vasculitis, cyclosphosphomide may be a most effective medication. Also, in the third world, this sort of therapy is readily available and is relatively cheap, two very important considerations. As with many other problems in medicine, this class of drugs presents a dual-edged sword, and their use should be considered only after long reflection.

**Antimetabolites.** Within this category of medications, azathioprine, which alters purine metabolism, and methotrexate, a folate analogue, are the two most widely used medications (Fig. 8-8).

***Azathioprine***

MODE OF ACTION. Azathioprine (Imuran) is thought to be a prodrug. Upon metabolism it is converted into the active agent, 6-mercaptopurine. Azathioprine is better absorbed, causes less gastrointestinal disturbance, and is less likely to be inactivated by liver enzymes than is 6-mercaptopurine. Once converted to its active form, it is thought to affect DNA and RNA metabolism by being converted to 6-thioinosine-5-phosphate (T-IMP) by the enzyme hypoxanthine guanine phosphoribosyltransferase. T-IMP is probably incorporated into nucleic acids, thus leading to false codes being generated. It appears that azathioprine has a greater effect on the afferent arm of the immune response when it is given before the antigenic challenge.

INDICATIONS AND DOSAGES. For putative autoimmune diseases such as rheumatoid arthritis, the suggested dosage of azathioprine is about 1 to 2.5 mg/kg/day,[26,27] with the average dose being 50 to 100 mg daily, given as one dose or in a divided dose[28] (see Table 8-2). The combination of azathioprine with low-dose steroid has been used in the treatment of uveitis by Andrasch and colleagues,[29] with about half of the 22 patients showing a positive therapeutic effect and the others having either no response or severe adverse effects. Other authors have used the drug for the treatment of sympathetic ophthalmia, the Vogt-Koyanagi-Harada syndrome, and pars planitis.[30] More than half the patients with Behçet's disease whom Aoki and Sugiura[31] treated with azathioprine appeared to have an improvement of their ocular disease. Yazici and coworkers[32] showed in a double-masked study that azathioprine (2.5 mg/kg/day) was superior to placebo in the prevention of new eye disease associated with Behçet's disease. Hooper and Kaplan[33] used an initial dosage of azathioprine of 1.5 mg/kg/day combined with steroid and cyclosporine for sight-threatening serpiginous choroidopathy (see Chapter 27). Certain drugs, such as allopurinol, can interfere with the metabolism of 6-mercaptopurine, and the dosage of the agent must be reduced accordingly.

SECONDARY EFFECTS. Antimetabolites can have serious side effects,[21] but in the past few years use of lower doses has prevented these unwanted effects from occurring or frequently has made them more tolerable. For azathioprine, perhaps the most problematic acute adverse effects are leukopenia, thrombocytopenia, and gastrointestinal disturbances. Of great long-term concern is that chronic immunosuppression increases the risk of neoplasia. Connell and colleagues[34] studied the risk of neoplasia in 755 patients with inflammatory bowel disease who were treated with azathioprine. These patients received a dosage of 2 mg/kg/day for a median time of 12.5 months, and no cases of non-Hodgkin's lymphoma were reported. There appeared to be no difference in cancer frequency between 86 patients with chronic ulcerative colitis who received azathioprine and 180 matched patients who did not. It appears that the risk of neoplasia is lower in those patients treated for autoimmune disorders, such as rheumatoid arthritis, as compared with those receiving therapy for the prevention of transplantation rejection.

***Methotrexate***

MODE OF ACTION. Methotrexate is a folate analogue, differing from folic acid only in that a hydrogen atom and hydroxyl group have been replaced by a methyl and amino group. Folate analogues are known to have profound effects on cellular metabolism by inhibiting dihydrofolate reductase activity. This enzyme is imperative for the production of tetrahydrofolate, an important coenzyme in cell metabolism. Tetrahydrofolate is needed for the production of thymidylate, an essential component of DNA, and mediates the production of purine nucleotides, also needed for RNA metabolism. Methotrexate demonstrates time-specific characteristics in that, under certain experimental conditions, an augmented immune response may be noted if the drug is given before antigenic challenge. Several effects on the immune system have been enumerated. Methotrexate has been shown to have an antiproliferative effect on endothelial cells,[35] can decrease the synthesis of leukotriene $B_4$ in neutrophils,[36] has been shown to decrease the concentration of interleukin–1 beta in synovial fluid,[37] and can suppress cell-mediated immunity.[38] An added action of methotrexate is its inhibition of histamine release.

INDICATIONS AND DOSAGES. Several dosage schedules have been suggested, with a weekly oral or intramuscular dose of 7.5 to 25 mg given until a therapeutic response is noted (see Table 8-2). Patients need to be told to abstain from all alcohol consumption. Patients with cyclitis, as well as sympathetic ophthalmia, have been reported to improve with the administration of this agent, but those with Behçet's disease and iridocyclitis have not.[39] Holz and colleagues[40] reported the use of low-dose methotrexate in the treatment of 14 patients with uveitis. Using a regimen of either 40 mg given intravenously once weekly followed by 15 mg/wk given orally or 15 mg oral methotrexate only, they found an improvement of visual acuity in 11 of the patients and an improvement in inflammatory disease in all. However, using the low dose of 12.5 mg/wk of methotrexate, Shah and colleagues[41] found that 16 patients with assorted ocular inflammatory conditions (including intermediate uveitis [9 patients] and retinal vasculitis [3 patients]) had a reduction in inflammatory activity and most of those could taper or discontinue their steroid therapy. However, when one looks at the success rate of those patients with chronic uveitis, only five of the nine responded, and improvement in visual acuity was not used as the criterion for success. Of the three patients with retinal vasculitis, two improved from moderate to mild disease and the other had no improvement.

Methotrexate has been used periocularly for the treatment of malignant conditions. Rootman and Gudauskas[42] used subconjunctival injections of methotrexate, cytarabine, and corticosteroids to successfully treat a leukemic infiltrate into the eye.

SECONDARY EFFECTS. The secondary effects of methotrexate are legion,[21] but the lower doses more recently used have given this agent a new therapeutic life. Severe toxic reactions have been reported with this medication, although usually at higher doses. A marked depression of the white blood cell count and thrombocytopenia can occur. Hepatotoxicity (liver atrophy, cirrhosis, and even necrosis) is one of the most worrisome side effects.[43] Up to one third of those receiving long-term weekly methotrexate will have elevated serum aminotransferase levels.[44] Liver enzymes twice that of normal warrant withholding or stopping the medication, with the levels usually rapidly returning to normal. Zachariae and coworkers[45] have reported that cirrhosis developed in 25% of patients with psoriasis who received long-term low-dose methotrexate therapy. The older the patient and the longer the methotrexate therapy are both independent predictors of possible toxicity. The question as to when to perform a liver biopsy still remains controversial. It has been suggested that a liver biopsy should be considered in patients before beginning methotrexate therapy if there is a history of excessive alcohol consumption, abnormal results of liver function tests, or chronic hepatitis. Liver biopsy should also be considered during therapy if there is a persistence of elevated liver function test results or a decrease in the serum albumin concentration.[13]

Another concern is an acute pneumonitis that can be accompanied with fever, progressive shortness of breath, and cough in up to 5% of patients treated with methotrexate.[46,47] This appears to be due to a drug hypersensitivity reaction, and it can occur early or late in the course of therapy. Because an x-ray film may reveal interstitial and alveolar infiltrative picture, sometimes bronchoalveolar lavage is needed to rule out an infectious process such as *Pneumocystis carinii.* In most cases the reaction disappears with discontinuation of therapy.

Methotrexate may also impair renal function. The agent has been noted in the tears of patients receiving high-dose therapy.[48] Methotrexate can have a high rate of toxicity, but this appears in part dose-related. In the low-dose study of Holz and colleagues,[40] slight elevations of transaminase levels were noted in 4 of 13 patients, partial alopecia in 2, and nausea in 3. A disturbing report from Zimmer-Galler and Lie[49] described the case of a patient with rheumatoid arthritis treated with low-dose methotrexate for 16 months who developed blurry vision. The blurry vision was noted to be due to choroidal nodules, which ultimately showed to be a large B-cell non-Hodgkin's lymphoma. It is always difficult to distinguish the underlying propensity that patients with autoimmune disease may have to developing neoplasms as opposed to a real risk from the therapy.

• • •

Many recommendations for cytotoxic agent therapy that the reader will find in the literature were written before the use of cyclosporine or FK506 in clinical practice, as well as the use of low-dose methotrexate or azathioprine. In our approach, cytotoxic agents are often used as third-line drugs—after corticosteroids and cyclosporine—for sight-threatening intraocular inflammatory disease. We would use cytotoxic agents if the side effects of steroid or cyclosporine were simply intolerable but the patient clearly was having an excellent therapeutic response to immunosuppressive therapy. We would make every effort to avoid alkylating agents in children inasmuch as the long-term effects of these agents make the risk sometimes ethically difficult to justify. It should be stressed that until recently no comparative clinical trials have been attempted to evaluate the true efficacy of these agents in the treatment of uveitis, nor are most of these agents listed in the *Physicians' Desk Reference* as indicated for the therapy of uveitis. There is, however, certainly no reason to doubt that in some cases these agents may be effective therapies—for example, their apparent profound positive effect on the ocular manifestations of Behçet's disease[16]; however, Tabbara has brought that assessment into question.[50]

In our experience, mostly with the alkylating agents, cytotoxic drugs have not been as effective in controlling the severe inflammatory conditions such as Behçet's disease as had been previously suggested. We have had patients with Behçet's disease discontinue cyclosporine because of toxicity and go on to alkylating agents with a very poor therapeutic result, necessitating a third therapeutic approach. However, others seem to have done well. Although alkylating agents are tolerated reasonably well, the side effects, such as leukopenia, may last for some time even after the discontinuance of the medication. We therefore advise caution when clinicians use these agents. The ophthalmologist should have someone well versed in this therapeutic approach actively involved in the care of the patient, should set strict goals that must be reached in terms of the therapeutic effect, and should avoid, to the extreme, using these agents in children, unless forced to and only with the in-depth understanding and permission of both the parents and the child.

One potential use for cytotoxic agents is local application to the eye. 5-Fluorouracil (5-FU) and mitomycin locally injected or topically applied at the time of filtering surgery on patients with uveitis may prove to be an important therapeutic tool in increasing the success of these procedures in what are usually patients at high risk. Local application of these agents carries significant ocular complications and potential systemic ones as well, and they should be used only within the context of an accepted clinical protocol. Locally administered methotrexate (or other agents) may prove to be a useful therapeutic approach to neoplastic disease with only a local reactivation in the eye.

## Cyclosporine

MODE OF ACTION. Cyclosporine is a natural product of several fungii. It was first investigated because of its potential antibiotic qualities, and indeed it is antibacterial but with a most limited spectrum. It was the unique immunomodulatory properties first observed by Jean Borel at Sandoz Ltd. in Basel, Switzerland, that altered immunotherapy principles and therapeutics in a profound way. Cyclosporin A, now termed *cyclosporine* (Sandimmune) is a neutral, lipophilic, cyclic endecapeptide with an unique amino acid side chain at the C1 position (Fig. 8-10). It is one of a large family of cyclosporines, some naturally occurring, some synthetically produced. This uncharged molecule, with a molecular weight of 1202, is insoluble in water. The original preparation for human use is an olive oil solution with 12.5% ethanol, which is taken by mouth with either milk or juice. The absorption of this oral preparation is variable, ranging from 4% to 60%, with probably about one third of the agent usually absorbed.[51,52] It is an agent that is concentrated in lipid-containing tissues such as breast, pancreas, liver, lymphoid tissue, and kidney. We found about 40% of the plasma concentration in the aqueous of patients with quiescent uveitis under therapy with cyclosporine and undergoing cataract surgery.[53] Cyclosporine tablets are now available but have not yet been as widely used in the United States as the oral solution.

The agent is metabolized in the liver by the cytochrome P-450 microsomal enzyme system. The ring structure is maintained throughout the metabolic process, with only 0.1% of the drug not undergoing metabolic changes. At least 15 metabolic products of cyclosporine are known. The parent structure appears to be the most active form. Drugs that interfere with cytochrome P-450 activity will slow cyclosporine metabolism and will affect cyclosporine levels. Ketoconazole is one such agent, permitting a reduction by up to 90% of the oral dose of cyclosporine.[54] Other medications that inhibit cyclosporine metabolism include oral contraceptives, androgens, and erythromycin.

Cyclosporine has been demonstrated to have a far more restricted effect on the immune system than any other immunosuppressive agent yet available. Although cyclosporine theoretically would affect any cell with its binding protein, its major clinical effect is directed against the factors that promote T-cell activation and recruitment. The exact point at

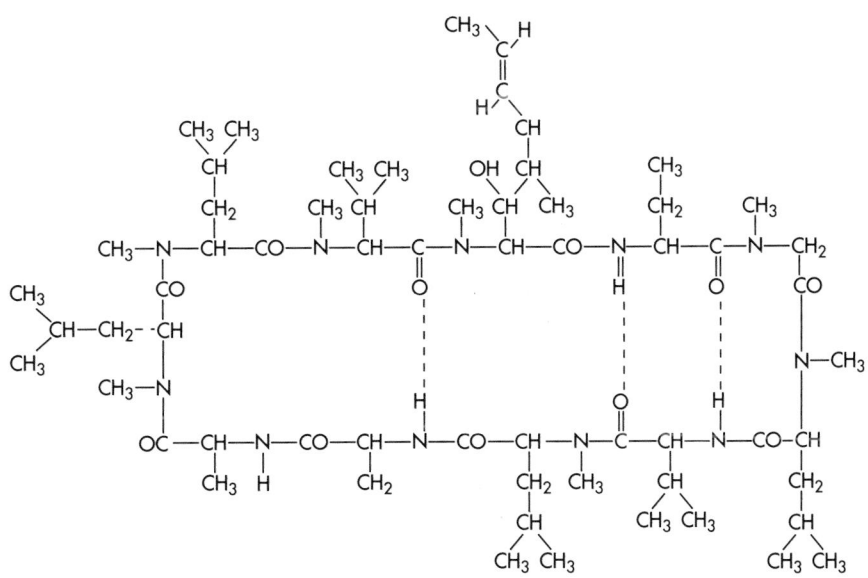

**Fig. 8-10.** Structure of cyclosporine (Sandimmune).

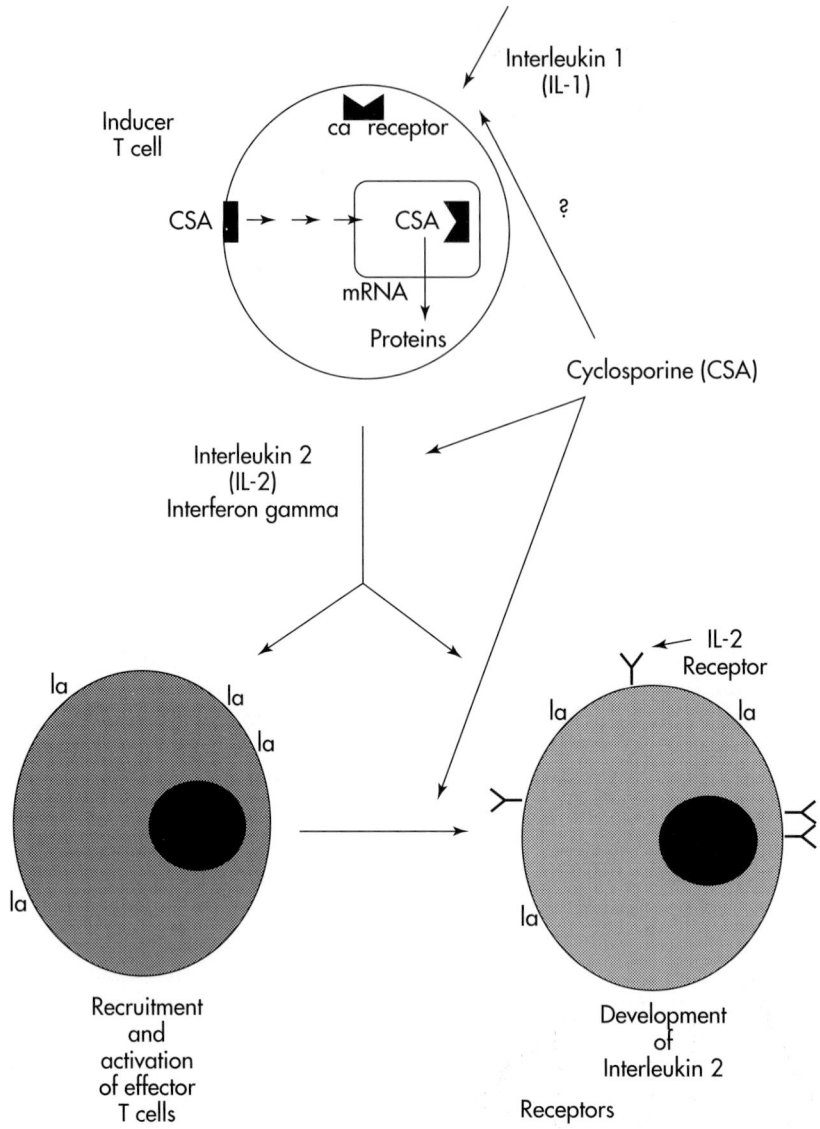


**Fig. 8-11.** Proposed mechanisms of cyclosporine on T-cell circuitry.

which cyclosporine intervenes in this scheme is debated (Fig. 8-11). It appears that cyclosporine enters the cell and is bound to an immunophilin (cyclophilin) meeting it at the cell membrane, similar to that seen with corticosteroids. It then is escorted into the nucleus, where it has an effect on messenger ribonucleic acid (mRNA) production and ultimately on protein synthesis. Although the mechanism still remains to be definitely shown, much has been elucidated.[55] Cyclosporine appears to block the activation of genes in T cells.[56] One intriguing notion is that cyclosporine binds to proteins binding to the IL-2 enhancer (such as NF-AT and octamer-associated protein [OAP]), which helps in the activation of the transcription of the IL-2 gene. These sites have been shown to be sensitive to cyclosporine.[57]

On the basis of several in vitro systems, different observations have been made concerning the mode of action of cyclosporine. Larsson[58] reported that cyclosporine blocked the acquisition of IL-2 receptors and therefore prevented resting cells from becoming activated and responding to IL-2. This theme has been less stressed in the more recent literature. Others, such as Bunjes and coworkers,[59] have suggested that cyclosporine affects the release of IL-2 but that the acquisition of these receptors was not inhibited by cyclosporine. The blockage of cyclosporine production was noted by Kaufman and colleagues[60] in a T-cell hybridoma that produces IL-2 but does not bear IL-2 receptors. It may be that cyclosporine's mode of action depends on the state of T-cell activation and the type of stimulus for T-cell activation.[61] It is clear, however, that cyclosporine was unique in mediating its action through the T-cell circuitry.

The T cell most affected seems to be the inducer T-cell subset. We have noted that recruitment of inducer T cells into the draining lymph node of a site of S-antigen immunization is markedly diminished with cyclosporine administration. Shifts in the kinetic T-cell and B-cell response are also noted when animals are given cyclosporine.

DOSAGES AND INDICATIONS. The dosage schedule for cyclosporine administration has undergone much change and remains in a state of flux.[62] In our initial studies[63] on the use of cyclosporine in ocular inflammatory disease patients were begun on a dosage of 10mg/kg/day, which at the time was thought to be a rather modest dose inasmuch as often two to two and a half times this dosage was being given to treat recipients of whole organ transplants. However, it became clear that dose-induced renal alterations made this starting dosage no longer acceptable (see later discussion of toxicity). Studies have suggested that a lower initiating dose of cyclosporine may not induce any or at least considerably lessen the possibility of renal toxicity[64] (to be discussed). It is usually suggested that cyclosporine be given at a starting dosage of 5 mg/kg/day (Fig. 8-12; see also Table 8-2), either as a single dose or a twice-daily regimen. The twice-daily regimen is more commonly the regimen employed to avoid large spikes in serum cyclosporine levels, which may predispose the patient to renal toxicity. A recommended maximum dosage of 7 mg/kg/day can be considered in special cases, such as in children or in patients with documented low cyclosporine serum levels. Cyclosporine is often used in combination with prednisone, usually at 10 to 20 mg/day, but for short periods, at even higher levels.

A relative contraindication for the initiation of therapy is the patient with poorly controlled hypertension or a history of renal disease accompanied by decreased creatinine clearance, or both. In addition, older patients (more than 55 years of age) must be evaluated

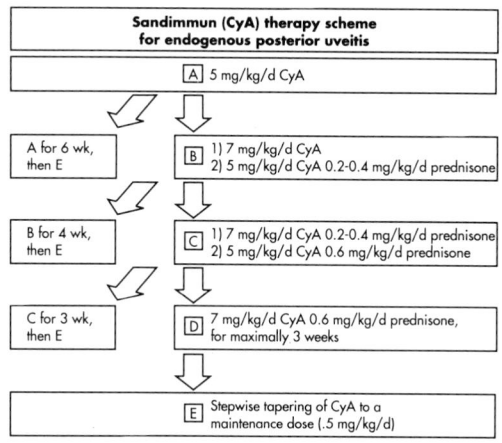


**Fig. 8-12.** Therapeutic scheme for treatment of sight-threatening bilateral endogenous uveitis with cyclosporine. (From Ben Ezra D, Nussenblatt RB, Timonen P: *Optimal use of Sandimmune in endogenous uveitis,* Springer-Verlag, Berlin, 1988.)

particularly closely because they lack an adequate renal reserve. If the patient is currently being treated with cytotoxic agents, we would discontinue the medication for at least 1 month before beginning cyclosporine. Those taking steroid orally continue to do so, with a slow taper to the 10 to 20 mg/day range. The ocular response to cyclosporine may be relatively slow (weeks to months), but preset goals should be established and they should be met by about 3 months of therapy. The serum creatinine level should not be permitted to rise 30% over baseline. Optimal decreases in cyclosporine dosages are usually between 50 and 100 mg/day at a time. It is ill advised to stop the medication abruptly because a rebound of the ocular disease may ensue.

The question of how long one needs to treat patients with cyclosporine is somewhat open-ended. It appears that an immunologically tolerant state is not induced with this medication, and therefore an extended therapeutic course is indicated in most patients. We have stopped the medication is some patients with no recurrence of their disease, which may be explained by the fact that the disease has run its course.

On the basis of our initial observations,[63,65,66] we believe that cyclosporine should be used in patients with active bilateral sight-threatening noninfectious uveitis, who are unable to tolerate systemic corticosteroid therapy at a moderate dosage (>25 mg prednisone) necessary for the treatment of their intraocular inflammatory disease.[67] Of special interest was the particularly positive clinical effect seen in patients with Behçet's disease who were treated with this medication.[68] This has been supported by a randomized, masked study in Japan[69] and in a study carried out by Diaz-Llopis and colleagues,[70] who found that with a dosage of 5 mg/kg/day and a maintenance dosage of 2 mg/kg/day, a good response was seen in 86% of patients, with a disappearance of attacks in 43%. This appears to be the one disease in which cyclosporine might be considered as an initial therapeutic agent combined with a moderate amount of prednisone, but only if specific criteria are met (see Chapter 25).

Several reports have appeared that support the use of cyclosporine in various types of intraocular inflammatory disease. Towler and coworkers[71] treated 13 patients with chronic intraocular inflammation with a mean cyclosporine dosage of 4.1 mg/kg/day, combined when needed with 15 mg or less of prednisone per day. They found that 10 patients had an improvement of visual acuity, and acuity remained stable in the other 3. One patient needed to return to an alternative form of immunosuppression. Secchi and colleagues,[72] in an open, noncontrolled, multicenter, long-term study of the use of cyclosporine, found it useful in the treatment of patients with posterior and intermediate uveitis, decreasing the number and severity of attacks while improving visual acuity and decreasing inflammation. Leznoff and coworkers[73] have reported a therapeutically positive response with cyclosporine in cases of sympathetic ophthalmia, as well as in a case of corneal transplantation, but a questionable response in patients with intermediate uveitis and serpiginous choroiditis. Pascalis and colleagues[74] have reported the use cyclosporine (initial dosage of 5 mg/kg/day) combined with fluocortolone and low-dose methotrexate in treating 32 patients with difficult-to-control noninfectious uveitis. They noted that 20 patients had a return to normal visual acuity, and all had a disappearance of ocular inflammatory activity. The follow-up period was from 6 to 18 months, during which they noted no signs of hepatic or renal toxicity.

It should be stressed that at this time no topical preparation of cyclosporine is commercially available as of yet, but one may be in the near future. Although perhaps of import to immune diseases involving the ocular surface, the physical properties of this medication are such that this method of application does not result in significant amounts of the drug entering the eye. Therefore, for the moment, this does not appear to a useful therapeutic approach with the formulations available today.

**Table 8-3.** Secondary effects associated with administration of cyclosporine (10 mg/kg/day) in patients with uveitis

| Effects | Incidence (%) |
|---|---|
| Symptoms | |
| Paresthesia/hyperesthesia | 40 |
| Epigastric burning | 20 |
| Fatigue | 24 |
| Hypertrichorism | 20 |
| Gingivitis | 20 |
| Decreased appetite | 5 |
| Breast tenderness/fibroadenoma | 8 |
| Hidradenitis | 4 |
| Signs | |
| Hypertension | 24 |
| Mild anemia | 24 |
| Hyperuricemia | 20 |
| Increased sedimentation rate | 75 |
| Abnormal liver function tests | 6 |
| Renal toxicity | ? |
| No opportunistic infections or lymphoma | |

SECONDARY EFFECTS. Table 8-3 lists the secondary effects we have noted with cyclosporine. However, these adverse effects were observed when cyclosporine was administered as the sole immunosuppressive agent at 10 mg/kg/day, which we no longer do. At lower dosages of cyclosporine the secondary effects noted by our patients have diminished considerably. In the main, when they occur, these side effects are well tolerated by this group of usually highly motivated patients. However, the two secondary problems that give the treating physician cause for most concern are hypertension and renal toxicity. Depending on one's definition of renal toxicity, renal toxicity develops in as many as 75% to 100% of the patients treated with cyclosporine.[53,75] It is not clear what the incidence (if any) of irreversible renal toxicity will be with the lower dosage of cyclosporine now recommended. At a higher dose the alterations we noted on renal biopsy, after an average of 2 years of therapy, were renal tubular atrophy and interstitital fibrosis, with the glomeruli in the main remaining intact.

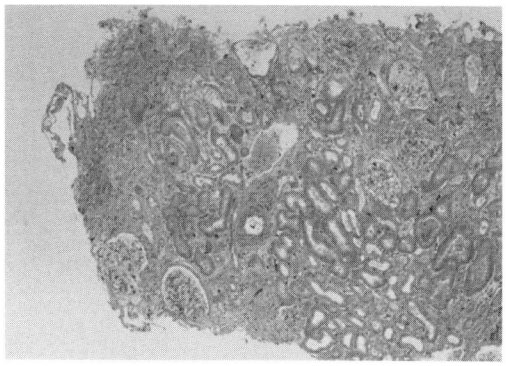

**Fig. 8-13.** Renal biopsy from patient receiving cyclosporine for uveitis. Interstitial fibrosis and marked patchy loss of renal tubules suggest toxicity due to this agent. Serum creatinine level was within normal limits at time of biopsy.

Renal vascular alterations can also appear[75] (Fig. 8-13). These alterations were noted histologically when the mean serum creatinine level of the patients undergoing biopsy was 1.5 mg/dl, within the upper limits of normal. It would appear that there is a reversible and irreversible component to the renal toxicity induced by cyclosporine. It may be that the initial starting dosage of 10 mg/kg/day sets into motion the mechanisms leading ultimately to the changes noted histologically. Some have found that even at lower starting doses of cyclosporine, changes in renal function can develop.[76] However, most recent reports from investigators treating autoimmune conditions (other than uveitis) with lower starting and maintenance dosages of cyclosporine have been heartening because little or no alterations in renal function associated with this agent have been noted.[64] Feutren and Mihatsch[77] reviewed 192 renal biopsy specimens from patients treated with cyclosporine for a variety of conditions, including diabetes mellitus, Sjögren's syndrome, and uveitis. It was found that three independent variables distinguished the 41 patients with cyclosporine-induced nephropathy from those free of nephropathy: a higher initial dose of cyclosporine, a larger maximal increase in the serum creatinine concentration above baseline, and age. Therefore it has been suggested that to decrease the risk of nephropathy a dosage of 5 mg/kg/day should be used and serum creatinine levels should not rise more than 30% above the patient's baseline. As well, a recent retrospective analysis of 1663 patients who had undergone renal transplantation and were receiving long-term cyclosporine therapy demonstrated that progressive toxic nephropathy did not occur.[78] The addition of steroid or bromocriptine[79] to the regimen permits a lower dose of cyclosporine to be used, with the hope that a similar therapeutic result with less toxicity will be achieved.

Opportunistic infections have not been a major problem in patients with uveitis who are treated with cyclosporine. Certainly, some risk is present if patients receive other immunosuppressive agents combined with cyclosporine. A trend was observed toward less renal toxicity in patients who receive combination cyclosporine/steroid therapy as opposed to cyclosporine alone.[80] We have noted that patients with uveitis treated with cyclosporine demonstrate appropriate immune responses to both new antigens and to old ones requiring a "recall" response.[81] Therefore vaccination apparently can be performed on patients treated with this medication, but preimmunization and postimmunization titers should be checked. Further, to date, no lymphomas or other cyclosporine-related neoplasms have been seen in our patients. The incidence of lymphoma observed in graft recipients treated with cyclosporine was 0.3%.[53] Most disease develops in the first few months and in the main has been associated with multiple-drug regimens.

• • •

In summary, the general approach to the use of immunosuppressive agents is to choose the least amount historically considered effective for the anatomic area affected (Fig. 8-14). However, it is important to establish control of the disease early with sufficient medication and to taper the medication after the inflammation resolves. Topical steroid administration for anterior segment disease can be most effective if given frequently. Periocular steroids are often overlooked, but they are effective for the patient with unilateral disease, or cystoid macular edema and for the child in whom one wishes to avoid the secondary effects of systemic corticosteroid administration. Systemic corticosteroid administration is still the mainstay of therapy in sight-threatening bilateral intermediate and posterior endogenous uveitis. In the patient with severe side effects due to steroid therapy, in children requiring high-dose corticosteroid therapy (1-1.5 mg/kg), or in the

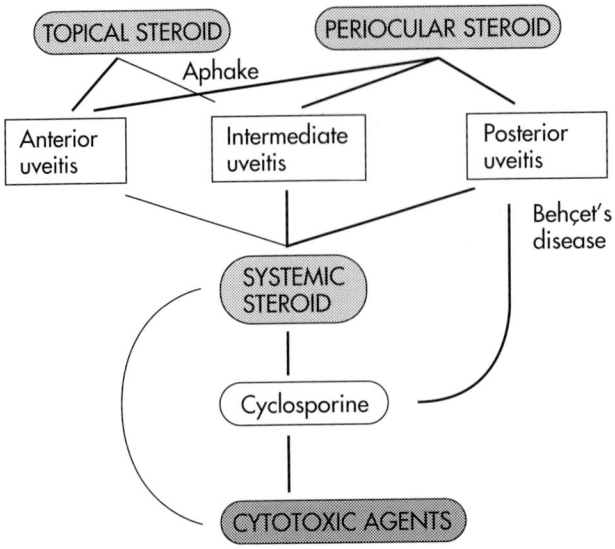


**Fig. 8-14.** Primary medical therapies for endogenous uveitis.

patient with Behçet disease (see Chapter 25), we would consider using cyclosporine with a moderate amount of prednisone. We reserve cytotoxic agents for therapeutic failures with the aforementioned agents. We would not use alkylating agents in children except under the most exceptional of circumstances. Both azathioprine (Imuran) and methotrexate, which are being used more frequently in both children and adults, are reasonable steroid- or cyclosporine-sparing agents. It is imperative that the therapeutic approach be reevaluated if the clinical course becomes worse (Fig. 8-15).

During the past few years cyclosporine therapy has been given in conjunction with an antimetabolite or steroid. Cyclosporine, prednisone, and azathioprine have been used in the treatment of patients undergoing renal transplantation. As well, the combination of cyclosporine, prednisone, and methotrexate has been found to be more effective in preventing acute graft-versus-host disease than was cyclosporine and prednisone alone.[82]

We have had the chance to compare the effects of cyclosporine G therapy with cyclosporine therapy in the treatment of noninfectious uveitis. Cyclosporine G varies from A by a small side-chain alteration and was thought to be possibly less nephrotoxic. In a masked, dose-escalation, randomization scheme, we noted that cyclosporine G and cyclosporine induced essentially the same degree of renal alterations at higher doses (7.5 and 10 mg/kg) but minimal changes at lower levels. We noted

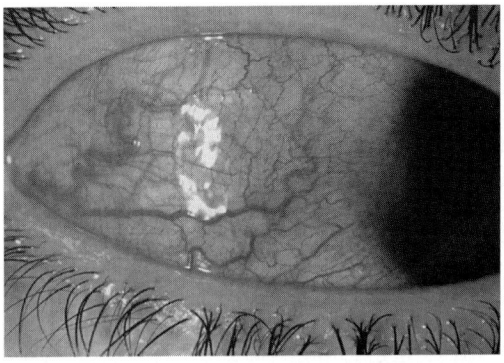

**Fig. 8-15.** Practitioner must always reevaluate therapeutic approach if no response or worsening of condition is seen. This patient was treated with high doses of immunosuppressive agents for scleritis. Therapy worsened the condition. Patient had a large ringlike toxoplasmosis lesion in retinal periphery, which was severe enough to cause secondary scleritis. Appropriate therapy led to disappearance of the lesion.

that cyclosporine G appeared to more effectively reduce or eradicate cystoid edema than did cyclosporine, although the relatively small number of patients prevented a definitive answer.[83] It would then seem that a lower dose of G could be as effective as a higher dose of A, thus decreasing the risk of nephrotoxicity.

## FK506

MODE OF ACTION. FK506, which is an immunosuppressive agent with a molecular weight of 822, was isolated from the broth of *Streptomyces tsukubaensis*[84,85] (Fig. 8-16). It is an agent

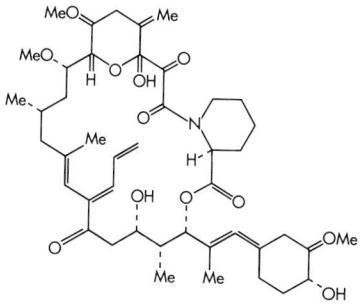


**Fig. 8-16.** Structure of FK506. (From Schreiber SL, Crabtree GR: The mechanism of action of cyclosporine A and FK506, *Immunol Today* 13:136, 1992.)

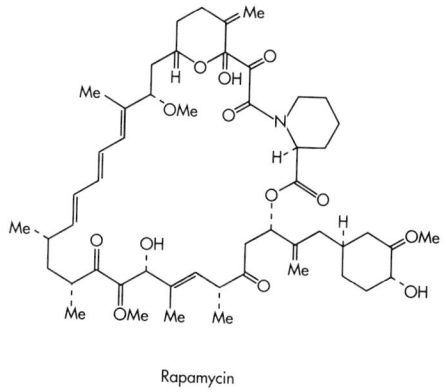


**Fig. 8-17.** Structure of rapamycin. (From Schreiber SL, Crabtree GR: The mechanism of action of cyclosporine A and FK506, *Immunol Today* 13:136, 1992.)

that is believed to have essentially the same mechanism of action as cyclosporine.[55] One difference is that the immunophilin that binds with FK506 is FKBP instead of cyclophilin. It suppresses the formation of mRNA for IL-2, as does cyclosporine, but at an effective in vitro therapeutic concentration of about 100 times less than that of cyclosporine.[86] With use of a dose of 10 to 30 times less than cyclosporine, FK506 was found to be effective in preventing the development of experimental autoimmune uveitis in rats,[87] as well as in monkeys.[88] However, the toxic effects (see later discussion) are seen at therapeutic doses, so that the decreased therapeutic dosage appears to have little benefit.

INDICATIONS AND DOSAGES. An open label clinical trial to evaluate the use of FK506 has been performed in Japan; 53 patients (most with Behçet's disease) were treated at varying doses. About three quarters of patients were thought to have benefited from this therapy.[89] A review of patients with Behçet's disease alone[90] confirmed these initial observations. A daily dosage of 0.10 to 0.15 mg/kg body weight/day has been suggested as an appropriate dosage. This drug has not been as yet widely used in the United States for uveitis, and only anecdotal reports have appeared, making it difficult to fully evaluate its usefulness in this country.

SECONDARY EFFECTS. With essentially the same mechanism of action as cyclosporine, one might assume similar secondary effects. Adverse affects include renal impairment, noted in 28% of patients reported by Mochizuki and colleagues.[89] Neurologic symptoms, including tremors, headache, ophthalmoplegia, and meningitis-like symptoms, have been noted. Gastrointestinal symptoms, usually manifested as nausea, loss of appetite, and abdominal pain, can occur. Hyperglycemia was reported by Mochizuki and colleagues to have occurred in 13% of patients.[89] In a recent report comparing the nephrotoxic effects of FK506 and cyclosporine in liver transplant recipients,[91] the early development of severe nephrotoxicity was noted only in some patients receiving FK506.[91]

## Rapamycin

MODE OF ACTION. Rapamycin is a macrolide immunosuppressant purified from isolates of *Streptomyces hygroscopicus* collected on Rapa Nui (Easter Island).[92] It blocks the proliferative signals of transduction in T cells[93,94] (Fig. 8-17). This blockage has been shown to prevent the expression of IL-2, Il-4, and IL-6. Of great interest and potential therapeutic importance are that rapamycin's effect occurs much later in the cell cycle ($G_1$ S-phase transition) than either cyclosporine or FK506. Rapamycin appears not to inhibit the expression of IL-2 receptors and IL-2 production, but it may interfere with the cell's ability to respond to interleukins, such as IL-2 and IL-4.[95,96] Rapamycin is bound in the cytoplasm to the same immunophilin as FK506 (FKBP), and therefore these two agents will competitively inhibit each other if placed in the same environment.

INDICATIONS AND DOSAGES. Rapamycin has not yet been used in patients with uveitis. At the moment it needs to be given intravenously, which would be a limiting factor. Rapamycin has been shown to be very effective in inhibiting the induction of experimental autoimmune uveitis (EAU) in Lewis rats[97] and to completely inhibit transfer of EAU[98] at a dosage of 0.1 mg/kg/day given as a continuous intravenous infusion. Studies have shown that cyclosporine and rapamycin may have a synergistic effect in vitro on T lymphocytes.[99] The combination of cyclosporine 2 mg/kg/day (one fifth the normal dose) plus intravenously administered rapamycin, 0.01 mg/kg/day (one tenth the normal therapeutic dose), will act synergistically to prevent the expression of EAU.[100]

**Toxicity.** Testing of rapamycin in humans is at an early phase. Animals have been reported to lose weight at a therapeutic dosage of 0.1 mg/kg/day.[94] Of concern have been reports of myocardial toxicity in rats,[101] occurring, however, at relatively high doses of the drug. Gastrointestinal vasculitis has been noted in dogs.[102] It is hoped that with combination rapamycin and cyclosporine therapy the markedly lowered doses may provide adequate immunosuppression with minimal or no risk of toxicity.

### Mycophenolate mofetil

Mycophenolate mofetil is a new immunosuppressive agent that has been used in humans. It has a molecular weight of 433.5. It metabolizes to MPA, which reversibly inhibits inosine monophosphate dehydrogenase, inhibiting a pathway of guanosine nucleotide synthesis without incorporation into DNA. In animal models mycophenolate mofetil has prolonged the survival of allogeneic transplants. It has been used in humans in combination with corticosteroids and cyclosporine for the prevention of organ rejection following allogeneic renal transplants. This agent has been used in preventing the expression of EAU (30 mg/kg/day) and even after immunization, but at higher dosages (60 mg/kg/day).[102a] It could be an alternative steroid/cyclosporine–sparing therapy for patients taking immunosuppressive drugs for uveitis.

### Monoclonal antibody therapy

Anti–T cell and antireceptor monoclonal antibodies have not yet been used in the treatment of human uveitis. However, such antibodies have been used for some time in other areas of medicine. Anti–T cell monoclonal antibodies, such as OKT3, have been recognized as effective immunosuppressive agents.[103] Their use in renal graft rejection has become well established.[104] Many regimens for the prevention of graft rejection call for OKT3 monoclonal antibody therapy, then followed by other immunosuppressive therapy. It was reported that two patients who underwent renal transplantation suffered marked visual loss after OKT3 therapy.[105] In the one patient tested, results of the electroretinogram (ERG) were flat.

Recently other antibodies, directed against specific receptors to lymphokines on T cells, have been developed and evaluated. One of the prime targets for such therapy has been the IL-2/IL-2 receptor complex. The 55-kd Tac subunit is expressed on T and B cells after lymphokine or antigen activation. Monoclonal antibodies directed against the 55-kd Tac subunit have been developed. These anti-Tac antibodies have been reported to be effective in prolonging allograft survival in monkeys and humans[106,107] and in decreasing incidence of graft-versus-host disease in humans.[108] Initial problems dealt with immune reactions against a foreign protein (i.e., mouse-produced antibody), but technology now has permitted these antibodies to be "humanized," so that they essentially are not recognized as "foreign."[109] Recently a mouse monoclonal antibody directed against the beta subunit of the IL-2 receptor has been developed. This Mikβ1 antibody, now humanized, appears to act synergistically with the humanized anti-Tac antibody.[110] Initial experiments with these humanized antibodies in uveitis induced in subhuman primates appear very promising (François Roberge, M.D., manuscript in preparation, 1995) and may provide a new approach to therapy in the future.

Adhesion molecules (see Chapter 2) are an area of great interest both for the basic researcher and those interested in interventional studies. Injections of anti–Mac-1 antibodies have been shown to inhibit endotoxin-induced uveitis.[111] In using several models of ocular inflammation, Rosenbaum and Boney[112] demonstrated that the time of administration was important. Whitcup and coworkers[113] have shown that monoclonal antibodies directed against intercellular adhesion molecule–1 (ICAM-1) and lymphocyte function-associated molecule–1 (LFA-1) inhibited EAU. Antibodies against ICAM are being used to prevent allograft rejection and to treat rheumatoid arthritis in humans.

### Oral tolerance

Oral tolerance is an approach that has received much clinical interest recently. A discussion of some of the basic mechanisms leading to the clinical application mentioned here can be found in Chapter 2. Feeding of antigens has been reported to be effective in the treatment of multiple sclerosis and rheumatoid arthritis.[114,115] A pilot study applied this approach to two patients with uveitis, one with pars planitis and one with the ocular complications of Behçet's disease.[116] The patients who entered into this pilot study had lymphocytes demonstrating in vitro proliferative responses to the retinal S-antigen. The patient with pars planitis had been treated with prednisone and was able to stop his medication completely once beginning the feeding with 30 mg of S-antigen three times a week. Of interest is the fact that because of the maintenance of good visual acuity with the feeding, continued oral dosing of the retinal S-antigen was stopped, with the hope that long-standing tolerance had been accomplished. However, the patient suffered a reactivation of his disease (Fig. 8-18). He was treated with systemic steroids and begun again on S-antigen feedings; he continues to be maintained on this regimen to date, without conventional immunosuppressive agents, and with a visual acuity of 20/20, 20/25 in each eye.

A randomized masked trial is currently underway to gain more information about this important mode of therapy. It could ultimately be helpful in at least two respects. The first is

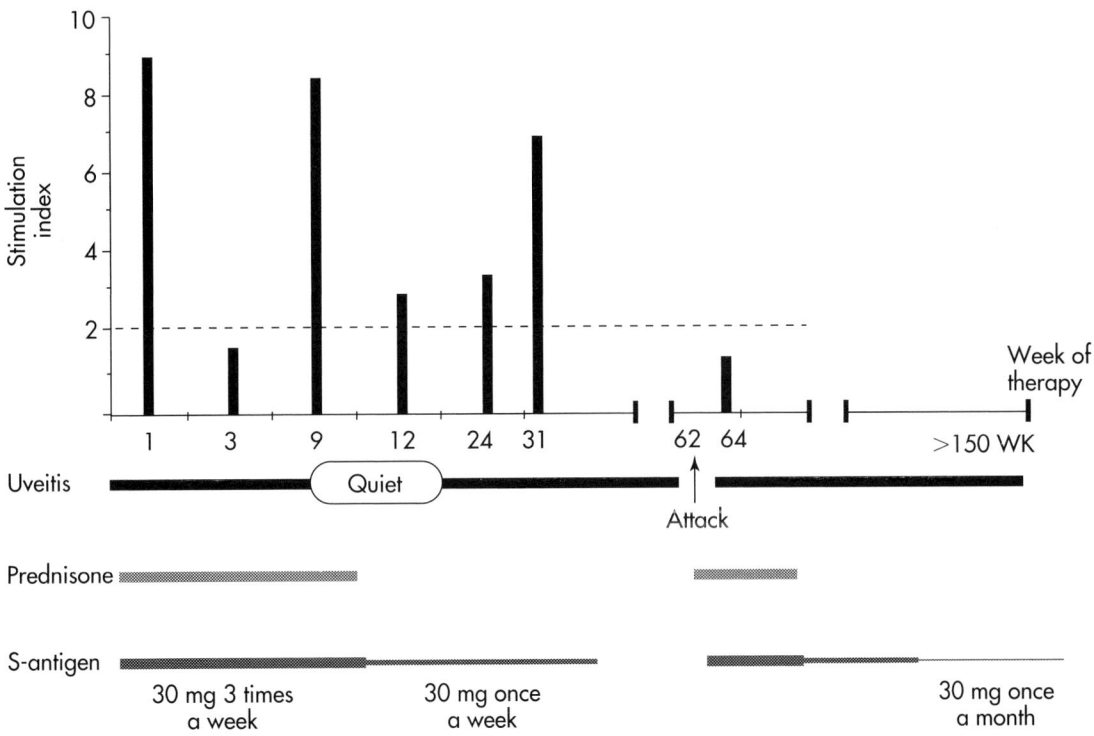


**Fig. 8-18.** Flow sheet of various clinical and immunologic parameters of patient with pars planitis discussed in text. This patient was given bovine retinal S-antigen orally in attempt to induce tolerance. Feeding began while he was taking prednisone. Prednisone was slowly tapered and then stopped while he continued taking S-antigen by mouth, ultimately once a week. He was without prednisone and without ocular activity for such an extended period that the feeding was stopped; recurrence of his ocular disease developed. Treatment with prednisone was then restarted, as was feeding, and he has remained free of ocular disease on a prednisone-free regimen to date, for 3 years, taking S-antigen only once a month. It is interesting to note that his peripheral lymphocytes' proliferative responses appear to be sensitive to changes in dose of immunosuppressive agent and to his taking retinal S-antigen by mouth. His vision is 20/20, 20/25. (For an excellent review, see Weiner HL: Oral tolerance, *Proc Natl Acad Sci USA* 91:10762-10765, 1994.)

to determine if this form of therapy is adequate as a sole therapeutic approach. The second is the possibility that it could be an immunosuppressant-sparing tool, permitting lower amounts of standard therapy to adequately control the intraocular inflammatory response.

### Antiviral therapy

It seems appropriate to mention the more frequently utilized agents for severe intraocular inflammatory disease due to virus. Perhaps in part pushed by the AIDS epidemic, the development of new antiviral agents, particularly against the herpes family, has been most impressive. It underlines the increasing importance of better diagnostic testing to rapidly identify the invading virus, which is still sometimes difficult to do and often based on clinical impression. The importance of quick and precise diagnosis will take on an even greater imperative as the armamentarium against these organisms continues to increase and become more specific.

**Acyclovir.** The development of acyclovir as an effective antiviral agent stems from the increased understanding of how the herpes family of viruses enters a cell and usurps the cell's control over itself. Nucleosides are needed for the building of new DNA. Nucleosides and acyclovir (Fig. 8-19) must be triphosphorylated to be incorporated into a DNA chain. These reactions are mediated by kinases. The diphosphate and triphosphate forms of the nucleoside and acyclovir are mediated through cellular kinases, but the initial phosphorylation of acyclovir is mediated through a kinase (thymidine kinase) specified by the herpesvirus gene. This enzyme is found only in infected cells. The human cellular kinase phosphorylates acyclovir to a very minimal degree, and therefore the drug is most active in those cells that are infected. Acyclovir will take its place in the growing DNA chain, but unlike the nucleoside, it lacks a sugar of its own, and therefore the DNA chain is terminated at this point. In addition, the DNA polymerase is bound at this point and unable to be used elsewhere. Although acyclovir is highly effective against herpes simplex virus, it is known that herpesviruses can develop drug resistance through mutational changes in the viral DNA polymerase, making acyclovir triphosphate a poorer substrate. Further, some viruses may mutate and develop a different type of thymidine kinase. In a similar fashion, acyclovir is a very poor substrate for the kinase elaborated by cytomegalovirus. Ganciclovir, di-hydroxypropoxymethylguanine (see Fig. 8-19), a molecule that closely resembles acyclovir is, however, very effective against this member of the herpes family (see later discussion).

For documented herpes simplex or zoster infections, the drug that is currently recommended for immunocompetent patients is acyclovir. The drug can initially be given intravenously to obtain high tissue levels. The initial dosage is 5 mg/kg every 8 hours for a patient with a normal serum creatinine level. Renal function should be followed up, and the dosage should be adjusted accordingly. Acyclovir can be given orally as well, but its oral absorption is not especially good. For herpes simplex infections, the dosage by mouth is recommended as 200 mg five times a day. For herpes zoster,

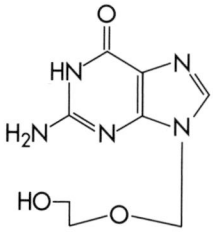


Acyclovir

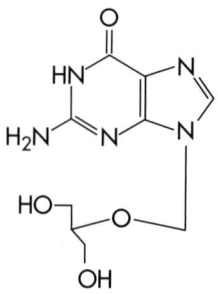


DHPG

**Fig. 8-19.** Structure of acyclovir and ganciclovir (DHPG). Minimal change in structure of ganciclovir permits it to be considerably more effective against cytomegalovirus infections.

higher concentrations of the drug are needed and four tablets (800 mg) taken five times a day is recommended. Intravenous acyclovir can suppress renal function, and hydration should be well maintained. Oral acyclovir is usually well tolerated with few significant side effects.

**Ganciclovir.** Ganciclovir is similar to acyclovir but is a much more effective substrate for cytomegalovirus (CMV). It has been shown to be effective in the treatment of CMV retinitis.[117] Generally, for the induction phase of therapy, an initial intravenous dosage of 5 mg/kg every 12 hours is given for 14 or 21 days (see Table 8-2). Because patients usually are wedded to this therapy once it has begun, an indwelling catheter (i.e., Hickman catheter) is placed to facilitate administration. The administration time is fairly long, and this therapy has an impact on the patient's quality of life. It is not frequently nephrotoxic, but like acyclovir, it is excreted by the kidneys and the dose should be adjusted for renal function. Bone marrow depression is problematic if patients are taking antiretroviral agents, such as azidothymidine (AZT), with similar toxicity. Ganciclovir causes significant granulocytopenia, and the dose must be decreased or stopped to keep the absolute granulocyte count above 500 to 1000/$mm^3$ or granulocyte stimulating factors can be given. Ganciclovir may have significant testicular toxicity, but this has not yet been studied in humans. After the induction period, a maintenance dosage of ganciclovir is given, usually 10 mg/kg/day, adjusted to any renal pathology.

Intravitreal injections of ganciclovir are effective in delaying the progression of CMV retinitis.[118] The injections are initially given twice a week and then weekly. There is an associated risk of endophthalmitis, retinal detachment, and vitreous hemorrhage.[119] An intraocular slow-release device for ganciclovir has been developed[120] (Fig. 8-20). Two rates of release have been developed, a 2-μg/hr device ( with an approximate life span of 4 months) and a 1 μg/hr device (with an approximate life span of 8 months). The 2 μg/hr device was evaluated in a consecutive case series and was shown to halt CMV progression in 27 patients, or 90% of the 30 eyes into which it was implanted.[121] A randomized controlled trial evaluating the 1 μg/hr device showed efficacy in a study of 26 (30 eyes) patients.[122] In that study the median time to progression of CMV retinitis in eyes with the device was 226 days; 12 implants were exchanged for new devices. A final visual acuity of 20/25 or better was obtained in 34 of 39 eyes. The estimated risk of developing CMV in the contralateral eye was 50% over the course of the study, and systemic CMV was documented in 31% of these patients who were not receiving systemic antiviral therapy. Of note was that in the patient group studied, seven late retinal detachments and one retinal tear without detachment occurred. Future studies will certainly deal with the retinal detachment risk and the use of the device in conjunction with oral systemic medications for the prophylactic treatment of patients with CMV infection, either viscerally or in the contralateral eye. The use of local therapy clearly benefits the patient's quality of life, because the hours of intravenous infusion previously needed are avoided. However, the lack of systemic coverage and the possible adverse effects still need to be examined.

An oral form of ganciclovir has been developed,[123] and it has been shown recently to impede the development of CMV retinitis.[124]

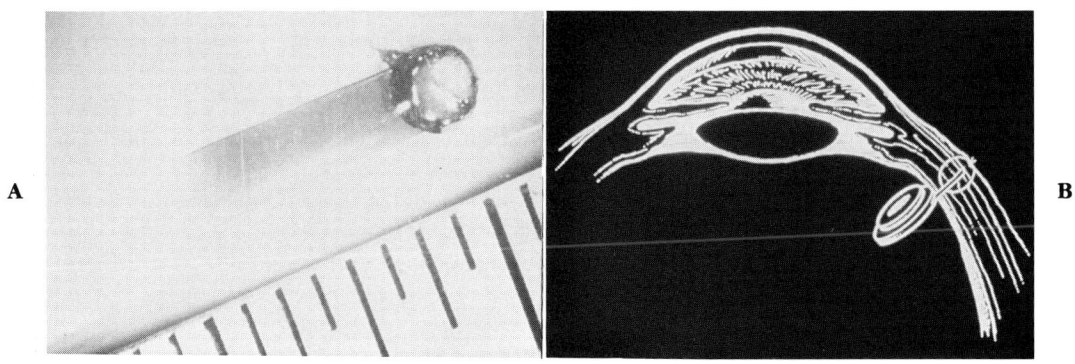


**Fig. 8-20. A,** Intraocular device used for delivery of ganciclovir. **B,** Position in vitreous after suturing into sclera at pars plana level. (Courtesy Chiron Corp.) (See Color Plate 7.)

This potentially will have an important effect on future therapeutic strategies for the treatment of CMV retinitis.

**Foscarnet.** Foscarnet (trisodium phosphonoformate) is a pyrophosphate analogue which has been shown to be effective in the initial treatment of CMV infection, as well as other herpes family viruses, in those patients undergoing renal and bone marrow transplantation.[125] Although effective, foscarnet-resistant herpes simplex viruses already have been reported.[126] Foscarnet is also effective against the human immunodeficiency virus when added to infected cultures.[127] Initially, a continuous intravenous infusion was used in treating CMV infections,[128,129] but now patients start with induction doses that are given twice daily, and then a maintenance dose is given once a day[130] (see Table 8-2). In a randomized comparative trial, retinitis progression occurred after 13 weeks with immediate foscarnet therapy as opposed to 3.2 weeks among those receiving no treatment.[131] As with ganciclovir, the drug is generally administered through an indwelling central line. In a study comparing the efficacy of ganciclovir versus foscarnet, the two drugs appeared to be equivalent in controlling CMV retinitis and visual acuity.[132] However, this study found that there was a longer survival among the patients receiving foscarnet as opposed to ganciclovir (12.6 months as opposed to 8.5 months).[133] Foscarnet has been shown to be a useful salvage therapy in patients with CMV retinitis who are intolerant or whose disease is resistant to ganciclovir.[134] Foscarnet has an associated nephrotoxicity, as well as metabolite alterations, that requires constant surveillance with eventual dosage reduction. Foscarnet has been licensed by the Food and Drug Administration (FDA) for the treatment of CMV retinitis.

Alternate means of administering foscarnet have been reported. Gumbel and coworkers[135] have reported the use of liposome-encapsulated foscarnet, and Sarraf and colleagues have used transscleral iontophoresis to deliver foscarnet into the rabbit eye.[136] The evaluation of intravitreal injections of foscarnet into rabbit eyes showed that intermittent injections appeared not to induce retinopathy.[137,138] Diaz-Llopis and colleagues[139] injected foscarnet (in a dose of 2400 μg) into the vitreous of 11 patients (15 eyes). Eight eyes had active CMV retinitis, with the rest in a quiescent stage of disease. These eyes received biweekly injections over a 3-week induction period, which was followed by weekly injections, as did the other eyes that were in a quiescent stage of disease. A total of 304 injections were given with a mean follow-up period of 16 weeks, and all cases appeared to respond therapeutically in the time period of the study.

**Combined ganciclovir and foscarnet.** This approach to therapy is one that is being used more and more, particularly as patient survival lengthens and the possibility of viral resistance increases. Jacobson and coworkers[140] evaluated this approach in 29 patients with AIDS and found that combination therapy appeared to provide better in vivo antiviral activity in suppressing CMV replication than did monotherapy. Weinberg and colleagues[141] treated seven patients (nine eyes) with combination therapy. All of these patients demonstrated progression of their retinitis on a monotherapy regimen, and many were intolerant to the induction doses usually given. The authors found that combination therapy was fairly well tolerated and that it prolonged the interval to progression. A recent Studies of Ocular Complications of AIDS (SOCA) randomized study[142] found that the time to progression in the group receiving combination therapy was statistically significantly longer than the time to progression seen in patients receiving either foscarnet or ganciclovir.

**HPMPC.** 1-(S)-[3-Hydroxy-2-(phosphonylmethoxy)propyl] cytosine dihydrate, known as *HPMPC* or Cidofovir, is a nucleotide analogue that has a broad spectrum against herpesvirus. The intracellular metabolite of HPMPC inhibits DNA polymerases from herpes viruses at a 50-fold lower concentration than that needed to inhibit human alpha DNA polymerase. It is of great interest as well because of the active metabolite's very long half-life, 30 hours.[143,144] HPMPC has been shown to have good anti-CMV activity, with a median infective dose ($ID_{50}$) for murine CMV of 0.02 μg/ml, as compared with 0.3 μg/ml for ganciclovir. Critical studies to look at the potential use of HPMPC as an anti-CMV retinitis agent have just begun. The optimal dosing schedule still needs to be developed, but most approaches use a dosage of 2.5 to 5.0 mg/kg/wk with probenecid (2-4 g total) administered at the same time. Nephrotoxicity, which appears to be dose dependent, is a major concern in the use of this drug. The concomitant dosing with probenecid is believed to prevent nephrotoxicity. The use of probenecid and good hydration, coupled with less frequent HPMPC dosing, may substantially reduce the incidence of the HPMPC-related nephrotoxicity.[145] Work in rats has shown that the drug may be carcinogenic, and patients have been apprised of these side effects. It is not clear, however, whether this presents a serious risk to humans. More definitive clinical trials to show drug efficacy and the full extent of toxicity are in progress. Work is also ongoing in the area of intravitreal instillation of HPMPC. Because of its long half-life, HPMPC would have the advantage (if is were proved effective) of needing less frequent administration than ganciclovir.

• • •

In summary, in immunocompetent persons, acyclovir remains the treatment of choice for infections caused by the herpesvirus family. However, this agent is, at best, weakly effective against CMV infections, including retinitis. Clearly, now the treating physician and the patient have some options. At present, most patients with CMV retinitis begin therapy with systemic ganciclovir rather than foscarnet, in spite of a randomized study to show that patients have a longer survival with the latter. The reasons for this are complex, but they include the facts that increased intravenous hydration is needed to prevent foscarnet-induced renal toxicity, that most physicians still have more experience with ganciclovir, that foscarnet requires more monitoring, and that patient complaints are more frequent with foscarnet, a problem that may reflect the treating physician's lack of experience with the drug. Patients respond differently to these medications, and some trial and error is sometimes unavoidable. Colony-stimulating factor to boost granulocyte production and generally overcome bone marrow toxicity helps in the use of ganciclovir at adequate dosages while antiretroviral therapy is continued. Both drugs still require a central line placement if patients are to receive these medications over any length of time, and these infusions must have a profound effect on patients' quality of life.

Several new factors need to be added into the equation. The first is the finding that combination therapy significantly prolongs progression of retinitis when compared with monotherapy. It may be that this will become the better alternative, but only further studies will tell the impact of very long infusion times on the quality of life of these patients.

Several other important factors need to be considered, including the introduction of sustained-release devices that deliver ganciclovir at a rate that provides therapeutic doses to the eye for up to 8 months. This approach, in our experience, has a profoundly positive effect on the life-style of patients. Avoiding the need for daily infusions of drug has been important for these patients. There is of course a tradeoff. There is a risk of late retinal detachment in the eye receiving an implant, and these patients are not being covered therapeutically for the prevention of CMV infection elsewhere, as in the contralateral eye. The use of oral ganciclovir (and other oral anti-CMV agents that may be developed) may be one alternative therapy that could be coupled with the local device. Other alternatives are systemic therapies that could be given once a week or less frequently. Such possibilities (but still to be shown) would include humanized anti-CMV antibodies and HPMPC. Finally, newer technologies, such as the use of antisense therapies, may be logical and powerful additions. It is clear that this area is developing quickly and that more effective therapies that improve the quality of life of our patients is an ongoing mission.

## Sorivudine

Sorivudine, also known as BV-ara-U, is an arabinofuranosyuracil analog. It is phosphorylated by both viral and cellular thymidine kinases to a form that inhibits varicella-zoster DNA synthesis. It is 1000 times more potent than acyclovir for zoster, similar to acyclovir's effect on type 1 herpes simplex, and poor for type 2. It is not effective for CMV infection. Pinnolis and coworkers[145a] have reported the effectiveness of this drug in the treatment of PORN.

## Colchicine

MODE OF ACTION. Colchicine, or acetyltrimethylcolchicinic acid, has poorly understood antiinflammatory characteristics. Colchicine suppresses lactic acid production in leukocytes and decreases phagocytosis. In addition, it decreases polymorphonuclear cell migration.

INDICATIONS AND DOSAGES. Heightened polymorphonuclear cell migration is a characteristic of patients with Behçet's disease (see Chapter 25) and may be a cause of the repeated ocular attacks seen in that disorder. Colchicine has been used in the treatment of Behçet's disease. It should be stressed that this agent is not employed to treat the active inflammatory condition but rather is used prophylactically in the person with multiple ocular attacks in order to decrease the frequency of these attacks, which can lead to blindness. This approach has not met with universal approval, being a more popular therapeutic mode in Japan than in other countries with a high incidence of this disease, such as Turkey. Many believe that this agent is not effective in treating white patients. Use of this agent might be considered in those fairly rare patients with Behçet's disease who have unilateral involvement and in whom one may not feel fully justified in starting more powerful immunosuppressive agents. The average dose of oral colchicine is 0.6 mg twice daily. Some clinicians have suggested that higher dosages may be helpful, but this is based on anecdotal information. Its effect on Behçet's disease has been at best marginal in our hands.

SECONDARY EFFECTS. Gastrointestinal reactions such as abdominal pain, diarrhea, nausea, and vomiting are quite common. Prolonged administration may cause bone marrow depression, with thrombocytopenia and aplastic anemia. Colchicine is contraindicated in pregnant women because it can harm the fetus.

### Bromocriptine

MODE OF ACTION. The neuroendocrine axis has been implicated in playing a natural immunomodulatory role.[146] Of particular import has been the anterior pituitary hormone, prolactin. Alterations in the prolactin levels of experimental animals have resulted in measurable changes of the immune response. Hypophysectomized rats have a marked antibody depression and a delayed type of hypersensitvity reactions,[147] but the addition of exogenous prolactin will restore the immune response.[148] Of further interest is the observation that prolactin stimulates lymphocyte activation and that it appears to compete with cyclosporine on the lymphocyte's cell surface. Prolactin secretion can be suppressed by the dopamine agonist, bromocriptine. Bromocriptine administration can diminish graft-versus-host reactions in mice and given in combination with low-dose cyclosporine may provide as effective a therapeutic response as seen with higher cyclosporine levels alone. Indeed, we have reported the effective treatment of the S-antigen–induced experimental uveitis model with combination bromocriptine and low-dose cyclosporine—using a dosage of cyclosporine that alone would not afford protection to most of the animals treated.[149]

INDICATIONS AND DOSAGES. There are to date no well-established uveitic indications for bromocriptine. However, the reader should be aware of several observations. Hedner and Bynke[150] noted the potentially effective control of recurrent anterior uveitis with bromocriptine. Further, the use of bromocriptine as a "cyclosporine sparing" agent was evaluated; 10 mg of bromocriptine given with cyclosporine, 4 to 5 mg/kg/day, may prove to be an effective therapeutic combination.[79]

SECONDARY EFFECTS. Light-headedness, nausea, and vomiting are the major complications associated with bromocriptine administration. It is most important to begin therapy slowly, giving an initial half tablet at bedtime and then slowly increasing the dosage to avoid these annoying side effects. The profound decrease in prolactin levels does not seem to lead to demonstrable endocrinologic problems nor to an increased risk of infection.

### Mydriatic and cycloplegic agents

The use of mydriatic and cycloplegic agents is an important adjunct to antiinflammatory or immunosuppressive therapy. The major indication for the use of dilatory agents is the presence of a "significant" anterior chamber inflammatory response. In those cases the addition of mydriatics helps prevent the development of posterior synechiae and, in the extreme, iris bombé. Further, cycloplegia will make the patient more comfortable and helps ensure the treating physician an unhindered view of the media and fundus. We generally do not use long-term dilating agents, such as atropine, except postoperatively. The shorter-acting agents, such as tropicamide (Mydriacyl), helps keep the iris moving and therefore decreases the possibility of posterior synechiae. One medication possibly to be avoided in patients with uveitis is cyclopentolate (Cyclogyl) in as much as it has been shown to be an effective chemoattractant for leukocytes.[151] Therefore the addition of this medication to the therapeutic regimen may prove problematic.

### Antitoxoplasmosis therapy

The therapeutic approach to treating ocular toxoplasmosis ideally consists of a combination of medications. Sulfadiazine (or trisulfapyrimidines, a mixture of sulfadiazine, sulfamerazine, and sulfamethazine) prevents the conversion of paraaminobenzoic acid (PABA) to folic acid, which is needed for the carbon metabolism of the *Toxoplasma* organism, and in human beings it is particularly needed for erythropoiesis (Fig. 8-21). Pyrimethamine (Daraprim) blocks the conversion of folic acid to folinic acid. Combination therapy, consisting of these agents, has been found to be synergistic in the killing of the *Toxoplasma* organism. Sulfadiazine can be given as a 1 to 2 g loading dose, followed by 0.5 to 1 g given orally four times daily. This is given in conjunction with a loading dose of 50 to 75 mg of pyrimethamine, followed by 25 mg twice daily. The therapy should be given for 3 to 4 weeks. Folic acid–containing vitamins should be stopped during this treatment period. Because of the potential serious depression of erythropoiesis that can be a consequence of pyrimethamine therapy, leucovorin 3 to 5 mg is given orally or intramuscularly two or three times a week. We obtain a baseline white blood cell count with differential and a platelet count at baseline and weekly thereafter. We give the leucovorin for 1 week after stopping the pyrimethamine. If there is a decrease in the platelet count ($< 100{,}000/mm^3$) or the appearance of hypersegmented polymorphonuclear lymphocytes, we discontinue the pyrimethamine. Pyrimethamine crosses the blood-brain barrier and is also used in the treatment of congenital toxoplasmosis. Sulfadiazine availability was very limited in the United States, with clinicians needing to contact the Centers for Disease Control and Prevention in Atlanta, Georgia, for access. This situation has been remedied and the drug is now readily available.

Clindamycin has been shown to be effective in killing the *Toxoplasma* organism[152] and has the added advantage of being readily absorbed into ocular tissues. It can be used as a therapeutic substitute for pyrimethamine. Evidence suggests that a synergistic effect may be seen when clindamycin is combined with sulfadiazine.[153] We have used clindamycin 150 to 300 mg four times daily orally or subconjunctivally, combined with the aforementioned sulfadiazine regimen. We treat for 3 to 4 weeks. We have noted that a large number of patients have suffered enough gastrointestinal distress as a result of this medication to warrant a decrease in the dosage or discontinuation. A pseudomembranous colitis is a serious side effect to this medication. Clindamycin does not cross the blood-brain barrier and is not effective for the treatment of congenital toxoplasmosis or encephalitis due to this organism. It should be remembered that this agent has not received FDA approval for this specific indication.

A new medication that has received much attention is atovaquone (Mepron). This hydroxynaphthoquinone has potent antiprotozoal activity. It appears to uncouple mitochondrial electron transport and in doing so inhibits pyrimidine and nucleic acid synthesis in the cell. In one animal study,[154] atovaquone (50 mg/kg/day) given for 15 days significantly ex-

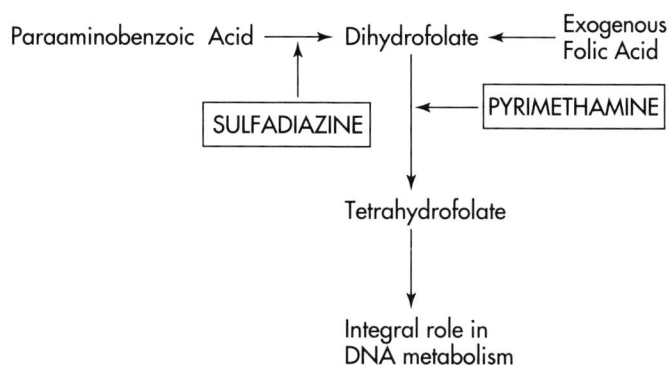


**Fig. 8-21.** Effects of sulfadiazine and pyrimethamine on carbon metabolism in *Toxoplasma* organism and in humans.

tended the life span of mice inoculated intraperitoneally with *Toxoplasma gondii* from 9 days to 26 days. Of great interest is the report of studies suggesting that the drug might have activity against *Toxoplasma* cysts,[155] which is of significant theoretic value because recurrences are thought to be due to the breaking down of cysts. Patients with AIDS suffering from toxoplasmic encephalitis have been treated with atovaquone.[156] The oral dose of atovaquone to date has been 750 mg four times daily. The medication seems to have been well tolerated, even when given concomitantly with AZT or ddI. In the main, most patients showed stabilization or improvement of their disease for at least some period. We had the opportunity to report the improvement of a toxoplasmic retinitis in a patient with AIDS after the initiation of atovaquone 750 mg four times daily.[157] Other patients with ocular toxoplasmosis (those with AIDS and immunocompetent patients) have now been treated in the United States as well as in France and Brazil. Patients appear to tolerate the medication well, and initial observations indicate a therapeutic effect. The major unanswered question is this medication's effect on the recurrence rate in this disease. If it effectively kills cysts, we presume that there would be a marked drop in the recurrence rate of ocular toxoplasmosis.

Other medications that have been used in the treatment of toxoplasmosis include minocycline, spiramycin, and sulfasoxazole. Minocycline positively alters the clinical course of animals infected with toxoplasmosis.[158] Spiramycin has been used with some success to treat human cases of ocular toxoplasmosis.[159] However, recurrences are very common. It is used in Latin America as a prophylactic agent because it is tolerated reasonably well; its prophylactic efficacy is yet to be evaluated, if indeed it is useful in such a role. Trimethoprim-sulfamethoxazole is perhaps less effective against the *Toxoplasma* organism than either sulfadiazine or trisulfapyrimidine but nonetheless has been used in the treatment of ocular toxoplasmosis.[160] Tetracycline can be considered in cases in which the more standard therapies cannot be used.

The use of corticosteroids as the sole therapeutic agent for toxoplasmosis is never indicated. However, there is a role for their judicious use in some cases in combination with antitoxoplasmosis therapy (see Chapter 14).

### Other therapeutic approaches

**Immunostimulators.** This therapeutic approach was quite popular several years ago for the treatment of endogenous uveitis. Levamisole was thought to boost immune responses and therefore might be useful in the treatment of uveitis. Others suggested the use of transfer factor, a leukocyte dialysate that was capable of transferring antigen-specific (such as purified protein derivative [PPD]) type IV hypersensitivity responses from a sensitized organism to a nonsensitized one. Transfer factor has been used to treat patients with cutaneous candidiasis. In uveitis the suggestion is that an exogenous factor to which the patient is unable to mount an immune response is causing the disease. All information to date suggests that patients with endogenous uveitis are fully immunocompetent, but rather there is a perturbation of their immunoregulatory system. One could frankly argue that the addition of an immunostimulatory agent may exacerbate the problem.

The role of immunostimulatory agents may, however, play an important role in the treatment of immunosuppressed patients, such as those with AIDS. Here immunostimulatory agents could theoretically be used in combination with specific antiviral drugs. The addition of colony-stimulating factors to the regimens of patients with AIDS has helped enormously because many medications, such as zidovudine, are bone-marrow toxic.

**Plasmapheresis.** The removal from the blood stream of toxic products is a concept that has its origin in the work performed by Abel and coworkers in 1914.[161] The first therapeutic success using plasmapharesis was for macroglobulinemia.[162] The rationale for this approach is that soluble products in the blood could be readily removed, and thus its use in diseases such as systemic lupus erythematosus, in which immune complexes were thought to play an important role in its pathogenesis, was tried. The exact mechanism still remains speculative. It is possible that even if humoral mechanisms are less important in the mechanism of intraocular inflammatory disease, this approach could remove cytokines important for the propagation or perpetuation of disease. The role in uveitis still is not clear. It has been reported as being effective in treating the acute attacks of Behçet's disease.[163] However, its continued use is unwieldy, and although initial success may be seen, a rebound of the disease may occur with time. Therefore, to maintain a more prolonged clinical effect, most studies have resorted to adding corticosteroids or cytotoxic agents.[162]

**Nonsteroidal antiinflammatory agents.** Prostaglandin inhibitors are agents well known to the ophthalmic community. They have been suggested as therapeutically helpful for various ocular conditions, including aphakic macular edema.[164] Some reports suggest that indomethacin decreases the severity and recurrences of anterior uveitis when used in conjunction with corticosteroids. Although isolated reports discuss the use of these agents in the treatment of uveitis,[165] they have not been demonstrated to be effective as sole agents in the treatment of endogenous intraocular inflammatory disease. Herbort,[166] however, has extensively looked at the use of diclofenac in the treatment of post-Nd:YAG capsulotomy inflammatory responses. He has reported that an effective therapeutic end point could be achieved with a combination of dexamethosone acetate 0.1% (Maxidex drops), diclofenac drops 0.1% (Voltaren-Ophtha), and systemic diclofenac (Voltaren). Diclofenac may be useful as a sole agent in treating postsurgical cataract inflammation.

• • •

***Caution:*** The drugs discussed in this chapter may have an important role in the treatment of various types of intraocular inflammatory disease. The reader should be reminded that not all of the drugs described here have been approved by the FDA for use in the treatment of uveitis. Others may be available under study protocols. It is the practitioner's duty to inquire as to the status of any medication and how the drug can be used within an accepted framework.

## REFERENCES


1. Whitcup SM, Nussenblatt RB: Treatment of autoimmune uveitis, *Ann NY Acad Sci* 696:307-318, 1993.
2. Wen S, Gao R, Hu Z: Comparison of Chinese traditional therapy combined with Western medicine and Western medicine alone in the treatment of uveitis, *Yen Ko Hsueh Pao* 7:205-208, 1991.
3. Gordon DM: Prednisone and prednisolone in ocular disease, *Am J Ophthalmol* 41:593-600, 1956.
4. Hench PS, Kendall EC, Slocumb CH et al: The effect of a hormone of the adrenal cortex (17-hydroxy-11-dehyrocorticosterone: compound E) and of pituitary adrenocorticotropic hormone on rheumatoid arthritis, *Proc Staff Meet Mayo Clinic* 24:181-197, 1949.
5. Clamen HN: Anti-inflammatory effects of corticosteroids, *Clin Immunol Allergy* 4:317-329, 1984.
6. Fauci AS: Clinical aspects of immunosuppression: use of cytotoxic agents and corticosteroids. In Bellanti JA, editor: *Immunology,* vol 2, Philadelphia, 1978, WB Saunders.
7. Schlaegel TF Jr: *Essentials of uveitis,* Boston, 1969, Little, Brown & Co.
8. Freeman WR, Green RL, Smith RE: Echographic localization of corticosteroids after periocular injection, *Am J Ophthalmol* 103:281-288, 1987.

8a. Smith RE, Nozik RA: *Uveitis: a clinical approach to diagnosis and management,* ed 2, Baltimore, 1989, Williams & Wilkins.

9. Fauci AS: Alternate-day corticosteroid therapy, *Am J Med* 64:729-731, 1978.
10. Fujikawa LS, Meisler DM, Nozik RA: Hyperosmolar hyperglycemic nonketotic coma: a complication of short-term systemic corticosteroids, *Ophthalmology* 90:1239-1242, 1983.
11. Wakakura M, Ishikawa S: Central serous chorioretinopathy complicating systemic corticosteroid treatment, *Br J Ophthalmol* 68:329-331, 1984.
12. Hemady R, Tauber J, Foster CS: Immunosuppressive drugs in immune and inflammatory ocular disease, *Surv Ophthalmol* 35:369-385, 1991.
13. Cash JM, Klippel JH: Second-line drug therapy for rheumatoid arthritis, *N Engl J Med* 330:1368-1375, 1994.
14. Dorr RT, Fritz WL: *Cancer chemotherapy handbook,* New York, 1980, Elsevier.
15. Buckley CE III, Gills JP Jr: Cyclophosphamide therapy of peripheral uveitis, *Arch Intern Med* 124:29-35, 1969.
16. Mamo JG, Azzam SA: Treatment of Behçet's disease with chlorambucil, *Arch Ophthalmol* 84:446-450, 1970.
17. Hoffman GS, Leavitt RY, Fleisher TA et al: Treatment of Wegener's granulomatosis with intermittent high-dose intravenous cyclophosphamide, *Am J Med* 89: 403-410, 1990.
18. Rosenbaum JT: Treatment of severe refractory uveitis with intravenous cyclophosphamide, *J Rheumatol* 21:123-125, 1994.
19. Godfrey WA, Epstein WV, O'Connor GR et al: The use of chlorambucil in intractable idiopathic uveitis, *Am J Ophthalmol* 78:415-428, 1974.
20. Tessler HH, Jennings T: High-dose short-term chlorambucil for intractable sympathetic ophthalmia and Behçet's disease, *Br J Ophthalmol* 74:353-357, 1990.
21. Nashel DJ: Mechanisms of action and clinical applications of cytotoxic drugs in rheumatic disorders, *Med Clin North Am* 69:817-840, 1985.
22. DeFronzo RA, Braine H, Colvin OM et al: Water intoxication in man after cyclophosphamide therapy, *Ann Intern Med* 78:861-869, 1973.
23. Kende G, Sirkin SR, Thomas PRM et al: Blurring of vision: a previously undescribed complication of cyclophosphamide therapy, *Cancer* 44:69-71, 1979.
24. Reeves BR, Casey G, Harris H et al: Long-term cytogenetic follow-up study of patients with uveitis treated with chlorambucil, *Carcinogenesis* 1615-1619, 1985.

25. Hoffman GS, Kerr GS, Leavitt RY et al: Wegener's granulomatosis: an analysis of 158 patients, *Ann Intern Med* 116:488-498, 1992.
26. Urowitz MB, Hunter T, Bookman AAM et al: Azathioprine in rheumatoid arthritis: a double-blind study comparing full dose to half dose, *J Rheumatol* 1:274-281, 1974.
27. Woodland J, Chaput-de-Saintonge DM, Evans SJ et al: Azathioprine in rheumatoid arthritis: double-blind study of full versus half doses versus placebo, *Ann Rheum Dis* 40:355-359, 1981.
28. O'Reilly TJ: Azathioprine in the treatment of refractory rheumatoid arthritis, *Ir Med J* 70:344-346, 1977.
29. Andrasch RH, Pirofsky B, Burns RP: Immunosuppressive therapy for severe chronic uveitis, *Arch Ophthalmol* 96:247-251, 1978.
30. Newell FW, Krill AE, Thomson A: The treatment of uveitis with 6-mercaptopurine, *Am J Ophthalmol* 61:1250-1255, 1966.
31. Aoki K, Sugiura S: Immunosuppressive treatment of Behçet's disease, *Mod Probl Ophthalmol* 16:309-313, 1976.
32. Yazici H, Pazarli H, Barnes CG et al: A controlled trial of azathioprine in Behçet's syndrome, *N Engl J Med* 322:281-285, 1990.
33. Hooper PL, Kaplan HJ: Triple agent immunosuppression in serpiginous choroiditis, *Ophthalmology* 98: 944-950, 1991.
34. Connell WR, Kamm MA, Dickson M et al: Long-term neoplasia risk after azathioprine treatment in inflammatory bowel disease, *Lancet* 343:1249-1252, 1994.
35. Cronstein BN: Molecular mechanism of methotrexate action in inflammation, *Inflammation* 16:411-423, 1992.
36. Sperling RI, Benincaso AI, Anderson RJ et al: Acute and chronic suppression of leukotriene $B_4$ synthesis ex vivo in neutrophils from patients with rheumatoid arthritis beginning treatment with methotrexate, *Arthritis Rheum* 35:376-384, 1992.
37. Thomas R, Carroll GJ: Reduction of leukocyte and interleukin-1 beta concentrations in the synovial fluid of rheumatoid arthritis patients treated with methotrexate, *Arthritis Rheum* 36:1244-1254, 1993.
38. Olsen NJ, Murray LM: Antiproliferative effects of methotrexate on peripheral blood mononuclear cells, *Arthritis Rheum* 32:378-385, 1989.
39. Wong VG: Immunosuppressive therapy of ocular inflammatory diseases, *Arch Ophthalmol* 81:628-637, 1969.
40. Holz FG, Krastel H, Breitbart A et al: Low-dose methotrexate treatment in noninfectious uveitis resistant to corticosteroids, *Ger J Ophthalmol* 1:142-144, 1992.
41. Shah SS, Lowder CY, Schmitt MA et al: Low-dose methotrexate therapy for ocular inflammatory disease, *Ophthalmology* 99:1419-1423, 1992.
42. Rootman J, Gudauskas G: Treatment of ocular leukemia with local chemotherapy, *Cancer Treat Rep* 69:119-122, 1985.
43. Rothenberg SP, Iqbal MP, da Costa M: Effect of folate compounds on the accumulation of methotrexate and the activity of dihydrofolate reductase in liver, kidney, and small intestine of the mouse, *J Pharmacol Exp Ther* 223:631-634, 1982.
44. Furst DE, Erikson N, Clute L et al: Adverse experience with methotrexate during 176 weeks of a long-term prospective trial in patients with rheumatoid arthritis, *J Rheumatol* 17:1628-1635, 1990.
45. Zachariae H, Kragballe K, Søgaard H: Methotrexate induced liver cirrhosis: studies including serial liver biopsies during continued treatment, *Br J Dermatol* 102:407-412, 1980.
46. Hargreaves MR, Mowat AG, Benson MK: Acute pneumonitis associated with low dose methotrexate treatment for rheumatoid arthritis: report of five cases and review of published reports, *Thorax* 47:628-633, 1992.
47. Carroll GJ, Thomas R, Phatouras CC et al: Incidence, prevalence and possible risk factors for pneumonitis in patients with rheumatoid arthritis receiving methotrexate, *J Rheumatol* 21:51-54, 1994.
48. Doroshow JH, Locker GY, Gaasterland DE et al: Ocular irritation from high-dose methotrexate therapy: pharmacokinetics of drug in the tear film, *Cancer* 48:2158-2162, 1981.
49. Zimmer-Galler I, Lie JT: Choroidal infiltrates as the initial manifestations of lymphoma in rheumatoid arthritis with low-dose methotrexate, *Mayo Clin Proc* 69:258-261, 1994.
50. Tabbara KF: Chlorambucil in Behçet's disease: a reappraisal, *Ophthalmology* 90:906-908, 1983.
51. Beveridge T, Gratwohl A, Michot F et al: Cyclosporin A: pharmacokinetics after a single dose in man and serum levels after multiple dosing in recipients of allogeneic bone-marrow grafts, *Curr Ther Res* 30:5-18, 1981.
52. Beveridge T: Pharmacokinetics and metabolism of cyclsporin A. In White DJG, editor: *Cyclosporin A*, New York, 1982, Elsevier.
53. Nussenblatt RB, Palestine AG: Cyclosporine: immunology, pharmacology, and therapeutic uses, *Surv Ophthalmol* 31:159-169, 1986.
54. de Smet MD, Rubin BI, Whitcup SM et al: Combined use of cyclosporine and ketoconazole in the treatment of endogenous uveitis, *Am J Ophthalmol* 113:687-690, 1992.
55. Schreiber SL, Crabtree GR: The mechanism of action of cyclosporin A and FK506, *Immunol Today* 13:136-142, 1992.
56. Cross SL, Halden NF, Lenardo MJ et al: Functionally distinct NF–kappa B binding sites in the immunoglobulin kappa and IL-2 receptor alpha chain genes, *Science* 244:466-469, 1989.
57. Granelli-Piperno A, Nolan P, Inaba K et al: The effect of immunosuppressive agents on the induction of nuclear factors that bind to sites on the interleukin 2 promotor, *J Exp Med* 172:1869-1872, 1990.
58. Larsson EL: Cyclosporin A and dexamethasone suppress T-cell responses by selectively acting at distinct sites of the triggering process, *J Immunol* 124:2828-2833, 1980.
59. Bunjes D, Hardt C, Rollinghoff M et al: Cyclosporin A mediates immunosuppression of primary cytotoxic T cell responses by impairing the release of interleukin 1 and interleukin 2, *Eur J Immunol* 11:657-661, 1981.
60. Kaufman Y, Chang AE, Robb RJ et al: Mechanism of action of cyclosporin A: inhibition of lymphokine

secretion studied with antigen-stimulated T-cell hybridomas, *J Immunol* 133:3107-3111, 1984.
61. DosReis GA, Shevach EM: Effect of cyclosporin on T-cell function in vitro: the mechanism of suppression of T cell proliferation depends on the nature of the T cell stimulus as well as the differentiation state of the responding T cell, *J Immunol* 129:2360-2367, 1982.
62. Nussenblatt R: The expanding use of immunosuppression in the treatment of non-infectious ocular disease, *J Autoimmun* 5(suppl A):247-257, 1992.
63. Nussenblatt RB, Palestine AG, Chan CC: Cyclosporin A therapy in the treatment of intraocular inflammatory disease resistant to systemic corticosteroids and cytotoxic agents, *Am J Ophthalmol* 96:275-282, 1983.
64. Miescher PA, Favre H, Chatelanat F et al: Combined steroid-cyclosporin treatment of chronic autoimmune diseases: clinical results and assessment of nephrotoxicity by renal biopsy, *Klin Wochenschr* 65:727-736, 1987.
65. Nussenblatt RB, Palestine AG, Rook AH et al: Treatment of intraocular inflammatory disease with cyclosporin A, *Lancet* 2:235-238, 1983.
66. Nussenblatt RB, Palestine AG, Chan CC: Cyclosporine therapy for uveitis: long-term followup, *J Ocular Pharmacol* 1:369-381, 1985.
67. de Smet MD, Nussenblatt RB: Clinical use of cyclosporine in ocular disease, *Int Ophthalmol Clin* 33:32-45, 1993.
68. Nussenblatt RB, Palestine AG, Chan CC et al: Effectiveness of cyclosporin therapy for Behçet's disease, *Arthritis Rheum* 28:671-679, 1985.
69. Masuda K, Nakajima A, Urayama A et al: Double-masked trial of cyclosporin versus colchicine and long-term open study of cyclosporin in Behçet's disease, *Lancet* 1:1093-1096, 1989.
70. Diaz-Llopis M, Cervera M, Menezo JL: Cyclosporin A treatment of Behçet's disease: a long-term study, *Curr Eye Res* 9(Suppl):17-23, 1990.
71. Towler HM, Whiting PH, Forrester JV: Combination low dose cyclosporin A and steroid therapy in chronic intraocular inflammation, *Eye* 4 (Pt 3):514-520, 1990.
72. Secchi AG, De Rosa C, Pivetti-Pezzi P et al: Open noncontrolled multicenter long-term trial with cyclosporin in endogenous non-infectious uveitis, *Ophthalmologica* 202:217-224, 1991.
73. Leznoff A, Shea M, Binkley KE et al: Cyclosporine in the treatment of nonmicrobial inflammatory ophthalmic disease, *Can J Ophthalmol* 27:302-306, 1992.
74. Pascalis L, Pia G, Aresu G et al: Combined cyclosporin A–steroid-MTX treatment in endogenous non-infectious uveitis, *J Autoimmun* 6:467-480, 1993.
75. Palestine AG, Austin HA, Balow JE et al: Renal histopathologic alterations in patients treated with cyclosporine for uveitis, *N Engl J Med* 314:1293-1298, 1986.
76. Deray G, Benhmida M, Le Hoang P et al: Renal function and blood pressure in patients receiving long-term, low-dose cyclosporine therapy for idiopathic autoimmune uveitis, *Ann Intern Med* 117:578-583, 1992.
77. Feutren G, Mihatsch MJ: Risk factors for cyclosporine-induced nephropathy in patients with autoimmune diseases (International Kidney Biopsy Registry of Cyclosporine in Autoimmune Diseases), *N Engl J Med* 326:1654-1660, 1992.
78. Burke JF Jr, Pirsch JD, Ramos EL et al: Long-term efficacy and safety of cyclosporine in renal-transplant recipients, *N Engl J Med* 331:358-363, 1994.
79. Palestine AG, Nussenblatt RB, Gelato M: Therapy for human autoimmune uveitis with low-dose cyclosporine plus bromocriptine, *Transplant Proc* 20(suppl 4):131-135, June 1988.
80. Whitcup SM, Salvo EC Jr, Nussenblatt RB: Combined cyclosporine and corticosteroid therapy for sight-threatening uveitis in Behçet's disease, *Am J Ophthalmol* 118:39-45, 1994.
81. Palestine AG, Roberge F, Charous BL et al: The effect of cyclosporine on immunization with tetanus and keyhole limpet hemocyanin (KLH) in humans, *J Clin Immunol* 5:115-121, 1985.
82. Chao NJ, Schmidt GM, Niland JC et al: Cyclosporine, methotrexate, and prednisone compared with cyclosporine and prednisone for prophylaxis of acute graft-versus-host disease, *N Engl J Med* 329:1225-1230, 1993.
83. Nussenblatt RB, de Smet MD, Rubin B et al: A masked randomized, dose response study between cyclosporine A and G in the treatment of sight-threatening uveitis of non-infectious etiology, *Am J Ophthalmol* 115:583-591, 1993.
84. Kino T, Hatanabe H, Hashimoto M et al: FK506, a novel immunosuppressant isolated from a *Streptomyces*. I. Fermentation, isolation, and physiochemical and biological characteristics, *J Antibiot* 40:1249-1255, 1987.
85. Kino T, Hatanaka H, Miyato S et al: FK506, a novel immunosuppressant isolated from a *Streptomyces*. II. Immunosuppressive effect of FK506 in vitro, *J Antibiot* 40:1256-1265, 1987.
86. Tocci MJ, Matkovich DA, Collier KA et al: The immunosuppressant FK506 selectively inhibits expression of early T cell activation genes, *J Immunol* 143:718-726, 1989.
87. Kawashima H, Fujino Y, Mochizuki M: Effects of a new immunosuppressive agent, FK506, on experimental autoimmune uveoretinitis in rats, *Invest Ophthalmol Vis Sci* 29:1265-1271, 1988.
88. Fujino Y, Mochizuki M, Chan CC et al: FK506 treatment of S-antigen induced uveitis in primates, *Curr Eye Res* 10:679-690, 1991.
89. Mochizuki M, Masuda K, Sakane T et al: A clinical trial of FK506 in refractory uveitis, *Am J Ophthalmol* 115:763-769, 1993.
90. Mochizuki M and Japanese FK506 Study Group on Refractory Uveitis in Behçet's Disease. In Wechsler B, Godeau P, editors: *Behçet's disease* (Proceedings of the Sixth International Conference on Behçet's Disease), Amsterdam, 1993, Excerpta Medica.
91. Porayko MK, Textor SC, Krom RAF et al: Nephrotoxic effects of primary immunosuppression with FK506 and cyclosporine regimens after liver transplantation, *Mayo Clin Proc* 69:105-111, 1994.
92. Sehgal SN, Baker H, Vézina C: Rapamycin (AY-22,989), a new antifungal antibiotic. II. Fermentation, isolation, and characterization, *J Antibiot* 28:727-732, 1975.
93. Dumont FJ, Staruch MJ, Koprak SL et al: Distinct mechanisms of suppression of murine T cell activation by the related macrolides FK506 and rapamycin, *J Immunol* 144:251-258, 1990.

94. Bierer EB, Mattila PS, Standaert RF et al: Two distinct signal transmission pathways in T lymphocytes are inhibited by complexes formed between immunophilin and either FK506 or rapamycin, *Proc Natl Acad Sci USA* 87:9231-9235, 1990.
95. Dumont FJ, Staruch MJ, Koprak SL et al: Distinct mechanisms of suppression of murine T cell activation by the related macrolides FK-506 and rapamycin, *J Immunol* 144:251-258, 1990.
96. Henderson DJ, Naya I, Bundick RV et al: Comparison of the effects of FK-506, cyclosporin A and rapamycin on IL-2 production, *Immunology* 73:316-321, 1991.
97. Roberge FG, Xu D, Chan CC et al: Treatment of autoimmune uveoretinitis in the rat with rapamycin, an inhibitor of lymphocyte growth factor signal transduction, *Curr Eye Res* 12:197-203, 1993.
98. Roberge FG, Kozhich A, Chan CC et al: Inhibition of cellular transfer of experimental autoimmune uveoretinitis by rapamycin, *Ocular Immunol Inflammation* 1:269-273, 1993.
99. Kahan BD, Gibbons S, Tejpal N et al: Synergistic interactions of cyclosporine and rapamycin to inhibit immune performances of normal human peripheral blood lymphocytes in vitro, *Transplantation* 51:232-239, 1991.
100. Martin DF, DeBarge LR, Nussenblatt RB et al: Synergistic effect of rapamycin and cyclosporin A in the treatment of experimental autoimmune uveoretinitis, *J Immunol* 154:922-927, 1995.
101. Whiting PH, Woo J, Adam BJ et al: Toxicity of rapamycin—a comparative and combination study with cyclosporine at immunotherapeutic dosage in the rat, *Transplantation* 52:203-208, 1991.
102. Calne RY, Collier DStJ, Llm S et al: Rapamycin for immunosuppression in organ allografting, *Lancet* 2:227-232, 1989.
102a. Chanaud NP III, Vistica BP, Eugui E et al: Inhibition of experimental autoimmune uveoretinitis by mycophenolate mofetil, an inhibitor of purine metabolism, *Exp Eye Res* (in press, 1995).
103. Chatenoud L, Bach J-F: Anti–T-cell monoclonal antibodies as immunosuppressive agents. In Rugstad HE, Endresen L, Førre Ø, editors: *Immunopharmacology in autoimmune diseases and transplantation,* New York, 1992, Plenum Press.
104. O'Connell PJ, Corpier CL et al: Monoclonal antibody therapy. In Thomson AW, editor: *Immunology of renal transplantation,* London, 1993, Edward Arnold.
105. Dukar OM, Barr CC: Visual loss complicating OKT3 monoclonal antibody therapy, *Am J Ophthalmol* 115:781-785, 1993.
106. Brown PS, Parenteau GL, Dirbas FM et al: Anti–Tac-H, a humanized antibody to the interleukin 2 receptor, prolongs primate cardiac allograft survival, *Proc Natl Acad Sci USA* 88:2663-2667, 1991.
107. Soulilou JP, Peyronnet P, Le Mauff B et al: Randomized controlled trial of a monoclonal antibody against the interleukin-2 receptor (33B3.1) as compared with rabbit antithymocyte globulin for prophylaxis against rejection of renal allografts, *N Engl J Med* 322:1175-1182, 1990.
108. Blaise D, Olive D, Hirn M et al: Prevention of acute GVHD by in vivo use of anti–interleukin-2 receptor monoclonal antibody (33B3.1): a feasibility trial in 15 patients, *Bone Marrow Transplant* 8:105-111, 1991.
109. Queen C, Schneider WP, Selick HE et al: A humanized antibody that binds to the interleukin 2 receptor, *Proc Natl Acad Sci USA* 86:10029-10033, 1989.
110. Hakimi J, Ha VC, Lin P et al: Humanized Mikβ1, a humanized antibody to the IL-2 receptor β-chain that acts synergistically with humanized anti-TAC, *J Immunol* 151:1075-1085, 1993.
111. Whitcup SM, DeBarge LR, Rosen H et al: Monoclonal antibody against CD11b/CD18 inhibits endotoxin-induced uveitis, *Invest Ophthalmol Vis Sci* 34:673-681, 1993.
112. Rosenbaum JT, Boney RS: Efficacy of antibodies to adhesion molecules, CD11a or CD18, in rabbit models of uveitis. *Curr Eye Res* 1993: 12:827-831.
113. Whitcup SM, DeBarge LR, Caspi RR et al: Monoclonal antibodies against ICAM-1 (CD54) and LFA-1 (CD11a/CD18) inhibit experimental autoimmune uveitis, *Clin Immunol Immunopathol* 67:143-150, 1993.
114. Weiner HL, Mackin GA, Matsui et al: Double-blind pilot trial of oral tolerization with myelin antigens in multiple sclerosis, *Science* 259(5099):1321-1324, 1993.
115. Trentham DE, Dynesius-Trentham RA, Orav EJ et al: Effects of oral administration of type II collagen on rheumatoid arthritis, *Science* 261(5129):1727-1730, 1993.
116. Nussenblatt RB, de Smet MD, Weiner HL et al: The treatment of the ocular complications of Behçet's disease with oral tolerization. In Wechsler B, Godeau P, editors: *Behçet's disease* (Proceedings of the Sixth International Conference on Behçet's Disease), Amsterdam, 1993, Excerpta Medica.
117. Palestine AG, Stevens G Jr, Lane HC et al: Treatment of cytomegalovirus retinitis with dihydroxy propoxymethyl guanine, *Am J Ophthalmol* 101:95-101, 1986.
118. Cantrill HL, Henry K, Melroe NH et al: Treatment of cytomegalovirus retinitis with intravitreal ganciclovir: long term results, *Ophthalmology* 96:367-374, 1989.
119. Cochereau-Massin I, Le Hoang P, Lautier-Frau M et al: Efficacy and tolerance of intravitreal ganciclovir in cytomegalovirus retinitis in acquired immune deficiency syndrome, *Ophthalmology* 98:1348-1353, 1991.
120. Smith TJ, Pearson PA, Blandford DL et al: Intravitreal sustained-release ganciclovir, *Arch Ophthalmol* 110: 255-258, 1992.
121. Anand R, Nightingale SD, Fish RH et al: Control of cytomegalovirus retinitis using sustained release of intraocular ganciclovir, *Arch Ophthalmol* 111:223-227, 1993.
122. Martin DF, Parks DJ, Mellow SD et al: Treatment of cytomegalovirus retinitis with an intraocular sustained-release ganciclovir implant: a randomized controlled clinical trial, *Arch Ophthalmol* (submitted).
123. Spector SA, Busch DF, Follansbee S et al: *Pharmacokinetic safety and antiviral profile of oral ganciclovir in HIV-infected persons (ACTG127).* Paper presented at the First National Conference on Human Retroviruses and Related Infections, Washington, DC, Dec 15, 1993.
124. Spector SA, McKinley G, Drew WL et al (for the Syntex Ganciclovir Study Group): A randomized, double-blind study of the efficacy and safety of oral ganciclovir for the prevention of cytomegalovirus disease in HIV-infected persons (*Late Breaker Abstracts,* No A/9,

p 7). Paper presented at the thirty-fourth meetings of Interscience Conference on Antimicrobial Agents and Chemotherapy (ICAAC), Orlando, Fla, Oct 1994.
125. Ringdén O, Wilczek H, Lönnqvist B et al: Foscarnet for cytomegalovirus infections, *Lancet* 1:1503, 1985.
126. Safrin S, Kemmerly S, Plotkin B et al: Foscarnet-resistant herpes simplex virus infection in patients with AIDS, *J Infect Dis* 169:193-196, 1994.
127. Sandstrom EG, Byington RB, Kaplin JC et al: Inhibition of human T-cell lymphotropic virus type III in vitro by phosphonoformate, *Lancet* 1:1480, 1985.
128. Palestine AG, Stevens G Jr, Lane HC et al: Treatment of cytomegalovirus retinitis with dihydroxy propoxymethyl guanine, *Am J Ophthalmol* 101:95-101, 1986.
129. Le Hoang P, Robinet M, Marcel P et al: Comparative study of foscarnet and DHPG in the treatment of CMV retinitis in AIDS, *Invest Ophthalmol Vis Sci* 29(suppl 3):42 1988 (abstract).
130. Lehoang P, Girard B, Robinet M et al: Foscarnet in the treatment of cytomegalovirus retinitis in acquired immune deficiency syndrome, *Ophthalmology* 96: 865-873, 1989.
131. Palestine AG, Polis MA, de Smet MD et al: A randomized controlled trial of foscarnet in the treatment of cytomegalovirus retinitis in patients with the acquired immunodeficiency syndrome, *Ann Intern Med* 115:665-673, 1991.
132. Foscarnet-ganciclovir cytomegalovirus retinitis trial. IV. Visual outcomes: studies of ocular complications of AIDS research group in collaboration with the AIDS clinical trials group, *Ophthalmology* 101:1250-1261, 1994.
133. Studies of the Ocular Complications of AIDS Research Group, in collaboration with the AIDS Clinical Trials Group: Mortality in patients with the acquired immunodeficiency syndrome treated with either foscarnet or ganciclovir for cytomegalovirus retinitis, *N Engl J Med* 326:213-220, 1992.
134. Jacobson MA, Wulfsohn M, Feinberg JE et al: Phase II dose-ranging trial of foscarnet salvage therapy for cytomegalovirus retinitis in AIDS patients intolerant of or resistant to ganciclovir (ACTG protocol 093) (AIDS clinical trials group of the National Institute of Allergy and Infectious Diseases), *AIDS* 8:451-459, 1994.
135. Gumbel HO, Ruckert DG, Cinatl J et al: In vitro anti-human cytomegalovirus activity of liposome-encapsulated foscarnet, *Ger J Ophthalmol* 3:5-8, 1994.
136. Sarraf D, Equi RA, Holland GN et al: Transscleral iontophoresis of foscarnet, *Am J Ophthalmol* 115:748-754, 1993.
137. Turrini B, Tognon MD, De Caro G et al: Intravitreal use of foscarnet: retinopathy of repeated injections in the rabbit eye, *Ophthalmic Res* 26:110-115, 1994.
138. Berthe P, Baudouin C, Garraffo R et al: Toxicologic and pharmacokinetic analysis of intravitreal injections of foscarnet, either alone or in combination with ganciclovir, *Invest Ophthalmol Vis Sci* 35:1038-1045, 1994.
139. Diaz-Llopis M, Espana E, Munoz G et al: High dose intravitreal foscarnet in the treatment of cytomegalovirus retinitis in AIDS, *Br J Ophthalmol* 78:120-124, 1994.
140. Jacobson MA, Kramer F, Bassiakos Y et al: Randomized phase I trial of two different combination foscarnet and ganciclovir chronic maintenance therapy regimens for AIDS patients with cytomegalovirus retinitis: AIDS clinical trials group protocol 151, *J Infect Dis* 170:189-193, 1994.
141. Weinberg DV, Murphy R, Naughton K: Combined daily therapy with intravenous ganciclovir and foscarnet for patients with recurrent cytomegalovirus retinitis, *Am J Ophthalmol* 117:776-782, 1994.
142. SOCA Research Group in collaboration with AIDS Clinical Trials Group: Combination foscarnet and gancyclovir therapy vs. monotherapy for the treatment of relapsed cytomegalovirus retinitis in patients with AIDS: the cytomegalovirus retinitis retreatment trial (in press).
143. Bronson JJ, Ghazzouli I, Hitchcock MJM et al: Synthesis and antiviral activity of the nucleotide analogue (S)-1-[3-hydroxy-2-(phosphonylmethoxy)propyl]cytosine, *J Med Chem* 32:1457-1463, 1989.
144. Hitchcock MJM, Woods K, Bronson J et al: Intracellular metabolism of the anti-herpes agent, (S)-1-[3-hydroxy-2-(phosphonylmethoxy)propyl]cytosine (HPMPC), *Mol Pharmacol* 41:197-202, 1992.
145. Polis MA, Spooner KM, Baird BF et al: Anti-cytomegaloviral activity and safety of cidofovir in patients with HIV infection and cytomegalogvirus vururia, *Antimicrob Agents Chemother* 39:882-886, 1995.
145a. Pinnolis MK, Foxworthy D, Kemp B: Treatment of progressive outer retinal necrosis with sorivudine, *Am J Ophthalmol* 119:516-517, 1995.
146. Grossman CJ: Regulation of the immune system by sex steroids, *Endocrinol Rev* 5:435-455, 1984.
147. Nagy E, Berczi I, Friesen HG: Regulation of immunity in rats by lactogenic and growth hormones, *Acta Endocrinol* 102:351-357, 1983.
148. Berczi I, Nagy E, Asa SL et al: Pituitary hormones and contact sensitivity in rats, *Allergy* 38:325-330, 1983.
149. Palestine AG, Muellenberg-Coulombre CG, Kim MK et al: Bromocriptine and low dose cyclosporine in the treatment of experimental autoimmune uveitis in the rat, *J Clin Invest* 79:1078-1081, 1987.
150. Hedner LP, Bynke G: Endogenous iridocyclitis relieved during treatment with bromocriptine, *Am J Ophthalmol* 100:618-619, 1985.
151. Tsai E, Till GO, Marak GE Jr: Effects of mydriatic agents on neutrophil migration, *Ophthalmic Res* 20:14-19, 1988.
152. Tate GW, Martin RG: Clindamycin in the treatment of ocular toxoplasmosis, *Can J Ophthalmol* 12:188-195, 1977.
153. Tabbara KF, O'Connor GR: Treatment of ocular toxoplasmosis with clindamycin and sulfadiazine, *Ophthalmology* 87:129-134, 1980.
154. Hudson AT, Randall AW, Ginger CD, et al: Novel anti-malarial hydroxynaphthoquinones with potent broad spectrum anti-protozoal activity, *Parasitology* 90:45-55, 1985.
155. Araujo FJ, Huskinson J, Remington JS: Remarkable in vitro and vivo activities of 566C80 against tachyzoites and tissue cysts of *Toxoplasma gondii, Antimicrob Agents Chemother* 35:293-299, 1991.
156. Kovacs JA: Efficacy of atovaquone in the treatment of toxoplasmosis in patients with AIDS, *Lancet* 340:637-638, 1992.
157. Lopez JS, de Smet MD, Masur H et al: Orally administered 566C80 for treatment of ocular toxoplasmosis in a patient with the acquired immunode-

ficiency syndrome, *Am J Ophthalmol* 113:331-333, 1992.
158. Rollins DF, Tabbara KF, Ghosheh R et al: Minocycline in experimental ocular toxoplasmosis in the rabbit, *Am J Ophthalmol* 93:361-365, 1982.
159. McCabe RE, Remington JS: Toxoplasmosis. In Warren KS, Mahmoud AAF, editors: *Tropical and geographical medicine,* New York, 1984, McGraw-Hill.
160. Opremcak EM, Scales DK, Sharpe MR: Trimethoprim-sulfamethoxazole therapy for ocular toxoplasmosis, *Ophthalmology* 99(6):920-925, 1992.
161. Abel JJ, Rowntree LG, Turner BB: Plasma removal with return of corpuscles, *J Pharm Exp Ther* 5:625-641, 1914.
162. Skoog WA, Adams WS: Plasmapheresis in a case of Waldenström's macroglobulinemia, *Clin Res* 7:96, 1959.
163. Saraux H, Le Hoang P, Audebert AA, et al: Intérêt de la plasmapherese dans le traitement du syndrome de Behçet, *Bull Soc Ophtalmol Fr* 82:41-44, 1982.
164. Yanuzzi LA: A perspective on treatment of aphakic cystoid macular edema, *Surv Ophthalmol* 28 (suppl): 540-553, 1984.
165. Monthey KF: Nonsteroid anti-inflammatory drugs in the treatment of intermediate uveitis, *Dev Ophthalmol* 23:158-162, 1992.
166. Herbort CP: Uveoscleritis after excessive neodymium: YAG laser posterior capsulotomy, *J Cataract Refract Surg* 20(1):80-81, 1994.

# CHAPTER 9

# Role of Surgery in the Patient With Uveitis

In spite of even optimal medical therapy to control ocular inflammation, structural damage will develop in many eyes with chronic inflammation, which can be repaired only by surgical intervention. In the past, surgery was often attempted hesitantly because of a high incidence of complications, including uncontrolled inflammation, hypotony, and phthisis. Two advances have contributed to safer surgical intervention in these eyes. The first is improved control of inflammation with steroids or other drugs, and the second is the rapid advances in microsurgical technique that have improved our ability to operate on the anterior segment, vitreous, and retina. This chapter discusses principles of ophthalmic surgery as they apply to the inflamed eye, both for therapy and for diagnosis. However, each eye with severe uveitis is unique in its anatomic alterations, and the approach to each case often must be individually altered.

## CONSIDERATIONS

In general, the indications for proceeding with surgery need to be more carefully considered in eyes with uveitis. Because of the possible increased risks, surgery is frequently not justified on eyes with slightly decreased—but functional—vision, which are not in danger of visual loss from a surgically repairable problem. On the other hand, we have observed many eyes in which surgery was delayed for so long that potentially treatable problems became hidden behind cataract or vitreous haze. Vision was then permanently lost during the attempt to be surgically conservative; the vision might have been saved if the inflammatory disease and its complications could have been directly viewed and treated. There is a tendency to not operate on an eye with dense opacities and light perception vision while unseen and untreated inflammation causes further permanent damage to the retina. In the end the eye does go blind, but there was a point in the course of the disease at which the potential benefits of surgical intervention, even if low, outweighed the resultant risk of nonintervention. In addition to visual rehabilitation, surgical procedures in eyes with uveitis are performed as part of a diagnostic evaluation. The relative risk versus the potential benefits is considered here.

Except for the few situations to be discussed in which it is necessary to operate on an acutely inflamed eye, surgery should be performed when the inflammation is quiescent. However, in some patients, it is impossible to clear every cell from the anterior chamber or vitreous. Furthermore, in patients with dense cataracts and primarily vitreoretinal inflammation, it is impossible to accurately assess the activity of the disease behind the opacity. Therefore an attempt should be made to quiet the inflammation as much as possible but not to delay surgery while the patient suffers long-term visual handicap because the inflammation never becomes completely quiescent. In the event that the inflammatory activity cannot be

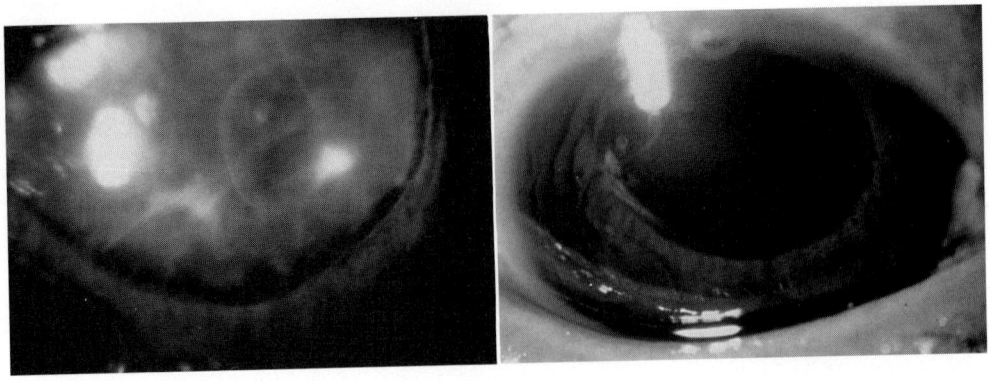


**Fig. 9-1. A,** Uveitic eye after extracapsular cataract extraction (ECCE) (phacoemulsification) and intraocular lens (IOL) placement. Postoperative inflammatory response was severe, with development of fibrin in anterior chamber. **B,** Clinical improvement occurred 24 hours after injection with tissue plasminogen activator (TPA). (Courtesy Rubens Belfort, Jr., M.D., Sao Paulo, Brazil.) (See Color Plate 8.)

assessed, the eye may be prophylactically treated for a few days as though active inflammation is present.

In our opinion, corticosteroids are still the best drug for the control of inflammation in the perioperative period. In a small study of 20 patients randomly selected to receive prednisone or cyclosporine before cataract surgery, we found that 3 of 10 patients treated with cyclosporine—but none of the steroid-treated patients—had severe postoperative inflammation that necessitated a change in medication to the other drug. Corticosteroids work at multiple points in the inflammatory process, as described in Chapter 8, and are able to affect inflammation mediated by neutrophils and macrophages, as well as by lymphocytes. Therefore they may prevent nonspecific postoperative inflammation that may occur in a previously inflamed eye, as well as inhibit the more specific pathways of inflammation. We prefer to begin steroid therapy on the day before or the day of surgery if the patient is not already receiving the drug and if there is no evidence of active inflammatory disease. Some practitioners prefer starting steroid several days before the scheduled surgical intervention. If there is no strong contraindication, it may not be unreasonable in some cases to do so, although it should be remembered that the effects of the daily steroid are gone 24 hours later. Usually 1 mg/kg/day of steroid is adequate. In addition, we give a subconjunctival corticosteroid injection at the time of surgery. If the patient has a history of severe intraocular inflammation, we also give an intravenous dose of corticosteroids, such as 50-100 mg methylprednisolone, at the time of surgery. The goal is clearly to prevent severe postoperative inflammation.

The surgeon should be aware that with the aforementioned perioperative therapy, the eye may appear relatively quiet for the first few days after surgery, but the inflammation may increase a few days later. It is therefore critical to examine patients with uveitis daily during the first 5 to 7 days after surgery. In young patients and in those with sarcoidosis, we have specifically noted marked postoperative flares of inflammation accompanied by significant fibrin and protein within the eye. At times the fibrin is so dense as to mimic vitreous bands, and the retina cannot be viewed. Tissue plasminogen activator (TPA) can be used to clear severe fibrin accumulation in the anterior chamber (Fig. 9-1). After surgery these eyes frequently have hypotony. Although these eyes appear to be in imminent danger of phthisis, continued treatment with steroids, combined with patience, usually results in marked clearing in 3 to 5 days without apparent additional ocular damage.

## REMOVAL OF BAND KERATOPATHY

Calcium hydroxyapatite accumulates in Bowman's membrane of the cornea in some patients with sarcoidosis or juvenile rheumatoid arthritis and occasionally in younger patients with a chronic uveitis such as pars planitis. Its location may be related to the local pH of the interpalpebral cornea. It can be removed by chelation if it is located centrally and interferes with vision because of opacity or glare or if it is the cause of recurrent corneal erosions. Although chelation with 1% to 2% ethylenediaminetetraacetic acid (EDTA) can be performed with use of local anesthesia, the age of

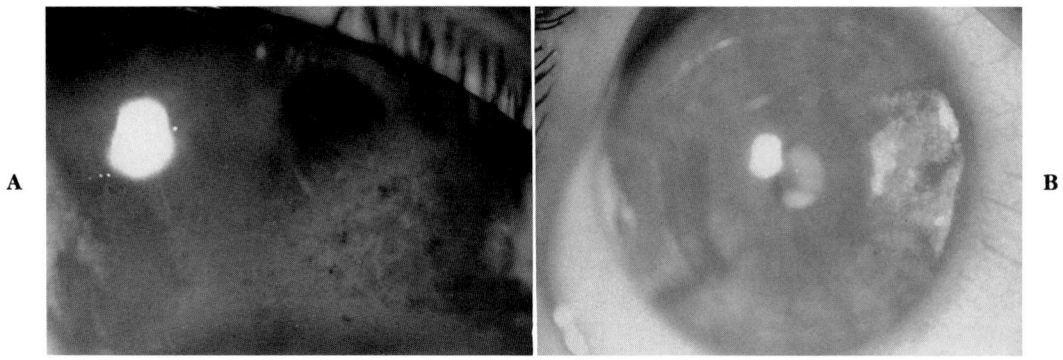


**Fig. 9-2. A,** Band keratopathy in 6-year-old boy with bilateral uveitis. **B,** Same eye 2 days after excimer laser surgery performed with use of topical anesthesia. (Courtesy Rubens Belfort, Jr., M.D., Sao Paulo, Brazil.) (See Color Plate 9.)

most patients with this condition makes general anesthesia necessary. Our procedure is to use a sterile 1.7% solution of EDTA in water or saline applied to the cornea with cotton or cellulose applicators. Gentle pressure and movement of the applicator result in removal of the corneal epithelium and gradual solubilization of the calcium deposits. This procedure can take up to 30 minutes and often must be performed before intraocular surgery. Occasionally, resistant deposits must be gently removed with a spatula or Tooke knife, but this may cause scarring of Bowman's membrane and should be avoided in the visual axis. The eye is then patched until the epithelial defect heals. Recently the removal of band keratopathy has been performed with use of the excimer laser (Fig. 9-2).

## CORNEAL TRANSPLANTATION

Although keratitic precipitates involve the corneal endothelial surface, endothelial decompensation is rare in our experience in patients with chronic uveitis. Thus corneal transplantation is rarely performed in this group because of corneal edema, but it may be necessary in patients with corneoscleral melting in association with systemic inflammatory disease and intraocular inflammation or in those patients with herpetic keratouveitis. If the intraocular inflammation has been severe, there may be coexistent glaucoma or cataract. The primary goal before corneal transplantation in these patients is to control the immune process, or the newly grafted tissue will melt as well. The ongoing inflammatory response suggests that corneal transplantation in any patient with active uveitis carries a high risk for rejection because there are already large numbers of cells in the eye that could present corneal antigens to the immune system and participate in the rejection event.

## CATARACT SURGERY

Much information has been acquired during the past years concerning cataract extraction in uveitic eyes. Yet there is still no clear consensus on the ideal method of cataract removal, especially in eyes that will continue to have chronic inflammation after surgery. Individual cases and various disorders often require different approaches. Summaries of cases performed 20 to 30 years ago suggested that the outcome of cataract surgery in eyes with uveitis was poor and that phthisis was frequent. This is clearly no longer the expected outcome in our hands, nor in the hands of a growing number of investigators. Today, intracapsular cataract extraction is rarely performed. The theoretic advantage of not leaving residual lens material in the eye seems to be outweighed by the larger incision and higher incidence of retinal detachment and cystoid macular edema in this approach as compared with other approaches. Cataracts in uveitis occur in relatively young patients, and we therefore reserve intracapsular extraction for mature lenses in those eyes with phacoantigenic uveitis or phacogenic glaucoma.

Extracapsular extraction, either via irrigation-aspiration or phacoemulsification, has the advantage of leaving the posterior capsule intact. By providing a barrier to diffusion of mediators from the anterior segment, the intact capsule reduces the incidence of cystoid macular edema in uveitis-free patients. We have observed two patients in whom the posterior capsule was not intact who had only anterior inflammation before cataract surgery but who, after surgery, developed cystoid macular edema with each episode of anterior inflammation. Other advantages include the containment of anhyphema to the anterior segment instead of spread of the blood into the posterior chamber. Postoperative hyphema is not uncommon in inflamed eyes. A disadvantage of this technique is the technical difficulty of dealing with posterior synechiae that frequently adhere to a pupillary membrane. The postoperative disadvantages of the extracapsular approach include the formation of posterior synechiae to the capsule, pupillary block glaucoma, the inability to remove vitreous debris, haze and vitreoretinal traction, and the possible opacification of the posterior capsule. Sometimes we prefer to perform a sector iridectomy in patients who have 360-degree posterior synechia, since active uveitis can cause occlusion of even the largest sector if the posterior capsule is intact. We have also observed patients in whom a neodynium: yttrium-aluminum-garnet (Nd:YAG) laser capsulotomy leads to an exacerbation of inflammation. Herbort[1] has reported the case of a patient in whom a severe and recurrent scleritis and uveitis developed after an Nd:YAG capsulotomy was performed 18 months after cataract extraction. A last theoretic disadvantage is the possible damage that may occur to the already compromised trabecular meshwork and corneal endothelium during anterior segment surgery. Extracapsular cataract surgery seems best suited to patients without vitritis and without possible vitreoretinal traction who have not had cystoid macular edema as a complication of their uveitis. This would include most patients with anterior uveitis such as HLA-B27–associated inflammatory disease.

### Anterior chamber

Our procedure has been to make a partial-depth 10 mm corneoscleral groove and then enter the anterior chamber with a No. 75 blade and a 3 mm incision. Rarely a sector iridectomy is performed because extracapsular cataract extraction in the eye with uveitis is complicated by posterior synechia. In addition, if the pupil is less than 2 to 3 mm, the surgeon is likely to encounter a dense fibrin membrane across the pupil. To widen the pupillary aperture we often use disposable iris retractors in the four quadrants. In rare cases, the pupil will not dilate until this membrane is cut with a Van Ness scissors after sodium hyaluronate (Healon) has been administered. Posterior synechiae not only may be present at the pupillary border but may extend over the entire surface of the lens. These extensive adhesions cannot be easily broken with an iris spatula, but with the aid of a sector iridectomy and pupillary membrane sectioning, an adequate anterior capsulotomy can be performed. In addition, an anterior surgical approach should be avoided if there are peripheral anterior synechiae extending onto clear cornea, because the surgical incision may not enter the anterior chamber but may go through the iris into the posterior chamber. With the use of iris retractors we have been able to perform phacoemulsification on many uveitic eyes requiring surgery. Many of these patients are young, and phacoemulsification time is quite low. Most of the nucleus can be removed by aspiration. We do, however, take a conservative approach to the use of phacoemulsification. In patients older than 50 years of age with extensive posterior synechiae, we often opt to perform a routine extracapsular cataract extraction.

The surgeon should expect uveitic eyes to bleed from the conjunctiva, Tenon's capsule, the corneoscleral wound, and the iris. Even eyes that have been quiet for several months appear to have an increased tendency to bleed during or after surgery. Bleeding can be controlled by careful cautery, by tamponade with the irrigating solution, and by patience.

### Pars plana lensectomy with vitrectomy

Pars plana lensectomy usually combined with a vitrectomy has been used by several authors to remove a cataract, reshape the pupil, and remove vitreous opacities and vitreoretinal traction in one operation.[2-6] The operation can be performed with use of the standard technique—three 1-mm incisions 3 or 3.5 mm posterior to the limbus. Trauma to the trabecular meshwork is avoided. Usually the use of disposable iris retractors will provide the surgeon with an adequate view initially, until the lens has been removed. However, if this is not the case, with the vitrectomy instrument, the pupilary aperture can be enlarged to be round and large enough to examine the retina after surgery. However, this technique can provoke bleeding from the edge of the iris. In addition, more conjunctiva can be left undisturbed for use in a future filtering operation. The main disadvantage is the removal of the posterior capsular barrier. Some surgeons have advocated keeping the anterior capsule intact to use as a possible support if a secondary implant is considered. We have had no experience with this approach. The possibility of retinal detachment shortly after surgery is less than 1% in our experience. This operation is difficult to perform in patients older than 50 years of age because, in our experience, the lens nucleus becomes rather hard, making it more difficult to remove. It has been suggested by several authors that pars plana vitrectomy reduces or eliminates recurrences of inflammation because it removes an antigen load from the vitreous. This has not been our experience. However, the removal of the vitreous can decrease the accumulation of cells and haze during an episode of inflammation, but the vision will still be affected by a new inflammatory episode. We therefore prefer this operation in patients younger than 50 years old who have had vitritis as part of their ocular inflammation, especially if the vitreous and retina cannot be visualized preoperatively because the pupil is small or there are other structural alterations in the anterior chamber.

Our technique for pars plana lensectomy/vitrectomy is to make three radial conjunctival incisions. The incisions are cleaned down to bare sclera, and scleral incisions are made 3 mm posterior to the limbus. An infusing cannula is inserted in one incision but is not turned on. An ultrasonic fragmenting instrument and an irrigating needle are introduced into the lens, and the lens material is removed within the capsular bag, using both the fragmenting instrument and the vitrectomy instrument. An alternative is to place the light pipe under the lens to help in visualization. Entry into the eye must be parallel to the iris or the posterior capsule will be broken prematurely (Fig. 9-3). After the lens material is removed, the vitreous cutter is used to remove the lens capsule and

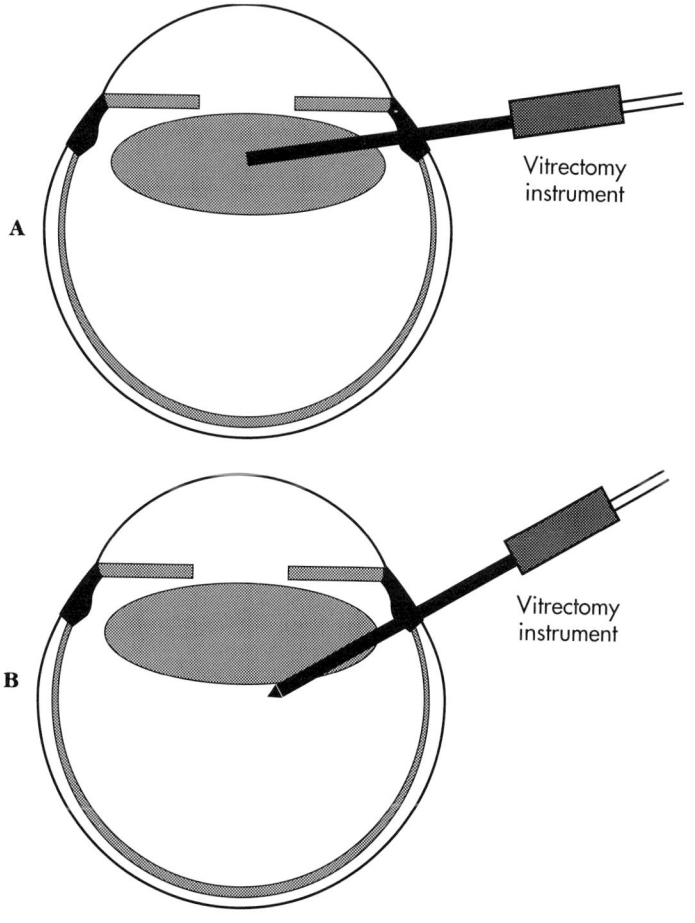


**Fig. 9-3. A,** Optimal position for entry of vitrectomy instrument or ultrasonic fragmenting instrument for pars plana lensectomy. **B,** If instrument is angled too steeply into eye, posterior capsule will break and cortex may fall toward retina during procedure, as illustrated here.

anterior vitreous and to reshape the pupil. A vitrectomy is then performed to remove opacities and any tractional abnormalities.

Results from cataract surgery have been reported to be favorable with both techniques (i.e., anterior chamber and pars plana) and depend more on previous damage from the inflammation than from surgical complications. Praeger and colleagues[7] reported excellent improvement after extracapsular surgery in patients with juvenile rheumatoid arthritis. Mackensen and Loeffler[8] reported that in 86 patients with chronic iridocyclitis who underwent extracapsular surgery, inflammation was reduced by 70% and recurrences were reduced by 94%. Vision improved in most patients. In a study by Smith and colleagues[2] 12 patients with chronic uveitis who underwent pars plana lensectomy/vitrectomy showed improved vision, but cystoid macular edema impaired the acuity in most of these patients. Girard and colleagues[3] reported that 5-year remissions of uveitis occurred in each of 23 patients, and 21 had improved vision after pars plana surgery. In the 39 patients Petrilli and coworkers[4] studied after pars plana surgery, 23% had vision better than 20/40 and 56% had vision worse than 20/100; 18% had cystoid macular edema. Other authors have had similar experiences.[5,6] In our experience the average vision after surgery in patients with long-standing chronic inflammation was 20/100 (Fig. 9-4). Phthisis occurred in approximately 2% of the eyes, and 90% of the patients had an improvement in vision.

Hypotony is often mentioned as a contraindication for cataract removal in these patients. However, if the cataract is dense and vision is hand motions or worse, surgery by the pars plana route can be considered in eyes with pressures below 3 mm Hg. Although phthisis may result, we have observed five eyes with preoperative hypotony in which there was an increase in intraocular pressure of several millimeters of mercury after pars plana lensectomy/vitrectomy. In many eyes with posterior inflammation, there is a dense anterior hyaloid that may be associated with ciliary body traction. Removal of this traction may result in improved ciliary body function.

Earlier anecdotal reports with both pars plana and extracapsular approaches suggested strongly that eyes with uveitis do survive cataract surgery and in fact may have a marked improvement of visual acuity.[2-8] In addition, a major question has been the indication to place an intraocular lens (IOL) at the time of surgery and if so what type. It is clear that a previous history of uveitis is a significant risk factor for an inflammatory response after cataract surgery and placement of a posterior chamber intraocular lens.[9]

### Intraocular lenses and uveitic eyes

It is imperative to use any means necessary to get the eye's inflammatory disease under strict control. Some would mandate even the absence of every cell, which for us is sometimes most difficult to obtain, but the message is one we fully support. The disease must be controlled, and it must be controlled for an

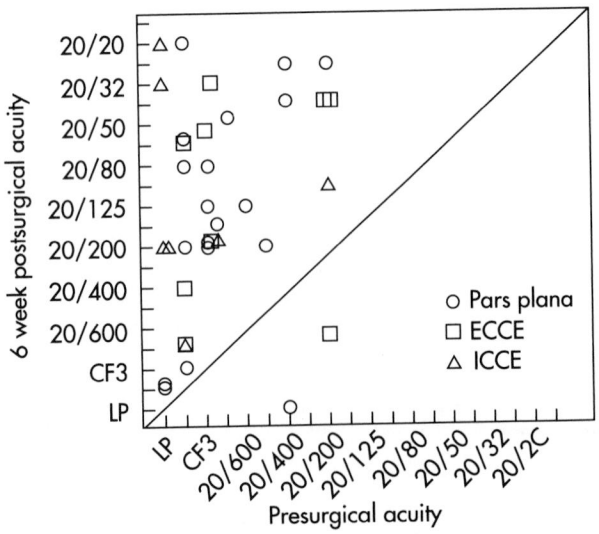


**Fig. 9-4.** Change in visual acuity after cataract removal in patients with uveitis.

extended period, usually 3 to 6 months before we would consider a surgical intervention. The patient should be informed about the possible need for continued and even more aggressive immunosuppressive therapy to control the disease postoperatively. An extracapsular cataract extraction (including phacoemusification) would be our general approach. This is often followed by a curtailed anterior vitrectomy. This sort of approach is outlined by Walker and colleagues.[10] The decision to place an IOL is a continuing question, and although there are no strict rules (how can there be in medicine?), certain guidelines have evolved. The presence of synechiae is a potential warning that a similar thing will happen postoperatively and could cause serious problems. Iris capture (Fig. 9-5)[11] is a real concern, and patients with posterior synechiae are at greater risk of this problem, as well as the capsule contraction syndrome, occurring postoperatively.[12] We will generally not place an IOL in children with uveitis for many reasons, including the Food and Drug Administration (FDA) requirements. As well, anecdotal evidence indicates that the type of uveitic diseases found in children has not responded well to an IOL insertion. A child's inflammatory response can be exuberant, causing serious difficulties postoperatively. A one-piece IOL without positioning holes placed in the posterior chamber (in the bag) would be the approach we would prefer. Much interest has been shown in surface-modified lenses and the possibility of their decreasing the postoperative inflammatory response. Although larger studies looking at this question are ongoing, it is interesting to note the observations of Percival and Pai,[13] who placed a heparin surface–modified one-piece lens into the posterior chamber of 36 patients with cataracts associated with past or chronic recurrent uveitis. They found that the recurrent inflammatory disease was present, including an acute postoperative fibrin reaction, but the heparin coating appeared to provide a cell-free IOL surface in most of the eyes (Figs. 9-6 and 9-7).

**Selected results from the literature.** Pleyer and colleagues[14] reported in a 5-year series that 71% of 28 eyes receiving an IOL had a postoperative visual acuity of 0.5 or better, as opposed to 54% of the 24 eyes that were aphakic. Because this was not a randomized study, it is difficult to compare the relative "success" rates. Foster and colleagues[15] reported that in 20 uveitic eyes, extracapsular cataract extraction with posterior chamber IOL and pars plana vitrectomy if needed achieved a 20/100 or better visual acuity in 60% of the eyes operated. Tessler and Farber,[16] comparing IOL placement to no IOL placement in uveitic eyes, believed that IOLs appeared to be relatively safe in patients with what was described as chronic iridocyclitis. However, a comment[17] and our interpretation of the paper would indeed suggest that the data would argue for the reverse—that is, eyes with IOLs had a poorer postoperative result. As Tessler and Farber state, only a larger study could definitively settle this question. On the other hand, it appears that eyes with Fuchs' heterochromic iridocyclitis do well after cataract surgery and IOL placement.[18]

Akova and Foster,[19] in a retrospective analysis of their patients with sarcoidosis, found that of 102 patients, 14 patients (21 eyes) came to surgery because of a visual acuity of 20/100 or less. In stressing the need for absolute control of the intraocular inflammatory disease, they

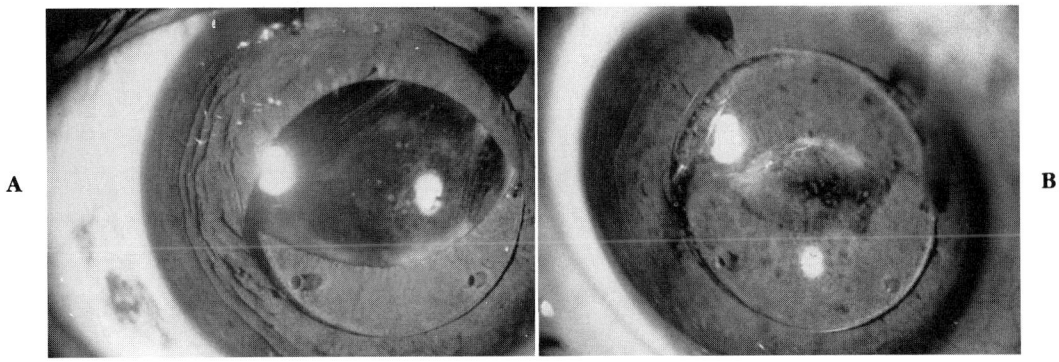


**Fig. 9-5.** Uveitic eye that underwent cataract surgery and posterior chamber IOL placement. **A,** Inferior portion of lens has migrated anterior to lens plane. **B,** Whole lens is now forward. This "iris capture" occurred without marked inflammatory disease. (Courtesy Rubens Belfort, Jr., M.D., Sao Paulo, Brazil.) (See Color Plate 10.)

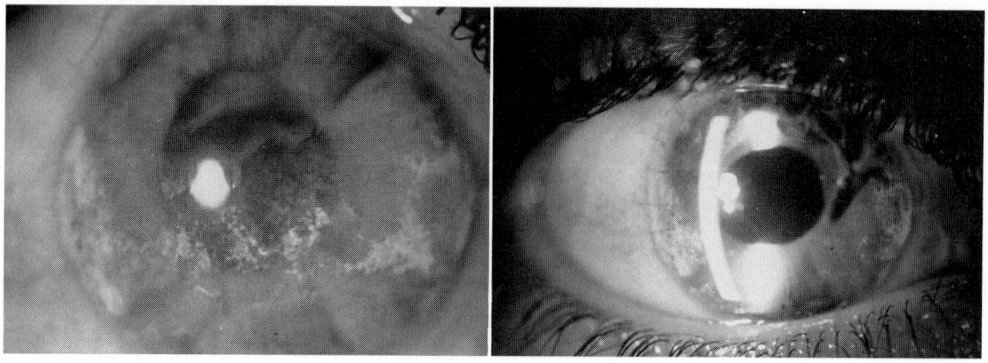


**Fig. 9-6.** When his disease was quiescent, an 11-year-old boy with anterior uveitis underwent cataract extraction and IOL placement. **A,** After multiple YAG capsulotomies and EDTA treatments, a persistent anterior chamber reaction required topical steroid therapy. **B,** After IOL removal and normalization of intraocular pressure, inflammation was absent, steroid therapy had been discontinued, and visual acuity was 20/100. (Courtesy Rubens Belfort, Jr., M.D., Sao Paulo, Brazil.) (See Color Plate 11.)

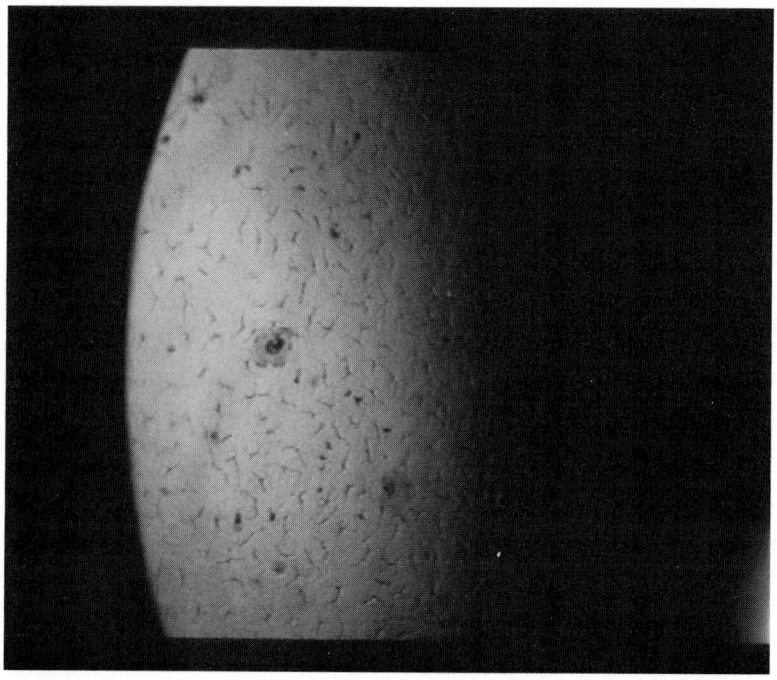

**Fig. 9-7.** With retroillumination, cells can be seen to accumulate on anterior surface of IOLs in uveitic eyes. Elongated cell bodies of smaller cells suggest macrophages. Larger cells with more substantial cytoplasm also appear.

found that 19 of the 21 patients received IOLs, and that 61% of the eyes had a stable visual acuity of 20/40 or better. In those who did not have a dramatic improvement of visual acuity, retinal pathologic conditions such as cystoid edema and epiretinal membranes, as well as glaucomatous optic nerve disease, were found.

Juvenile rheumatoid arthritis is a disorder in which IOL placement has not been recommended. In a review of the 16 eyes of 10 patients with juvenile rheumatoid arthritis, Fox and colleagues[20] found that after pars plana lensectomy and vitrectomy the short-term visual acuity was 20/70 or better in 13 of 16 eyes (81%), but a longer follow-up showed that the final visual acuity was 20/70 or better in 9 of 16 eyes (56%). This drop was attributed to glaucoma and retinal disease such as cystoid edema.

## GLAUCOMA SURGERY

Secondary glaucoma that cannot be controlled by medical therapy is sometimes a consequence of severe anterior segment in-

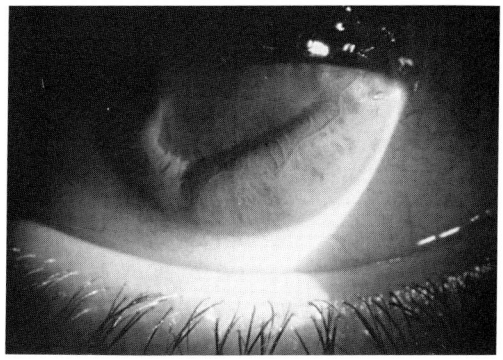

**Fig. 9-8.** Slit-lamp photograph of patient with uveitis and pupillary block glaucoma. Iris bombé, due to broad iris-lens synechiae, localized from 3 to 6 o'clock position. (See Color Plate 12.)

flammation. It is important to differentiate between pupillary block glaucoma and secondary angle closure by peripheral anterior synechiae. The two processes may coexist in the eye with uveitis. Active inflammation may suppress ciliary body function and also decrease trabecular filtration. Thus intraocular pressure in the actively inflamed eye may be higher or lower than in the uninflamed one. Although patients with long-standing chronic inflammation have poor outflow, increased inflammation will lead to decreased aqueous production and a pressure decrease. If treatment with corticosteroids is accompanied by a rise in pressure, it does not necessarily mean that the patient is a "steroid responder."

It may be difficult to distinguish pupillary block glaucoma in a patient with chronic inflammation and posterior synechiae that involve the entire lens surface. These patients do not show a classic iris bombé pattern but may have a subtle shallowing of the anterior chamber with a low, peripheral iris bombé. The iris elevation may be localized only to areas where the iris and the lens are not adherent (Fig. 9-8). If the diagnosis is suspected but is unclear, a laser iridectomy will be diagnostic and therapeutic. If the laser iridectomy fails to lower the intraocular pressure, pupillary block can be ruled out as a mechanism.

Filtering surgery such as trabeculectomy or a Scheie procedure has a lower chance of success in patients with ongoing uveitis because of the younger age of such patients and because the inflammatory mediators promote fibrous tissue growth and closure of the filtering bleb. However, not all filtering blebs will fail in these patients, and an attempt at this type of surgery appears to be warranted inasmuch as the alternative is blindness from glaucoma or an attempt at a procedure to destroy the ciliary body. A normal response on the part of the treating physician is frequently to practice restraint. An insidious loss of visual function can ensue due to the glaucoma even with excellent control of the uveitis. The operation should be done when the eye is quiet at a site that has not had previous surgery. Because these eyes frequently need repeated surgical procedures, combining a filtering operation with cataract removal if appropriate seems justified to reduce the number of possible interventions.

Drugs such as 5-fluorouracil (5-FU) and mitomycin are used to improve the success of filtering surgery by slowing the growth of fibrous tissue. Patitsas and colleagues[21] have used 5-FU combined with filtering surgery in treating patients with both uveitis and glaucoma. They found that intraocular pressure was controlled in 71% of 21 eyes over a median time of 35 months. Control was better achieved in phakic eyes (90%) than in aphakic or pseudophakic (55%) eyes. Complications that have been associated with 5-FU use occurred. These need further evaluation in patients with uveitis; although 5-FU therapy may keep the bleb open in the initial few weeks or months after surgery, recurrent inflammation could still threaten to destroy a functional filtering bleb. Indeed, there has been one report of an idiosyncratic anterior granulomatous uveitis in a patient who received one injection of subconjunctival 5-FU.[22]

Alternative approaches include a modified goniotomy or trabeculodialysis. Kanski and McAllister[23] reported on 23 such operations and found a 60% success rate in patients with juvenile rheumatoid arthritis. However, in only five patients could control be achieved without additional antiglaucoma medication. Williams and colleagues[24] reported a success rate in 56% of 25 uveitic eyes undergoing trabeculodialysis, with aphakic eyes doing no worse than those that were phakic. Ultrasonic filtering surgery has not yet been used in enough patients with uveitis to suggest whether this approach may be helpful.

Another approach that we have used and find worth considering in difficult uveitis cases is the use of an aqueous draining device. We have had experience with the Molteno implant

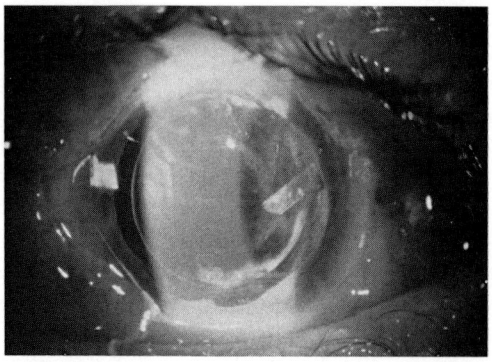

**Fig. 9-9.** Uveitic eye with secondary glaucoma that could not be controlled with maximum medication or trabeculectomy surgery. Tube from single-plate Molteno implant can be seen in anterior chamber at 2 o'clock position. (See Color Plate 13.)

(Fig. 9-9). Although in our experience patients will demonstrate a severe intraocular inflammatory response combined with hypotony the first days after surgery, on a long-term basis there appears to be good control of the intraocular pressure. Hill and coworkers[25] reviewed 45 patients with both uveitis and glaucoma and found that an aqueous drainage device was more likely to control the intraocular pressure in those patients who would suffer significant, immediate, or chronic postoperative inflammation. However, they also believed that trabeculectomy gave surprisingly good results as well. Freedman and Rubin[26] have also reported good results with a single-plate Molteno.

Other devices include the anterior chamber tube shunt to encircling band (ACTSEB) procedure. Although initial results with this procedure are reported to compare favorably with the Molteno implant,[27,28] it is still too early to truly evaluate the relative advantages or disadvantages of the two devices. Newer drainage devices control aqueous flow to protect against hypotony.

If the aforementioned surgical approaches fail, the only alternative is to try to decrease aqueous formation. Cyclocryotherapy and laser destruction are both possible methods of achieving this goal. Cyclocryotherapy is best performed in sequential treatments 4 to 8 weeks apart. We begin treating from the 6 to 8 o'clock positions with 1-minute freezes. If this fails to lower the pressure after several weeks, 6 more clock-hour positions are treated, with 3 of the clock hours overlapping the first treatment. Further treatments may be required but should be approached cautiously. The operation is accompanied by significant postoperative pain and does not work immediately. Preoperative anterior chamber paracentesis has been suggested to prevent an immediate cryotherapy-induced rise in intraocular pressure. Cryotherapy can be useful if properly titrated in view of the other options for the patient. Laser destruction of the ciliary processes allows more careful titration of the destructive process but requires a widely dilated pupil so that the ciliary body can be visualized and directly treated. This dilation is difficult to achieve in patients with chronic uveitis.

## TREATMENT OF VITREORETINAL DISEASE

Significant vitreous opacities, areas of vitreoretinal traction, or epiretinal membranes sometimes develop in patients who have severe posterior inflammation, and newer techniques have permitted these problems to be approached with a reasonable hope for success.[29] If the opacities and membranes appear to be the major source of a decrease in vision or if there is a significant tractional retinal detachment, then vitrectomy without lensectomy is indicated. In general, the surgical management of these eyes does not differ from eyes with vitreous opacities or traction from other causes.

Bacskulin and Eckardt[30] have found that in 13 children with uveitis who underwent either vitrectomy alone or combined with lensectomy, their disease was easier to treat and in some there was resolution of macular edema. In our hands we have found vitrectomy useful in helping to observe the posterior pole and thus follow the course of disease, and the procedure appears to make it easier for steroid to penetrate intraocularly. However, we have not found it to be an effective therapy when used alone, as has been suggested by Kaplan.[31] Bovey and colleagues[32] performed a vitrectomy or cataract extraction, or both, in 30 eyes and found an improvement in visual acuity but not an improvement in the inflammatory process, nor did Nolle and Eckardt[33] in nine patients with multifocal chorioretinitis who underwent vitrectomy.

The prognosis for visual improvement after epiretinal membrane removal is lower in eyes with uveitis than in eyes with idiopathic membranes.[34] In addition, after repair of a rhegmatogenous retinal detachment by standard scleral buckling procedures, there is probably a higher risk of proliferative vitreoretinopathy (PVR) in eyes with ongoing chronic inflammation, because the inflammatory mediators stimulate fibrous tissue proliferation. The development of PVR usually necessitates additional surgery with membrane stripping and gas-fluid exchange. After this procedure, control of the inflammation is critical or the membranes may reform.

The repair of giant retinal tears that may complicate viral retinitis, such as acute retinal necrosis or cytomegalovirus retinitis, frequently is not best managed by scleral buckling. The retina in these diseases has become necrotic and areas may be ischemic. The use of a high buckle might increase this ischemia, leading to retinal neovascularization. An alternative solution has been to perform a pars plana vitrectomy and to reattach the retina with gas or silicone oil tamponade and laser photocoagulation.[35]

## LASER TREATMENT

Lasers can be used to perform peripheral iridectomies and posterior capsulotomies, to cut pupillary membranes, to clear deposits off the anterior surface of an IOL, and to treat retinal or subretinal neovascularization. The use of the laser, however, does not eliminate the possibility of inducing inflammation.

In the anterior segment either the YAG or argon laser can be used to perform an iridotomy. Although the procedure is probably technically easier with the YAG laser, there is the theoretic possibility that the incidence of hyphema from the vascular, inflamed iris may be greater after YAG laser therapy than after argon laser treatment because the YAG laser does not coagulate tissue. This has not been studied in patients with uveitis. Posterior capsulotomy is easily performed with the YAG laser unless there has been a significant fibrous reaction or calcification as a result of the inflammation. Pupillary membranes can occasionally be so dense that the laser procedure becomes very long, necessitates the use of high energies, or cannot be successfully performed at all (Fig. 9-10). In addition, although an uncomplicated capsulotomy can be performed with only a few bursts of laser energy—and at

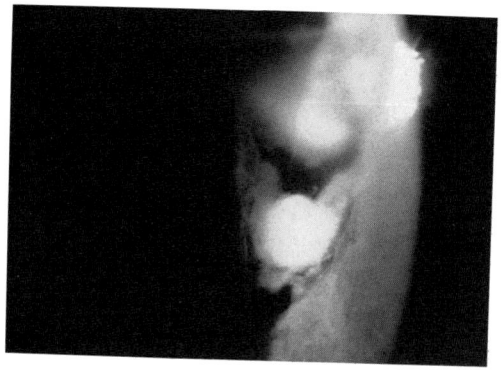

**Fig. 9-10.** YAG laser membrane discission in patient with dense post–cataract surgery pupillary membrane. (See Color Plate 14.)

the time of the procedure it appears that little has been disrupted within the eye—the energy delivered by the YAG laser does alter the blood-aqueous barrier.[36] We have observed several patients with chronic uveitis who have had severe flare-ups of inflammation associated with a marked temporary decrease in acuity 1 day after YAG laser capsulotomy. Therefore, use of the YAG laser in patients with severe inflammatory disease should be treated with the same concern as an invasive surgical procedure and the patient should be pretreated with corticosteroids to prevent recurrence of the inflammation.

The photocoagulation of the retina for surface or subretinal neovascularization may also be accompanied by bouts of inflammation. Panretinal or sector argon photocoagulation for surface neovascularization is indicated if the new vessels have not regressed on antiinflammatory therapy. Patients with sarcoidosis and neovascularization of the optic disc often show regression of the vessels with steroid therapy. In contrast, patients with retinal neovascularization due to Behçet's disease rarely show resolution because the retinal ischemia remains even when the eye is quiet. These eyes usually respond to panretinal photocoagulation. Retinal laser therapy may lead to increased intraocular inflammation not only because of the alterations in the blood-retinal barrier related to the laser energy but because there may be significant amounts of retinal antigens released during the destruction of the retina. We have seen one patient who had previous ocular surgeries in the right eye but developed sympathetic ophthalmia in both eyes shortly after a retinal hole in the left eye was treated with laser. The Dalen-Fuchs nodules began around the site of laser therapy and expanded to involve the rest of that eye (see Chapter 22). This implies that the release of antigen in an already primed patient triggered an autoimmune response.

Subretinal neovascular membranes are not often seen in uveitis, except in the presumed ocular histoplasmosis syndrome. Because alterations in Bruch's membrane are widespread in some types of uveitis, these membranes can occur in a variety of locations. If they are threatening the macula, it is reasonable to treat them with argon or krypton laser, but in extramacular lesions the physician must balance the potential visual loss from the membrane with the potential increase in inflammation that could result from the therapy. If treated, the response to therapy would not be expected to differ from the response in other, more common causes of the subretinal membranes, but because of the relative rarity of this condition in patients with uveitis, it has not been specifically studied.

## DIAGNOSTIC SURGERY

Surgical procedures frequently are the only method of distinguishing a disease of presumed autoimmune etiology from an infectious or malignant ocular process. The clinical appearance of many ocular infections and some malignant conditions are not always diagnostic. For example, a patient with cytomegalovirus retinitis may have lesions that are consistent with Behçet's syndrome during a certain period in the course of the disease. The overall course of the two diseases is different, but at the time the physician examines the patient, the two may appear similar. In this example, a careful history would probably suggest that, if the patient were immunosuppressed, a viral retinitis was more likely than an autoimmune disease. Infection with *Propionibacterium acnes* (see Chapter 18) and large cell lymphoma of the vitreous (see Chapter 29) are other examples of diseases that are not autoimmune but that may appear similar. In addition, if an infectious or malignant process is suspected, the appropriate therapy usually cannot begin until the diagnosis is confirmed by histologic or microbiologic examination.

The indication for any intraocular diagnostic procedure in an inflamed eye is that, in the physician's experience, the course of the uveitis or its appearance is not typical for the suspected autoimmune disease and that an infectious or malignant process is suspected. It is unusual for such a suspicion to be strong at the time of the first examination. However, as the patient's disease fails to respond to therapy in an expected manner, the physician begins to suspect that the original diagnosis may be incorrect and other diagnoses need to be considered. Once these alternate diagnoses are proposed, the appropriate diagnostic surgical procedure may be the only way to reliably exclude these possibilities.

### Anterior chamber paracentesis

Anterior chamber paracentesis is an easily performed technique that yields a small amount of fluid for analysis. The procedure can be performed with use of local anesthesia. The eye can be fixated by a forceps firmly holding the limbus. The eye is entered with a 30-gauge needle on a tuberculin syringe, and at least 200 to 250 μL of fluid can usually be obtained. A small hyphema may occur if the eye is actively inflamed, but this will clear as the anterior chamber rapidly reforms. This small amount of fluid must be handled carefully by means of a plan established for handling the specimen before the procedure is begun. In general we spin the fluid, separate the cells, and prepare slides for immunohistologic examination. The supernatant can then be analyzed for antibodies. Serum should be obtained on the same day for comparison. However, if an infectious organism is suspected, the unspun fluid must be cultured. Because of the small amount of fluid, only one or two types of cultures can be set up and the clinician must chose the tests that will be most helpful. If too many tests are attempted, the amount of fluid may produce negative results because of an inadequate sample size. We therefore prefer to use aqueous for cell studies and antibody measurement. If an infection is suspected, the vitreous provides more material for culture. In addition, even in postoperative endophthalmitis, the vitreous has a higher yield of positive culture results and more types of cultures can be set up with the material.

Aqueous specimens should therefore be cultured in their entirety if an infectious organism is suspected and there is no other sample. Otherwise, they should be centrifuged at approximately 1000 rpm and the supernatant carefully removed. The cells that remain can be resuspended in 50 to 100 μL of buffered saline, and samples of 10 to 15 μL can be placed on gelatinized glass slides. This provides a sufficient number of slides for monoclonal antibody studies or other special stains. In cases of pseudophakia or aphakia and after a vitrectomy, a communication between the vitreous cavity and the anterior chamber exists and the aqueous specimen may be positive for lymphomatous cells.

Vitreous specimens may be obtained either by vitrectomy or by direct vitreous aspiration. We prefer to perform a vitrectomy because more material can be obtained and the posterior ocular structures can be better visualized after the surgery. In addition, this procedure provides more control over the amount of vitreous traction produced during surgery. In some situations it is useful to obtain an undiluted vitreous sample. This can be accomplished by aspirating directly with a syringe and needle or by using the vitrectomy instrument on low suction without turning on the infusion until 0.5 to 1 ml of vitreous is obtained. This latter method prevents pulling on the vitreous base and prevents prolonged hypotony in the eye. The sample can be aspirated directly into a syringe. For cases in which lymphoma is suspected, we put a small amount of culture fluid (such as Roswell Park Memorial Institute [RPMI] medium–1640) into the vitrectomy cassette. This material is immediately sent to the laboratory before the surgical procedure has been completed. When one uses the vitreous fluid that is diluted with irrigating solution, it is sometimes useful to pass a portion through a Millipore filter. The Millipore filter can be cut up for culture for fungus or can be studied by the cytologist. Direct application onto gelatinized slide is also useful for cytologic study and monoclonal antibody staining. If the cells are trapped in cut pieces of dense vitreous, a portion of the sample can be incubated with hyaluronidase to digest the vitreous and free the cells. The cells can be also cultured or typed by immunohistologic or cell-sorting techniques. The fluid can be analyzed for antibodies or inflammatory factors,[37] and these findings can be a valuable diagnostic tool in adjusting therapy.[38]

## Chorioretinal biopsy

Occasionally neither aqueous nor vitreous specimens will provide a useful answer. Certain pathogens may not "spill over" into the vitreous if the disease involves the retina or choroid only. For example, cytomegalovirus, which is difficult to culture from the vitreous, can be cultured from or seen on electron microscopic examination of the retina. In diseases in which the vision is threatened and the physician seems sure that continuation of the present therapy will not be effective, it may be reasonable to consider a chorioretinal biopsy.[39] This procedure provides a small piece of tissue that, if handled carefully, can provide a diagnosis. This procedure is probably useful only when the diagnostic possibilities include diseases for which there is specific therapy. In general, this has been performed in cases with progressive chorioretinal lesions of unknown cause.[15] The indications for the biopsy include macular-threatening lesions unresponsive to therapy or suspicion of either a malignant process or an infection. In the eyes on which we have performed chorioretinal biopsy, the preoperative visual acuity was 20/200 or worse.

Our procedure for chorioretinal biopsy is similar to that described by Peyman and colleagues[40] except that we have not used an external support ring and we perform the vitrectomy before the biopsy incision. If the vitrectomy is completed first, the localization of an area of active disease to be biopsied is more accurate. A biopsy specimen of normal retina or retina in which the disease is quiescent will rarely provide diagnostic information. A flap-door approach rather than a full-thickness eye wall resection is used. A scleral flap 6 by 6 mm is made beginning 4 mm from the limbus and is hinged posteriorly (Fig. 9-11). As thick a flap as possible is made. The inner bed is surrounded by diathermy. An inner rectangle of remaining sclera, choroid, and retina, 4 by 2 to 3 mm, is removed with use of a microblade and sharp Van Ness scissors. The blade must be inserted fully to sever the retina cleanly. The specimen should be gripped in only one corner with fine-toothed forceps so as not to damage the tissue. It is important to attempt to keep the specimen together so that the correct anatomic relationships are preserved. After the specimen is removed, any vitreous around the wound is removed. The scleral flap is then sutured over the bed with nylon suture, and the eye is reinflated with either air or balanced salt solution. This procedure is used to obtain a biopsy specimen from a process involving the peripheral retina near the ora serrata. The incision may be moved somewhat posteriorly to obtain tissue anterior to the equator. It is not suitable for lesions found in the posterior pole.

An alternate method of biopsy is endoretinal biopsy. This has been used by Freeman and colleagues[35] to obtain a specimen from the edge of detached retina during retinal reattachment procedures. If the retina is detached with a large tear, an intraocular scissors can be used to obtain a sample of the tissue. If the retina is not detached, a piece of retina could conceivably be removed from the eye after photocoagulation without disturbing the choroid. This latter technique has not yet been applied to human tissue.

The retinal or chorioretinal biopsy specimen should be divided as shown in Fig. 9-12. This permits culture, histologic examination, and monclonal antibody studies and maximizes the chance of gleaning useful information. There is sufficient specimen for only limited numbers of cultures, and therefore the piece should be sent for either viral or fungal culturing. Inasmuch as most fungal pathogens that involve the choroid and retina can be cultured from the vitreous—but in viral retinitis viral cultures of the vitreous may indicate negative results because of neutralizing antibodies or low viral shedding—we prefer to send most specimens for viral studies if an infectious cause is suspected. PCR can be performed on the retinal tissue as well. Additional studies using monoclonal antibodies can aid in identifying the type of fungus or virus that is present, and the results may be available much faster than the time needed to culture the organism.

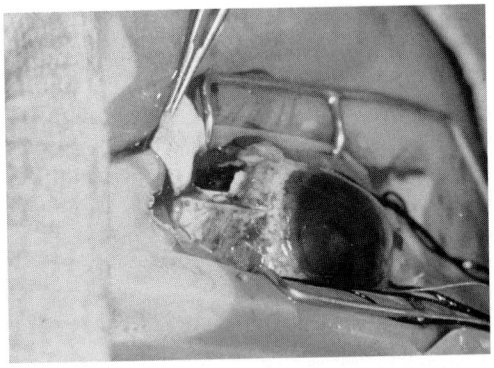

**Fig. 9-11.** Scleral flap incision during chorioretinal biopsy procedure of lesion near ora serrata.

The careful handling of ocular specimens obtained for diagnostic purposes is essential if they are to be of use. Advanced planning and notification of the laboratories that will be involved in processing the specimen are useful in ensuring that the specimen is expected and will be processed correctly.

### Subretinal surgery

Much interest has recently centered around the development of new surgical and diagnostic

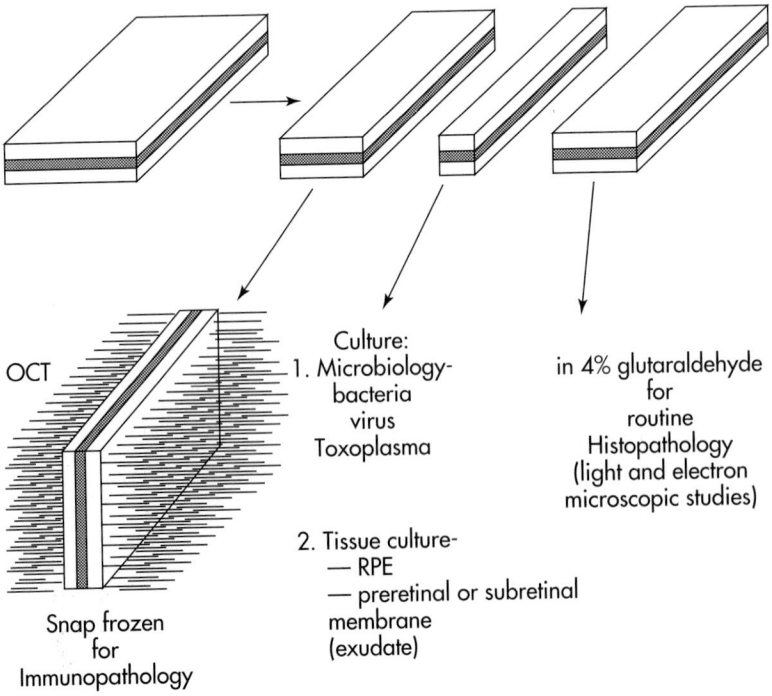


**Fig. 9-12.** Schematic drawing of approach to subdivide and analyze chorioretinal biopsy specimen.

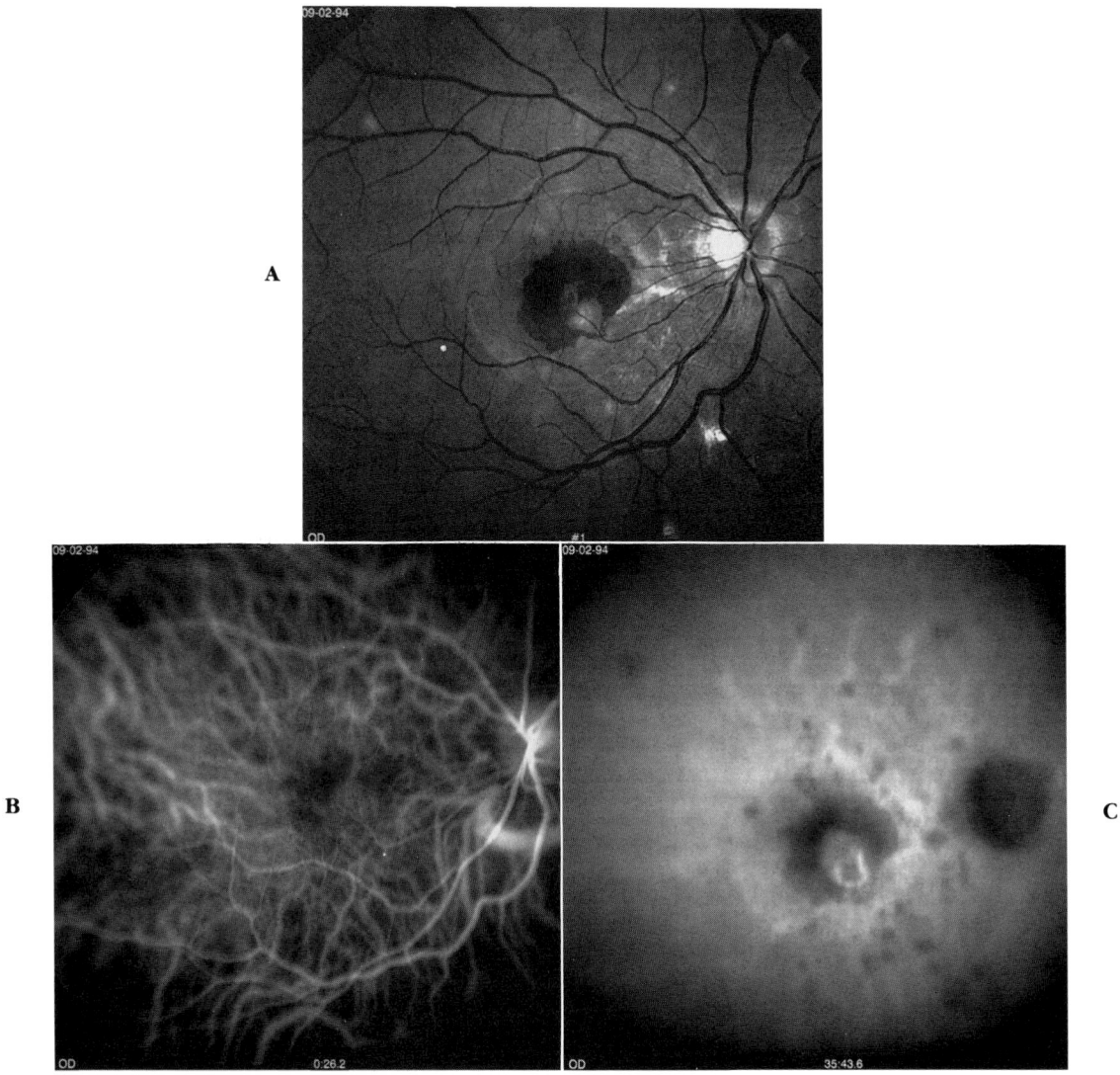


**Fig. 9-13.** Indocyanine green (ICG) angiogram showing position of submacular neovascular net. **A,** Fundus photograph showing submacular hemorrhage with marked reduction in visual acuity. Because of blood, fluorescein angiogram was difficult to interpret. **B,** ICG early photograph shows feeder vessel to net. **C,** Later photograph outlines extent of net, which was successfully treated with laser photocoagulation and not removed by surgery.

techniques for subretinal (submacular) surgery (Fig. 9-13). The implications of these techniques would seem to go beyond the surgery itself and will also influence future work in retinal pigment epithelium (RPE) transplantation. The removal of subfoveal neovascular membranes[41] in the eyes of patients with the presumed ocular histoplasmosis syndrome paves the way for an exciting new area of therapy (Fig. 9-14). This is in contradistinction to patients with age-related maculopathy, who have not consistently had such an improvement in vision. In a report by Thomas and colleagues,[42] they found that after subretinal surgery in eyes with the ocular histoplasmosis syndrome, visual acuity was stabilized or improved in 56 or 83% of eyes, whereas 20/40 or greater was achieved in 21 or 31% of eyes (mean follow-up 10.5 months). The results are quite different in eyes with age-related maculopathy, in which visual acuity was improved in 5 (12%) of the eyes operated, and 20/40 or better occurred in two eyes (5%), with a mean follow-up of 15 months. Of interest is Gass's

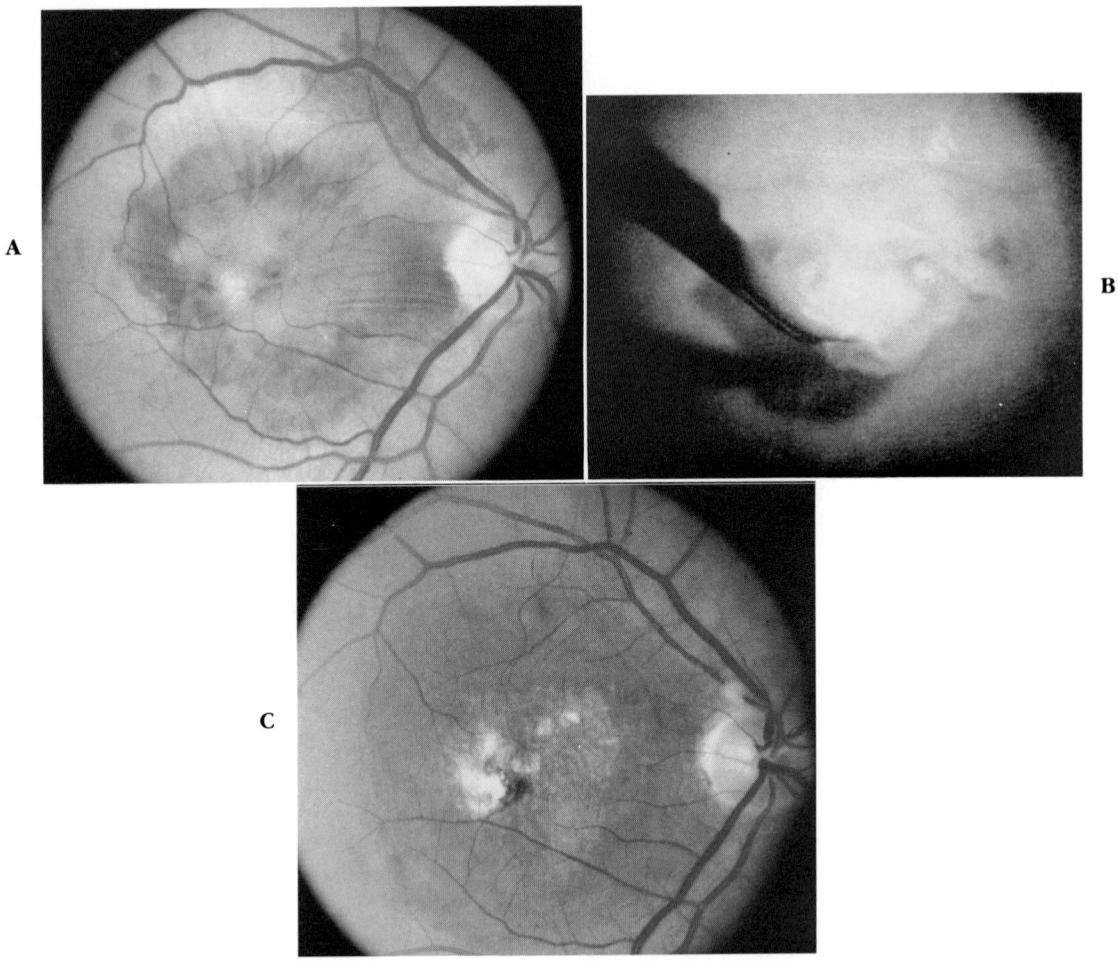


**Fig. 9-14. A,** Subretinal neovascular lesion in macular region. **B,** Removal of lesion with special subretinal forceps. **C,** Fundus as it appears after surgery. (Courtesy Antonio Capone Jr., M.D., and Daniel Martin, M.D., Emory University, Atlanta, Ga.) (See Color Plate 15.)

hypothesis[43] that the membranes removed from patients with histoplasmosis grew in the subsensory retinal space and not under the RPE as did those from patients with age-related maculopathy. In addition, the membranes from patients with histoplasmosis are covered with a redundant layer of RPE, and therefore removal may aid in the normal apposition of the retinal elements. Other questions still remain as to how widely applicable subretinal surgery will be for patients with uveitis in general. Recurrence rates of membranes still need to be determined. Newer techniques such as subretinal endophotocoagulation may help to deal with some of these problems.[44] However, the removal of the membrane alone may not be sufficient to restore vision inasmuch as defective RPE cells, as well as damaged or lost photoreceptors, may be the major problem. This may then represent just the first step of a whole series of rehabilitation measures that will be needed.

**Case 9-1**

A middle-aged African-American man with a history of glaucoma and cataract surgery in his right eye had decreased vision in that eye and, subsequently, in the left eye. Ocular examination showed peripheral choroidal detachments, as well as multiple, subretinal yellow-white lesions, strewn througout the fundus (see Fig. 29-9). HLA typing showed HLA-A29 positivity. An extensive work-up failed to help in making a diagnosis, except that the patient showed purified protein derivative (PPD) positivity and a monoclonal band in the urine. The differential diagnosis included miliary tuberculosis, lymphoma, other systemic neoplastic metastases, an undetected infectious process, and birdshot retinochoroidopathy. After extensive discussion, it was believed that a chorioretinal biopsy was indicated. The results of the biopsy showed the ocular condition to be reactive lymphoid hyperplasia, which resolved with oral prednisone therapy. (For a more detailed description of this case, see Cheung MK et al: Diagnosis of reactive lymphoid hyperplasia by chorioretinal biopsy, *Am J Ophthalmol* 118: 457-462, 1994.

## REFERENCES


1. Herbort CP: Uveoscleritis after excessive neodynium: YAG laser posterior capsulotomy, *J Cataract Refract Surg* 20:80-81, 1994.
2. Smith RE, Kokoris N, Nobe JR et al: Lensectomy-vitrectomy in chronic uveitis, *Trans Am Ophthalmol Soc* 81:261-275, 1983.
3. Girard LJ, Rodriguez J, Mailman ML et al: Cataract and uveitis management by pars plana lensectomy and vitrectomy by ultrasonic fragmentation, *Retina* 5:107-114, 1985.
4. Petrilli AM, Belfort R, Abreu MT et al: Ultrasonic fragmentation of cataract in uveitis, *Retina* 6:61-65, 1986.
5. Diamond JG, Kaplan HJ: Uveitis: effect of vitrectomy combined with lensectomy, *Ophthalmology* 86:1320-1328, 1979.
6. Dangel ME, Stark WJ, Michels RG: Surgical management of cataract associated with chronic uveitis, *Ophthalmic Surg* 14:145-152, 1983.
7. Praeger DL, Schneider HA, Sakowski AD Jr et al: Kelman procedure in the treatment of complicated cataract of the uveitis of Still's disease, *Trans Ophthalmol Soc UK* 96:168-172, 1976.
8. Mackensen G, Loeffler K: Cataract extraction in chronic iridocyclitis: long-term follow-ups, *Klin Monatsbl Augenheilkd* 183:7-9, 1983.
9. Drolsum L, Davanger M, Haaskjold E: Risk factors for an inflammatory response after extracapsular cataract extraction and posterior chamber IOL, *Acta Ophthalmol (Copenh)* 72:21-26, 1994.
10. Walker J, Rao NA, Ober RR et al: A combined anterior and posterior approach to cataract surgery in patients with chronic uveitis, *Int Ophthalmol* 17:63-69, 1993.
11. Belfort R, Nussenblatt RB: Surgical approaches to uveitis, *Int Ophthalmol Clin* 30:314-317, 1990.
12. Davison JA: Capsule contraction syndrome, *J Cataract Refract Surg* 19:582-589, 1993.
13. Percival SP, Pai V: Heparin-modified lenses for eyes at risk for breakdown of the blood-aqueous barrier during cataract surgery, *J Cataract Refract Surg* 19:760-765, 1993.
14. Pleyer U, Pawlikowska J, Zierhut M et al: Clinical aspects, follow-up and results of cataract extraction in uveitis, *Ophtalmologie* 89:295-300, 1992.
15. Foster RE, Lowder CY, Meisler DM et al: Combined extracapsular cataract extraction, posterior chamber intraocular lens implantation, and pars plana vitrectomy, *Ophthalmic Surg* 24:446-452, 1993.
16. Tessler HH, Farber MD: Intraocular lens implantation versus no intraocular lens implantation in patients with chronic iridocyclitis and pars planitis, *Ophthalmology* 100:1206-1209, 1993.
17. Letter to editor, *Ophthalmology* 101:625-626, 1994.
18. Daus W, Schmidbauer J, Buschendorff P et al: Results of extracapsular cataract extraction with intraocular lens implantation in eyes with uveitis and Fuchs' heterochromic iridocyclitis, *Ger J Ophthalmol* 1:399-402, 1992.
19. Akova YA, Foster CS: Cataract surgery in patients with sarcoidosis-associated uveitis, *Ophthalmology* 101: 473-479, 1994.
20. Fox GM, Flynn HW Jr, Davis JL et al: Causes of reduced visual acuity on long-term follow-up after cataract extraction in patients with uveitis and juvenile rheumatoid arthritis, *Am J Ophthalmol* 114:708-714, 1993.
21. Patitsas CJ, Rockwood EJ, Meisler DM et al: Glaucoma filtering surgery with postoperative 5-fluorouracil in patients with intraocular inflammatory disease, *Ophthalmology* 99:594-599, 1992.
22. Mohan M, Kumar H, Rana S: Acute granulomatous iritis following 5-fluorouracil therapy for failed trabeculectomy, *Indian J Ophthalmol* 39:125-126, 1991.
23. Kanski JJ, McAllister JA: Trabeculodialysis for inflammatory glaucoma in children and young adults, *Ophthalmology* 92:927-930, 1985.
24. Williams RD, Hoskins HD, Shaffer RN: Trabeculodialysis for inflammatory glaucoma: a review of 25 cases, *Ophthalmic Surg* 23:36-37, 1992.
25. Hill RA, Nguyen QH, Baerveldt G et al: Trabeculectomy and Molteno implantation for glaucomas associated with uveitis, *Ophthalmology* 100:903-908, 1993.
26. Freedman J, Rubin B: Molteno implants as a treatment for refractory glaucoma in black patients, *Arch Ophthalmol* 109:1417-1420, 1992.
27. Smith MF, Sherwood MB, McGorray SP: Comparison of the double-plate Molteno drainage implant with the Schocket procedure, *Arch Ophthalmol* 110:1246-1250, 1992.
28. Omi CA, De Almeida GV, Cohen R et al: Modified Schocket implant for refractory glaucoma: experience of 55 cases, *Ophthalmology* 98:211-214, 1991.
29. Freeman WR: Application of vitreoretinal surgery to inflammatory and infectious disease of the posterior segment, *Int Ophthalmol Clin* 32:15-33, 1992.
30. Bacskulin A, Eckardt C: Results of pars plana vitrectomy in chronic uveitis in childhood, *Ophthalmologie* 90: 434-439, 1993.
31. Kaplan HJ: Surgical treatment of intermediate uveitis. In Böke WRF, Manthey KF, Nussenblatt RB, editors: *Intermediate uveitis*, vol 23, pp 185-189, Karger Basel, 1992.
32. Bovey EH, Gonvers M, Herbort CP: Pars plana vitrectomy in uveitis, *Klin Monatsbl Augenheilkd* 200:464-467, 1992.
33. Nolle B, Eckardt C: Vitrectomy in multifocal chorioretinitis, *Ger J Ophthalmol* 2:14-19, 1993.
34. Michels RG: Vitrectomy for macular pucker, *Ophthalmology* 91:1384-1388, 1984.
35. Freeman WR, Henderly DE, Wan WL et al: Prevalence, pathophysiology, and treatment of rhegmatogenous retinal detachment in treated cytomegalovirus retinitis, *Am J Ophthalmol* 103:527-536, 1987.
36. Forster RK, Zachary IG, Cottingham AJ et al: Further observations on the diagnosis, cause and treatment of endophthalmitis, *Am J Ophthalmol* 81:52-56, 1976.
37. Davis JL, Solomon D, Nussenblatt RB et al: Immunocytochemical staining of vitreous cells: indications,

techniques, and results, *Ophthalmology* 99:250-256, 1992.

38. Baarsma GS, Luyendijk L, Kijlstra A et al: Analysis of local antibody production in the vitreous humor of patients with severe uveitis, *Am J Ophthalmol* 112:147-150, 1991.
39. Martin DF, Chan CC, de Smet MD et al: The role of chorioretinal biopsy in the management of posterior uveitis, *Ophthalmology* 100:705-714, 1993.
40. Peyman GA, Juarez CP, Raichand M: Full-thickness eye-wall biopsy: long-term results in 9 patients, *Br J Ophthalmol* 65:723-726, 1981.
41. Thomas MA, Kaplan HJ: Surgical removal of subfoveal neovascularization in the presumed ocular histoplasmosis syndrome, *Am J Ophthalmol* 111:1-7, 1991.
42. Thomas MA, Dickinson JD, Melberg NS et al: Visual results after surgical removal of subfoveal choroidal neovascular membranes, *Ophthalmology* 101:1384-1396, 1994.
43. Gass JDM: Biomicroscopic and histopathologic considerations regarding the feasibility of surgical excision of subfoveal neovascular membranes, *Am J Ophthalmol* 118:285-298, 1994.
44. Thomas MA, Ibanez HE: Subretinal endophotocoagulation in the treatment of choroidal neovascularization, *Am J Ophthalmol* 116:279-285, 1993.

# PART 4

# INFECTIOUS UVEITIC CONDITIONS

# CHAPTER 10

# Bacterial and Fungal Diseases

Half a century ago, bacterial diseases such as tuberculosis and syphilis were thought to cause the majority of cases of uveitis. Even today, a number of infectious diseases remain important causes of uveitis. Furthermore, because specific antimicrobial therapy can be curative and prevent long-term visual sequelae, early diagnosis of infectious causes of uveitis should be a priority for all practitioners.[1]

Infections may elicit a uveitis by a number of pathogenic mechanisms. Direct infection of ocular tissues usually leads to an inflammatory response manifested by signs and symptoms of uveitis. Injection of bacterial endotoxins at sites far from the eye will also elicit intraocular inflammation in the absence of ocular infection. Endotoxins generate a number of harmful biologic effects including fever, hypotension, disseminated coagulation, and shock. In the same year that Murray Shear elucidated the basic structure of endotoxin, Ayo[1] demonstrated that a single intravenous injection of endotoxin could induce ocular inflammation, and this inflammatory response was ascribed to "Schwartzman toxins." Although this endotoxin-induced uveitis (EIU) was easily elicited in dogs, cats, and rabbits, smaller laboratory animals were resistant to developing the disease. In 1980, Rosenbaum and colleagues[2] demonstrated EIU in Lewis rats after intravenous, intraperitoneal, or intrafootpad injection of lipopolysaccharide (LPS)[2], and Forrester and colleagues[3] showed EIU after intraocular LPS injection in Columbia-Sherman rats. More recently, EIU has also been described in C3H/HeN mice.[4] EIU is now a useful animal model for the study of acute ocular inflammation and is characterized by iris hyperemia, miosis, increased aqueous humor protein, and inflammatory cell infiltration into the anterior uvea and anterior chamber (Fig. 10-1). Inflammatory cell infiltration into the vitreous in the area of the optic nerve head also occurs. As you read in the chapter on anterior uveitis, uveitis can follow bacterial infections such as bacterial

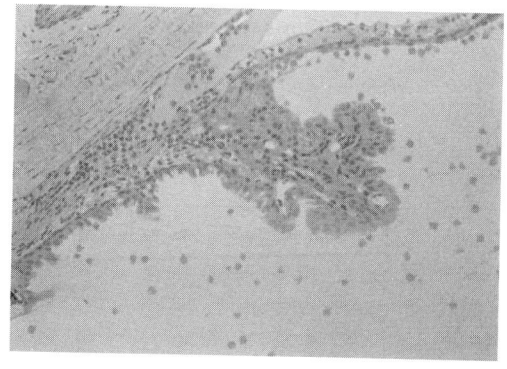

**Fig. 10-1.** Histologic section of anterior chamber of mouse with endotoxin-induced uveitis shows infiltration with neutrophils, macrophages, and occasional lymphocytes. (Hematoxylin and eosin, ×200.)

Parts of this chapter are modified from Whitcup SM, Raizman MB: Spirochetal infections and the eye. In Albert DM, Jakobiec FA, editors: *Principles and practice of ophthalmology*, vol 5, Philadelphia, 1994, WB Saunders, pp 3078–3092, with permission.

dysentery and the mechanism of some of these cases may be the result of an immunologic response to endotoxin.

This chapter will focus on uveitis caused by ocular infection from bacteria or fungus. Although a number of infectious agents can invade the eye and lead to ocular inflammation, we will concentrate on the most common bacterial and fungal causes of uveitis including leprosy, tuberculosis, spirochetal diseases, including syphilis, Lyme disease, relapsing fever, and leptospirosis, brucellosis, candidal infections, and aspergillosis. Postsurgical bacterial and fungal endophthalmitis are discussed separately in Chapter 18.

## LEPROSY

Leprosy was the first documented bacterial infection in human beings. The etiologic agent of leprosy, *Mycobacterium leprae,* is a gram-positive intracellular bacillus that was first identified by Hansen in 1874[5]; however, the disease has been a scourge to society for thousands of years. It is estimated that from 10 to 15 million people have leprosy[6] and that from 500,000 to 700,000 persons have been blinded by this condition.[7] The organisms have a tropism for parts of the body with low temperatures, particularly organs of ectodermal origin such as skin, peripheral nerves, nasal mucosa, and the eye. The mode of transmission of leprosy remains unclear. Although most of the population is exposed to the bacillus in endemic areas, over 90% are immune to the disease and do not develop symptoms. Leprosy is often divided into two major subtypes: tuberculoid leprosy and lepromatous leprosy. In patients with tuberculoid leprosy, the organism induces a strong cell-mediated immune response, and few organisms are found invading organ tissues. Little immunity follows the infection in patients with lepromatous leprosy, and a plethora of organisms are found throughout the body. Borderline forms of the disease also exist in some classification systems.[8]

### Clinical findings

From 50% to 70% of patients with leprosy have the tuberculoid form of the disease, which tends to be localized to the skin and nerves.[9] The disease in these patients is characterized by granuloma formation and the absence of a large number of bacilli because of their active cell-mediated immune response. The skin test with lepromin is highly positive (Mitsuda reaction). The lepromatous form of the disease is characterized by a severe generalized condition with massive bacterial infection. In contrast to patients with tuberculoid leprosy, these patients have a poor cellular immune response, and macrophages are predominantly found on histologic examination. Intraocular inflammatory disease occurs more commonly in this form of leprosy. In addition, the severe disfiguring changes of the limbs and face are associated with lepromatous leprosy. Patients with borderline groupings of leprosy can shift suddenly to the lepromatous state.

A list of the ocular complications of leprosy can be found in Box 10-1. Structural damage to the eyelids, poor lid closure as a result of facial nerve involvement, and impaired corneal sensation often lead to exposure of the cornea. Loss of the temporal portion of the eyebrows (madarosis) is a typical finding and a stigma to those afflicted. It is important to remember, however, that trachoma can exist in the same population with leprosy and can compound the external disease in these patients.[10] The keratitis associated with leprosy starts superiorly and first appears as subepithelial chalky infiltrates surrounded by gray stromal opacifications.[11] Corneal exposure predisposes patients to development of corneal ulcers (Fig. 10-2) that are often difficult to manage.

Intraocular inflammatory disease is a known complication of leprosy. The organisms can directly invade the iris and ciliary body, and chronic anterior uveitis is commonly seen in these patients. If the uveitis is not aggressively treated, cataract and hypotony frequently re-

**Box 10-1**
**Ocular manifestations of leprosy**

- Prominent corneal nerves
- Conjunctivitis
- Granulomatous anterior uveitis
- Iris pearls
- Facial nerve palsy (tuberculoid leprosy)
  - Ptosis
  - Exposure keratitis
- Trigeminal nerve involvement
  - Corneal anesthesia
- Lid lesions and deformities (lepromatous leprosy)
- Choroidal lesions

sult. Less frequently, patients present with an acute anterior uveitis. In a study of 100 leprosy patients in Brazil, 72 had ocular complications.[12] Seventeen had a chronic anterior uveitis, whereas only two had an acute anterior uveitis. In a study in Nepal, 8% of patients with tuberculoid leprosy had uveitis, whereas 16% of patients with lepromatous leprosy had anterior chamber inflammatory disease.[13] Spaide and colleagues found that uveitis was uncommon in leprosy patients in the United States, which possibly reflects the results of more aggressive treatment with antilepromatous and antiinflammatory agents.[13a]

Granuloma form in the iris and appear like iris "pearls" on the anterior surface (Fig. 10-3). Iris atrophy also occurs in many patients (Fig. 10-4).

Although less common, retina changes have been described in leprosy patients. Patients with long-standing lepromatous leprosy can have large numbers of organisms that invade not only the anterior segment but the adjoining peripheral pars plana and retina. Pars planitis has been reported in patients with leprosy.[14] Chovet and colleagues[15] demonstrated segmental vasculitis in the posterior pole on fluorescein angiography of patients with lepromatous disease.

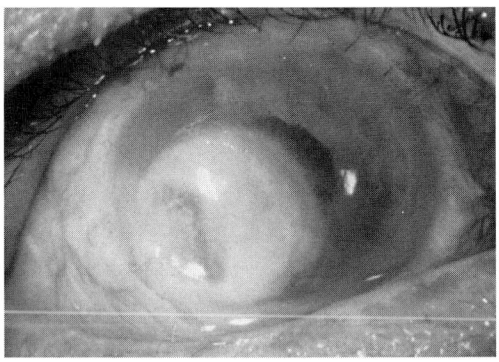

**Fig. 10-2.** Severe bacterial corneal ulcer in patient with leprosy. (Courtesy R. Christopher Walton, M.D.)

## Immunology and pathology

Human beings are the only natural host for *M. leprae.* After entering the host, the organism reproduces in mononuclear cells, particularly skin histiocytes. The doubling time for the organisms is extraordinarily long, about 20 days, and attempts at culturing the organism in a cell-free environment have not been successful. Recent work has centered on the use of the 9-banded armadillo as an experimental model.[16] This animal has a low basal temperature that seems to permit large numbers of *M. leprae* to propagate.

The immune characteristics of patients with this disorder have been extensively studied. Imbalances in T cells,[17] antigen-specific suppressor T cells,[18] and defective production of monocyte-activating cytokines have all been described.[19] $CD4^+$ T cells predominate in tuberculoid lesions, but $CD8^+$ T cells are almost exclusively found in lepromatous lesions.[20] Family studies with HLA typing have suggested that there is an HLA-linked recessive gene that may predispose patients to the tuberculoid form of the disease.[21]

## Therapy

Dapsone, rifampin, and clofazimine are the principal antileprosy agents used. The World Health Organization recommends multidrug treatment regimens because of dapsone-resistant strains of *M. leprae.*[22] Attempts to develop a vaccine are currently underway. Ocular care

A

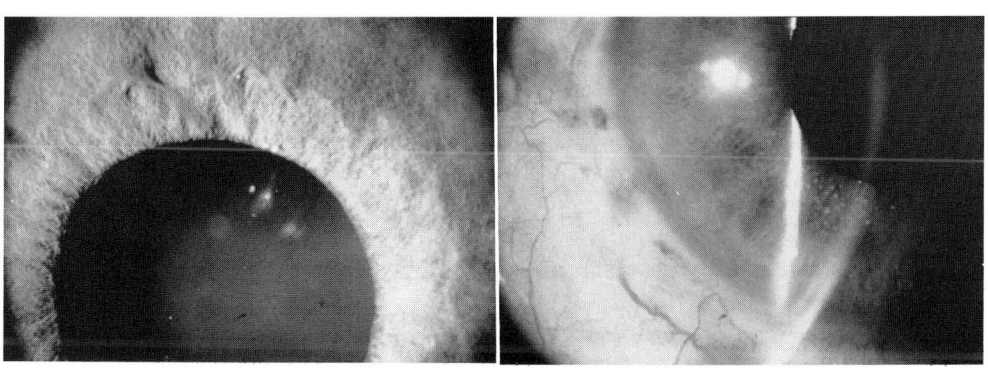

B

**Fig. 10-3. A,** Iris "pearl" of leprosy seen as small white object on iris edge. In **B,** many of these can be seen just right of slit beam. (Courtesy Khalid Tabbara, M.D.)

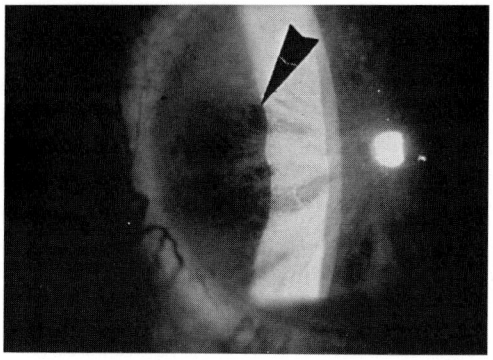

**Fig. 10-4.** Multiple areas of iris atrophy *(arrowhead)* in patient with iritis caused by leprosy. (Courtesy Fernando Oréfice, M.D.)

**Box 10-2**
**Ocular manifestations of tuberculosis**

Tubercle formation of eyelids
Conjunctivitis
Interstitial keratitis
Anterior uveitis
Scleritis
Choroidal granulomas
Posterior uveitis
Retinal vasculitis

of patients with leprosy requires careful management of the external disease including surgical management of eyelid deformities and judicial use of ocular lubrication. If intraocular surgery is planned, great care must be taken to be sure that the eye is quiet and that postoperative problems can be adequately managed.

## TUBERCULOSIS

Woods and Guyton identified tuberculosis (TB) as the most common underlying disease in the vast majority of granulomatous uveitis cases seen by them in the 1940s.[23] It is now clear that many of these patients actually had other conditions, such as ocular histoplasmosis, that caused the uveitis. Although the rates of incidence, mortality, and morbidity from TB have declined since the 1940s, 25,000 to 30,000 new cases of TB are still reported annually in the United States.[24] Furthermore, reported cases of TB have risen during the past 10 years, predominantly because of infection of patients with AIDS and immigration from endemic countries.[25] However, 25,313 cases of TB (9.8 cases per 100,000 population were reported to the Centers for Disease Control and Prevention in 1993, a 5.1% decrease from 1992.[26]

### Systemic disease

Infection in the United States is predominantly transmitted in aerosolized droplets. Most patients develop an asymptomatic, self-limited pneumonia that usually heals with granuloma formation. Sensitization develops 2 to 10 weeks after infection and is manifested by a positive skin test to an extract of the tuberculous bacillus (purified protein derivative, PPD). The granulomas usually calcify and remain inactive. However, onset of symptoms can occur after a breakdown of the patient's immune system associated with age, disease, or the use of immunosuppressive therapy for other conditions.

### Ocular disease

Ocular involvement occurs in about 1% to 2% of patients with TB.[27] The ocular manifestations of tuberculosis are listed in Box 10-2. Tuberculosis can involve both the anterior and posterior segments of the eye as well as the ocular adnexae and orbit. In miliary TB, tubercles can be seen in the choroid, giving the impression of a unifocal or multifocal choroiditis (Fig. 10-5). Choroidal tubercles have also been associated with the development of subretinal neovascularization.[28] More rarely, tubercles occur in the anterior chamber and may elicit a severe inflammatory response (Fig. 10-6). In addition, tubercle formation of the lids conjunctiva, cornea, and sclera have been reported.[29] Granulomatous iritis is the inflammatory condition most often associated with TB.[30] Coles[30a] wrote that TB should be suspected not only in cases of granulomatous uveitis but also in cases of intense nongranulomatous anterior uveitis of short duration, mild relapsing uveitis, or chronic smoldering inflammatory disease.

Interstitial keratitis and phlyctenular keratoconjunctivitis are common findings in patients with ocular TB; but they are not thought to result from direct invasion of organisms but instead to represent an immunologic response to the mycobacteria. Eales' disease, a disorder characterized by retinal vasculitis and vitreous hemorrhage, is also associated with TB (see Fig. 26-1, *A* and *B*). Finally, optic nerve involvement and cataracts have also been reported in

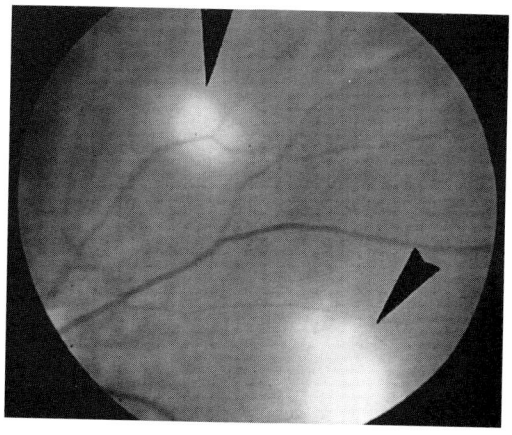

**Fig. 10-5.** Two large choroidal lesions *(arrowheads)* caused by miliary tuberculosis. (Courtesy Fernando Oréfice, M.D.)

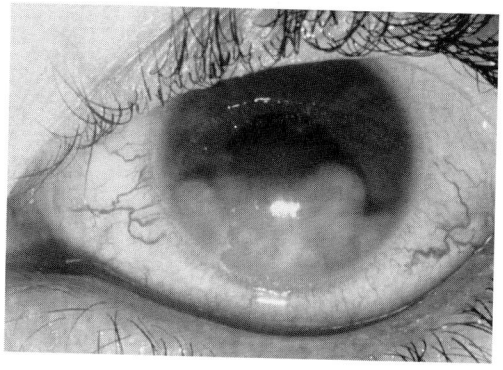

**Fig. 10-6.** Patient with systemic tuberculosis who presented with large floccular mass in anterior chamber. (Courtesy Roberto Neufeld, M.D.)

patients with ocular TB.[27,29] A number of infectious and noninfectious disorders may cause ocular disease similar to TB. For example, the retinal periphlebitis that results from tuberculosis can mimic the ocular disease associated with sarcoidosis and syphilis. Finally, an underlying immunosuppressive state, such as AIDS, should always be considered in patients with ocular TB.

## Diagnosis

The diagnosis of ocular TB is usually difficult to make. We have spent countless hours debating the diagnostic approach to patients with possible TB-associated uveitis. Definitive diagnosis requires the identification of *M. tuberculosis* organisms in ocular tissues or fluids, but samples are often difficult to obtain, and biopsy may be hard to justify in a patient who has only a small chance of having the disease. Patients with suspected ocular TB should have a systemic evaluation for evidence of the disease. A chest x-ray should be obtained, and tuberculin skin tests should be performed. An intermediate tuberculin skin test should be used for most patients. However, if a patient has a history of TB or a positive PPD in the past, an intermediate strength PPD may cause a severe dermatologic response, and a lower strength PPD should be used. In addition, a patient with numerous tubercle bacilli in the eye was reported to have a negative strength PPD and no systemic manifestations of disease.[31] Importantly, a positive PPD in a patient with uveitis does not mean that the uveitis is caused by TB, as TB is a very rare cause of inflammatory eye disease. In fact, without other signs of TB, a positive PPD in a patient with uveitis is probably more misleading than helpful.

Although many patients with ocular TB will have evidence of systemic disease, TB infection limited to specific organs, including the eye, may occur. Microscopic examination of ocular tissues or fluids may show bacilli; however, culture is more sensitive. Recently, polymerase chain reaction has been used to diagnose TB infection,[32] but this is only experimental in most laboratories at this time.

## Therapy

The previously recommended treatment of TB used to include regimens including isoniazid and ethambutol for 1.5 to 2 years. Since the late 1960s, however, a number of studies have demonstrated that short-course treatment regimens can be effective. Most regimens contain isoniazid and rifampin for 9 months. A third drug, ethambutol, streptomycin, or pyrazinamide, is usually added for the first 3 months to prevent resistance. Clearly, therapy would be administered by a practitioner well versed with the current treatment recommendations.[33]

The difficult decision is whether antituberculous therapy is warranted for the patient with an uveitis compatible with TB, no evidence of systemic disease, and a positive PPD. Schlaegel and Weber[34] have recommended an isoniazid therapeutic test for these patients. The test involves giving isoniazid at 300 mg per day and examining the patient every week. If ocular inflammation improves after 1 to 2 weeks of therapy, the patient is considered to have a positive test response. Schlaegel and Weber suggested that in these positive cases, the patient should then receive a full course of therapy. There are several problems with this test. From a practical point of view, many patients with presumed tubercuolous uveitis are concomitantly treated with corticosteroids, which makes it difficult to determine whether the antituberculous or antiinflammatory therapy had the principal effect. The disease course may wax and wane; therefore, improvement may be due to the natural course of the disorder and be unrelated to antituberculous drugs. Importantly, a randomized double-masked study of isoniazid in the treatment of uveitis showed no significant difference between the treated and placebo groups.[35] It is currently our recommendation to treat only patients with uveitis and a positive PPD if there are other findings to support the diagnosis of TB. Although the hematogenous seeding of organisms from the lung is the most common mode of ocular infection, the chest x-ray may be normal, and disease is occasionally limited to a specific organ. A history of exposure to TB, a history of inadequately treated TB, a positive PPD with a large area of induration, or positive culture results all greatly increase the likelihood of disease. Once a decision to treat is made, the patient should receive at least two drugs for at least 3 to 6 months before a decision about efficacy is made.

## SPIROCHETAL DISEASE

This section devoted to spirochetal diseases covers a historic gamut of infectious diseases with ocular manifestations, including syphilis, bejel, pinta, yaws, Lyme disease, relapsing fever, and leptospirosis. We will first discuss treponemal infections, with syphilis by far the most common and important to the practicing ophthalmologist. Syphilis remains an important cause of eye disease and blindness in the United States, and it is diagnosed with increasing frequency in patients with the acquired immunodeficiency syndrome (AIDS). Sections on endemic syphilis (bejel) and nonvenereal treponemal infections (yaws and pinta) are also included.

The second part of the section contains information on two infections caused by spirochetes of the genus *Borrelia* and a section on leptospirosis. Whereas the cause of syphilis was identified at the beginning of this century, the causative agent for Lyme disease was not discovered until 1982. Interestingly, Lyme disease and syphilis share a number of clinical features and should be considered together in the differential diagnosis of infectious diseases with ophthalmologic involvement. The section also reviews relapsing fever, an additional infection caused by *Borrelia* that is often misdiagnosed. Leptospirosis is discussed at the end of this chapter and may be an important cause of uveitis of unknown causes.

### Syphilis

**Etiology and epidemiology.** Syphilis was originally called the great pox but acquired its current name from the title character of a poem written by the Veronese physician and poet Girolamo Fracastoro in 1530. The poem was entitled *Syphilis, sive Morbus Gallicus,* which means *Syphilus, or the French Disease.* In the poem, the name of this dreaded venereal disease is an altered form of the hero's name, Syphilus. The hero was a shepherd and is supposed to have been the first victim of the disease. Syphilis has also been called the "great imitator," because of the myriad of symptoms and signs in its repertoire and its ability to mimic a number of other illnesses. Although clinical descriptions of syphilis date back at least half a millennium, it was not until 1905 that Schaudinn and Hoffman[36] isolated the spirochete *Treponema pallidum* from skin lesions of patients with syphilis.

After initial infection there is both a humoral and cellular immune response. In 1910, Wasserman introduced a complement fixation test to detect nonspecific antibodies that react against cardiolipins, antibodies that are commonly found in patients with syphilis. The next milestone in the history of syphilis was the use of arsenic derivatives to treat the disease. The coup de grâce in the war against syphilis came in 1943 with the discovery of penicillin, still the mainstay of therapy today.[37] Unfortunately, syphilis is again becoming a prominent adversary to those who battle infectious diseases. There has been a substantial increase in primary and secondary syphilis and an increased incidence in congenital syphilis, especially in the inner city.[38,39] In 1986, only 57 cases of congenital syphilis were reported in New York City, but in 1989, over 1000 cases were documented.[40] Syphilis is also a problem in patients coinfected with HIV. These patients may not mount a serologic response to the treponemal infection and thus elude diagnosis. In addition, standard therapy may be insufficient to eradicate the infection in these immunocompromised patients.[41,42]

*T. pallidum* cannot survive long out of the body; it can be cultured and remain viable for several days. Syphilis is transmitted almost exclusively by sexual contact, including sexual intercourse, orogenital and anorectal contact, and occasionally by kissing. Patients with untreated primary syphilis or secondary syphilis with skin lesions are the most infectious. Disease can also be transmitted by patients with early latent syphilis, especially if they have mucocutaneous involvement; however, patients with late latent syphilis and tertiary syphilis are not infectious. Congenital syphilis occurs with transplacental spread of the spirochete. Interestingly, infection with syphilis does not confer lasting immunity, especially if treatment is received early in the course of the disease.

*T. pallidum* can penetrate intact mucous membranes or abraded skin. The period of incubation varies from 10 to 90 days but averages 3 weeks.[43] Before primary skin lesions appear, the spirochete spreads through the lymphatics to the bloodstream where it then disseminates.

As with many of the spirochetal diseases, the clinical course of syphilis is divided into stages: primary, secondary, and tertiary syphilis.

**Clinical manifestations**

***Primary syphilis.*** The chancre is the predominant lesion of primary syphilis. It appears about 4 weeks after infection and heals in about 1 to 2 months in untreated persons. The lesion begins as an erythematous papule at the inoculation site and later erodes to form a painless ulcer. Multiple chancres can occur, especially in patients coinfected with HIV.[44] Serous fluid from these lesions is teeming with spirochetes. Lesions occur on the penis, anus, and rectum in men, and on the cervix, vulva, and perineum in women. Small lesions may also occur on the lips, tongue, buccal mucosa, and skin, and chancres of the eyelids and conjunctiva have also been described.[45]

***Secondary syphilis.*** If untreated, patients with primary syphilis will progress to secondary syphilis 4 to 10 weeks after initial manifestations of the disease. A generalized rash is characteristic of secondary syphilis and may be maculopapular or pustular. The rash commonly occurs on the flexor and volar surfaces of the body, typically the palms and the soles. The rash usually resolves without scarring, but some patients are left with areas of hyperpigmentation or hypopigmentation. Mucous membranes become eroded forming erythematous patches. Condylomata lata are another characteristic dermatologic manifestation of secondary syphilis. They are papules that develop at the mucocutaneous junctions and in moist areas of the skin and appear as dull pink or gray hypertrophic lesions. Systemic symptoms of secondary syphilis include fever, malaise, headache, nausea, anorexia, and joint pain.[46] A generalized lymphadenopathy is found in both primary and secondary syphilis. Syphilitic infiltration of the kidneys, liver, and gastrointestinal tract also occurs in secondary syphilis, and about 10% of patients will have ocular involvement. Anterior uveitis is the predominant eye finding in early secondary syphilis and may be the most common ocular lesion in syphilis.[47] A number of patients may demonstrate a cerebrospinal fluid (CSF) pleocytosis, and a few of these will develop acute syphilitic meningitis with headache, neck stiffness, cranial nerve palsies, and disc edema.

***Latent syphilis.*** In the first year after initial infection, patients may have recurrence of infectious mucocutaneous lesions. This period of the disease is called early latent syphilis. The late latent phase of syphilis occurs after 1 year after infection, and during this stage of the disease infectious relapses are rare. Most patients who have not been treated will remain in this late latent phase of the disease; however, about 30% of patients will go on to develop tertiary syphilis.

***Tertiary syphilis.*** Tertiary syphilis is also called late syphilis and is often subdivided into three groups: benign tertiary syphilis, cardiovascular syphilis, and neurosyphilis.

***Benign tertiary syphilis.*** The gumma is the typical lesion of benign tertiary syphilis and is a chronic granulomatous lesion that heals with scarring and fibrosis. It is a rare finding and responds rapidly to treatment. The gummas tend to develop in the skin and mucous membranes but can occur in almost any tissue and have even been found in the choroid of the eye.[48]

***Cardiovascular syphilis.*** The lesions of cardiovascular syphilis include aortitis and aortic aneurysms, aortic valvular insufficiency, and narrowing of the coronary ostia. Disease starts about 5 to 10 years after infection, but symptoms of cardiovascular syphilis may not be clinically evident for over 20 years.

***Neurosyphilis.*** Neurosyphilis is said to occur in 5% to 10% of untreated patients with syphilis. Asymptomatic neurosyphilis is found in some patients who have a positive CSF Venereal Disease Research Laboratory (VDRL) test, but no symptoms of central nervous system (CNS) disease. In addition, invasion of the central nervous system by *T. pallidum* may be more common in early syphilis than once thought. Lukehart and colleagues[49] isolated *T. pallidum* from the CSF of 12 (30%) of 40 patients with untreated primary and secondary syphilis, and an additional four patients had a reactive CSF VDRL test in which no *T. pallidum* was isolated.

One type of neurosyphilis, meningovascular syphilis, presents as an aseptic meningitis that can occur at any time after primary syphilis. Unilateral or bilateral cranial nerve palsies are common, and headache, neck stiffness, dizziness, lassitude, and blurred vision occur. The classic neuroophthalmic finding of neurosyphilis is the Argyll Robertson pupil.[50] The Argyll Robertson pupil is a small irregular pupil that is unreactive to light but normally reactive to accommodation; it is frequently seen in cases of meningovascular syphilis when the base of the brain is involved. The spinal cord may also be involved.

*T. pallidum* may also invade the substance of the brain. Parenchymatous neurosyphilis is a meningoencephalitis with progressive loss of cortical function. Patients can develop altered mental status and even a syphilitic psychosis. Pathologically, the brain parenchyma is infiltrated with spirochetes, and the meninges are inflamed and thickened. The CSF is abnormal with a positive VDRL. Cranial nerve palsies, however, are uncommon, and optic atrophy is rare. Although pupillary abnormalities may be seen, complete Argyll Robertson pupil is not characteristic. Neurosyphilis should still be considered in the differential diagnosis of advanced neurologic disease with generalized paresis, although this finding is rare in the United States.

Tabes dorsalis is a form of neurosyphilis with involvement of the posterior columns and posterior roots of the spinal cord resulting in pain, ataxia, sensory changes, decreased tendon reflexes, and frequent ocular findings. Severe stabbing pain of the lower extremities heralds this form of neurosyphilis. Charcot's joints are destructive changes that occur in the large joints devoid of sensation. Argyll Robertson pupils are common in this form of neurosyphilis, and optic atrophy is frequently found.

***Congenital syphilis.*** Congenital syphilis results from the transplacental transmission of *T. pallidum* from the mother to the fetus. Untreated primary or secondary syphilis is almost invariably transmitted to the fetus, although transmission in later stages of the disease occurs less frequently. Congenital syphilis is preventable with proper treatment of the mother; therefore all expectant mothers should be tested with a VDRL at the beginning and near the end of pregnancy. In fact, screening at the time of delivery is now mandated in New York state.[40]

Signs and symptoms of early congenital syphilis may not appear until several days after birth, and a recent study by Dorfman and Glaser[51] states that congenital syphilis may be missed if serologic tests are not performed for both the mother and her infant at the time of delivery. A generalized rash develops and resembles the rash of secondary syphilis except that in the infant, the rash may be vesicular or bullous. Rhinitis (also called the snuffles), jaundice, hepatosplenomegaly, anorexia, and pseudoparalysis may also be found. Osteochondritis and pathologic fractures are common, and radiographic changes on bone films are present in over 90% of patients. Chorioretinitis is often evident in the first few months of life.

Congenital syphilis may mimic a number of other congenital infections such as rubella, cytomegalovirus, and toxoplasmosis. A positive serologic test for syphilis may result from passive transfer of antibody from the mother; therefore diagnosis of congenital syphilis is based on a positive fluorescent treponemal antibody absorption (FTA-ABS) test and a rising VDRL titer. Serologic tests performed in infants and their mothers may be negative at the time of delivery if syphilis is acquired toward the end of the pregnancy.

After 2 years, the child is defined as having late congenital syphilis. Like syphilis in adults, late congenital syphilis may remain latent with few sequelae, although cardiovascular involve-

**Box 10-3**
**Ocular manifestations of syphilis**

**PRIMARY SYPHILIS**

Chancres of eyelid and conjunctiva

**SECONDARY SYPHILIS**

Blepharitis
Madarosis
Conjunctivitis
Dacryocystitis
Dacryoadenitis
Keratitis
Iris nodules
Iridocyclitis
Episcleritis
Scleritis
Chorioretinitis
Vitritis
Neuroretinitis
Disc edema
Exudative retinal detachment
Perivasculitis

**TERTIARY SYPHILIS**

Gummas of eyelids
Unilateral interstitial keratitis
Punctate stromal keratitis
Bilateral periostitis of the orbital bones
Episcleritis
Scleritis
Anterior and posterior uveitis
Chorioretinitis
Vasculitis
Venous and arterial occlusive disease
Exudative retinal detachment
Macular edema
Neuroretinitis
Vitritis
Pseudoretinitis pigmentosa
Chorioretinal neovascular membrane
Lens dislocation
Argyll Robertson pupil
Oculomotor palsies

**CONGENITAL SYPHILIS**

Bilateral interstitial keratitis
Pigmentary retinitis
Glaucoma
Keratouveitis

Modified from Whitcup SM, Raizman MB: Spirochetal infections and the eye. In Albert DM, Jakobiec FA, editors: *Principles and practice of ophthalmology,* vol 5, Philadelphia, 1994, WB Saunders, pp 3078-3092.

ment does occur and meningovascular syphilis with neurologic manifestations including eighth cranial nerve deafness is not uncommon. Acute syphilitic meningitis, generalized paresis, and tabes dorsalis are less common. Interstitial keratitis is the classic ophthalmologic sign of congenital syphilis and occurs in 10% of patients.

Deformities of the permanent teeth occur after early syphilitic infection. The characteristic "Hutchinson's teeth" are notched thin upper incisors with abnormal spacing. Hutchinson's triad is the occurrence of Hutchinson's teeth, interstitial keratitis, and deafness, but the occurrence of all three in the same patient is unusual. The bone lesions of early congenital syphilis tend to progress in late congenital syphilis with the development of syphilitic arthritis. Finally, gummas may develop in the subcutaneous tissue and produce ulcerative skin lesions.

**Ocular manifestations.** Box 10-3 lists some of the more common eye manifestations of the different stages of syphilis. Ophthalmologic manifestations of primary syphilis are limited to chancres of the eyelid and conjunctiva. A primary syphilitic lesion in the lacrimal gland is extremely rare but reported.[52]

The eyelids are commonly involved with the rash of secondary syphilis, with the frequent occurrence of blepharitis and loss of lashes and eyebrows. Conjunctivitis mimicking trachoma has also been seen in secondary syphilis, but dacryocystitis and dacryoadenitis are rare. Keratitis, iris nodules (Fig. 10-7), iridocyclitis, episcleritis, and scleritis have all been reported in secondary syphilis. Late in the secondary stage, a chorioretinitis and vitritis may develop (Fig. 10-8). A diffuse neuroretinitis may occur and is often localized to the peripapillary area.[53] This neuroretinitis is followed by a pigmentary retinopathy simi-

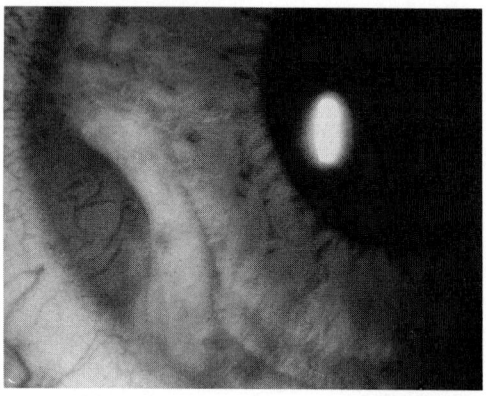

**Fig. 10-7.** Iris nodule caused by syphilis. (From Weekly clinicopathological exercises, *N Engl J Med* 310: 972-981, 1984.)

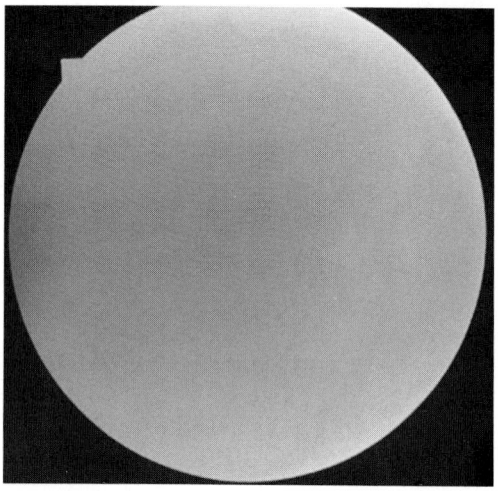

**Fig. 10-8.** Dense vitritis in patient with syphilis. Optic disc and retinal vasculature are barely visible. Patient was treated with course of intravenous penicillin with resolution of vitritis (see Fig. 10-9).

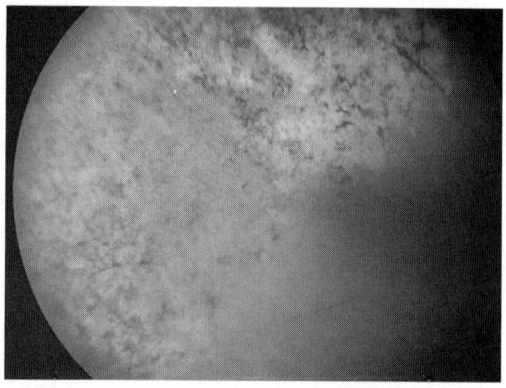

**Fig. 10-9.** Patient with syphilis shown in Fig. 10-8 after intravenous penicillin therapy. Vitritis and retinal infiltrates have resolved, and pigmentary retinopathy characteristic of old ocular syphilis is noted.

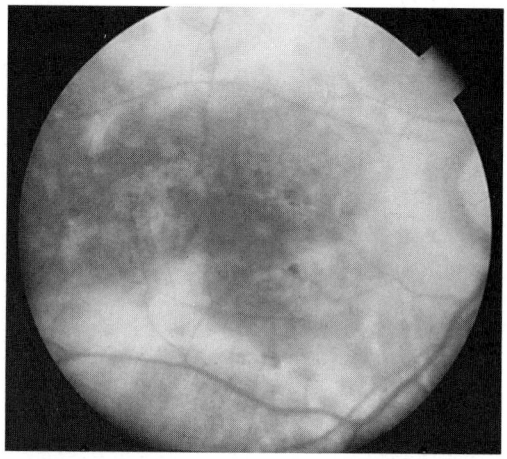

**Fig. 10-10.** Extensive subretinal fibrosis caused by ocular syphilis. (Courtesy Rubens Belfort, Jr., M.D.)

lar in appearance to retinitis pigmentosa (Fig. 10-9). In some cases, the pigmentary retinopathy is associated with diffuse areas of subretinal fibrosis (Fig. 10-10). Disc edema (Fig. 10-11), exudative retinal detachment, and vasculitis (Fig. 10-12) are less common findings.[54,55]

The gummas of tertiary syphilis can involve the lids and, if extensive, cause destructive ulceration, but gummatous dacryoadenitis and infiltration of the lacrimal sac have only rarely been reported. Conjunctival vascular changes occur, but gummas of the conjunctiva almost never occur. As seen in secondary syphilis, syphilitic blepharitis with madarosis is not uncommon. A diffuse bilateral periostitis is the most frequent orbital finding of tertiary syphilis. A uniocular interstitial keratitis is the most common corneal finding in tertiary syphilis, but a punctate stromal keratitis can occur with iritis. Episcleritis and scleritis occur, but discrete gummas of the sclera are rare. Uveitis is a frequent finding in late tertiary syphilis. Halperin and colleagues[56] state that the main posterior segment complications of acquired syphilis include chorioretinitis, vasculitis, venous and arterial occlusive disease, retinal detachment with choroidal effusion, macular edema, neuroretinitis, optic neuritis, vitritis, and pseudoretinitis pigmentosa. They also report five cases of choroidal neovascular membranes associated with acquired syphilis. Vitreous opacities are common, and lens dis-

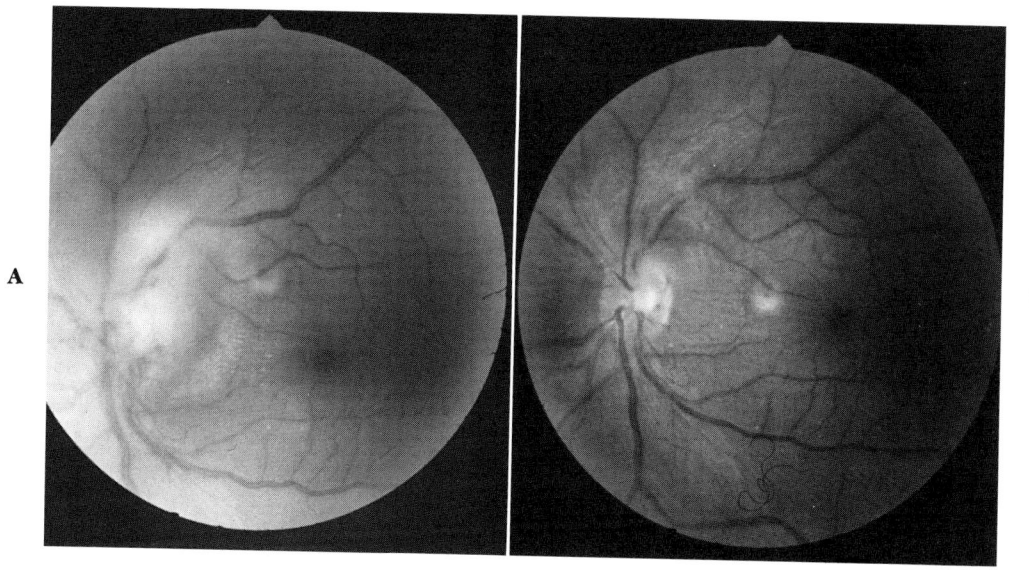


**Fig. 10-11.** Patient with acquired syphilis who presented with papillitis and retinitis **(A).** Patient was treated vigorously with antibiotics, and resolution of lesion was noted **(B).** (Courtesy Phuc Le Hoang, M.D.)

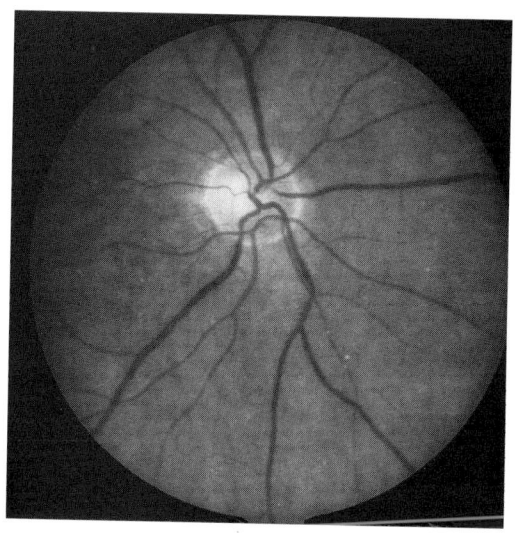

**Fig. 10-12.** Nodular arteritis in patient with secondary syphilis that cleared with appropriate therapy. (Courtesy N. Le Van, M.D., and Phuc Le Hoang, M.D.)

location has been reported in a number of patients.

The most typical manifestation of congenital syphilis is bilateral interstitial keratitis that appears later in life. A pigmentary retinitis and glaucoma can also occur as a result of congenital syphilitic keratouveitis.

The Argyll Robertson pupil and disc edema are most frequently seen in meningovascular syphilis along with oculomotor palsies and other pupillary abnormalities. Later in the course of meningovascular syphilis, optic atrophy is found. Complete Argyll Robertson pupil is rare in cases of general paresis, but as with optic atrophy, it is more common in cases of tabes dorsalis.

**Diagnosis.** The diagnosis of syphilis is based on the clinical history, physical examination, and laboratory tests. Confusion often arises in determining when to order a VDRL versus FTA-ABS and in interpreting the results. In this section the various diagnostic tests for syphilis will be explained, and a strategy for ordering tests will be outlined.

Darkfield microscopy can be used to identify spirochetes present in tissue fluids. *T. pallidum* is difficult to distinguish from other spirochetes; thus darkfield examination requires expertise. In clinical practice, greater reliance is placed on the serologic tests for syphilis.

The two most commonly used screening tests for syphilis are the Venereal Disease Research Laboratory (VDRL) test and the rapid plasma reagin (RPR) test. Infection with *T. pallidum* stimulates nonspecific antibodies against cardiolipin. The VDRL test quantitates these antibodies with slide flocculation. The VDRL test is well standardized and is reported as reactive, weakly reactive, borderline, or nonreactive. The RPR is a similar test to detect anticardiolipin antibody.

The sensitivity and specificity of the VDRL test varies depending on the stage of disease (Table 10-1). The VDRL test starts to become

**Table 10-1.** Patients With Positive Results to VDRL and FTA-ABS Tests

| Test | Primary syphilis (%) | Secondary syphilis (%) | Late or latent syphilis | |
|---|---|---|---|---|
| | | | Treated (%) | Untreated (%) |
| VDRL | 70 | 99 | 1 | 70 |
| FTA-ABS | 85 | 100 | 98 | 98 |

Modified from Whitcup SM, Raizman MB: Spirochetal infections and the eye. In Albert DM, Jakobiec FA, editors: *Principles and practice of ophthalmology,* vol 5, Philadelphia, 1994, WB Saunders, pp 3078-3092.

positive about 1 to 2 weeks after the appearance of the primary chancre and is positive in 99% of patients with secondary syphilis.[57] In later stages of the disease, however, the VDRL test reactivity decreases, and only about 70% of patients with cardiovascular or neurosyphilis have a positive VDRL test. In addition, the VDRL test will often become nonreactive after treatment for syphilis.

The serologic tests for syphilis are not 100% specific, and a number of false-positive results can occur, especially with other spirochetal diseases and connective tissue diseases (Box 10-4). Any weakly reactive or reactive VDRL needs to be confirmed with a more specific test. The tests used for this purpose are the treponemal tests for syphilis such as the *Treponema pallidum* immobilization (TPI) test or the more commonly used FTA-ABS test. The TPI test is almost completely specific for syphilis, but it is expensive and difficult to perform and is thus used less frequently than the FTA-ABS test. The microhemagglutination assay for antibodies to *T. pallidum* is another specific test for syphilis, but is also used less frequently than the FTA-ABS tests. In the FTA-ABS test, the patient's serum is absorbed with extracts of nonpathogenic treponemes to remove possible cross-reacting antitreponemal antibody not specific for *T. pallidum.* The absorbed serum is then reacted against *T. pallidum,* and specific antibodies are detected by the addition of fluorescein-labeled antihuman gamma globulin. Results are reported as nonreactive or as 1 to 4+ positive, on the basis of the intensity of the fluorescence.

A weakly reactive FTA-ABS test may not be reproducible. The FTA-ABS test is more sensitive than the VDRL at all stages of syphilis, but it is more expensive and difficult to perform. The FTA-ABS is also not entirely specific for syphilis, as false-positive results are seen in patients with systemic lupus erythematosis, biliary cirrhosis, and some connective tissue diseases such as rheumatoid arthritis (Box 10-4).

Because serologic tests for syphilis may take several weeks to become reactive, immediate diagnosis requires demonstration of treponemes in tissue fluid by darkfield microscopy. The VDRL test is an excellent screening test for patients with later primary and secondary syphilis. The sensitivity of the VDRL test is 99% for patients with secondary syphilis; however, all positive results should be confirmed with an FTA-ABS test.

Because the sensitivity of the VDRL test may be only 70% in patients with latent or late syphilis, an FTA-ABS test should be ordered if later stage syphilis is suspected. From the ophthalmologic standpoint, many patients with uveitis or disc edema are suspected of having late syphilis, and many uveitis specialists and neuroophthalmologists routinely order both a VDRL and FTA-ABS test in the evaluation of these patients.

In addition, all patients who may have had syphilis for more than a year should have a lumbar puncture to examine CSF. A cell count, differential, protein, and VDRL test should be performed on the CSF to look for evidence of neurosyphilis. As stated previously, CNS invasion by *T. pallidum* may be common in early syphilis.[49] The finding of CNS involvement is important because the recommended therapy is different than for patients without CNS involvement.

Infants born with congenital syphilis will have a positive VDRL and FTA-ABS test from the passive transfer of IgG antibodies across the placenta; therefore, an IgM FTA-ABS test is used to diagnose congenital syphilis, because IgM antibodies do not cross the placenta, and a positive test would indicate actual infection in the infant.[40]

Patients with undiagnosed interstitial keratitis should be suspected of having late congeni-

**Box 10-4**
**Causes of false-positive serologic test results for syphilis**

**Spirochetal infections**

Endemic syphilis/bejel
Yaws and pinta
Leptospirosis
Lyme disease
Relapsing fever

**Other infections**

Chancroid
Chickenpox
Hepatitis
HIV
Infectious mononucleosis
Leprosy
Malaria
Measles
Mycoplasma pneumonia
Pneumococcal pneumonia
Scarlet fever
Subacute bacterial endocarditis
Trypanosomiasis

**Noninfectious diseases/states**

Blood transfusions
Chronic liver disease
Connective tissue disease
Narcotic addiction
Pregnancy
Vaccination

Modified from Whitcup SM, Raizman MB: Spirochetal infections and the eye. In Albert DM, Jakobiec FA, editors: *Principles and practice of ophthalmology,* vol 5, Philadelphia, 1994, WB Saunders, pp 3078-3092.

tal syphilis. A thorough history of previous therapy should be elicited, and patients should then be given VDRL and FTA-ABS tests and a CSF examination. If the CSF VDRL is positive, some experts recommend that the patient be treated for latent syphilis (see Table 10-1). Patients with a positive serum VDRL or FTA-ABS but a negative CSF examination are treated for primary or secondary syphilis.

**Prognosis.** Most patients recover without long-term sequelae when syphilis is recognized and treated early. If untreated, about 25% of patients with syphilis will have one or more relapses with mucocutaneous lesions. Eventually, most untreated patients will remain in a latent stage of the disease; however, about one third of patients will go on to develop tertiary syphilis. Benign tertiary syphilis occurs in about 15% of untreated patients. Cardiovascular syphilis occurs in 10% and CNS involvement is seen in about 8% of untreated patients.

**Box 10-5**
**Treatment of syphilis**

Primary and secondary syphilis
Procaine penicillin, 2.4 million units, and probenecid 1.0 g po qd × 10 days.
If penicillin allergies exist, treat with erythromycin or tetracycline 500 mg po q 6 hours × 15 days or doxycycline 200 mg po qd × 15 days.
Latent and tertiary syphilis including neurosyphilis
Aqueous crystalline penicillin G 2.0 to 4.0 million units IV q4 hours × 10 days.
Congenital syphilis in the infant
Procaine penicillin 50,000 units/kg/day IM × 10 days or aqueous crystalline penicillin G 50,000 units/kg/day IM or IV in two divided doses × 10 days.

Modified from Whitcup SM, Raizman MB: Spirochetal infections and the eye. In Albert DM, Jakobiec FA, editors: *Principles and practice of ophthalmology,* vol 5, Philadelphia, 1994, WB Saunders, pp 3078-3092.

**Treatment**

***General recommendations.*** Although guidelines for the treatment of syphilis exist, controversy persists. Before treating a patient with syphilis, one should refer to the most current recommendations for therapy, and consultation with an infectious disease specialist may be helpful. Coinfection with HIV should be ruled out because standard therapy may be insufficient to eradicate disease in these patients. Recommendations for therapy are based on the stage of disease and are presented in Box 10-5.[57] Unfortunately, the ideal therapy for patients with uveitic syphilis has not been determined. Persistent virulent *T. pallidum* have been reported to persist in the eye despite treatment with penicillin; therefore many experts suggest that patients with any ocular inflammation as a result of syphilis be treated as for neurosyphilis, even if the CSF examination is normal.

In addition to treating the patient, the physician has a responsibility to report the disease to the local health department to ensure that all sexual contacts over at least the past 3 months are contacted, examined, and treated as necessary.

Patients with syphilis should have their VDRL test repeated at 3, 6, and 12 months after treatment because titers should become nonreactive within a year after successful therapy. In addition, patients with CSF involvement should have a repeat CSF examination at 6-month intervals for at least 3 years. Patients should be retreated if clinical evidence of syphilis occurs, if a previously nonreactive VDRL test again becomes reactive, or if an initially high-titer VDRL test does not decrease fourfold within a year.

Finally, patients who receive therapy for syphilis, especially intravenous therapy, should be monitored for a Jarisch-Herxheimer reaction. This is a hypersensitivity response to treponemal antigens. This reaction may exacerbate preexisting ocular inflammation such as uveitis and interstitial keratitis, and prophylaxis with corticosteroids may be helpful in some cases.

***Approach to syphilis in patients with AIDS.*** Recognition of concurrent infection with HIV in patients with syphilis is important to the clinician because the diagnostic and therapeutic approach to syphilis may differ in these patients. A number of reports suggest that uncharacteristic clinical manifestations of syphilis may be seen in patients with concomitant HIV infection.[42,58] Unusual cases of ocular syphilis in HIV-infected patients have been reported with findings of panuveitis and retinal detachment, and some authors[59–61] state that the incidence of ocular complications of syphilis may be increased in HIV-infected patients. In addition, acute retinal necrosis and acute retinitis have been associated with syphilis in patients coinfected with HIV.[55,59] Despite some unique symptoms and signs, these patients usually also develop the characteristic clinical manifestations of syphilis. Patients with both HIV infection and syphilis may have an accelerated course with a greater likelihood of uveitis and progression to neurosyphilis.[42,60,62] In the study by Lukehart and colleagues,[49] there was no difference in the detection of *T. pallidum* in the CSF in patients with or without concurrent HIV infection; nevertheless, it appears that treatment failures are more common in HIV-infected patients.[41,63,64] In addition, serologic evidence of syphilis may be delayed. Hicks and colleagues[65] reported a patient with AIDS and skin manifestations consistent with secondary syphilis in whom VDRL and FTA-ABS test results were negative on two separate occasions. A skin biopsy demonstrated spirochetes with Warthin-Starry staining of the tissue, and later the results of the patient's VDRL and FTA-ABS tests became positive, suggesting a delayed immunologic response.

A number of patients with HIV infection and CNS involvement with syphilis do not have positive results to CSF VDRL tests and may only manifest CSF leukocytosis or elevated CSF protein concentration, findings that are seen in HIV patients without syphilis.[66] These findings have prompted some clinicians to treat all patients with concurrent HIV infection and syphilis with high dosage antibiotics to cover the possibility of CNS involvement. The Centers for Disease Control and Prevention in Atlanta is currently studying the question of appropriate antibiotic therapy for patients with syphilis and concurrent HIV infection. For now, recommendations include the careful evaluation of all patients with syphilis for underlying HIV infection. Patients with AIDS should also be monitored for clinical signs of syphilis, and the diagnosis pursued despite negative serologic test results early in the course of the disease.

Patients with syphilis and HIV infection should have a lumbar puncture to look for evidence of neurosyphilis. Because treatment failures are common, some infectious disease consultants suggest that all patients be treated with a regimen adequate for neurosyphilis. After treatment a VDRL test is suggested every month for at least 3 months with close observation for evidence of recurrence.[67]

## Nonvenereal treponematoses

### Endemic syphilis

***Etiology and epidemiology.*** Endemic syphilis, yaws, and pinta are three nonvenereal treponemal infections that are spread by body contact and are endemic in certain geographic areas. Endemic syphiis, also known as bejel, is caused by *T. pallidum II,* a spirochete that is morphologically and serologically indistinguishable from the *T. pallidum* that causes syphilis. Bejel is endemic in a number of arid

**Box 10-6**
**Ocular manifestations of endemic syphilis**

Anterior uveitis
Iris atrophy
Cataract
Vitreous opacity
Optic atrophy
Choroiditis
Chorioretinitis
Attenuated retinal arterioles
Patchy choroidal atrophy

Modified from Whitcup SM, Raizman MB: Spirochetal infections and the eye. In Albert DM, Jakobiec FA, editors: *Principles and practice of ophthalmology*, vol 5, Philadelphia, 1994, WB Saunders, pp 3078-3092.

countries, mostly in the Middle East and Africa.[68]

***Clinical manifestations.*** Onset of bejel usually occurs in childhood and typically presents with a mucous patch on the buccal mucosa. Mucosal lesions are followed by papulosquamous and erosive papular lesions of the trunk and extremities. Latency can occur if early stages of the disease are not treated. Periostitis of the bones of the legs and gummatous lesions of the nose and soft palate are seen in later stages. Neurologic and cardiovascular involvement, and congenital transmission of endemic syphilis are uncharacteristic of endemic syphilis. Similarly, chancres, typical of primary syphilis, are not found as early signs of endemic syphilis.

***Ocular manifestations.*** Although neurologic involvement is uncharacteristic of endemic syphilis, ocular manifestations have been reported. Tabbara and colleagues[69] studied 17 patients with clinical findings and serologic studies consistent with endemic syphilis, who also had ocular complaints. Eye findings included uveitis in nine patients, optic atrophy in six patients, and chorioretinal scars in six patients. Additional findings are presented in Box 10-6.

***Diagnosis.*** Serologic tests do not distinguish endemic syphilis from venereal syphilis. Both the VDRL and FTA-ABS are typically positive in endemic syphilis, and spirochetes can be isolated from skin lesions. Differentiation of venereal and nonvenereal syphilis is therefore made on clinical grounds.

***Prognosis.*** Most patients with bejel respond well to antibiotic therapy. The prognosis of untreated bejel is unknown. Patients can develop neurologic or cardiovascular sequelae late in the course of their disease; however, symptoms are usually mild in comparison to tertiary syphilis.

***Treatment.*** Patients with early lesions are treated with one dose of benzathine penicillin, 1.2 million units given intramuscularly. Patients with late manifestations of endemic syphilis are treated with two doses of penicillin separated by 7 days. After treatment, most patients will become seronegative and should be monitored for this.

**Yaws and pinta.** Yaws, also called frambesia, is a nonvenereal treponematosis endemic in humid countries near the equator.[70] After an incubation period of 3 to 4 weeks, the first manifestation of the disease is a skin papule often on the lower extremities. The lesion enlarges, ulcerates, and becomes crusted, often with regional lymphadenitis. A secondary, generalized rash occurs as the initial lesion heals. Soft granulomas then erupt on the face, legs, and buttocks, often at mucocutaneous junctions. Hyperkeratotic lesions also develop, and may occur on the soles of the feet. Later in the course of the disease, periostitis, exostoses of the maxillary bone, juxtaarticular nodules, and gummatous skin lesions may appear.

Pinta is the third nonvenereal treponematosis and is endemic among the Indians of Mexico, Central America, and South America. Similar to yaws, pinta begins as a small papule at the inoculation site with regional lymphadenitis followed by a generalized maculopapular eruption. One to several years after healing of the initial skin lesion, large blue or brown macules are found over the extremities, face, and neck. They later become depigmented and may be misdiagnosed as vitiligo. Also, as in yaws, hyperkeratotic lesions on the soles of the feet are found.

***Ocular manifestations.*** J. Lawton Smith and colleagues[71] headed a cooperative study to determine whether neuroophthalmologic involvement occurs in late yaws or pinta. A group of 71 patients with late yaws, 11 patients with late pinta, and 41 matched positive and negative controls were examined. Ocular and neurologic abnormalities were not found in cases of late pinta, although one patient had a bilateral interstitial keratitis. Nevertheless, several patients with late yaws had neuroophthalmic abnormalities including light-near dissociation of the pupillary response, perivascular pigmentation, and sheathing of the retinal vessels, and moderate optic atrophy.

***Diagnosis.*** As in endemic syphilis, spirochetes may be isolated from skin lesions at the site of inoculation. Two weeks after inoculation, both the VDRL and FTA-ABS are positive, and the diagnosis of yaws and pinta is based on clinical findings in the setting of positive syphilis serologies.

***Prognosis.*** Yaws may undergo spontaneous clinical and serologic resolution at any stage of the disease without therapy; however, antibiotic treatment improves the cure rate. Untreated patients may develop periarticular ulcers that cause crippling contractures and osteomyelitis. Patients with untreated pinta develop depigmented patches of the skin that may lead to their social ostracization, the major consequence of pinta.

***Treatment.*** The treatment of yaws and pinta parallels the therapy outlined for endemic syphilis.

**Lyme disease**

***Etiology and epidemiology.*** In the spring and summer of 1975 there was a group of children living in Lyme, Conn., that presented with an inflammatory arthropathy similar to juvenile rheumatoid arthritis.[72] A characteristic rash was associated with the illness as well as neurologic and cardiac abnormalities. Steere and colleagues labeled this illness as Lyme disease in 1977. Epidemiologic studies implicated ticks as the vector for the disease, but the etiologic agent for Lyme disease remained elusive.

Similar rashes called erythema migrans or erythema chronicum migrans had been associated with tick bites and systemic disease in Europe, and spirochete-like structures had been found in skin specimens from several patients.[73] In the United States, evidence was accumulating that patients with Lyme disease treated with penicillin fared better than untreated patients. A tick-borne organism was suspected as the causative agent, and in 1982 Dr. Willy Burgdorfer found spirochetes in *Ixodes dammini* ticks while looking for the cause of Rocky Mountain Spotted Fever in his Montana laboratory.[74] Spirochetes were later isolated from patients with Lyme disease in the United States as well as from patients in Europe with erythema migrans and Bannwarth's syndrome (a chronic lymphocytic meningitis associated with erythema chronicum migrans).[75] The previously unrecognized spirochete was isolated by Burgdorfer and Barbour, and named *Borrelia burgdorferi.*[76]

Along with *Leptospira* and *Treponema, Borrelia* belongs to the eubacterial phylum of spirochetes.[77] They are usually more loosely coiled than other spirochetes, but if coiled, they have a cork-screw appearance and look exactly like *Treponema pallidum. Borrelia* are easy to isolate from infected ticks, but are difficult to isolate from infected patients. *Borrelia burgdorferi* is transmitted by certain *Ixodes* ticks. In the United States the preferred host for the larval and nymphal forms of the tick is the white-footed mouse,[78] whereas the preferred host for the adult form of the tick is the white-footed deer.[79] The ticks have now been found on at least 30 species of animals and 49 species of birds.[80] Lyme disease also occurs in domestic animals including cats, dogs, and horses. *Ixodes* ticks are multitalented and also transmit babesiosis and tularemia in addition to Lyme disease.

There were 13,795 cases of Lyme disease reported in the United States from 1980 to 1988.[81] These cases occurred mostly in three areas: the northeast from Massachusetts to Maryland, the midwest in Wisconsin and Minnesota, and on the west coast in California and Oregon, although sporadic cases have been reported in 43 states. Lyme disease is thought to be the most common vector-borne infection in the United States, and it has also been reported in Europe, the Soviet Union, China, Japan, and Australia. The rapid spread of the disease has been attributed to an increase in forested areas that house the tick-infested deer and the migration of susceptible residents into these areas. For example, 35% of 190 residents living adjacent to a nature preserve in Ipswich, Mass., developed Lyme disease over a 7-year period.[82] The number of cases of Lyme disease continues to grow as awareness of the disease by both physicians and patients increases.

***Clinical manifestations.*** Lyme disease is usually described as occurring in stages. Early infection is divided into stage 1 (local) and

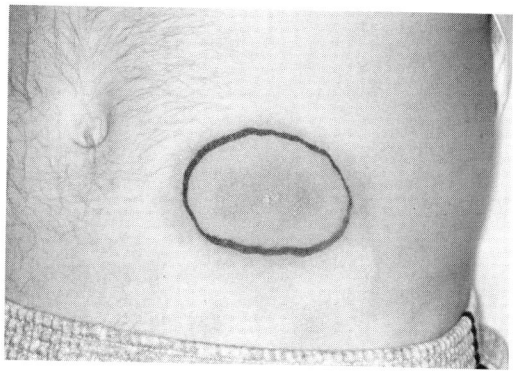

**Fig. 10-13.** Erythema migrans, rash characteristic of Lyme disease, is seen on abdomen of patient. Rash is usually oval or annular with expanding borders. Black circle was drawn to outline border of rash 24 hours before time of this photograph. Note that borders of rash have expanded substantially since previous day. (Courtesy Stephen Katz, M.D.) (See Color Plate 16.)

stage 2 (disseminated). Late infection is categorized as stage 3 (persistent). After infection, the spirochete spreads locally in the skin in 60% to 80% of patients and causes the characteristic rash, erythema migrans.[80,83] Erythema migrans is an oval or annular, erythematous lesion with expanding borders that usually fades in 3 to 4 weeks in untreated patients but may recur later in the disease (Fig. 10-13). Patients will recall being bitten by a tick about half of the time. Specific antibody to *Borrelia burgdorferi* is often lacking at this stage of the disease during which patients may have minor flu-like constitutional symptoms and regional lymphadenopathy. The most common eye finding in early Lyme disease is conjunctivitis.[83]

Stage 2 disease occurs within days to weeks after infection. During this time, the spirochete can spread to many organs via the blood, causing a multitude of signs and symptoms. These systemic manifestations are mainly characterized by cardiac and neurologic involvement, although patients may develop secondary annular skin lesions. Neurologically, patients develop severe headache and mild stiffness of the neck. The CSF is normal early on in the disease but later reveals a lymphocytic pleocytosis with a cell count in the range of 100 cells/mm$^3$, elevated protein concentration, and a normal CSF glucose.[84] Peripheral neuropathies, intermittent arthralgia, and musculoskeletal pain are common, and unilateral and bilateral Bell's palsy is the most common cranial neuropathy.[85]

Four to eight percent of patients have cardiac involvement with fluctuating atrioventricular block.[86] Fewer patients have been reported with acute myopericarditis. About 6 months after infection patients can develop oligoarticular arthritis with a white blood cell count in joint fluid from 500 to 110,000 cells/mm$^3$. Other manifestations of stage 2 Lyme disease include hepatitis, nonproductive cough, microscopic hematuria or proteinuria, and orchitis.[80] The most commonly reported eye findings in stage 2 disease are conjunctivitis and uveitis.

Stage 3 infection is characterized by prolonged episodes of arthritis. Chronic neurologic manifestations include ataxia, chronic encephalomyelitis, spastic paraparesis, and dementia. Patients often complain of chronic fatigue, and erythema migrans can be seen late in the disease. Bilateral keratitis is described as a characteristic finding in late infection with Lyme disease.[85–89]

Transplacental transmission of *Borrelia burgdorferi* has been reported in two infants whose mothers had Lyme disease in the first trimester of pregnancy,[90–92] although a recent study of 463 infants from endemic or nonendemic areas showed no association between congenital malformations and the presence of detectable antibody to *Borrelia burgdorferi* in cord blood.[93]

***Ocular manifestations.*** In initial reports, the only consistently reported eye finding in Lyme disease was transient conjunctivitis, which occurred in 11% of persons with Stage I disease.[83] Other ocular findings reported in the early stages of Lyme disease include episcleritis, iridocyclitis with posterior synechiae, and retinal vasculitis.[94,95] Steere and colleagues[96] reported a case of a 45-year-old white woman who, 4 weeks after the onset of erythema migrans, developed unilateral iritis followed by panophthalmitis, and spirochetes were found in specimens of vitreous debris obtained at surgery.

In March 1987, Bertuch and colleagues[87] reported three patients with eye findings of Lyme disease. The first patient presented with a bilateral Bell's palsy and a late occurring optic neuritis. The other two patients developed patchy intrastromal infiltrates of the cornea from Bowman's layer to Descemet's membrane. These corneal infiltrates caused decreased vision but no pain and occurred late in the course of disease. There was dramatic

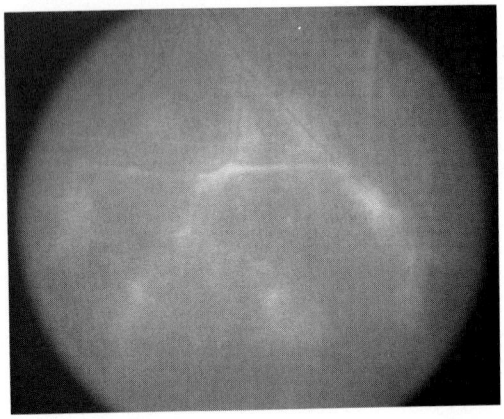

**Fig. 10-14.** Sheathing of peripheral retinal vessels is seen in patient with Lyme disease. Other ocular findings included vitritis and mild scleritis. Ocular findings resolved after treatment with intravenous ceftriaxone.

resolution of the keratitis after treatment with topical corticosteroids suggesting an immune mechanism rather than a direct infection with the spirochete. Baum and colleagues[88] has reported three patients who developed bilateral keratitis long after Lyme disease was diagnosed and treated; they also noted the effectiveness of topical corticosteroid therapy. Since then several other articles[89,94,95] have documented keratitis late in the course of Lyme disease.

Less common eye findings associated with Lyme disease, including vitritis and peripheral retinal vasculitis (Fig. 10-14), have been reported. Bialasiewicz and colleagues[97] described a patient with meningeal symptoms and diffuse choroiditis, cystoid macular edema, and exudative retinal detachments initially misdiagnosed as Vogt-Koyanagi-Harada syndrome. Immunofluorescent tests for Lyme disease were positive, and the patient improved markedly after treatment with doxycycline. Scholes and Teske[98] tested 19 patients with intermediate uveitis for Lyme disease, and 7 of 19 patients had positive antibody titers suggesting a possible association between Lyme disease and pars planitis. Copeland and colleagues[99] reported two patients with intermediate uveitis only partially responsive to steroids who were later diagnosed with Lyme disease after positive Lyme titers were obtained. The uveitis in both patients cleared rapidly with systemic antibiotic treatment. In a report by Winward and colleagues,[100] patients with intermediate uveitis associated with Lyme disease demonstrated more significant anterior segment inflammation. Recently, Karma and colleagues[101] diagnosed 10 cases of ocular lyme borreliosis out of 236 uveitis patients seen over a 2-year period. Diagnosis was based on the medical history, clinical findings, and serologic tests results. Abnormalities of the posterior segment of the eye, including vitritis, retinal vasulitis and neuroretinitis, were seen in six of the patients. Bilateral paralytic mydriasis, interstitial keratitis, episcleritis, and anterior uveitis were seen in one patient each.

Neuroophthalmologic findings in Lyme disease are not uncommon.[73,102] Involvement of the CNS by Lyme disease causes a number of cranial nerve palsies. Unilateral and bilateral Bell's palsies are the most frequent cranial nerve palsies, often resulting in exposure keratitis. Diplopia caused by cranial nerve VI, IV, and III palsies can occur. Wu and colleagues[103] described a 7-year-old child who developed bilateral disc edema in association with Lyme disease. A similar patient was described by Jacobson and Frens,[104] and that condition was diagnosed as pseudotumor cerebri syndrome associated with Lyme disease. Other reported neuroophthalmic manifestations of Lyme disease include optic neuritis, cortical blindness, and orbital myositis.[105–107] The association of some of these ocular findings with Lyme disease stems from one or two case reports in which the diagnosis of Lyme disease is based predominantly on positive serologic tests for Lyme disease. Because serologic tests for Lyme disease may be falsely positive, some of the cases may have been wrongly diagnosed as Lyme disease. A list of the ophthalmologic manifestations associated with Lyme disease is presented in Box 10-7.

***Diagnosis.*** Currently, available techniques for the diagnosis of Lyme disease are not ideal. A patient with a history of a tick bite who later develops erythema migrans most surely has Lyme disease; however, a tick bite is recalled in only about 50% of cases, and a pathognomonic rash may be overlooked or not occur in a significant number of patients. Because of the difficulty in culturing *B. burgdorferi* from patients, laboratory diagnosis is currently based on the results of serologic testing. Most patients have elevated antibody titers to *Borrelia burgdorferi* several weeks after infection. Both immunofluorescent assay (IFA) and enzyme-linked immunosorbent assay (ELISA) tests

**Box 10-7**
**Ocular manifestations of Lyme disease**

**EARLY INFECTION**

Conjunctivitis
Episcleritis
Iridocyclitis
Retinal vasculitis
Optic disc edema
Panophthalmitis
Choroiditis
Pars planitis
Exudative retinal detachment
Exposure keratitis
Diplopia
Cortical blindness
Orbital myositis

**LATE INFECTION**

Keratitis
Episcleritis

Modified from Whitcup SM, Raizman MB: Spirochetal infections and the eye. In Albert DM, Jakobiec FA, editors: *Principles and practice of ophthalmology,* vol 5, Philadelphia, 1994, WB Saunders, pp 3078-3092.

are used in the diagnosis of Lyme disease, although the ELISA test is more sensitive in all stages of the disease. Unfortunately, serologic testing has not been standardized, and interlaboratory variability is significant although improving.[108–110] Currently, the sensitivity of the ELISA for Lyme disease in several laboratories approaches 90% after the first few weeks of infection. Many laboratories will confirm positive ELISA results with Western blots. Nevertheless, the clinician must be aware of false-negative and false-positive results. False-negative results occur during the first few weeks of infection when antibody titers may be low and missed by serologic tests of lower sensitivities. Early antibiotic therapy may also cause false-negative test results, and cases of seronegative Lyme disease have been reported.[111]

False-positive results may also occur as a result of cross-reaction between *B. burgdorferi* and other spirochetes such as *T. pallidum*. Cross-reactivity between a Lyme IFA and a FTA-ABS is reported in 11% to 54% of patients.[112–114] In a study by Hunter and colleagues,[115] 22% of patients with Lyme disease had reactive FTA-ABS at a dilution of 1:5, but all of these samples were negative at a dilution of 1:10. Nevertheless, the rapid serum reagin (RPR) test and microhemagglutination assay to *T. pallidum* (MHA-TP) are usually negative in patients with Lyme disease.[112] False-positive results have also been reported in a number of autoimmune disorders, Rocky Mountain spotted fever, infectious mononucleosis, and neurologic disorders.[114,116–118] Importantly, in most areas of the country the prevalence of Lyme disease is quite low. Even with a sensitivity and specificity of 90%, the predictive value of a positive ELISA for Lyme disease is probably less than 20% in patients with a clinical picture atypical for the disease.

A fourfold increase in serial anti-*Borrelia burgdorferi* IgM antibody levels in patients with a clinical history compatible with Lyme disease remains the most specific laboratory indicator, but this increase is not often documented by serial tests. Western blot analysis and other molecular biology techniques are being developed for the diagnosis of Lyme disease but are occasionally difficult to interpret.

Current recommendations for laboratory screening for Lyme disease include obtaining an ELISA test using both IgM and IgG specific or a polyvalent antiimmunoglobulin.[116] Persistence of the specific IgM response throughout infection is an unusual feature of the antibody response seen in some patients with Lyme disease and may be the result of an impairment in the helper-T-cell function needed to switch from IgM to IgG production.[119] Because the clinical appearance of Lyme disease and syphilis are similar, an FTA-ABS test should be done on all patients tested for Lyme disease, and infectious mononucleosis should also be considered as a possible cause of false-positive results. Finally, the importance of pursuing a history of tick bites, residence in or travel to endemic areas for Lyme disease, rash, chronic joint complaints, or facial nerve palsy cannot be overemphasized.

***Prognosis.*** From 10% to 40% of patients with untreated erythema chronicum migrans will progress to second stage Lyme disease. From 3% to 10% of patients will develop chronic arthritis, acrodermatitis chronica atrophicans, or neurologic disease. Once it occurs, arthritis

**Box 10-8**
**Treatment of Lyme disease**

**EARLY INFECTION**

**Adults**

Tetracycline 250 mg po qid × 10 to 30 days
or
doxycycline 100 mg po bid × 10 to 30 days
or
amoxicillin 500 mg po qid × 10 to 30 days

**Children**

Amoxicillin or penicillin V 250 mg po tid or 20 mg/kg/day in divided doses × 10 to 30 days
If penicillin allergies exist, use erythromycin 250 mg po tid or 30 mg/kg/day in divided doses × 10 to 30 days

**SEVERE UVEITIS OR NEUROLOGIC ABNORMALITIES**

Ceftriaxone 2 g/day IV × 14 days or
penicillin G 20 to 24 million units/day IV × 10 to 14 days

Modified from Whitcup SM, Raizman MB: Spirochetal infections and the eye. In Albert DM, Jakobiec FA, editors: *Principles and practice of ophthalmology,* vol 5, Philadelphia, 1994, WB Saunders, pp 3078-3092.

does not always respond to antibiotic therapy. Similarly, it is not known whether neurologic involvement is prevented by oral antibiotic therapy for early Lyme disease.

***Treatment.*** Current recommendations for the treatment of Lyme disease were recently reviewed by Steere[80] and can be found in Box 10-8. Patients with mild ocular disease may respond well to oral antibiotics, but in cases with more severe ocular manifestations such as posterior uveitis, intravenous antibiotic therapy with ceftriaxone is probably the treatment of choice, and prolonged treatment may be required. Some data suggest that prior treatment with corticosteroids may predispose the patient to antibiotic failure; therefore the use of topical corticosteroids should be limited to patients with anterior segment inflammation who are also being treated with antibiotics.[99,100] Topical corticosteroids are also used to treat Lyme keratitis.[88] Finally, if the suspicion for Lyme disease is high, a therapeutic trial of antibiotics seems warranted even in seronegative patients.

### Relapsing fever

**Etiology and epidemiology.** Relapsing fever is an acute infectious disease caused by spirochetes of the genus *Borrelia* and characterized by recurrent bouts of fever separated by relatively asymptomatic periods.[120–122] Relapsing fever is divided into two epidemiologic types: epidemic or louse-borne and endemic or tick-borne. Epidemic or louse-borne relapsing fever is transmitted from person to person by the human body louse, *Pediculus humanus,* which previously ingested blood infected with *B. recurrentus.*[122] Infection occurs when the hemolymph from infected body lice contaminates abraded or even normal skin, usually with scratching when lice are crushed and come into contact with previously excoriated bites. The epidemic form of relapsing fever is currently found in parts of Africa, South America, and China where crowding, poor sanitation, and famine foster louse infestation.[123]

Endemic or tick-borne relapsing fever was first documented in the United States in 1915 after five persons contracted the disease in Bear Creek Canyon, Colo.[124] This form of the disease is caused by at least 15 species of *Borrelia,* and the tick vectors have now been identified as several species of the genus *Ornithodorus* with a rodent reservoir.[120,125] Transmission to human beings occurs when infected saliva from the tick contaminates the site of the bite. In the United States, tick-borne relapsing fever occurs mostly in western states usually between May and September.[126]

**Clinical manifestations.** After inoculation, the spirochetes multiply in the blood and invade most tissues of the body. Onset of the disease occurs 3 to 12 days after infection and is marked by fever to 39° to 40° C, chills, severe headache,[121] and frequently eye pain, blurred vision, and photophobia. Other symptoms include myalgias and joint pain, meningismus, anorexia, abdominal pain, nonproductive cough, and neurologic symptoms including facial paralysis and altered mental status. Hepatosplenomegaly, jaundice, myocarditis, and heart failure are sometimes seen late in the disease. The course of louse-borne relapsing fever tends to be more severe than tick-borne

**Box 10-9**
**Ocular manifestations of relapsing fever**

Conjunctivitis
Subconjunctival and retinal hemorrhages
Iridocyclitis (usually after several relapses of disease)
Vitritis
Ptosis (as result of facial nerve paralysis)
Mydriasis
Optic neuritis
Retinal venous occlusion

Modified from Whitcup SM, Raizman MB: Spirochetal infections and the eye. In Albert DM, Jakobiec FA, editors: *Principles and practice of ophthalmology*, vol 5, Philadelphia, 1994, WB Saunders, pp 3078-3092.

relapsing fever. Bleeding is common in both forms of the disease and often manifests as purpura, petechiae, or epistaxis.[127] Subconjunctival and retinal hemorrhages have been described. In more severe cases of relapsing fever, gastrointestinal or cerebral hemorrhage and disseminated intravascular coagulation may result in death.

The initial attack of relapsing fever lasts 3 to 6 days and is followed by an afebrile period of 6 to 9 days. Defervescence may be accompanied by hypotension. Relapses tend to become shorter and less severe as the disease progresses. Mortality in relapsing fever ranges between 2% and 5% in treated cases and as high as 40% in untreated cases.[121]

Eye pain and photophobia are common, and conjunctivitis and iridocyclitis have both been reported in approximately 15% of cases of relapsing fever usually after several relapses.[128] Cases of more severe uveitis with vitritis have been reported but apparently respond well to therapy.[129] Neuroophthalmic manifestations of relapsing fever are mostly limited to ptosis caused by paralysis of the facial nerve, but pupillary dilation and optic neuritis have also been documented. Retinal venous occlusion with retinal hemorrhage and exudate has been documented in one case.[120] The ocular manifestations of relapsing fever are listed in Box 10-9.

**Diagnosis.** Definitive diagnosis of relapsing fever is based on the presence of *Borrelia* on a thick smear of peripheral blood obtained during a febrile episode. *Borrelia* is best seen with Giemsa or Wright's stain.[121] Repeat smears or use of an acridine orange fluorescent stain will increase the sensitivity of the smears.[121,130] If direct methods of diagnosis fail, blood from the patient may be injected into mice or rats; and the blood from these animals is then examined for spirochetes.

IFA and ELISA tests are being developed, but serologic testing is not yet useful in diagnosing relapsing fever.[124] Nonspecific laboratory abnormalities include anemia, elevated erythrocyte sedimentation rate, a platelet count less than 150,000 per cubic millimeter, and a prolonged bleeding time. Serologic tests for syphilis may be positive in as many as 10% of patients tested. In patients with CNS involvement, analysis of the CSF usually reveals a pleocytosis with an elevated protein concentration but normal glucose.[121]

**Prognosis.** Of patients with relapsing fever, 95% recover with current therapy; however, untreated louse-borne relapsing fever is frequently fatal. Rare complications include respiratory disease, nephritis, endocarditis, neurologic disease, and bleeding diatheses. Uveitis may lead to permanent visual disability.

**Treatment.** The treatment of choice for tick-borne relapsing fever in adults is tetracycline 500 mg orally every 6 hours for 10 days. Penicillin, erythromycin, and chloramphenicol are also effective. In louse-borne relapsing fever, the treatment of choice in adults is one dose of erythromycin 500 mg given orally or intravenously. Therapy should be given during the early part of a febrile episode to diminish the possibility of a Jarisch-Herxheimer reaction.[131] The Jarisch-Herxheimer reaction is caused by release of a nonendotoxin pyrogen as *Borrelia* are killed and is characterized by rigors, fever, and elevated blood pressure followed by hypotension and possible shock.

### Leptospirosis

**Etiology and epidemiology.** Leptospirosis is a zoonosis caused by spirochetes of the genus *Leptospira* whose natural reservoir is wild animals, mostly rodents. Weil[132] first recognized a severe form of leptospirosis as a distinct clinical entity in 1886, and the spirochetal cause of Weil's disease was discovered by Inada and colleagues in 1915.[133] Leptospirosis can affect domestic animals including livestock and dogs. Human beings are accidental hosts who acquire the disease through contact with infected urine, tissues, or water. The spirochetes invade human beings through abraded skin or mucous membranes, although penetration through intact skin occasionally occurs. The disease is often occupational, occurring in farmers, veterinarians, and abattoir workers.[134,135] Most cases of leptospirosis in the United States are acquired during water sports, and predominantly occur in young adult males in the late summer and early fall.[133,135]

Currently 207 different leptospiral serovars have been identified with pathologic leptospires belonging to the species *Leptospira interrogans.*[134] Approximately 40 to 100 cases of leptospirosis are reported annually, but because the signs and symptoms of the disease are not distinct, many cases go undiagnosed. Once inside the host, leptospires enter the bloodstream, can penetrate tissues, and are found in almost all organs within 24 hours. The mechanism by which leptospires cause tissue damage is not entirely clear, although toxic factors have been isolated in some culture supernatants.

**Clinical manifestations.** The incubation period for leptospirosis ranges from 2 to 26 days with the usual period extending from 7 to 13 days. The disease is often biphasic and the first or leptospiremic phase is abrupt in onset and characterized by severe frontal, bitemporal, or retroorbital headaches, fever and chills, and severe muscle aches. Conjunctival suffusion is a characteristic finding that usually appears on the third or fourth day of the disease but is frequently overlooked.[136,137] Hepatosplenomegaly and jaundice are uncommon in the first stage of leptospirosis but occur later in the course of more severe forms of the disease. The leptospiremic phase lasts from 4 to 9 days with recurrent fever spikes exceeding 39° C.

For 8 to 10 days after infection leptospires can be isolated from blood and cerebrospinal fluid but disappear as patients defervesce and enter the second or immune phase of the disease. The immune phase of leptospirosis begins on the sixth to twelfth day of the illness and corresponds to the time when antibodies appear in the serum. The clinical course of the immune phase is variable, and some patients develop few symptoms. High fever and meningismus, however, may occur in half the patients, and examination of CSF after the seventh day postinfection will reveal pleocytosis in 50% of patients often with a mildly elevated CSF protein level. Other manifestations of the disease include encephalitis, optic neuritis, cranial nerve paresis involving cranial nerves VI, VII, and VIII, and peripheral neuropathies. Spontaneous abortion may result from leptospirosis acquired during pregnancy.

A severe form of leptospirosis, called Weil's disease, occurs with jaundice, azotemia, hemorrhages, anemia, persistent fever, and altered mental status. Renal and hepatocellular dysfunction usually occur on the 3rd to 6th day after infection. Mortality from leptospirosis occurs only in patients with jaundice and approaches 15% in younger patients and 30% in patients older than 60 years of age.

Ocular findings in leptospirosis have been reported in 3% to 92% of patients.[138] Bulbar and palpebral conjunctival hyperemia with engorged conjunctival and episcleral vessels is the most common and characteristic ophthalmologic finding in leptospirosis. This hyperemia usually occurs without discomfort, lacrimation, or discharge; however, if ocular discharge is present, it can harbor leptospires and be a source of further infection.[139]

In Weil's disease with hepatic involvement, scleral icterus is present, and in patients with severe disease, subconjunctival and retinal hemorrhages may occur. Less commonly, during the immune phase of the disease with CNS involvement, patients may develop palpebral herpes, optic neuritis, and facial nerve paresis. Between 10% and 44% of patients with leptospirosis develop uveitis,[140] which is typically an acute often bilateral iridocyclitis with fine keratic precipitates, posterior synechiae, occasional vitreous opacities, and rarely retinal exudates. Patients often complain of blurred vision and mild ocular irritation, but respond well to treatment with mydriatics and topical steroids. More severe cases of uveitis have been reported and may occur long after the disease has appeared to subside. Barkay and Garzozi[137] reported 16 patients with predominantly anterior uveitis as a result of leptospirosis with positive serologic tests. Leptospirosis can be considered as a possible cause of uveitis of unknown cause, especially in patients with

**Box 10-10**
**Ocular manifestations of leptospirosis**

Leptospiremic phase
- Conjunctival suffusion

Immune phase
- Iridocyclitis
- Optic neuritis
- Facial nerve palsy
- Palpebral herpes
- Posterior uveitis (with retinal exudates)
- Scleral icterus
- Subconjunctival hemorrhages
- Retinal hemorrhages

Modified from Whitcup SM, Raizman MB: Spirochetal infections and the eye. In Albert DM, Jakobiec FA, editors: *Principles and practice of ophthalmology,* vol 5, Philadelphia, 1994, WB Saunders, pp 3078-3092.

occupational or recreational risk factors for the disease. The ocular manifestations of leptospirosis are listed in Box 10-10.

**Diagnosis.** The white blood cell count is normal to slightly elevated in most cases of leptospirosis; values above 15,000 suggest hepatic disease. Differential counts usually reveal greater than 70% neutrophils that may differentiate leptospirosis from viral infection. In patients with liver involvement, intravascular hemolysis may cause anemia and elevated serum bilirubin.

Definitive diagnosis of leptospirosis requires isolation of the spirochete from a clinical specimen, usually blood or CSF, or seroconversion (a fourfold or greater rise in antibody titer) in the presence of clinical illness. The organism is only present in blood and CSF for 8 to 10 days after infection, and the spirochete quickly disappears as antibodies appear in the serum. The leptospires can be identified in darkfield examination, but this technique requires expertise. Leptospiuria occurs during the immune phase, although leptospires are easily confused with cellular debris in urine sediment. Tissue samples may also be examined, but tissue analysis for leptospires is predominantly limited to postmortem examination.

In practice, laboratory diagnosis of leptospirosis is usually made serologically. The macroscopic slide agglutination test uses a boiled suspension of leptospires and is used mostly as a screening test. The microscopic agglutination test uses live or formalin-treated antigens, is more specific, and can be used to determine both antibody titer and serotype. Recently, sensitive and specific complement fixation tests and ELISA techniques for the detection of IgM antibody against leptospiral antigens have been developed. They are both inexpensive and easy to use and are playing an increasing role in the diagnosis of leptospirosis. Agglutinins appear on the 6th to 12th day of illness, and the maximum titer is reached during the 3rd and 4th weeks. Early treatment with antibiotics may delay or suppress development of the antibody response, but if initial serologic tests are negative, they should be repeated in 2 weeks.

**Prognosis.** Patients with anicteric leptospirosis usually recover uneventfully in 2 to 6 weeks, although convalescence may extend up to 1 month. Deaths occur in 5% to 30% of untreated patients and are usually attributable to acute renal failure. Uveitis occurs in 10% of patients from 2 weeks to 1 year after initial infection, but the prognosis for these patients is generally good.

**Treatment.** Chemotherapeutic trials were conducted during recent outbreaks of leptospirosis in military personnel training in Panama. Doxycycline at a dosage of 200 mg orally once a week and at the end of training prevented infection.[141] Antibiotics have been shown to decrease disease complications if given by the fourth day of infection, but they are still recommended for severe infections even if diagnosis is made after 4 days postinfection.

In severe cases of leptospirosis recommended therapy is penicillin 1.5 million units or ampicillin 500 to 1000 mg administered intravenously every 6 hours for 10 days. Less severe cases may be treated with doxycycline 100 mg orally twice a day or ampicillin 500 mg orally every 6 hours for a total of 7 days.[142] Supportive therapy is given for renal failure, hypotension, and hemorrhage.

Prevention of leptospirosis centers around the elimination of large animal reservoirs of disease including livestock and pets. In fact, cattle-associated leptospirosis is a current problem in the British Isles with at least 4% of all British dairy workers at risk for infection.[135]

The ophthalmologist must be diligent in pursuing the clinical history for evidence of previous or persistent low-grade infection suggestive of leptospirosis when evaluating patients with a uveitis of unknown cause, especially in dairy farmers. Because many cases are unrecognized, it is not possible to definitively state how many cases of uveitis are caused by leptospirosis; however, a recent report states that only 17% of 483 proven cases of leptospirosis were initially correctly diagnosed.[143] Watt[144] in a recent editorial suggests that a history of water or animal contact in a patient with severe myalgias and conjunctival suffusion suggests leptospirosis, particularly in someone returning from travel in Asia or Latin America. Diagnosis can be confirmed by sending a serum sample to a reference laboratory for the microscopic agglutination test or for an ELISA test for leptospirosis.

### Brucellosis

Brucellosis is a bacteria that infects the genitourinary tract of cattle *(Brucella abortus)* and pigs *(Brucella suis)*. Human beings become infected after exposure to infected animals or contaminated meat or dairy products. The disease in human beings is characterized by fever, chills, headache, arthralgias, lymphadenopathy, and splenomegaly. Diagnosis can be difficult but is based on positive blood cultures or cultures of usually sterile fluids. Serologic tests are available for brucellosis and assist with the diagnosis.

The organism has been reported to affect all the ocular structures, but optic nerve involvement appears to be the most serious ocular manifestation.[145] Box 10-11 lists the ocular manifestations of the disease. Uveitis has been described in patients with brucellosis. Recurrent iritis, localized thickening of the iris, and multiple irregular choroidal exudates associated with little inflammation and retinal detachment have all been ascribed to brucellosis.[146,147] Walker and colleagues[148] recently published a case of a patient with well-circumscribed lesions in the periphery of the choroid in a patient with brucellosis (Fig. 10-15). However, brucellae have never been cultured from the eye in uveitis,[147] and with current health measures including pasteurization, the incidence of this disease has declined dramatically. It is not clear whether antibiotic therapy is helpful for uveitis associated with brucellosis. Nevertheless, therapy with combinations of tetracyclines cephalosporins and other antibiotics appears effective for systemic disease and indicated for patients with possible brucellosis-associated uveitis.

**Box 10-11**
**Ocular manifestations of brucellosis**

- Disc edema
- Optic neuritis
- Keratitis
- Corneal ulcers
- Conjunctivitis
- Chronic anterior uveitis
- Multifocal choroiditis
- Eyelid edema
- Posterior uveitis
- Cranial nerve palsies
- Endophthalmitis
- Retinal detachment

Modified from Whitcup SM, Raizman MB: Spirochetal infections and the eye. In Albert DM, Jakobiec FA, editors: *Principles and practice of ophthalmology*, vol 5, Philadelphia, 1994, WB Saunders, pp 3078-3092.

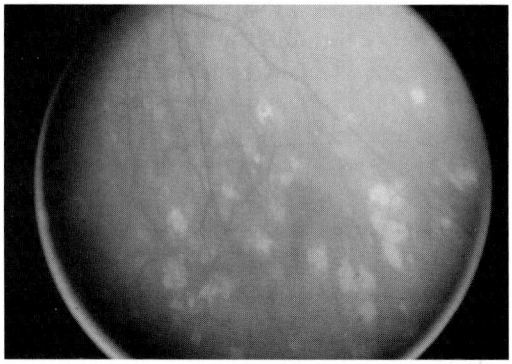

**Fig. 10-15.** Well-circumscribed lesions in periphery of choroid in patient with brucellosis. (Courtesy Narsing A. Rao, M.D.) (See Color Plate 17.)

## CHRONIC GRANULOMATOUS DISEASE

Chronic granulomatous disease (CGD) is an inherited disorder that predisposes affected children to pyogenic infections. Currently, an X-linked recessive and autosomal recessive form of the disease have been identified. A number of ocular findings are associated with this disease including blepharokeratoconjunctivitis with pannus formation and inflammatory chorioretinal lesions that lead to extensive scarring (Fig. 10-16).[149] We recently found

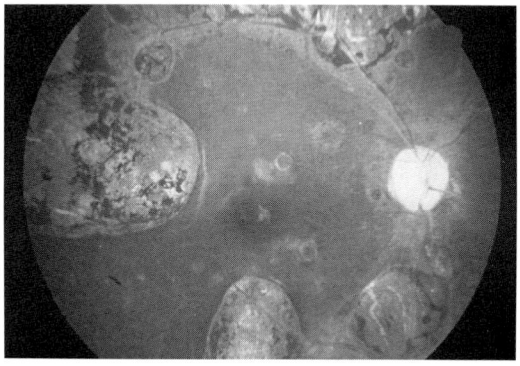

**Fig. 10-16.** Chorioretinal lesions in young patient with chronic granulomatous disease. Macular involvement resulted in decreased visual acuity. (See Color Plate 18.)

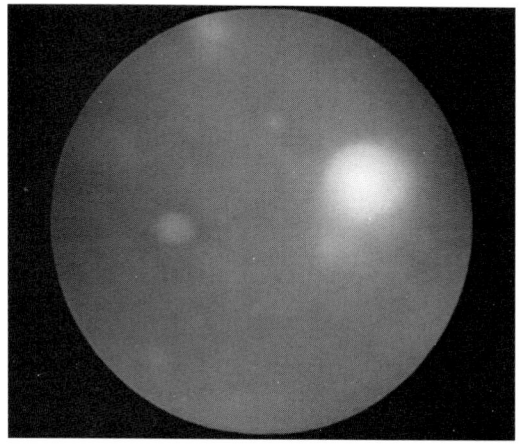

**Fig. 10-17.** Fundus of eye of known intravenous drug abuser who complained of floaters and decrease in vision. Multiple small choroidal lesions were present in addition to large white fluffy mass in vitreous that contained *Candida* sp.

chorioretinal lesions in 7 (37%) of 19 patients of patients with X-linked CGD but in 0 of 6 patients with autosomal recessive disease. Three of the patients with chorioretinal lesions had visual acuity less than 20/400 and abnormal electrooculograms. Usually by the time these lesions are discovered in these young children who rarely complain of problems with their vision, there is no active inflammatory disease. It is unclear whether treatment with corticosteroids or antibiotics alters the course of the lesions; however, therapy is probably indicated if acute inflammatory disease is noted. In any event, sight-threatening disease is a frequent complication of CGD and appears to be associated with the x-linked form of the disease; periodic eye examinations in these patients are warranted.[150]

## FUNGAL DISEASE

The most common fungal disease associated with uveitis is histoplasmosis. Ocular histoplasmosis and presumed ocular histoplasmosis syndrome are described in Chapter 28 on white-dot syndromes. In general, fungal infection of the choroid, retina, and vitreous occurs in several types of patients: postoperative patients, immunosuppressed patients with systemic mycotic infections, immunocompetent patients with systemic mycotic infection, intravenous drug users, and in patients with ocular trauma. Occasionally a patient without a known risk factor may develop a fungal endophthalmitis.

Fungal endophthalmitis usually present as a chronic panuveitis. Fluffy deep yellow-white retinal or choroidal lesions are frequently present, and the vitreous often contains "fluff balls" (Fig. 10-17). Posttraumatic cases of fungal endophthalmitis are easily differentiated from other forms of uveitis because of the clear history of trauma and the presence of uniocular disease, unlike sympathetic ophthalmia that would be a bilateral uveitis after trauma. Postsurgical fungal endophthalmitis may, however, mimic a chronic idiopathic uveitis and is discussed more fully in the chapter on postsurgical uveitis (see Chapter 18). This chapter will focus on endogenous fungal infections that cause a uveitis.

*Candida* species are the fungal organisms that most frequently cause fungal endophthalmitis.[151] *Candida albicans* is the most common of the *Candida* organisms, but other organisms such as *C. tropicalis, C. parapsilosis,* and *C. stellatoidea* also cause fungal disease in human beings. *Candida* endophthalmitis usually occurs in chronically ill patients with an indwelling catheter who are receiving antibiotics or immunosuppressive agents including corticosteroids.[152] The disorder is also a frequent complication of intravenous drug use.[153]

Patients with fungal endophthalmitis may complain of floaters. However, the disease is sometimes asymptomatic and detected only on ophthalmologic screening of patients with positive fungal cultures or fever of unknown origin, although the diagnostic yield from these examinations is not well established. Later in the course of the disease, redness, pain, decreased vision, hypopyon, dense vitritis, and dense retinal and choroidal lesions may occur. The diagnosis of *Candida* endophthalmitis is usually straightforward in a chronically ill patient with positive blood cultures. The usual assumption is that the same organisms in the blood is responsible for the ocular disease. Nevertheless, multiple organisms may be present in the blood and eye of severely immunocompromised patients. In addition, some intravenous drug users who develop a candidal infection from emboli do not develop a systemic infection. These patients frequently develop multiple yellow-white deep retinal or choroidal lesions associated with vitreous fluff balls and retinal hemorrhage (Fig. 10-17).

Histopathologic examination of a vitreous specimen from patients with *Candida* endophthalmitis shows neutrophils, macrophages, and lymphocytes along with either yeast forms or pseudohyphae consistent with *Candida*. Culture of the vitreous or aqueous confirms the diagnosis. The cellular infiltrate of the vitreous can be influenced by the patient's immune status, and patients with AIDS frequently have a diminished inflammatory response, especially when their CD4 T cell counts are severely diminished.

The optimal treatment of candida endophthalmitis remains controversial. Animal studies show that ocular infection spreads from the blood vessels in the retina and choroid and suggests that with breakdown of the blood-retinal barrier that intravenously administered antibiotics should adequately penetrate the eye.[154] Some experts have suggested that vitrectomy should only be performed in patients with dense vitreous opacities.[155] If vitrectomy is performed, 5 to 10 μg of amphotericin B should be injected into the vitreous at the end of the procedure. Systemic amphotericin B remains the mainstay of therapy. Because most patients with fungal endophthalmitis have systemic disease, a total dose of at least 1 g appears warranted. Unfortunately, the drug is toxic and can result in renal dysfunction, anemia, electrolyte imbalances, and hypotension. In addition to amphotericin B, flucytosine, and miconazole have also been used for the treatment of *Candida* endophthalmitis. Flucytosine at 150 mg/kg per day is effective in some patients, but because many strains of *Candida* are resistant to this drug, other antifungal agents are often used in combination with flucytosine. Oral administration and minimal toxicity are major advantages of this drug. Miconazole appears to penetrate the eye well but does not seem to be useful for treating ocular disease until a dosage of 2400 mg per day was used.[155] Recently, a few patients with fungal ocular disease have been treated with ketaconazole, usually in combination with other antifungal agents.[156] Initiation of therapy early in the course of the disease before macular involvement occurs improves the prognosis.[155]

Aspergillosis is the second most common disseminated fungal infection.[151] It has been reported as a cause of endophthalmitis in immunosuppressed patients and intravenous drug users.[157,158] *Aspergillus* infection of the eye presents as a vitritis with fluff balls and yellow-white lesions in the retina similar to those seen with candidal infections. Also similar to *Candida* endophthalmitis, redness, pain, hypopyon, retinal hemorrhages, and decreased vision can also occur. *Aspergillus* may be difficult to culture from the blood.[159] In one case report, there was no evidence of systemic infection in an intravenous drug user with *Aspergillus* endophthalmitis.[158] This patient was successfully treated with vitrectomy, intravitreal and subconjunctival amphotericin B, and oral flucytosine. A 15-day-old infant without any risk factors for infection was diagnosed with bilateral *Aspergillus* endophthalmitis on enucleation of one eye. Systemic amphotericin B resulted in good visual outcome in the other eye.[160] Unfortunately, many patients with ocular involvement caused by *Aspergillus* species have had poor visual outcomes.

Endogenous fungal endophthalmitis can occur from a variety of these organisms including *Coccidioides immitis,*[161] *Cryptococcus neoformans,*[162] *Histoplasma capsulatum,*[163] *Sporotrichum schenckii,*[164] and *Blastomyces dermatitidis.*[165] The risk factors and ocular characteristics of endogenous fungal infections are listed in Table 18-1. These infections are all less common than disease caused by either *Candida* or *Aspergillus* infection and therefore represent a diagnostic challenge to the clinician. It is interesting to note that histopathologic examination of an eye with coccidioidomycosis had both choroidal and retinal granulomatous lesions that did not overlap anatomically suggesting hematogenous spread

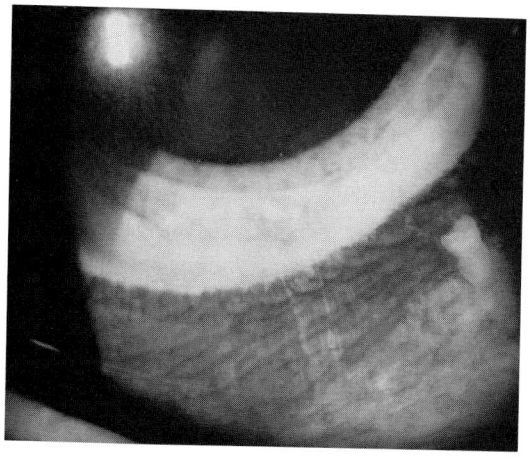

**Fig. 10-18.** Hypopyon uveitis in patient with syphilis (see Case 10-1).

through both the retinal and choroidal circulation.[161] Finally, *Nocardia asteroides* is a weakly acid-fast bacteria that causes a disease that appears similar to fungal ocular infections. This disease, however, is resistant to antifungal agents but sensitive to antibiotic therapy, which makes prompt and accurate diagnosis imperative.

Advances in therapy for cancer, autoimmune disease, and other chronic diseases have increased the number of chronically immunosuppressed patients. In addition, HIV infection has lead to an increase in immunosuppressed patients prone to opportunistic infections. It is therefore of increasing importance that clinicians become well versed in the diagnosis and treatment of endogenous fungal disease.

### Case 10-1

A 59-year-old HIV-positive white man developed a sudden decrease in vision in both eyes. Visual acuity was 20/400 OU. Examination revealed bilateral hypopyons (Fig. 10-18), vitritis, and patchy areas of retinal infiltrates in both eyes (Fig. 10-8). The patient was referred to the National Institutes of Health with a diagnosis of presumed cytomegalovirus retinitis. Laboratory evaluation at the National Institutes of Health revealed a positive VDRL and FTA-ABS. A diagnosis of syphilis was made, and the patient was treated with intravenous penicillin G. Within 2 weeks visual acuity improved to 20/40 OU. The retinal infiltrates also resolved and the patient was left with a pigmentary retinopathy characteristic of resolved syphilitic retinitis (see Fig. 10-9).

## REFERENCES


1. Ayo C: A toxic ocular action: new property of Schwartzman toxins, *J Immunol* 46:113-132, 1943.
2. Rosenbaum JT, McDevitt HO, Guss RB et al: Endotoxin-induced uveitis in rats as a model for human disease, *Nature* 286:611-613, 1980.
3. Forrester JV, Worgul BV, Merriam GR Jr: Endotoxin-induced uveitis in the rat. *Albrecht von Graefes Arch Klin Ophthalmol* 213:221-233, 1980.
4. Tanouchi Y, Kogiso M, Miki S et al: Endotoxin-induced uveitis in LPS-susceptible C3H/HeN mice, *Invest Ophthalmol Vis Sci* 32(suppl):792, 1991.
5. Hansen GHA: Investigations concerning the etiology of leprosy, *Norsk Magazin Laegevidenskaben* 4:76-79, 1874.
6. Binford C, Meyers W, Walsh G: Leprosy, *JAMA* 247: 2283-2292, 1982.
7. Blindness in leprosy, *Br J Ophthalmol* 65:221-222, 1981.
8. Ridley DS, Jopling WH: Classification of leprosy according to immunity, a five group system, *Int J Lepr Other Mycobact Dis* 34:255-273, 1966.
9. Sansonetti P, LaGrange PH: The immunology of leprosy: speculations on the leprosy spectrum, *Rev Infect Dis* 3:422-469, 1981.
10. Schwab IR, Nassar E, Malaty R et al: Leprosy in a trachomatous population, *Arch Ophthalmol* 102:240-244, 1984.
11. Hornblass A: Ocular leprosy in South Vietnam, *Am J Ophthalmol* 75:478-480, 1973.
12. Shields JA, Waring GO III, Monte LG: Ocular findings in leprosy, *Am J Ophthalmol* 77:880-890, 1974.
13. Brandt F, Malla OK: Ocular findings in leprous patients: a report of a survey in Malunga/Nepal, *Albrecht von Grafes Arch Klin Ophthalmol* 217:27-34, 1981.

13a. Spaide R, Nattis R, Lipka A et al: Ocular findings in leprosy in the United States, *Am J Ophthalmol* 100:411-416, 1985.

14. Vedy J, Graveline J: *Précis d'Ophtalmologie Tropicale,* Marseille, 1979, Diffusion Generale de Librairie, p 125.
15. Chovet M, Metge P, Fauxpoint B et al: Uvéite postérieure lépreuse, *Bull Soc Ophtalmol Fr* 12:1215-1217, 1976.
16. Kircheimer WF, Storrs EE: Attempts to establish the armadillo (*Drasypus novemcentus* Linn.) as a model for study of leprosy, *Int J Lepr* 39:693-702, 1971.
17. Wallach D, Cottenot F, Bach M-A: Imbalances in T-cell subpopulations in lepromatous leprosy, *Int J Lepr* 50:282-290, 1982.
18. Stoner GL, Atlaw T, Touw J et al: Antigen-specific suppressor cells in subclinical leprosy infection, *Lancet* 2:1372-1377, 1981.
19. Horwitz MA, Levis WR, Cohn ZA: Defective production of monocyte-activating cytokines in lepromatous leprosy, *J Exp Med* 159:666-678, 1984.
20. Van Voorhis WC, Kaplan G, Nunes Sarno E et al: The cutaneous infiltrates of leprosy: cellular characteristics and the predominant T-cell phenotypes, *N Engl J Med* 307:1593-1597, 1982.
21. De Vries RRP, van Eden W, van Rood JJ: HLA-linked control of the course of *M. leprae* infection, *Lepr Rev* 52 (suppl):109-119, 1981.

22. WHO Study Group: Chemotherapy of leprosy for control programmes. *WHO Tech Rep Ser* 675, 1982.
23. Schlaegel TF Jr: *Essentials of uveitis,* Boston, 1969, Little Brown.
24. Glassroth J, Robins AG, Snider DE: Tuberculosis in the 1980s, *N Engl J Med* 302:1441-1450, 1980.
25. Barnes PF, Bloch AB, Davidson PT et al: Tuberculosis in patients with human immunodeficiency virus infection, *N Engl J Med* 324:1644-1650, 1991.
26. Centers for Disease Control and Prevention: Expanded tuberculosis surveillance and tuberculosis morbidity-United States, 1993, *MMWR* 43:361-366, 1994.
27. Donahue HC: Ophthalmologic experience in a tuberculosis sanatorium, *Am J Ophthalmol* 64:742-748, 1967.
28. Massaro D, Katz S, Sachs M: Choroidal tubercles: a clue to hematogenous tuberculosis, *Ann Intern Med* 60:231-241, 1964.
29. Helm CJ, Holland GN: Ocular tuberculosis, *Surv Ophthalmol* 38:229-256, 1993.
30. Darrell RW: Acute tuberculous panophthalmitis, *Arch Ophthalmol* 78:51-54, 1967.
30a. Coles RS. Uveitis associated with systemic disease, *Surv Ophthalmol* 8:377-392, 1963.
31. Smith RE: Tuberculoma of the choroid, discussion, *Ophthalmology* 87:257-258, 1980.
32. Musial CE, Tice LS, Stockman L et al: Identification of mycobacteria from culture by using the Gen-Probe Rapid Diagnostic System for *Mycobacterium avium* complex and *Mycobacterium tuberculosis* complex, *J Clin Microbiol* 26:2120-2123, 1988.
33. Schlaegel TF Jr, O'Connor GR: Tuberculosis and syphilis, *Arch Ophthalmol* 99:2206-2207, 1981.
34. Schlaegel TF Jr, Weber JC: Double-blind therapeutic trial of isoniazid in 344 patients with uveitis, *Br J Ophthalmol* 53:425-427, 1969.
35. Oksala A, Salminen A: Leptospiral uveitis, *Acta Ophthalmol* 34:185-194, 1956.
36. Schaudinn FR, Hoffman E: Vorlaüfger Bericht über das Vorkommen von Spirochaeten in Syphilitschen Krakheitsproducten und bei papillomen, *Arbeiren aus dem k Gesundheitsamte* 22:527, 1905.
37. Mahoney JF, Arnold RC, Harris A: Penicillin treatment of syphilis: a preliminary report, *J Vener Dis Inform* 24:355-357, 1943.
38. Continuing increase in infectious syphilis—United States, *MMWR* 37:35-38, 1988.
39. Relationship of syphilis to drug use and prostitution—Connecticut and Philadelphia, Pennsylvania, *MMWR* 37:755-764, 1988.
40. Congenital syphilis treatment and follow-up recommendations, *MMWR* 37:1-13, 1988.
41. Berry CD, Hooton TM, Collier AC et al: Neurologic relapse after benzathine penicillin therapy for secondary syphilis in a patient with HIV infection, *N Engl J Med* 316:1587-1589, 1987.
42. Johns DR, Tierney M, Felsenstein D: Alteration in the natural history of neurosyphilis by concurrent infection with the human immunodeficiency virus, *N Engl J Med* 316:1569-1572, 1987.
43. Sparling PF: Natural history of syphilis. In Holmes KK, Per-Anders M, Sparling PF, Wiesner PJ, editors: *Sexually transmitted diseases,* New York, 1990, McGraw-Hill, p 214.
44. Chapel TA: The variability of syphilitic chancres, *Sex Transm Dis* 5:68-70, 1978.
45. Pulido JS: Syphilis. In Gold DH, Weingeist TA, editors: *The eye and systemic disease,* Philadelphia, 1990, Lippincott, p 234.
46. Chapel TA: The signs and symptoms of secondary syphilis, *Sex Transm Dis* 7:161-164, 1980.
47. Woods AC: Syphilis of the eye, *Am J Syph Gonor Vener Dis* 27:133-186, 1943.
48. Wilhelmus KR: Syphilis. In Insler MS, editor: *AIDS and other sexually transmitted diseases and the eye,* Orlando, 1987, Grune & Stratton, pp 73-104.
49. Lukehart SA, Hook EW, Baker-Zander SA et al: Invasion of the central nervous system by *Treponema pallidum:* implications for diagnosis and treatment, *Ann Intern Med* 109:855-862, 1988.
50. Lowenfeld IE: The Argyll Robertson pupil, 1869-1969: a critical survey of the literature, *Surv Ophthalmol* 14:199-299, 1969.
51. Dorfman DH, Glaser JH: Congenital syphilis presenting in infants after the newborn period, *N Engl J Med* 323:1299-1302, 1990.
52. Duke-Elder S: The ocular adnexa. II. Lacrimal, orbital, and paraorbital diseases, *System of ophthalmology,* vol 13, St Louis, 1974, Mosby.
53. Arruga J, Valentines J, Mauri F et al: Neuroretinitis in acquired syphilis, *Ophthalmology* 92:262-270, 1983.
54. Morgan CM, Webb RM, O'Connor GR: Atypical syphilitic chorioretinitis and vasculitis, *Retina* 4:225-231, 1984.
55. Mendelsohn AD, Jampol LM: Syphilitic retinitis: a cause of necrotizing retinitis, *Retina* 4:221-234, 1985.
56. Halperin LS, Lewis H, Blumenkranz MS et al: Choroidal neovascular membrane and other chorioretinal complications of acquired syphilis, *Am J Ophthalmol* 108:554-562, 1989.
57. Tramont EC: *Treponema pallidum* (syphilis). In Mandell GL, Douglas RG Jr, Bennett JE, editors: *Principles and practice of infectious diseases,* New York, 1990, Churchill Livingstone, p 1803.
58. Tramont EC: Syphilis in the AIDS era, *N Engl J Med* 316:1600-1601, 1987.
59. Stoumbos VD, Klein ML: Syphilitic retinitis in a patient with acquired immunodeficiency syndrome–related complex, *Am J Ophthalmol* 103:103-104, 1987.
60. Passo MS, Rosenbaum JT: Ocular syphilis in patients with human immunodeficiency virus infection, *Am J Ophthalmol* 106:1-6, 1988.
61. Levy JH, Liss RA, Maguire AM: Neurosyphilis and ocular syphilis in patients with concurrent human immunodeficiency virus infection, *Retina* 9:175-180, 1989.
62. Zaidman GW: Neurosyphilis and retrobulbar neuritis in a patient with AIDS, *Ann Ophthalmol* 18:260-261, 1986.
63. Markowitz DM, Beutner KR, Maggio RP et al: Failure of recommended treatment for secondary syphilis, *JAMA* 255:1767-1768, 1986.
64. Richards BW, Hessburg TJ, Nussbaum JN: Recurrent syphilitic uveitis, *N Engl J Med* 320:62, 1989.
65. Hicks CB, Benson PM, Lupton GP et al: Seronegative secondary syphilis in a patient infected with the human immunodeficiency virus (HIV) with Kaposi sarcoma, *Ann Intern Med* 107:492-495, 1987.

66. Hollander H: Cerebrospinal fluid normalities and abnormalities in individuals infected with human immunodeficiency virus, *J Infect Dis* 158:855-858, 1988.
67. Recommendations for diagnosing and treating syphilis in HIV-infected patients, *MMWR* 37:600-608, 1988.
68. Pace JL, Csonka GW: Endemic non-venereal syphilis (Bejel) in Saudi Arabia, *Br J Vener Dis* 60:293-297, 1984.
69. Tabbara KF, Al Kaff AS, Fadel T: Ocular manifestations of endemic syphilis (Bejel), *Ophthalmology* 96:1087-1091, 1989.
70. Smith JL: Neuro-ophthalmological study of late yaws: I. an introduction to yaws, *Br J Vener Dis* 47:223-225, 1971.
71. Smith JL, David NJ, Indgin S et al: Neuro-ophthalmological study of late yaws and pinta: II. the Caracas project, *Br J Vener Dis* 47:226-251, 1971.
72. Steere AC, Malawista SE, Snydman DR et al: Lyme arthritis: an epidemic of oligoarticular arthritis in children and adults in three Connecticut communities, *Arthritis Rheum* 20:7-17, 1977.
73. MacDonald AB: A neuro-ophthalmologic view, *J Clin Neurol Ophthalmol* 7:185-190, 1987.
74. Burgdorfer W, Barbour AG, Hayes SF et al: Lyme disease: a tick-borne spirochetosis? *Science* 216:1317-1319, 1982.
75. Berger BW, Kaplan MH, Rothenberg IR et al: Isolation and characterization of the Lyme disease spirochete from the skin of patients with erythema chronicum migrans, *J Am Acad Dermatol* 13:444-449, 1985.
76. Barbour AGA: Isolation and cultivation of Lyme disease spirochetes, *Yale J Biol Med* 57:521-525, 1984.
77. Barbour AG, Hayes SF: Biology of *Borrelia* species, *Microbiol Rev* 50:381-400, 1986.
78. Levine JF, Wilson ML, Spielman A: Mice as reservoirs of the Lyme disease spirochete, *Am J Trop Med Hyg* 34:355-360, 1985.
79. Wilson ML, Adler GH, Spielman A: Correlation between abundance of deer and that of the deer tick, *Ixodes dammini* (Acari: Ixodidae), *Ann Entomol Soc Am* 23:172-176, 1986.
80. Steere AC: Lyme disease, *N Engl J Med* 321:586-596, 1989.
81. Tsai TS, Bailey RE, Moore PS: National surveillance of Lyme disease 1987–1988, *Conn Med* 53:324-326, 1986.
82. Lastavica CC, Wilson ML, Berardi VP et al: Rapid emergence of a focal epidemic of Lyme disease in coastal Massachusetts, *N Engl J Med* 320:133-137, 1989.
83. Steere AC, Bartenhagen NH, Craft JE et al: The early clinical manifestations of Lyme disease, *Ann Intern Med* 99:76-82, 1983.
84. Pachner AR, Steere AC: The triad of neurologic manifestations of Lyme disease: meningitis, cranial neuritis, and radiculoneuritis, *Neurology* 35:47-53, 1985.
85. Clark JR, Carlson RD, Sasaki CT et al: Facial paralysis in Lyme disease, *Laryngoscope* 95:1341-1345, 1985.
86. Steere AC, Batsford WP, Weinberg M et al: Lyme carditis: cardiac abnormalities of Lyme disease, *Ann Intern Med* 93:8-16, 1980.
87. Bertuch AW, Rocco E, Schwartz EG: Eye findings in Lyme disease, *Conn Med* 51:151-152, 1987.
88. Baum J, Barza M, Weinstein P et al: Bilateral keratitis as a manifestation of Lyme disease, *Am J Ophthalmol* 105:75-77, 1988.
89. Orlin SE, Lauffer JL: Lyme disease keratitis, *Am J Ophthalmol* 107:678-680, 1989.
90. Schlesinger PA, Duray PH, Burke BA et al: Maternal-fetal transmission of the Lyme disease spirochete, *Borrelia burgdorferi, Ann Intern Med* 103:67-69, 1985.
91. Weber K, Bratzke HJ, Neubert U et al: *Borrelia burgdorferi* in a newborn despite oral penicillin for Lyme borreliosis during pregnancy, *Pediatr Infect Dis* 7:286-289, 1988.
92. Markowitz LE, Steere AC, Benach JL et al: Lyme disease during pregnancy, *JAMA* 255:3394-3396, 1986.
93. Williams CL, Benach JL, Curran AS et al: Lyme disease during pregnancy: a cord blood serosurvey, *Ann N Y Acad Sci* 539:504-506, 1988.
94. Aaberg TM: The expanding ophthalmologic spectrum of Lyme disease, *Am J Ophthalmol* 107:77-80, 1989.
95. Flack AJ, Lavoie PE: Episcleritis, conjunctivitis, and keratitis as other manifestations of Lyme disease, *Ophthalmology* 97:973-975, 1990.
96. Steere AC, Duray PH, Kauffmann DJ et al: Unilateral blindness caused by infection with the Lyme disease spirochete, *Borrelia burgdorferi, Ann Intern Med* 103:382-384, 1985.
97. Bialasiewicz AA, Ruprecht KW, Naumann GOH et al: Bilateral diffuse choroiditis and exudative retinal detachments with evidence of Lyme disease, *Am J Ophthalmol* 105:419-420, 1988.
98. Scholes GN, Teske M: Lyme disease and pars planitis, *Ophthalmology* 107 (Suppl):126, 1989.
99. Copeland RA Jr, Nozik RA, Shimokaji G: Uveitis in Lyme disease, *Ophthalmology* 107 (Suppl):127, 1989.
100. Winward KE, Smith JL, Culbertson WW et al: Ocular Lyme borreliosis, *Am J Ophthalmol* 108:651-657, 1989.
101. Karma A, Seppälä I, Mikkilä H et al: Diagnosis and clinical characteristics of ocular lyme borreliosis, *Am J Ophthalmol* 119:127-135, 1994.
102. Logigian EL, Kaplan RF, Steere AC: Chronic neurologic manifestations of Lyme disease, *N Engl J Med* 323: 1438-1444, 1990.
103. Wu G, Linoff H, Ellsworth RM et al: Optic disc edema and Lyme disease, *Ann Ophthalmol* 18:252-255, 1986.
104. Jacobson DM, Frens DB: Pseudotumor cerebri syndrome associated with Lyme disease, *Am J Ophthalmol* 107:81-82, 1989.
105. Schecter SL: Lyme disease associated with optic neuropathy, *Am J Med* 81:143-145, 1986.
106. Reik L Jr, Burgdorfer W, Donaldson JO: Neurologic abnormalities in Lyme disease without erythema chronicum migrans, *Am J Med* 81:73-78, 1986.
107. Seidenberg KB, Leib M: Orbital myositis with Lyme disease, *Am J Ophthalmol* 109:13-16, 1990.
108. Schwartz BS, Goldstein MD, Ribeiro JMC et al: Antibody testing in Lyme disease, *JAMA* 262:3431-3434, 1989.
109. Luger SW, Krauss E: Serologic tests for Lyme disease: interlaboratory variability, 1990, 150:761-763, 1990.
110. Barbour AG: The diagnosis of Lyme disease: rewards and perils. *Ann Intern Med* 110:501-502, 1989.
111. Dattwyler RJ, Volkman DJ, Lugt BJ et al: Seronega-

tive Lyme disease dissociation of specific T- and B-lymphocyte responses to *Borrelia burgdorferi*, *N Engl J Med* 319:1441-1446, 1988.
112. Russell H, Saampson JS, Schmid GP et al: Enzyme-linked immunosorbent assay and indirect immunofluorescence assay for Lyme disease, *J Infect Dis* 149:465-470, 1984.
113. Craft JE, Grodzicke RL, Steere AC: The antibody response in Lyme disease: evaluation of diagnostic tests, *J Infect Dis* 149:789-795, 1984.
114. Magnarelli LA, Anderson JF, Johnson RC: Cross-reactivity in serological tests of Lyme disease and other spirochetal infections, *J Infect Dis* 156:183-188, 1987.
115. Hunter EF, Russell H, Farshy CE et al: Evaluation of sera from patients with Lyme disease in the fluorescent treponemal antibody test for syphilis, *Sex Transm Dis* 13:232-236, 1986.
116. Duffy J, Mertz LE, Wobig FH et al: Diagnosing Lyme disease: the contribution of serologic testing, *Mayo Clinic Proc* 63:1116-1121, 1988.
117. Grodzicki RL, Steere AC: Comparison of immunoblotting and indirect enzyme-linked immunosorbent assay using different antigen preparations for diagnosing early Lyme disease, *J Infect Dis* 157:790-797, 1988.
118. Mandell H, Steere AC, Reinhardt BN et al: Lack of antibodies to *Borrelia burgdorferi* in patients with amyotrophic lateral sclerosis, *N Engl J Med* 320:255-256, 1989.
119. Steere AC, Grodzicke RL, Kornblatt AN et al: The spirochetal etiology of Lyme disease, *N Engl J Med* 308:733-740, 1983.
120. Bryceson ADM, Parry EHO, Perine PL et al: Louse-borne relapsing fever, *Q J Med* 39:129-170, 1970.
121. Southern PM Jr, Sanford JP: Relapsing fever: a clinical and microbiological review, *Medicine* 48:129-149, 1969.
122. Johnson WD Jr: *Borrelia* species (relapsing fever). In Mandell GL, Douglas RG, Bennett JE, editors: *Principles and practice of infectious diseases,* ed 3, New York, 1990, Churchill Livingstone, pp 1816-1819.
123. Bryceson ADM, Parry EHO, Perine PL et al: Louse-borne relapsing fever: a clinical and laboratory study of 62 cases in Ethiopia and a reconstruction of the literature, *Q J Med* 39:129-170, 1969.
124. Meader CN: Five cases of relapsing fever originating in Colorado, with positive blood findings in two, *Colo Med* 12:365-368, 1915.
125. Burgdorfer W: The enlarging spectrum of tick-borne spirochetoses: R. R. Parker memorial address, *Rev Infect Dis* 8:932-940, 1986.
126. Horton JM, Blaser MJ: The spectrum of relapsing fever in the Rocky Mountains, *Arch Intern Med* 145:871-875, 1985.
127. Perine PL, Parry EHO, Vukotich D et al: Bleeding in louse-borne relapsing fever I. clinical studies in 37 patients, *Trans R Soc Trop Med Hyg* 65:776-781, 1971.
128. Quin CE, Perkins ES: Tick-borne relapsing fever in East Africa, *J Trop Med* 49:30-32, 1946.
129. Hamilton JB: Ocular complications in relapsing fever, *Br J Ophthalmol* 27:68-80, 1943.
130. Sciotto CG, Lauer BA, White WL et al: Detection of *Borrelia* in acridin orange-stained blood smears by fluorescence microscopy, *Arch Pathol Lab Med* 107: 384-386, 1982.
131. Warell DA, Perine PL, Krause DW et al: Pathophysiology and immunology of the Jarisch-Herxheimer-like reaction in slow-borne relapsing fever: comparison of tetracycline and slow-release penicillin, *J Infect Dis* 147:898-908, 1983.
132. Weil A: Über eine eigentümliche, mit milztumor. Ikterus and nephritis einhergehende, akute infektionskrankheit, *Deutsches Arch Klin Med* 39:209-232, 1886.
133. Barkay S, Garzozi H: Leptospirosis. In Gold DH, Weingeist TA, editors: *The eye in systemic disease,* Philadelphia, 1990, JB Lippincott, pp 226-228.
134. Palmer MF: Laboratory diagnosis of leptospirosis, *Med Lab Sci* 45:174-178, 1988.
135. Waitkins SA: Update on leptospirosis, *BMJ* 290:1502-1503, 1985.
136. Bernard N, Moshe H: Human leptospirosis associated with eye complications, *Isr Med J* 22:182, 1963.
137. Barkay S, Garzozi H: Leptospirosis and uveitis, *Ann Ophthalmol* 16:164-168, 1984.
138. Duke-Elder S: *Diseases of the uveal tract, system of ophthalmology,* London, 1966, Henry Kimpton, pp 322-325.
139. Duke-Elder S: *Diseases of the outer eye, system of ophthalmology,* London, 1965, Henry Kimpton, pp 201-203.
140. Murdoch D: Leptospiral uveitis, *Trans Ophthal Soc* 32:73-75, 1980.
141. Takafuji ET, Kirkpatrick JW, Miller RN: An efficacy trial of doxycycline chemoprophylaxis against leptospirosis, *N Engl J Med* 310:497-500, 1984.
142. Farrar WE: *Leptospira* species (Leptospirosis). In Mandell GL, Douglas RG Jr, Bennett JE, editors: *Principles and practice of infectious diseases,* ed 3. New York, 1990, Churchill Livingstone, pp 1813-1816.
143. Heath CW Jr, Alexander AD, Galton MM: Leptospirosis in the United States, *N Engl J Med* 273:857-922, 1965.
144. Watt GW: Leptospirosis as a cause of uveitis, *Arch Intern Med* 150:1130-1132, 1990.
145. Puig-Solanes M, Heatley J, Arenas F et al: Ocular complications in brucellosis, *Am J Ophthalmol* 36: 675, 1953.
146. Tabbara KF, al Kassimi H: Ocular brucellosis, *Br J Ophthalmol* 74:249, 1990.
147. Rolando I, Carbone A, Haro D et al: Retinal detachment in chronic brucellosis, *Am J Ophthalmol* 99:733, 1985.
148. Walker J, Sharma OP, Rao NA: Brucellosis and uveitis, *Am J Ophthalmol* 114:374-375, 1992.
149. Palestine AG, Meyers SM, Fauci AS et al: Ocular findings in patients with neutrophil dysfunction, *Am J Ophthalmol* 95:598-604, 1983.
150. Parks DJ, Walton RC, Cheung MK et al: Sight-threatening complications of chronic granulomatous disease, *Ophthalmology* 101(Suppl):132, 1994.
151. Abe F, Tateyama M, Shibuya H et al: Disseminated fungal infection, *Acta Pathol Jpn* 34:1201-1208, 1984.
152. Edwards JE, Foos RY, Montgomerie JZ et al: Ocular manifestations of candida septicemia: review of seventy-six cases of hematogenous candida endophthalmitis, *Medicine* 53:47-75, 1974.
153. Gallo J, Playfair J, Gregory-Roberts J et al: Fungal endophthalmitis in narcotic abusers, *Med J Aust* 142:386-388, 1985.
154. Cohen M, Edwards JE Jr, Hensley TJ et al: Experimen-

tal hematogenous *Candida albicans* endophthalmitis: electron microscopy, *Invest Ophthalmol Vis Sci* 16:498-511, 1977.

155. Blumenkranz MS, Stevens DA: Therapy of endogenous fungal endophthalmitis, *Arch Ophthalmol* 98:1216-1220, 1980.
156. Goodman DF, Stern WH: Oral ketoconazole and intraocular amphotericin B for treatment of postoperative Candida parapsilosis endophthalmitis, *Arch Opthalmol* 105:172-173, 1987.
157. Naidoff MA, Green WR: Endogenous aspergillus endophthalmitis occurring after kidney transplant, *Am J Ophthalmol* 79:502-509, 1975.
158. Roney P, Barr CC, Chun CH et al: Endogenous aspergillus endophthalmitis, *Rev Infect Dis* 8:955-958, 1986.
159. Young RC, Bennett JE, Vogel CL et al: Aspergillosis: the spectrum of the disease in 98 patients, *Medicine* 49:147-173, 1970.
160. Sihota R, Agarwal HC, Grover AK et al: Aspergillus endophthalmitis, *J Ophthalmol* 71:611-613, 1987.
161. Glasgow BJ, Brown HH, Foos RY: Miliary retinitis in coccidiodomycosis, *Am J Ophthalmol* 104:24-27, 1987.
162. Hiles DA, Font RL: Unilateral intraocular cruptococcosis with unilateral spontaneous regression, *Am J Ophthalmol* 65:98-108, 1968.
163. Goldstein BG, Buellner H: Histoplasmic endophthalmitis: a clinicopathologic correlation, *Arch Ophthalmol* 101:774-777, 1983.
164. Font RL, Jakobiec FA: Granulomatous necrotizing retinochoroiditis caused by sporotrichum schenkii, *Arch Ophthalmol* 94:1513-1519, 1976.
165. Font RL, Spaulding AG, Green WR: Endogenous mycotic panophthalmitis caused by *Blastomyces dermatitidis, Arch Ophthalmol* 77:217-222, 1967.

# CHAPTER 11

# Acquired Immunodeficiency Syndrome

## HUMAN IMMUNODEFICIENCY VIRUS

Since the first clinical recognition, in 1981, of the acquired immunodeficiency syndrome (AIDS), new, complex clinical problems have emerged in all medical specialties. The epidemic of infection with human immunodeficiency virus (HIV) and its subsequent fatal consequence of AIDS have produced a variety of clinical ocular disease. Until effective treatment and preventive therapy are available, we will continue to see an increasing number of patients with AIDS and HIV-related disorders.

HIV is a retrovirus and therefore has only RNA in its genome. It can infect many types of human cells, but much of its pathologic effect is secondary to infection of the helper/inducer T cell ($OKT4^+$, $CD4^+$).[1] Because this cell is crucial for the development of cell-mediated immune responses, infection of this cell type and subsequent cell death result in severe immunosuppression. The HIV virion binds to the $CD4^+$ cell, and once in the cell, its RNA is translated into DNA by viral reverse transcriptase (Fig. 11-1). This DNA then enters the nucleus and incorporates into the cell genome. The viral DNA is then capable of directing protein synthesis of new viral proteins using the infected cell's apparatus. These viral particles are then shed from the cell, and the infected cell eventually dies.

HIV infection can be detected by the presence of antibody to viral antigens, which usually occurs 4 to 12 weeks after infection. A commercial enzyme-linked immunosorbent assay (ELISA) is used and can be confirmed by Western blot analysis.[2,3] However, some patients will not develop antibodies for many months after exposure to HIV, but they will be infected. The antibodies do not contain the infection nor prevent its sequelae. The virus can also be cultured from blood, semen, saliva, and tears, as well as from solid tissues. In the eye, the virus has been found in the cornea,[4] vitreous, and retina.[5]

HIV infection in the United States is most common in homosexual men with multiple partners and in intravenous drug users.[2,3] However, there is increasing infection among heterosexuals as the virus spreads throughout the population through sexual contact and intravenous drug use. Before the availability of a serologic test for HIV antibody, large numbers of patients, including hemophiliacs, were exposed to the virus through blood product transfusion.

AIDS is the most severe manifestation of HIV infection and occurs at a point at which the immune system is so damaged by the HIV infection that opportunistic infections such as *Pneumocystis carinii, Cryptococcus neoformans,* cytomegalovirus (CMV), oral candidiasis, or unusual malignant processes such as Kapo-

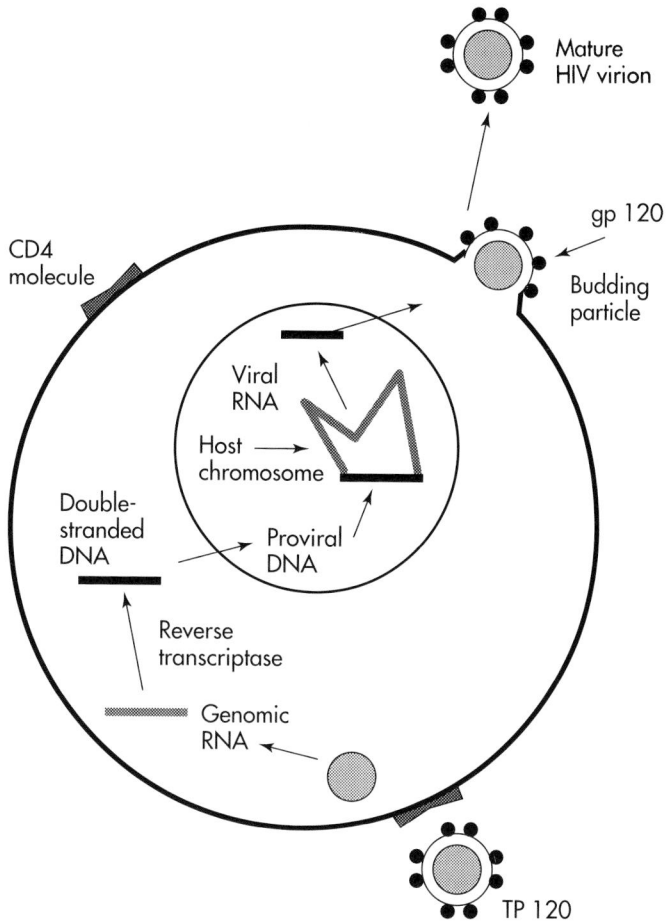


**Fig. 11-1.** Diagram of life cycle of human immunodeficiency virus (HIV).

si's sarcoma can emerge.[2,3] There is also an encephalopathy caused by direct HIV infection of the brain. Before AIDS or any of its symptoms develop, the HIV-infected patient can live for a number of years as a symptom-free carrier. Some patients experience an AIDS-related complex (ARC) of weight loss, fatigue, fever, lymphadenopathy, and lymphopenia before AIDS develops.

Although direct HIV infection in the brain appears to produce a severe encephalopathy, there is still no definitive evidence that HIV infection of ocular tissue leads to clinically important pathologic effects. However, subclinical infection of retinal neural and endothelial cells has been reported.[5] The noninfectious retinopathy of AIDS may be caused by interaction between viral antigens and antibodies that circulate in the blood and then deposit in the eye; however, this has not been clearly shown. This retinopathy consists primarily of cotton-wool spots that are seen in 25% to 92% of AIDS patients and much less frequently in ARC or in symptom-free HIV patients.[6-9] The incidence increases with the degree of immunosuppression. The presence of the p24 antigen, a surface HIV antigen, in the blood also increases with advancing disease, and it is possible that this antigenemia may yet be related to the cause of this retinopathy, with immune complex formation in the retinal vasculature. Superficial and deep retinal hemorrhages, retinal perivasculitis, and possibly vascular occlusions also may occur. Small symptomless peripheral blot hemorrhages can be found as well and appear to be more common with decreasing CD4 counts. Electron microscopy studies of these lesions reveal swollen endothelial cells and degenerating pericytes.[10] Inflammatory cell infiltrates and infectious organisms are not seen in cotton-wool spots; however, the microvascular abnormalities are widespread throughout the retina and may be the entrance for opportunistic viral infections of the retina.

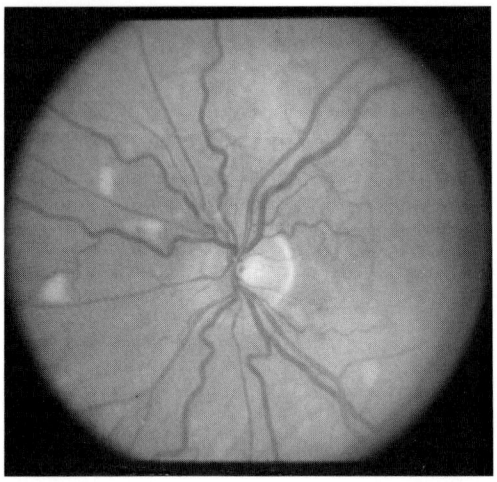

**Fig. 11-2.** Multiple nerve fiber layer infarcts (cotton-wool spots) in patient with AIDS. (See Color Plate 19.)

Clinically, cotton-wool spots are seen as superficial white fluffy lesions in the retina (Fig. 11-2). There may be small dilations of the microvasculature nearby. Visual symptoms are rarely associated with the presence of a cotton-wool spot. A cotton-wool spot cannot occur in the foveal avascular zone inasmuch as there is no nerve fiber layer to become infarcted in this part of the retina. Perifoveal cotton-wool spots may be recognized by the patient as a relative, but not absolute, scotoma, which can be useful in distinguishing a cotton-wool spot from an early area of viral retinitis. In AIDS patients these lesions can sometimes be more than 0.5 disc diameters in size. They are distinguished from infectious retinitis by the fact that they do not enlarge. Although individual lesions will disappear over a period of several months, new lesions often appear.

CMV retinitis is the most common ocular infection in AIDS and is discussed in the next section. Other intraocular infections that may occur in AIDS patients include syphilis, toxoplasmosis, tuberculosis, candidal infection, and cryptococcosis.[11-15] These have been discussed in previous chapters and must be differentiated from CMV infection. Herpes zoster ophthalmicus in a young, healthy homosexual man is an early sign of HIV infection.[16] Herpes zoster retinitis accompanied by acute retinal necrosis (see Chapter 12) and herpes simplex retinitis has occasionally been seen in patients with AIDS.[10] These viral retinal infections are often difficult to differentiate clinically from CMV retinitis. Autopsy studies have shown that more than 95% of viral retinitis in AIDS is due to CMV infection.[6,10] However, these studies were completed early in the history of the AIDS epidemic, and the percentages may have changed.

## CYTOMEGALOVIRUS RETINITIS

CMV is a herpes class virus and therefore contains double-stranded DNA. Systemic infection is common and causes a heterophil, antibody-negative mononucleosis syndrome. Therefore many adults have CMV antibodies because of previous infection. Approximately 50% of heterosexual men and 95% of homosexual men have evidence of a previous CMV infection. However, with the exception of a few unusual cases, CMV infection of the retina occurs as an opportunistic infection only in immunosuppressed persons or in infants with congenital CMV infection. The disease was first recognized in congenital infection in 1947. In the past, organ transplantation and chemotherapy were the most common causes of CMV retinitis.[17] It is interesting to note that CMV retinitis is much more frequent after renal transplantation than after bone marrow transplantation. In the current era, however, the increasing number of patients with AIDS has led to a marked increase in the number of cases. CMV retinitis tends to occur in those patients who are the most significantly immunosuppressed by HIV infection,[6,18] rarely occurring if the CD4 count is greater than 100 cells/μL. CMV retinitis has been reported in 7% to 40% of AIDS patients in several series, but it probably occurs clinically in 15% to 20% of these patients at some time.[6,7,10,11] CMV retinitis probably reaches the eye via the blood stream although the possibility of reactivation of latent virus has not been ruled out. Evidence of hematogenous spread includes that fact that one eye frequently develops retinitis several months before the other eye and that new foci of retinitis can appear in an affected eye. It is unusual to see more than three separate of areas of CMV retinitis in an eye, and most eyes contain one initial focus that then spreads across the retina.

CMV retinitis begins as small white retinal infiltrates that if seen early may resemble a large cotton-wool spot. Two types of clinical appearances may be seen. The first is a perivascular fluffy white lesion with many scattered hemorrhages (Fig. 11-3). Another manifestation is a more granular-appearing lesion that has few associated hemorrhages and often has a central area of clearing, with atrophic retina and stippled retinal pigment epithelium (Fig. 11-4).

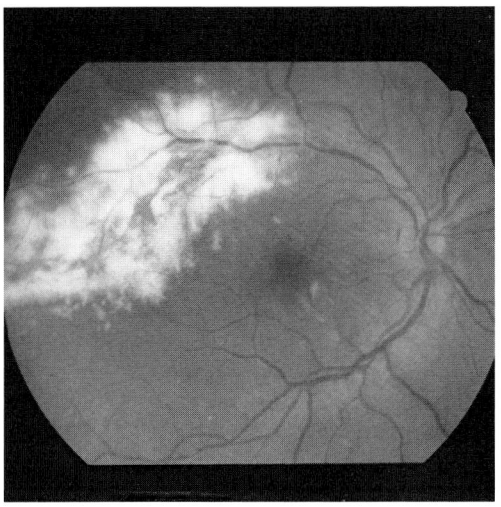

**Fig. 11-3.** Cytomegalovirus retinitis in vascular distribution characterized by fluffy-white retinal infiltration and small area of retinal hemorrhage. (See Color Plate 20.)

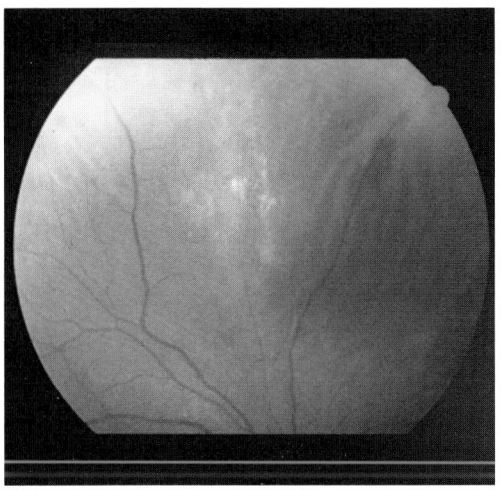

**Fig. 11-4.** Cytomegalovirus retinitis may also have granular appearance with mottling of retinal pigment epithelium and little associated retinal hemorrhage. (See Color Plate 21.)

In autopsy studies CMV has been identified in both types of lesions in AIDS patients. However, because we do not understand what factors predispose a person to one type of lesion, we cannot exclude the possibility that some of these lesions may be other viral retinal infections. It is possible that the underlying immune status of the patient influences the clinical appearance of the lesion. However, local factors also must be important inasmuch as an occasional patient will have different-appearing lesions. Both types of lesions respond to the therapeutic approach that will be discussed later, which is consistent with herpes class viral infections of the retina.

The diagnosis of CMV retinitis is based on clinical criteria. Although it is possible to confirm the diagnosis with a polymerase chain reaction performed on a vitreous specimen or by culture of the virus from the vitreous or retina, this is rarely done in practice. As the number of treatment options grows and becomes more specific, accurate diagnosis will be increasingly important. Active CMV retinitis always has a faint granular border of intraretinal infiltrates that represent the new foci of viral activity in normal retina. In addition, the disease grows at approximately 250 μm/wk, and therefore there are usually areas that have begun to atrophy as denoted by retinal pigment epithelial stippling. This is in contrast to acute retinal necrosis in which the disease spreads rapidly, and one is less likely to find active retinitis surrounding an atrophic center. There is always a low-grade vitritis with CMV retinitis, frequently less than might be expected for the degree of retinal necrosis. Often this is barely noticeable trace vitreal cells, and rarely is the view obscured by vitreal haze. There may be fine anterior-chamber keratic precipitates (KP), although most patients have no anterior chamber reaction. Vision is normal unless the optic disc or fovea is involved.

CMV retinitis is often symptomless because the lesions begin in the periphery or because the patient does not notice an increase in floaters or a new scotoma. Therefore it may make clinical sense to screen patients who are at risk with CD4 counts less than 50 to 100 cells/μL. A reasonable screening frequency is every 3 or 4 months for this population, although this may need to be modified as oral prophylactic therapies enter widespread usage. Because children more rarely complain of visual symptoms, ophthalmologic screening should be performed at least every 3 months when the CD4 count is less than 50 cells/μL.

### Progression

CMV retinitis progresses in two ways. New lesions may form that are not physically near an old lesion, probably by hematogenous spread. Second and most common, an old lesion spreads at its borders to involve new, previously uninfected retina. In this latter situation, the center of the old lesion eventually ceases to be white because the white color is due to scattering of light by edematous and necrotic retina. Once retinal cell death has occurred and only a glial scar remains, the atrophic retina is again transparent with underlying retinal pigment epithelial stippling (see Fig. 11-4). Therefore, in assessing the progression and resolution of CMV retinitis, it is most important to pay attention to the edge of the lesions to look for advancement of the border and to not look at the center of the lesion and interpret a decrease in whiteness as improvement.

Visual loss in CMV retinitis occurs in several ways. Most commonly, the infected retina develops an absolute scotoma due to retinal necrosis. As the macula is involved, the central vision is lost. Macular involvement can be either a presenting sign or a late sign. However, until the macula is involved by active retinitis, the vision can be nearly normal unless there is secondary macular edema from a nearby area of retinitis. Patients can retain normal central vision with only a few degrees of visual field in this disease, and they can be significantly disabled by the peripheral retinal destruction. The optic disc can also become involved, and the vision can be lost even when the amount of retinitis is still minimal. In some patients, paramacular CMV will produce macular edema, which is a reversible cause of visual loss if it can be treated before the active virus progresses through the fovea. Last, the retina can develop a rhegmatogenous retinal detachment because there is vitreous traction on the thin, atrophic retina.

Retinal detachment develops in approximately 20% of patients with retinitis, with 50% of these patients developing detachment in the second eye if it is involved with retinitis. Approximately 11% of patients with retinitis will experience a retinal detachment 6 months after diagnosis, and 24% will have detachment over the first year after diagnosis in the first eye.[19] The greater the amount of peripheral retinal involvement, the greater the risk of retinal detachment. Compared with eyes with 10% of the peripheral retina involved, eyes with greater than 25% had a fivefold increase in detachment rate. This risk increased to 24-fold if active retinitis also was present.

The mechanism of retinal detachment in CMV retinitis is vitreous traction on the thinned, atrophic retina. Multiple retinal breaks are usually present, and large, relatively posterior breaks can be seen. Tears can occur at the edge of the normal retina but also throughout the atrophic areas. The risk of retinal detachment is increased if the patient with CMV retinitis is myopic. The posterior vitreous is usually adherent to the retina, and the combination of low-grade vitritis with a thinned retina allows the vitreous to pull the retina forward, causing the retina to detach. The rate of growth of the detachment is variable and depends on the extent of traction and location within the eye.

The standard surgical approach for retinal detachment is not optimal for eyes with CMV retinitis. Scleral buckling is appropriate when retinal breaks are located near the vitreous base. The breaks in eyes with CMV retinitis often are more posterior and multiple. Scleral buckling may be successful in selected cases, but a more effective approach is vitrectomy, endolaser surgery, and application of a long-lasting retinal tamponade. In CMV-free patients these detachments are often approached with use of a long-acting intraocular gas tamponade. This requires the patient to keep a face-down position for 10 to 21 days for the gas bubble to be effective. In patients with limited long-term survival who have other medical illnesses, compliance is a difficult problem. In addition, vision with a gas bubble is limited to perceiving only hand motions until the bubble resorbs.

### Treatment

Some of the problems in the treatment of retinal detachment in patients with CMV retinitis can be circumvented with the use of a silicone oil tamponade. Head position can be more normal, although the patient still cannot lie on his or her back. Vision can be rehabilitated in a few days. Most important, the chance of retinal redetachment in CMV retinitis repaired with a sulfur hexafluoride bubble is more than 60% whereas it is less than 5% with silicone oil. The surgery can be performed as a local, outpatient procedure with minimal postoperative discomfort.

The major disadvantage of silicone oil is the induced hyperopia of 5 to 6 diopters, which, unless a contact lens is worn, will produce diplopia if only one eye has had surgery. Both gas bubbles and silicone oil are associated with an increased risk of cataract formation. These cataracts commonly become visually significant 1 year after the surgery. Older patients may have a greater chance of cataract development than do younger patients. Because the silicone oil is rarely removed in patients with AIDS, further progression of the retinitis and addi-

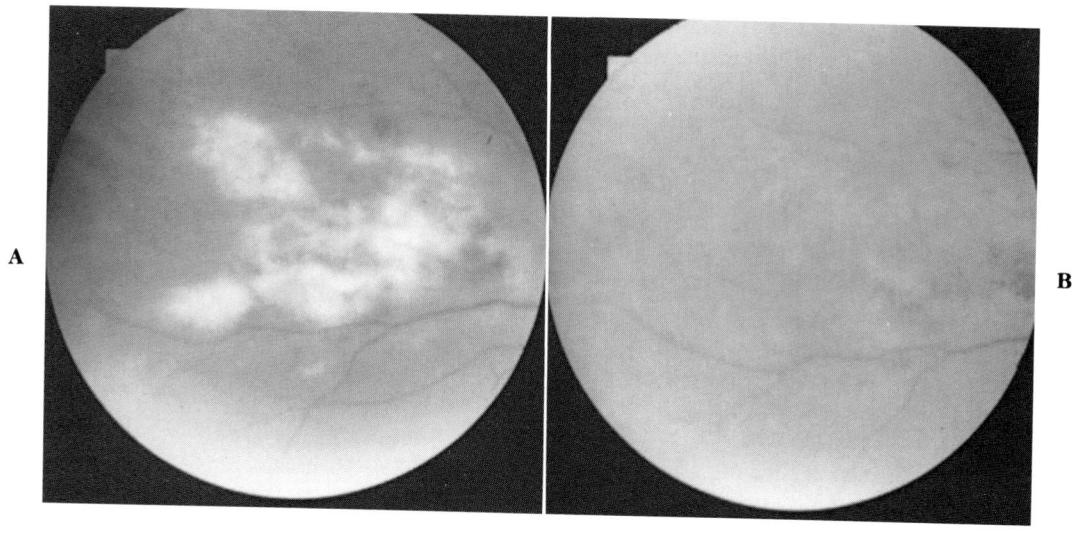


**Fig. 11-5. A,** Retinal photograph of area of cytomegalovirus retinitis in patient with immunosuppression secondary to chemotherapy. **B,** Same area after 2 weeks of therapy with 5 mg/kg ganciclovir given twice daily.

tional retinal breaks rarely cause redetachment. In AIDS-free patients the oil is commonly left in for several years and then removed. In addition, the chance of cataract formation increases greatly when silicone oil is left in the eye for more than 1 year. As survival with CMV retinitis increases, more cataracts will need to be removed in this patient population. Of interest is that the oil causes a hyperopic shift of approximately 1 to 2 diopters with a posterior chamber intraocular lens (IOL) as opposed to the 5- to 6-diopter change in the phakic eye. One additional potential disadvantage of silicone oil is that the use of intravitreal drug injections is difficult and the therapeutic result unpredictable.

The use of laser surgery to demarcate areas of retinitis and thereby prevent detachment has been suggested. A similar approach is often used in acute retinal necrosis due to herpes zoster infection.[20] Although there is literature supporting this approach, it is not uniformly successful, and inasmuch as CMV retinitis often continues to progress through a barrier of laser burns, this approach will not prevent either spread or detachment in all patients.[21] It is unclear whether this approach should be widely utilized, but it may be possible to study this question and identify high-risk groups for whom prophylactic laser will be useful.

The goal of repair of the retinal detachment is to preserve vision in patients with a limited life span but with a high risk of bilateral blindness. Because it is not possible to predict which eye will have a better treatment outcome or will develop drug resistance, it appears sensible to attempt to repair and salvage vision in both eyes. As life expectancy increases, the risk of visual loss from progressive CMV, as well as other causes such as cryptococcal meningitis or optic neuropathy, increases. The goal of antiviral drug therapy is to prevent viral growth. Inasmuch as there are currently no methods for removing CMV viral DNA from retinal cells, all current therapies are virostatic and slow or eliminate viral replication. Thus, whenever therapy is discontinued or the virus develops a mechanism of resistance, the viral growth resumes in the retina.

**Ganciclovir.** Effective therapy of CMV retinitis was not possible before the advent of ganciclovir (DHPG) [9-(1,3,dihydroxy-2-propoxymethyl) guanine] in 1984. We attempted laser destruction of the infected retina without success in stopping the progression of the disease.[21] Whereas acyclovir is not sufficiently active against CMV infection, ganciclovir is virostatic in vitro and in vivo. Ganciclovir is triphosphorylated in the cell and then inhibits viral DNA polymerase. Therapy with 5 mg/kg intravenously twice daily for 14 days will result in halting progression and the development of a less active lesion in more than 90% of patients[22-24] (Fig. 11-5). However, because the drug is virostatic, recurrences are common unless the underlying immunosuppression can be altered. In AIDS patients the median time to progression of retinitis without treatment is 21 days. Intravenous administration of ganciclovir, 5 mg/kg/day, 7 days per week prolongs the median time to relapse to 56 days, and many patients go significantly longer without a relapse.[25] A dosage of 6 mg/kg/day also has been used with little apparent increase in toxicity. Maintenance dosages lower than 25 mg/kg/wk are associated with a higher relapse rate. It is probable that maintenance therapy in its current form does not completely suppress viral replication but slows it sufficiently so that remission is maintained for a period of time. After treatment, visual loss due to macular edema often improves, but visual loss due to retinal necrosis does not.

The main toxicity of ganciclovir therapy is neutropenia.[22-25] Neutrophil counts must be maintained above 500/μl. A decreasing count is often seen in the second week of therapy or during maintenance therapy. In addition, there is evidence of gonadal toxicity in animal testing, but this has not been evaluated in human beings. Neutropenia was a major contraindication to continued ganciclovir therapy until the development of granulocyte colony-stimulating factor (GCSF; Nupogen). Injection of the biologic compound one to three times per week will increase blood neutrophil counts as well as neutrophil function. This allows the use of long-term ganciclovir therapy and even permits long-term dosing at 5 mg/kg intravenously twice daily. There are no comparative data on the use of long-term, twice-daily, intravenously administered ganciclovir, but this approach does allow for more consistent antiviral drug levels.

Foscarnet was the second drug approved for the treatment of CMV retinitis. It inhibits DNA polymerase in a manner different from that of ganciclovir. In addition to being inhibitory to CMV and other herpesviruses, it inhibits reverse transcriptase and the replication of the HIV virus. It is also administered intravenously with a 2-week induction dosage of either 60 mg/kg three times daily or 90 mg/kg twice daily, followed by 90 mg/kg or 120 mg/kg daily.[26] There is some suggestion that the higher maintenance dose is more effective. Foscarnet is less toxic to the bone marrow than is ganciclovir, but it is nephrotoxic and leads to electrolyte abnormalities in serum calcium, phosphate, and magnesium levels. It cannot be used with other nephrotoxic drugs such as amphotericin B. Other symptoms of toxicity include nausea, gastrointestinal disturbance, and fatigue. The nausea can be avoided by pretreatment with antiemetic agents before infusion. Nephrotoxicity can be reduced by intravenous hydration therapy associated with each dose. A current investigation focuses on whether oral hydration may be as effective as intravenous hydration if the patient can consume sufficient oral fluid to promote diuresis during infusion. This reduces renal accumulation of the drug.

Ganciclovir and foscarnet were compared in the multicenter trial conducted by Studies of Ocular Complications of AIDS (SOCA).[25,27] Both drugs were found to be equally effective in preventing progression of CMV retinitis, with a median time to progression of approximately 8 weeks for each; 85% of patients showed progression within 17 weeks. However, foscarnet was shown to increase survival to 12 months after diagnosis compared with 8 months for ganciclovir in patients with normal renal function.

The SOCA study also demonstrated several other aspects of treatment with either foscarnet or ganciclovir. The time to relapse after each subsequent reinduction with either drug decreases with subsequent relapses. In other words, both drugs become less effective in slowing retinal destruction. The rate of visual field loss was 30 degrees per month (or 5% of the visual field), and the rate of three lines of visual loss in an involved eye was 94/100 persons per year. However, because CMV was bilateral in only 41% of patients at the start of the study, 91% of patients maintained 20/40 or better in the best eye after 6 months of therapy. Inasmuch as the ocular effects of ganciclovir and foscarnet appear to be similar, the choice of initial agent is based largely on systemic factors and tolerance.

CMV retinitis can have either an indolent appearance as defined by a granular active edge of retinitis or a more fulminant appearance with extensive areas of edema and hemorrhage. The indolent-appearing lesion may have a better prognosis, but it is unclear whether this is related to the higher likelihood of a fulminant lesion being located in the posterior pole or whether viral and immune factors mediate the appearance and severity of the disease.

Initial relapses of retinitis should be treated with reinduction using the same drug, especially if the patient had a reasonable response to the first course of therapy. Because the second relapse will occur sooner than the first,[27] eventually most patients receive foscarnet as well as ganciclovir. In some patients clinical resistance to therapy develops as evidenced by shortening of response duration and eventually lack of control of the retinitis even on induction dosing. Some patients may be ganciclovir-resistant in one eye and foscarnet-resistant in the other.

**Combined therapy.** Combined therapy with intravenous foscarnet and ganciclovir, each given once daily, has been well tolerated and is useful in situations in which either drug alone is not effective.[28] In addition, current clinical trials are in progress to determine if this combination therapy is superior to therapy with either drug alone in terms of treating CMV retinitis and improving survival. The drugs work at different sites of DNA polymerase inhibition, and by giving each 12 hours apart, 24-hour antiviral levels can be obtained. This approach is rarely used as primary therapy because of the extended amount of time required for infusion, but it may be useful for immediately life-threatening disease.

Another approach that has been used in the treatment of CMV retinitis is intravitreal injection of ganciclovir[29] or foscarnet.[30] Two injections per week may result in prolonged remission in the treated eye as long as the injections are continued. The initially suggested dose of ganciclovir was 200 μg given in 0.1 ml. The pH of the available solution is fairly alkaline, but no adverse reactions have been reported with the use of this drug in the eye. The pharmacokinetics in the vitreous suggest that therapeutic levels are present for 62 hours after each injection, with an intraocular drug half-life of 13.3 hours. Higher levels of ganciclovir can be used in patients who are developing resistance, and doses of 1 or 2 mg/0.05 ml can be given once or twice a week. Often once-a-week therapy is effective at these higher doses, and the lower volume decreases the risk of central retinal artery closure. Foscarnet is usually used at 1.2 mg/0.05 ml although 2.4 mg/0.1 ml is also tolerated by the eye. This approach with either drug is most useful when systemic therapy is not possible because of neutropenia or the use of other drugs. With repeated injections, the risk of vitreal hemorrhage, infection, and retinal detachment increases. In addition, intravitreal therapy does not treat possible systemic infection with CMV such as CMV colitis. Some AIDS patients prefer the intravitreal route of therapy because there is no intravenous infusion and quality of life is improved. The injections can be given painlessly if a small subconjunctival lidocaine injection is given 10 minutes before the intravitreal injection. Many patients can also tolerate the injection with administration of only topical anesthesia.

Oral ganciclovir is being developed for both prophylaxis and maintenance therapy. A dosage of 3000 mg/day given after 3 weeks of intravenously administered ganciclovir therapy leads to slightly faster progression with oral therapy than with intravenous therapy. Although some patients have long remissions, the median time to progression is only 29 days. In contrast, oral ganciclovir given to patients with CD4 counts less than 100 cells/μL resulted in a 50% decrease in CMV-related events, either colitis or retinitis. This approach seems to be a promising method of reducing the incidence of CMV retinitis; however, requires prophylactic therapy for the 80% of AIDS patients who were never destined to develop retinitis. An effective oral preparation of foscarnet is not yet available.

An interesting approach to anti-CMV therapy is the ganciclovir implant. This is a slow-release device, which releases 1 μg of drug per hour for 8 months. It is surgically implanted through the pars plana after a local vitrectomy is performed. The mean time to progression with this implant is 226 days, with about 50% of the untreated contralateral eyes developing CMV retinitis during the study.[31] The efficacy of this device for treating local CMV retinitis is clear, but again, this local therapy does not treat systemic CMV infection. Combinations of the ganciclovir implant with systemic therapy, such as oral ganciclovir, may treat both local and systemic infection while avoiding daily systemic infusions. The relative benefits of this therapeutic approach needs further exploration.

A CMV-specific monoclonal antibody has also been developed, which when given with concomitant maintenance ganciclovir therapy, was reported to increase the time to progression to approximately 200 days. This drug is administered by injection every 2 weeks and is under development at this time. Another novel therapy is the ISIS 2922 antisense drug. This is a 21-monomer nucleotide chain with a phosphothio backbone in which the oxygens are replaced by sulfur to resist DNase. This drug is injected intravitreally every 1 to 2 weeks at a dose of 300 μg. It has been effective in cases of CMV resistant to antiviral drug therapy. Some patients have experienced anterior and posterior segment inflammation, most of which has been treatable with topical or periocular steroids and that sometimes have disappeared with continued therapy. Changes in the RPE have also been noted at higher doses.[32] Cidofovir (HPMPC) is another compound with anti-CMV effect that is being tried in clinical trials for CMV retinitis. This drug is administered intravenously, but it can be given every 1 to 2 weeks, obviating the need for daily infusions and central venous access. Renal toxicity develops in many patients but may be controlled by coadministration of probenicid. Intravitreol injection of cidofovir is also under investigation for CMV retinitis.[33]

Survival in patients with CMV retinitis has been increasing during the past decade. This effect is probably a combination of antiretroviral and anti-herpesvirus therapy combined with prophylaxis and aggressive treatment for other opportunistic infections. A median survival of 14 to 18 months is currently seen, with only the rare patient surviving 3 years after diagnosis. In large part the preservation of useful vision in at least one eye is based on the fact that survival for most patients is limited. As survival increases, current ganciclovir and foscarnet therapies will be increasingly inadequate in preserving vision because their effect is only to decrease the time to progression by 50% compared with no treatment. Emerging strategies, including the ganciclovir implant and monoclonal antibody therapy, may be more successful.

## HERPES ZOSTER

Herpes zoster ophthalmicus occurs more frequently in HIV-positive patients and may often be the presenting sign of the disease, but it is not an opportunistic infection. Cutaneous zoster occurring in a severely immunosuppressed patient with AIDS is more likely to disseminate and may be more difficult to treat with acyclovir compared with its effectiveness in the immunocompetent patient. Intravenously administered acyclovir sometimes is required for cutaneous dermatomal zoster and certainly is needed for disseminated zoster.

Varicella-zoster virus (VZV)-retinitis in the HIV-positive patient has a somewhat more varied clinical spectrum than is seen in immunocompetent patients. Although the clinical picture in some patients is identical to acute retinal necrosis, other clinical appearances have been described. In one study 17% of HIV-positive patients with herpes zoster ophthalmicus subsequently developed acute retinal necrosis.[34] A form of retinitis, which has been termed *progressive outer retinal necrosis* (PORN), appears as multifocal areas of retinitis with good preservation of the inner retina and retinal vasculature in the early clinical stages[35] (discussed in detail in Chapter 12). The areas of necrosis occasionally appear similar to those in acute retinal necrosis. In punctate outer retinal necrosis, the lesions are small, often multifocal, and consist of multiple punctate white retinal dots located in the outer retina (see Fig. 12-6). Still other patients may initially manifest multiple retinal vascular occlusions with areas of retinitis (see Fig. 12-5).

The response to systemic acyclovir is inconsistent in these immunosuppressed patients. Approximately half of the patients have a good response to intravenous acyclovir followed by oral acyclovir, with resultant quieting of the retinitis. Some of these patients can be weaned from the oral acyclovir, but others have recurrences without maintenance therapy.[36] In contrast, other patients have progressive retinitis despite intravenous acyclovir. Although intravenous foscarnet may also be tried in these patients, the course of their disease may be relentlessly progressive. Because this process can be bilateral, severe visual disability can result. The risk of retinal detachment appears similar for immunosuppressed and immunocompetent patients with VZV retinitis, and repair techniques are similar.

The major differential diagnosis in the HIV-positive patient is between CMV and VZV retinitis. This is important because acyclovir is considerably less toxic than either ganciclovir or foscarnet. CMV retinitis is at least 20 times more common than VZV retinitis, and the differential diagnosis is based primarily on clinical criteria, taking into account the rate of progression and the multifocality.

## *PNEUMOCYSTIS CARINII* CHOROIDITIS

*P. carinii* choroiditis was first reported by Macher et al.[37] It is characterized by multifocal white plaques in the choroid with little evidence of intraocular inflammation (Fig. 11-6).[38] It is an extrapulmonary form of pneumocystic

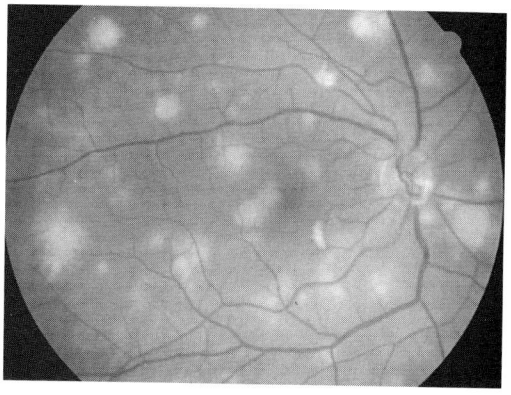

**Fig. 11-6.** Fundus photograph of patient with AIDS and *Pneumocystis carinii* pneumonia shows multiple yellow deep choroidal lesions. Histopathologic examination revealed not only *P. carinii* cysts but also cytomegalovirus (see Fig. 11-7) and *Mycobacterium avium–intracellulare* (see Fig. 11-8). (From *Retina* 12:331-335, 1992.) (See Color Plate 22.)

disease usually seen in patients using a prophylactic inhalant for this condition, which prevents pulmonary involvement but does not provide systemic prophylaxis. This has become a less common problem as the use of aerosolized pentamidine has decreased. Histopathologic examination in these cases shows numerous cysts in the choroid (Fig. 11-7).

The lesions rarely cause visual loss because they are located beneath the retinal pigment epithelium (RPE) and have no associated inflammation. They respond to therapy with intravenously administered pentamidine. Histologic examination has demonstrated large numbers of cysts with no host response. It is important to identify this disease so that the internist can be aware of the potential for an extrapulmonary pneumocystic involvement. The ocular disease is associated with prophylactic aerosolized pentamidine and appears to be less common as aerosolized pentamidine use has decreased.

### *MYCOBACTERIUM AVIUM-INTRACELLULARE* CHOROIDITIS

*Mycobacterium avium-intracellulare* manifests as infiltrates, usually 50 to 100 μm in size and scattered throughout the fundus.[39,40] It usually causes no visual symptoms but, as in the case of pneumocystic disease, is evidence of disseminated systemic infection. *M. avium-intracellulare* choroiditis is a common pathogen in patients with AIDS, which often involves the bone marrow and leads to marrow failure.

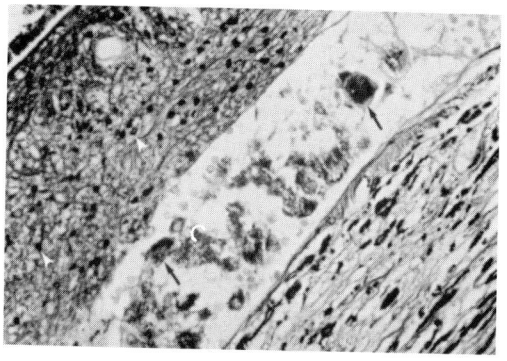

**Fig. 11-7.** Photomicrograph of choroidal lesion of right eye shows numerous *Pneumocystis carinii* cysts *(white arrowheads)* and cytomegalovirus cells in choroidal blood vessel *(arrows)*. (Gomori's methenimine-silver stain; ×400.) (From *Retina* 12: 331-335, 1992.) (See Color Plate 23.)

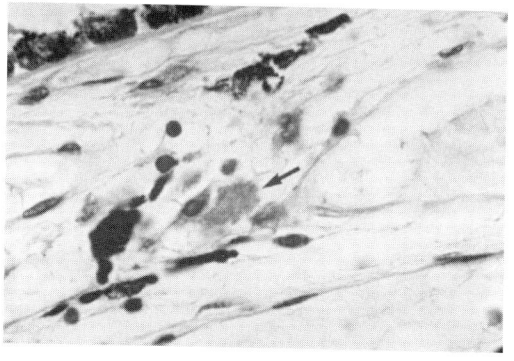

**Fig. 11-8.** Photomicrograph of choroid adjacent to area infiltrated with *Pneumocystis carinii* shows cluster of acid-fast bacilli *(arrow)*. (Ziehl-Neelsen stain; ×100.) (From *Retina* 12:331-335, 1992.) (See Color Plate 24.)

## OTHER DISEASES

Multiple infections in a single eye may be present in patients with AIDS. Choroidal lesions such as those caused by *Pneumocystis* organisms can be seen concurrently with other organisms such as CMV and *M. avium-intracellulare* (Figs. 11-7 and 11-8), but the greatest concern is a CMV infection combined with herpes zoster or herpes simplex. In this situation the retinitis response can be atypical, and if the zoster infection is treated with acyclovir, the CMV will continue to progress. Toxoplasmosis, which is discussed in Chapter 14, is also seen as a retinal infection with a vitritis and should be managed with an antitoxoplasmosis regimen.[40] In addition, B cell lymphoma can occur in AIDS, manifesting as choroidal, retinal, or vitreous lesions.[41] A pos-

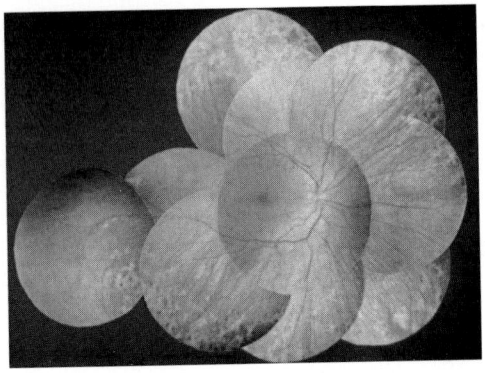

**Fig. 11-9.** Photographic montage of patient with didanosine-related retinal lesions. Atrophic areas of RPE hypopigmentation and hyperpigmentation are seen in midperiphery of fundus. (See Color Plate 25.)

terior ocular process that fails to respond to the therapy chosen on the basis of the clinical presentation may require a biopsy to ascertain the presence of lymphoma. Finally, syphilis is becoming increasingly common in HIV-infected patients and is discussed in detail in Chapter 10.[42]

## DRUG-RELATED OCULAR INFLAMMATION

Several reports have identified both anterior and posterior uveitis occurring in patients treated with rifabutin.[43] These inflammations can occur months after the initiation of therapy. Rifabutin is used to treat *M. avium–intracellulare* infection. A severe uveitis can result that often, but not necessarily, is bilateral. The inflammation responds to appropriate steroid therapy or to reduction in rifabutin dosage. The mechanism of this inflammation is unclear and may either be direct drug hypersensitivity or a response to mycobacterial death with subsequent inflammatory response. In addition, we have described retinal lesions in patients treated with the antiretroviral agent didanosine (ddl) that appear to predominantly involve the RPE (Fig. 11-9).[44]

Although research in AIDS is progressing, the disease will continue to spread and a definitive cure does not appear likely in the next decade. We will continue to see an evolving spectrum of clinical ocular disease as patients with profound immunosuppression survive for extended periods of time.

### Case 11-1

A 42-year-old man with a diagnosis of AIDS reported a 2-week history of decreased vision in the right eye. He had no light perception in the right eye and 20/20 in the left eye. The right eye contained 1+ vitreous cells and had a significant area of necrotic retinitis surrounding and involving the optic disc. Blood cultures were positive for cytomegalovirus. The left eye had a small white infiltrate with an associated hemorrhage near the superior vascular arcade.

Over the next few weeks the area of involvement in the left eye increased in size. Treatment with ganciclovir was begun, with a marked improvement of the retinitis in both eyes. Vision did not return in the right eye. Ganciclovir therapy was discontinued after 3 weeks, and the vision remained 20/20 for 2 weeks. The vision in the left eye then fell to 20/300 because of macular edema. The necrotic retinitis was larger. A second-course ganciclovir regimen was begun, and the retinitis again resolved and the vision returned to 20/25. The patient was placed on maintenance therapy but, because of neutropenia, could not tolerate 5 mg/kg 5 days per week. The patient lost all vision in the left eye approximately 2 months later and died several weeks later.

## REFERENCES


1. Gallo R: The AIDS virus, *Sci Am* 256:46-56, 1987.
2. Curran JW, Morgan WM, Hardy AM et al: The epidemiology of AIDS: current status and future prospects, *Science* 229:1352-1357, 1985.
3. Layon J, Warzynski M, Idus R: Acquired immunodeficiency syndrome in the United States—a selective review, *Crit Care Med* 14:819-827, 1986.
4. Salahuddin SZ, Palestine AG, Heck E et al: Isolation of the human T-cell leukemia/lymphotropic virus type III from the cornea, *Am J Ophthalmol* 101:149-152, 1986.
5. Pomerantz RJ, Kuritzkes DR, de la Monte SM et al: Infection of the retina by human immunodeficiency virus type I, *N Engl J Med* 317:1643-1647, 1987.
6. Palestine AG, Rodrigues MM, Macher AM et al: Ophthalmic involvement in the acquired immune deficiency syndrome, *Ophthalmology* 91:1092-1099, 1984.
7. Freeman WR, Lerner CW, Mines JA et al: A prospective study of the ophthalmologic findings in the acquired immune deficiency syndrome, *Am J Ophthalmol* 97: 133-142, 1984.
8. Newsome DA, Green WR, Miller ED et al: Microvascular aspects of acquired immune deficiency syndrome retinopathy, *Am J Ophthalmol* 98:590-601, 1984.
9. Kestelyn P, Van de Perre P, Rouvroy D et al: A prospective study of the ophthalmologic findings in the acquired immune deficiency syndrome in Africa, *Am J Ophthalmol* 100:230-238, 1985.
10. Pepose JS, Holland GN, Nestor MS et al: Acquired immune deficiency syndrome: pathogenic mechanisms of ocular disease, *Ophthalmology* 92:474-484, 1985.
11. Schuman JS, Friedman AH: Retinal manifestations of the acquired immune deficiency syndrome, *Trans Ophthalmol Soc UK* 103:177-189, 1983.

12. Weiss A, Margo CE, Ledford DK et al: Toxoplasmic retinochoroiditis as an initial manifestation of the acquired immune deficiency syndrome, *Am J Ophthalmol* 101:248-249, 1986.
13. Stoumbos VD, Klein ML: Syphilitic retinitis in a patient with acquired immunodeficiency syndrome–related complex, *Am J Ophthalmol* 103:103-104, 1987.
14. Croxatto JO, Mestre C, Puente S et al: Nonreactive tuberculosis in a patient with acquired immune deficiency syndrome, *Am J Ophthalmol* 102:659-660, 1986.
15. Macher A, Rodrigue MM, Kaplan W et al: Disseminated bilateral chorioretinitis due to *Histoplasma capsulatum* in a patient with the acquired immunodeficiency syndrome, *Ophthalmology* 92:1159-1164, 1985.
16. Sandor EV, Millman A, Croxson TS et al: Herpes zoster ophthalmicus in patients at risk for the acquired immune deficiency syndrome (AIDS), *Am J Ophthalmol* 101:153-155, 1986.
17. Egbert PR, Pollard RB, Gallagher JG et al: Cytomegalovirus retinitis in immunosuppressed hosts. II. Ocular manifestations, *Ann Intern Med* 93:664-670, 1980.
18. Kupperman BD, Petty JG, Richman DD et al: Correlation between CD4+ counts and the prevalence of cytomegalovirus retinitis and human immunodeficiency virus-related noninfectious retinal vasculopathy in patients with acquired immunodeficiency syndrome, *Am J Ophthalmol* 115:575-582, 1993.
19. Freeman WR, Friedberg DN, Berry C et al: Risk factors for the development of rhegmatogenous retinal detachment in patients with cytomegalovirus retinitis, *Am J Ophthalmol* 116:713-720, 1993.
20. Sternberg P, Han DP, Yeo JH et al: Photocoagulation to prevent retinal detachment in acute retinal necrosis, *Ophthalmology* 95:1389-1393, 1988.
21. Stevens G, Palestine AG, Rodrigues MM et al: Failure of argon laser to halt cytomegalovirus retinitis, *Retina* 6:119-122, 1986.
22. Palestine AG, Stevens G, Lane HC et al: Treatment of cytomegalovirus retinitis with dihydroxy propoxymethyl guanine, *Am J Ophthalmol* 101:95-101, 1986.
23. Holland GN, Sakamoto MJ, Hardy D et al: Treatment of cytomegalovirus retinopathy in patients with acquired immunodeficiency syndrome, *Arch Ophthalmol* 104: 1794-1800, 1986.
24. D'Amico DJ, Talamo JH, Felsenstein D et al: Opthalmoscopic and histologic findings in cytomegalovirus retinitis treated with BW-B759U, *Arch Ophthalmol* 104:1788-1793, 1986.
25. Studies of Ocular Complications of Aids Research Group: Mortality in patients with the acquired immunodeficiency syndrome treated with either foscarnet or ganciclovir for cytomegalovirus retinitis, *N Engl J Med* 326:213-220, 1992.
26. Palestine AG, Polis MA, De Smet MD et al: A randomized controlled trial of foscarnet in the treatment of cytomegalovirus retinitis in patients with AIDS, *Ann Intern Med* 115:665-673, 1991.
27. Studies of Ocular Complications of Aids Research Group: Foscarnet-ganciclovir cytomegalovirus retinitis trial. IV. Visual outcomes, *Ophthalmology* 101:1250-1261, 1994.
28. Flores-Aquilar M, Kuppermann B, Quiceno JI et al: Pathophysiology and treatment of clinically resistant cytomegalovirus retinitis, *Ophthalmology* 100:1022-1031, 1993.
29. Henry K, Cantrill H, Fletcher C et al: Use of intravitreal ganciclovir (dihydroxy propoxymethyl guanine) for cytomegalovirus retinitis in a patient with AIDS, *Am J Ophthalmol* 103:17-23, 1987.
30. Diaz-Llopis M, Chipont E, Sanchez S et al: Intravitreal foscarnet of cytomegalovirus in a patient with acquired immunodeficiency syndrome, *Am J Ophthalmol* 114: 742-747, 1992.
31. Martin DF, Parks DJ, Mellow SD et al: Treatment of cytomegalovirus retinitis with an intraocular sustained-release ganciclovir implant—a randomized controlled clinical trial, *Arch Ophthalmol* 112:1531-1539, 1994.
32. Palestine AG, Cantrill H, Ali E, Lieberman R: Treatment of cytomegalovirus (CMV) retinitis with Isis 2922, *Invest Ophthalmol Vis Sci* 36:S181, 1995.
33. Kirsch L, Arevalo JF, Chavez de la Pax E et al: Intravitreal cidofovir (HPMPC) treatment of cytomegalovirus retinitis in patients with acquired immune deficiency syndrome, *Ophthalmology* 102:533-543, 1995.
34. Sellitti TP, Huang AJ, Schiffman J et al: Association of herpes zoster ophthalmicus with the acquired immunodeficiency syndrome and acute retinal necrosis, *Am J Ophthalmol* 116:297-301, 1992.
35. Forster DJ, Dugel PU, Frangieh GT et al: Rapidly progressive outer retinal necrosis in the acquired immunodeficiency syndrome, *Am J Ophthalmol* 110: 341-348, 1990.
36. Johnston WH, Holland GN, Engstrom RE et al: Recurrence of presumed varicella zoster virus retinopathy in patients with the acquired immunodeficiency syndrome, *Am J Ophthalmol* 116:42-50, 1993.
37. Macher AM, Bardenstein DS, Zimmerman LE et al: *Pneumocystis carinii* choroiditis in a male homosexual with AIDS and disseminated pulmonary and extrapulmonary *P. carinii* infection, *N Engl J Med* 316:1092, 1987.
38. Sha BE, Benson CA, Deutsch T et al: *Pneumocystis carinii* choroiditis in patients with AIDS: clinical features, response to therapy and outcome, *J Acquir Immune Defic Syndr* 5:1051-1058, 1992.
39. Whitcup SM, Fenton RM, Pluda JM et al: *Pneumocystis carinii* and *Mycobacterium avium–intracellulare* infection of the choroid, *Retina* 12:331-335, 1992.
40. Morinelli EN, Dugel PU, Riffenburgh R et al: Infectious multifocal choroiditis in patients with acquired immune deficiency syndrome, *Ophthalmology* 100:1014-1021, 1993.
41. Stanton CA, Sloan B III, Slusher MM et al: Acquired immunodeficiency syndrome–related primary intraocular lymphoma, *Arch Ophthalmol* 110:1614-1617, 1992.
42. Johns DR, Tierney M, Felsenstein D: Alteration in the natural history of neurosyphilis by concurrent infection with the human immunodeficiency virus, *N Engl J Med* 316:1569-1572, 1987.
43. Shafran SD, Deschenes J, Miller M et al: Uveitis and pseudojaundice during a regimen of clarithromycin, rifabutin and ethambutol, *N Engl J Med* 330:438-439, 1994.
44. Whitcup SM, Butler KM, Caruso R et al: Retinal toxicity in human immunodeficiency virus–infected children treated with 2′,3′-dideoxyinosine, *Am J Ophthalmol* 113:1-7, 1992.

CHAPTER 12

# Acute Retinal Necrosis and Progressive Outer Retinal Necrosis

Despite many advances in the diagnosis and treatment of ocular disease, viral infections affecting the eye remain difficult to diagnose and difficult to treat. Many cases of uveitis, including multifocal choroiditis, acute posterior multifocal placoid pigment epitheliopathy (APMPPE), and multiple evanescent white-dot syndrome (MEWDS), are presumed to be caused by viral infection. Nevertheless, antiviral agents rarely are used in their treatment because the evidence supporting the viral etiology is anecdotal. For example, Epstein-Barr virus (EBV) infection has been associated with multifocal choroiditis and panuveitis[1,2]; however, because EBV infection is such a ubiquitous infection, it is difficult to prove a definite causal relationship between the virus and the choroidal disease. Many viral infections associated with uveitis are discussed in the chapter on white-dot syndromes (see Chapter 28). This chapter focuses on two disorders associated with herpes virus infections: acute retinal necrosis and progressive outer retinal necrosis. Two other viral infections causing uveitis, herpes simplex virus, and herpes zoster virus infection are discussed in Chapter 13.

## ACUTE RETINAL NECROSIS

The evolution in our understanding of the etiology and pathophysiology of acute retinal necrosis (ARN) is an example of how scientific knowledge can improve our ability to accurately diagnose and treat inflammatory eye disease. ARN was initially described in 1971 in a report by Urayama and colleagues[3] that described six patients with intraocular inflammation, retinal vascular sheathing, and large white confluent retinal infiltrates in one eye. The disease was called *Kirisawa's uveitis,* and these patients, in whom rhegmatogenous retinal detachments subsequently developed, were left with poor visual acuity. No etiologic agent was identified, and no therapy appeared to affect the outcome of the disease.

Additional cases of retinitis with rhegmatogenous retinal detachment were reported in the late 1970s,[4,5] and these retinal detachments were difficult to repair because of both tractional and rhegmatogenous components. Cases of bilateral acute retinal necrosis (BARN) were also described.[6] In 1982 the finding of herpes virus in the retina of ARN patients by Culbertson and colleagues[7] led the way for specific antiviral therapy for the disease. Nevertheless, late retinal detachment remains a serious complication of the disease despite the use of prophylactic laser photocoagulation and modern vitreoretinal surgical techniques.

Is ARN a new disease, or just newly recognized? Few if any similar cases were reported before 1971. Yet almost 100 reports on the topic have appeared in the literature since that

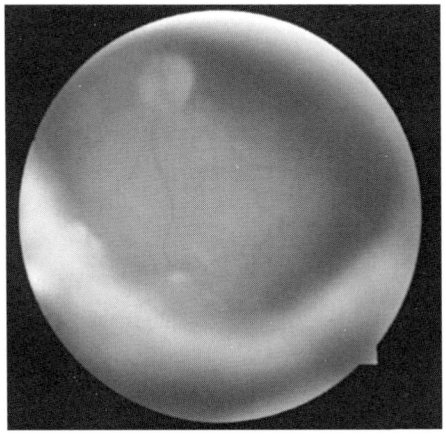

**Fig. 12-1.** Acute retinal necrosis with dense white retinal infiltrate in retinal periphery. (See Color Plate 26.)

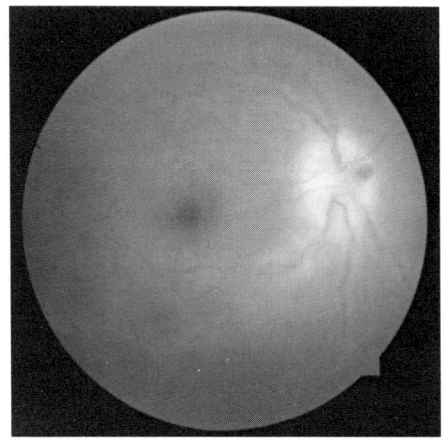

**Fig. 12-2.** Posterior pole of retina in patient 1 week after onset of symptoms of acute retinal necrosis and after vitrectomy had been performed demonstrating optic disc swelling and retinal perivascular sheathing.

time. Many investigators believe that ARN is a new disease, possibly due to mutations in the virus or changes in host susceptibility. Others believe that our improved diagnostic techniques and awareness of the disease have led to increased recognition.

### Epidemiology

Initially reported in Japan, ARN has now been reported throughout Europe and North America. ARN can occur in either sex and at any age, although there may be a slight male preponderance. The youngest patient reported with ARN was 13 years of age[8]; however, the disease has been reported in elderly patients as well. Although this disease was initially described in immunocompetent patients, ARN has now been documented in patients with immunosuppression such as AIDS.[9,10]

### Clinical features

The disease may affect one or both eyes; most cases begin with unilateral disease.[8] The second eye becomes involved in almost one third of cases, usually within 1 to 6 weeks; however, disease in the second eye has been reported to occur more than 10 years after disease in the first eye.[11] Most patients have a history of pain, redness, floaters, and blurred vision. An anterior uveitis with or without keratic precipitates often occurs early in the disease, and although a plasmoid aqueous has been described in these patients, hypopyon is rare. Occasionally there is an associated herpes infection at another site,[4,12] but most patients are healthy, immunocompetent, and without systemic symptoms.

With the onset of vitritis, patients report floaters and diminished visual acuity. Vitritis tends to worsen as cellular immunity to the virus occurs, and the infiltrating inflammatory cells are predominantly lymphocytes and plasma cells.[7] The earliest retinal lesions are small, patchy, white-yellow areas that tend to enlarge, increase in number, and coalesce over time (Fig. 12-1). The lesions usually start in the midperiphery; they occasionally occur in the posterior pole but do not follow the architecture of the retinal vessels. After several weeks the lesions begin to resolve with areas of clearing forming a Swiss cheese pattern. At this time perturbation of the retinal pigment epithelium (RPE) also develops. Retinal vasculitis is another manifestation of ARN (Fig. 12-2). Patients often demonstrate a severe retinal arteritis. Capillary nonperfusion can be documented on fluorescein angiography, and periphlebitis and venous occlusions have been described less commonly. Retinal hemorrhage can occur, especially in cases of venous occlusive disease. In contrast to other venous occlusive diseases, neovascularization of the iris or retina is uncommon but reported.[13,14] The choroidal vasculature is also involved in this disease, and fluorescein angiography has shown areas of early hypofluorescence and late staining consistent with ischemia-induced inflammatory changes.

Optic neuropathy also occurs in patients with ARN. Disc edema is a common finding early in the course of the disease,[8] and Sergott and colleagues[15] described two patients with intraorbital optic nerve enlargement. Optic nerve involvement should be suspected in patients with an afferent pupillary defect and severe visual loss with few retinal findings. Visual field testing and color vision assessment can be instructive. Visual loss may be caused by vascular occlusive disease, viral infiltration of the nerve, or optic nerve distention. Optic nerve sheath fenestration has been proposed as a possible therapeutic intervention,[16] but its effect has been unproved in well-controlled clinical trials.

The acute inflammatory disease tends to resolve with or without therapy in several months. In untreated patients the acute phase of the disease usually resolves in 2 to 3 months, and this may be shortened by 4 to 6 weeks with acyclovir therapy, although this has not been shown in a well-controlled, masked, randomized clinical trial. The course of the disease can also be predicted by the number of clock hours of initial retinal involvement. Unfortunately, within the next several months, tractional and rhegmatogenous retinal detachments with many large breaks develop in up to 86% of patients.[8,17] Despite control of the active viral replication in the retina, cellular infiltration into the vitreous and the formation of vitreal membranes composed of RPE and fibroblasts develop and contribute to the tearing and detachment of an already thinned retina.[18]

Recently, the Executive Committee of the American Uveitis Society published a set of standard diagnostic criteria for the ARN syndrome.[19] The criteria state that the designation of ARN syndrome should be based solely on clinical appearance and the course of infection. Clinical characteristics that must be seen include (1) one or more foci of retinal necrosis with discrete borders in the peripheral retina, (2) rapid progression of disease if antiviral therapy has not been given, (3) circumferential spread of disease, (4) evidence of occlusive vasculopathy with arteriolar involvement, and (5) a prominent inflammatory reaction in the vitreous and anterior chamber. Optic nerve involvement, scleritis, and pain support but are not required for the diagnosis, and macular lesions, although less common, do not preclude a diagnosis of ARN if peripheral lesions are present.

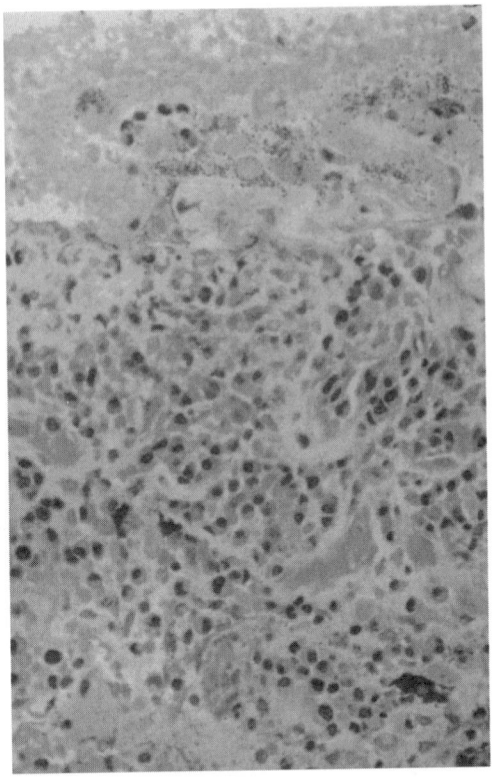

**Fig. 12-3.** Histologic section of chorioretinal biopsy specimen from patient with acute retinal necrosis showing lymphocytic infiltration and areas of necrosis. (Hematoxylin-eosin stain; ×400). (Courtesy Chi-Chao Chan, M.D.)

## Etiology

ARN was initially believed to be an autoimmune disease.[18] In 1982 Culbertson and colleagues[7] described the first case of an enucleated eye in a patient with ARN, in which herpesvirus particles were noted in the retina on electron microscopy study. However, virus was not cultured from the eye, and serum antibodies were found to herpes simplex, herpes zoster, cytomegalovirus (CMV), and EBV. Histologic examination showed prominent retinal arteritis and marked retinal necrosis with abrupt demarcation between normal and necrotic retina. Optic nerve inflammation was also noted. A similar histologic picture was seen in a retinal biopsy specimen we obtained from a patient with ARN in 1983, which revealed inflammatory cell infiltration and necrosis of the retina (Fig. 12-3). There was a predominance of T lymphocytes in the vitreous, but the retina contained many B lymphocytes, which suggested that antibody to the virus could be produced locally in the retina. Finally, results of electron microscopy study showed herpes class

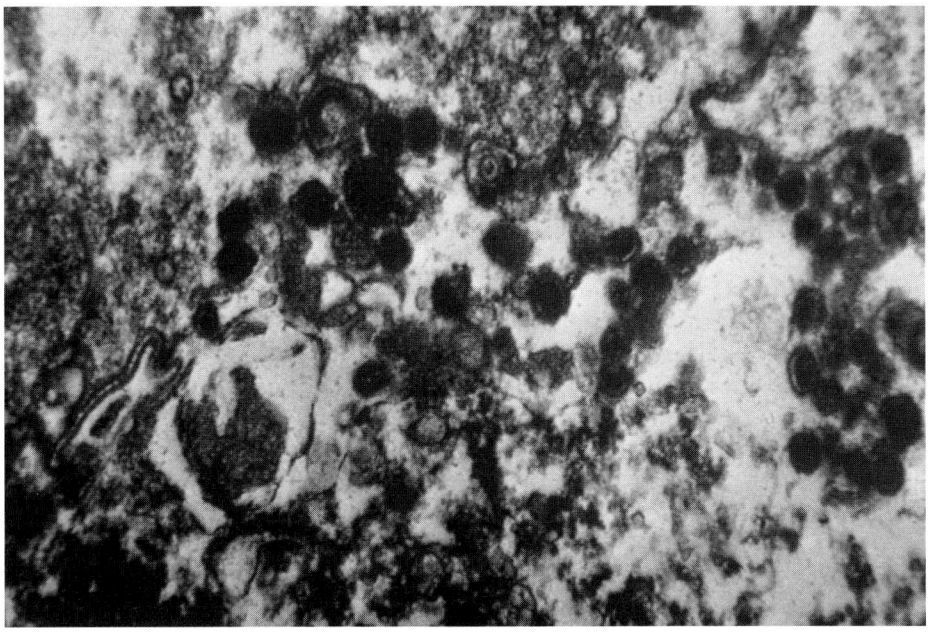

**Fig. 12-4.** Electron micrograph demonstrating herpes class virions in retinal biopsy specimen of patient with acute retinal necrosis.

viral particles (Fig. 12-4), although virus was not cultured from the specimen. In 1986 Culbertson and colleagues[20] used immunohistochemical staining to reveal herpes zoster in two eyes with ARN and also succeeded in culturing the virus from one of the two eyes. Although the herpes zoster–varicella virus group is thought to account for most of the typical cases of ARN, herpes simplex, types 1 and 2, and rarely CMV have also been implicated as a cause of the disease.[21-25] Herpes simplex virus has also been implicated in ARN because of serially increasing serum and intraocular antibody levels, as well as by the plasma clearance rate (PCR). However, these may result from a nonspecific polyclonal activation of B cells in the inflammatory process rather than a humoral immune response against a specific virus involved in the current disease. In addition, PCR is so sensitive that viral DNA from a previous infection years earlier may yield confusing results, especially because viral infection with herpes simplex, CMV, and herpes zoster are quite common. Although vitreous biopsy might be expected to provide material for viral culture so that therapy could be tailored to the correct virus for each patient, virus may be difficult to culture from the vitreous of a patient with ARN because of the presence of intravitreal antibodies or insufficient intact virions shed from the infected retina into the vitreous.

Injection of herpes simplex virus, type 1, in Balb/c mice produces a necrotizing retinitis in the contralateral eye in about 10 days.[26] This animal model has similarities to ARN in human beings and has yielded interesting immunologic insight into the pathophysiology of the disease. The necrotizing retinitis develops only in immunocompetent animals. In addition, disease develops in the contralateral eye only if it is infected with virus via the optic nerve. Thus as in other inflammatory eye diseases, retinal damage, initially induced by an infectious agent, leads to a secondary immune response against previously sequestered retinal antigens. This secondary immune response can then propagate the inflammatory damage to the retina.

Other factors may play a role in the pathogenesis of ARN. Holland and colleagues[27] showed an association between ARN and HLA-DQw7 and phenotype Bw62, DR4. These data suggest that some persons may have a genetically determined predisposition to mounting an immune response against certain infectious agents that promotes the development of ocular inflammatory disease.

## Differential diagnosis

Because ARN can often begin as an anterior uveitis, examination of the peripheral retina is important in all patients with a new onset of

**Box 12-1**
**Differential diagnosis of acute retinal necrosis syndrome**

Exogenous bacterial endophthalmitis
Fungal endophthalmitis
Behçet's disease
Pars planitis
Toxoplasmosis
Syphilis
Cytomegalovirus retinitis
Sarcoidosis
Intraocular lymphoma
Progressive outer retinal necrosis syndrome

anterior inflammation. The differential diagnosis of ARN is listed in Box 12-1. In general, only Behçet's disease and endophthalmitis mimic the rapid progression and severity of ARN. The lesions of Behçet's disease rarely begin as uniformly in the periphery and are often associated with systemic symptoms and signs such as arthritis, mouth and genital ulcers, and skin lesions. A vitrectomy may be needed to rule out endophthalmitis.

### Therapy

Many patients appear to benefit from treatment with acyclovir. Acyclovir has good activity against herpes simplex virus and, at slightly higher concentrations, is effective against herpes zoster. Although acyclovir is not as good a drug as ganciclovir or foscarnet for treating CMV infection, inasmuch as CMV is rarely a cause of ARN and acyclovir is an easier and a safer drug, acyclovir is the best initial therapy for the disease. Our current therapeutic regimen is to treat patients with newly diagnosed ARN with a 10- to 14-day course of intravenously administered acyclovir, 500 mg/m$^2$ every 8 hours. Oral acyclovir, 800 mg five times a day is then continued for an additional 6 weeks. The goal of therapy is to hasten the resolution of disease in the infected eye and to prevent contralateral spread. Severe side effects of acyclovir are relatively rare. A reversible rise in the serum creatinine level and elevation in liver function test results may occur. The most commonly reported side effects include nausea, vomiting, and headache, but most of these occur in fewer than 3% of patients.

Unfortunately there have been no randomized prospective clinical trials of acyclovir for the treatment of ARN. In a retrospective study by Palay and colleagues[28] 87.1% of patients treated with acyclovir did not develop contralateral disease compared with 35.1% of patients not receiving the drug. Other case series seem to show that retinal lesions resolve quickly after initiation of acyclovir, but therapy does not appear to diminish the vitritis or to prevent subsequent retinal detachment.[17,29] Patients with severe and progressive disease despite acyclovir therapy may be treated with ganciclovir or foscarnet. In addition, systemic corticosteroids such as prednisone 0.5 to 1.0 mg/kg can be added after the patient has received 24 to 48 hours of intravenous acyclovir. Steroids can be slowly tapered based on the amount of vitritis. Because of the extensive retinal arteritis and development of retinal vascular occlusions, some have suggested aspirin therapy,[30] but again this therapy has not been scrutinized in a clinical trial.

Retinal detachment and optic neuropathy remain the causes of severe visual loss in this disease. Laser photocoagulation to demarcate a zone between involved and uninvolved retina has been tried as a prophylactic therapy to prevent retinal detachment. Sternberg and colleagues[31] showed that retinal detachments occurred in 2 of 12 eyes receiving laser therapy and in 4 of 6 eyes not receiving laser therapy. However, this retrospective analysis may be biased because the condition of patients with the most severe disease and worst vitritis may not have been amenable to laser therapy. Others have suggested prophylactic vitrectomy, scleral buckling, and endolaser for eyes at high risk for detachment, but there are little data to support this therapy.[32]

Clearly, surgery is warranted to repair retinal detachments in patients with ARN, although these detachments are difficult to repair and proliferative vitreoretinopathy is common.[17] Vitrectomy, fluid-gas exchange, and endolaser have been suggested for cases of complicated detachments.[33] Whether this therapy is better than vitrectomy with scleral buckling is unknown. Use of silicone oil has also been employed with success in some patients.

Less well studied is the effect of therapy on optic nerve disease. Optic nerve fenestration and corticosteroids have been used for treating optic neuropathy in ARN, but no well-controlled data are available to support the effectiveness of these therapeutic interventions.

With the discovery of the viral etiology of ARN, specific therapy has been employed for the treatment of this disease. Nevertheless, many questions about the disease remain. We still do not know why certain individuals are more susceptible to developing the disease, because ARN is relatively rare but herpesvirus infection is quite common. Finally, although acyclovir and corticosteroids are used to treat patients with ARN, there are still no randomized, masked, clinical trials definitively showing the benefits of therapy.

## PROGRESSIVE OUTER RETINAL NECROSIS

During the last several years a syndrome characterized by rapidly progressive outer retinal necrosis (PORN) has been described in immunocompromised patients. This syndrome seems to be different from the other cases of ARN in immunocompromised patients and carries an extremely poor prognosis. Unfortunately it is thought to be the second most frequent opportunistic retinal infection in AIDS patients in North America.[34]

### Diagnosis

PORN is thought to be a variant of a necrotizing herpetic retinopathy in immunocompromised patients. The syndrome was described by Forster and colleagues in 1990.[35] Margolis and coworkers[36] then described varicella-zoster virus retinitis in patients with AIDS and also noted a rapidly progressive necrotizing retinitis with early patchy choroidal and deep retinal lesions, which progressed relentlessly until patients were left with atrophic and necrotic retinas and pale optic nerves. Unlike typical ARN there is little or no vasculitis and less vitritis, and in many cases, posterior pole involvement occurs early in the course of disease (see Fig. 12-5).

Engstrom and colleagues[34] recently reviewed the cases of 38 AIDS patients with PORN. A definite history of cutaneous herpes zoster was documented in 22 of 33 (67%) patients. The median CD4 lymphocyte count in these patients was 21/mm$^3$ with a range of 0 to 130/mm$^3$. Most patients had a unilateral decrease in visual acuity, although about one fourth of the patients had a presenting complaint of decreased peripheral vision or constriction of visual field. Seven patients (11%) were symptom-free at the time of diagnosis. The median visual acuity at presentation was 20/30, but some patients had NLP vision at presentation. Anterior chamber and vitreous inflammation were minimal or absent in all patients. Multifocal, deep retinal lesions were typically found in the periphery; however, macular lesions were noted in 21 eyes (32%) at the time of diagnosis. Optic nerve involvement was present in 11 of 65 eyes (17%), and an afferent pupillary defect was noted in 11 of 29 patients (38%). Characteristic of this syndrome, the lesions rapidly progressed to confluence. Interestingly, although the syndrome is described as involving the outer retina, Rao has presented pathologic evidence that the disease causes substantial destruction of the inner retina.

### Differential diagnosis

The differential diagnosis for PORN is similar to that of ARN, and a comparison of their diagnostic criteria is noted in Table 12-1. It is important to differentiate these two disorders. Retinal lesions in PORN appear to predominantly involve the deep retina, whereas lesions in ARN appear full-thickness. Posterior retinal lesions are more common in PORN, whereas anterior chamber inflammation and dense vitritis are characteristic of ARN but rare in PORN. Similarly, vascular inflammation is also rare in PORN but common in ARN. Finally, lesions progress rapidly to confluence despite therapy in PORN but are usually controlled with acyclovir therapy in ARN.

### Therapy

We have tried various combinations of induction doses of intravenous ganciclovir and foscarnet, as well as intravitreal foscarnet, with little to no success. High-dose intravenous acyclovir at a dosage of 10 mg/kg every 8 hours for 2 weeks has also been used with inconsistent success. Others have reported that initial intravenous antiviral therapy appeared to reduce disease activity in 17 of 32 eyes (53%), but final visual outcome was not altered by therapy.[34] In this study, final visual acuity was NLP in 67% of eyes within 4 weeks after diagnosis. Complications of the disorder included retinal detachment in 70% of eyes, despite prophylactic laser retinopexy in some eyes. Unfortunately the number of cases with this syndrome appears to be increasing,

**Table 12-1.** Diagnostic criteria

| Progressive outer retinal necrosis syndrome | Acute retinal necrosis syndrome |
|---|---|
| Multifocal lesions characterized by deep retinal opacification without granular borders; there may be areas of confluent opacification | One or more foci of full-thickness retinal necrosis with discrete borders |
| Lesions located in the peripheral retina with or without macular involvement | Lesions located in the peripheral retina* |
| Extremely rapid progression of lesions | Rapid progression of disease† |
| No consistent direction of disease spread | Circumferential spread of disease around the peripheral retina |
| Absence of vascular inflammation | Evidence of occlusive vasculopathy, with arteriolar involvement |
| Minimal or absent intraocular inflammation | Prominent inflammatory reaction in the vitreous and anterior chamber |
| Characteristics that support, but are not required, for diagnosis<br>Perivenular clearing of retinal opacification | Characteristics that support, but are not required, for diagnosis<br>Optic neuropathy/atrophy<br>Scleritis<br>Pain |

From Engstrom RE Jr, Holland GN, Margolis TP et al: The progressive outer retinal necrosis syndrome: a variant of necrotizing herpetic retinopathy in patients with AIDS, *Ophthalmology* 101:1488-1502, 1994.
*Involving the area adjacent to, or outside, the major temporal vascular arcades.
†Progression can be successfully halted in most cases with intravenous acyclovir therapy.

making the search for an effective therapy critical.

**Case 12-1**

A 22-year-old woman developed sudden blurring of vision in the right eye, which was red and accompanied by a right-sided headache. She saw an ophthalmologist 1 week later who diagnosed an anterior uveitis that was treated with topical corticosteroids. Three days later she developed a herpes simplex lesion on her lip, but an initial medical evaluation was uneventful. Two weeks after the initial symptoms, peripheral white lesions in the retina were noted. Vision in the right eye had decreased to 20/125. There were 3+ cells and 3+ flare in the anterior chamber and 4+ cells in the vitreous, and a diagnosis of acute retinal necrosis was made.

A vitrectomy was performed to improve visualization of the retinal lesions and for viral cultures. Viral culture results were negative; however, intravenous acyclovir was started after surgery. The white retinal lesions began to resolve. After 10 days the intravenous acyclovir was discontinued, and the patient was treated with 200 mg of oral acyclovir five times daily. Laser photocoagulation was applied to the posterior edge of the white retinal lesions in an attempt to prevent retinal detachment. Two weeks later there was increased ocular inflammation and fibrin in the vitreous and the retina. Intravenous acyclovir was restarted and the inflammation slowly resolved. Vision 2 months later was 20/25 and remained stable without retinal detachment for more than a year.

**Case 12-2**

A 32-year-old African-American woman was diagnosed with HIV infection in December 1990. Two years later she developed an immunoblastic B cell non-Hodgkin's lymphoma involving the lung and nasopharynx. She was treated with six cycles of chemotherapy, which was completed in June 1993. In October 1993 the patient reported a 3-day history of blurry vision in the left eye. Visual acuity was 20/16 in both eyes, and results of slit-lamp biomicroscopy were normal. There were 1+ vitreous cells but no haze in the left eye, and funduscopic examination revealed multifocal lesions of the outer retina with no posterior pole involvement. The patient was immediately started on induction doses of ganciclovir; however, the patches of retinitis continued to progress and coalesce. Induction doses of intravenous foscarnet were added to the regimen and seemed to halt progression of the retinitis. Nevertheless, 1 month later visual acuity had decreased to 5/125, with spread of the retinitis into the posterior pole (Fig. 12-5), and a localized retinal detachment developed inferiorly. The CD4 lymphocyte count at this time was less than 10 cells/mm$^3$. A diagnosis of PORN was made, and the patient was placed on maintenance doses of ganciclovir and foscarnet, with follow-up.

One week later the visual acuity had decreased to hand motions at a distance of 1 foot. The retinitis appeared to involve the deep retina; the retinal vessels were relatively spared. The patient was placed back on induction doses of foscarnet and maintenance doses of ganciclovir. In January 1994 visual acuity remained limited to light

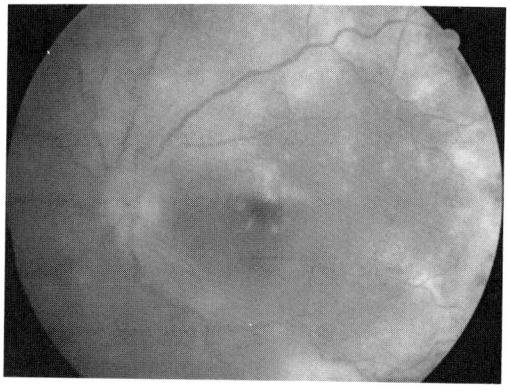

**Fig. 12-5.** Diffuse retinitis involving posterior pole in patient with progressive outer retinal necrosis. Retinitis appears to involve outer retina with little evidence of retinal vasculitis. (Courtesy Chris Walton, M.D.) (See Color Plate 27.)

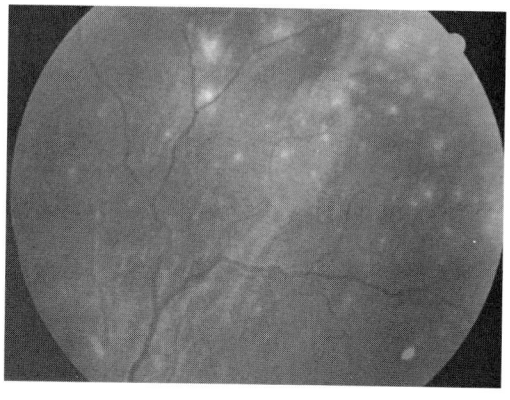

**Fig. 12-6.** Multifocal punctate lesions involving outer retina early in course of progressive outer retinal necrosis. These lesions quickly spread and coalesced despite therapy. (Courtesy Chris Walton, M.D.) (See Color Plate 28.)

perception in the left eye, but now multifocal lesions of the outer retina in the right eye developed (Fig. 12-6), which progressed rapidly. The patient was then treated with intravenous ganciclovir and intravitreal injections of foscarnet. Disease progression appeared to be halted in the right eye for the next 2 months, but she lost vision in that eye in March 1994. At that time visual acuity was limited to light perception in the right eye and no light perception in the left eye. Funduscopic examination showed a cherry-red spot in the right macula with a diffuse areas of retinitis and a large retinal detachment. The patient opted to stop therapy and died in July 1994.

## REFERENCES


1. Tiedeman JS: Epstein-Barr viral antibodies in multifocal choroiditis and panuveitis, *Am J Ophthalmol* 103:659-663, 1987.
2. Weber DJ, Hoffman KL, Thoft RA et al: Endophthalmitis following intraocular lens implantation, *Rev Infect Dis* 8:12-20, 1986.
3. Urayama A, Yamada N, Sasaki T et al: Unilateral acute uveitis with periarteritis and detachment, *Jpn J Clin Ophthalmol* 25:607-619, 1971.
4. Willerson D, Aaberg TM, Reeser FH: Necrotizing vaso-occlusive retinitis, *Am J Ophthalmol* 84:209-219, 1977.
5. Young NJA, Bird AC: Bilateral acute retinal necrosis, *Br J Ophthalmol* 62:581-590, 1978.
6. Price FW, Schlaegel TF: Bilateral acute retinal necrosis, *Am J Ophthalmol* 89:419-424, 1980.
7. Culbertson WW, Blumenkranz MS, Haines H et al: The acute retinal necrosis syndrome. II. Histopathology and etiology, *Ophthalmology* 89:1317-1325, 1982.
8. Fisher JP, Lewis ML, Blumenkranz M et al: The acute retinal necrosis syndrome. I. Clinical manifestations, *Ophthalmology* 89:1309-1316, 1982.
9. Jabs DA, Schachat AP, Liss R et al: Presumed varicella-zoster retinitis in immunocompromised patients, *Retina* 7:9-13, 1987.
10. Friberg TR, Jost BF: Acute retinal necrosis in an immunosuppressed patient, *Am J Ophthalmol* 98:515-517, 1984.
11. Saari KM, Boke W, Manthey KF et al: Bilateral ARN, *Am J Ophthalmol* 93:403-411, 1982.
12. Ludwig IH, Zegarra H, Zakov ZN: The acute retinal necrosis syndrome: possible herpes simplex retinitis, *Ophthalmology* 91:1659-1664, 1984.
13. Han DP, Abrams GW, Williams GA: Regression of disc neovascularization by photocoagulation in the ARN syndrome, *Retina* 8:244-246, 1988.
14. Wang CL, Kaplan HJ, Waldrep JC et al: Retinal neovascularization associated with acute retinal necrosis, *Retina* 3:249-252, 1983.
15. Sergott RC, Belmont JB, Savino PJ et al: Optic nerve involvement in the acute retinal necrosis syndrome, *Arch Ophthalmol* 103:1160-1162, 1985.
16. Sergott RC, Anand R, Belmont JB et al: Acute retinal necrosis neuropathy: clinical profile and surgical therapy, *Arch Ophthalmol* 107:692-696, 1989.
17. Blumenkranz MS, Culbertson WW, Clarkson JG et al: Treatment of the acute retinal necrosis syndrome with intravenous acyclovir, *Ophthalmology* 93:296-300, 1986.
18. Topilow HW, Nussbaum JJ, Freeman HM et al: Bilateral acute retinal necrosis: clinical and ultrastructural study, *Arch Ophthalmol* 100:1901-1908, 1982.
19. Holland GN and the Executive Committee of the American Uveitis Society: Standard diagnostic criteria for the acute retinal necrosis syndrome, *Am J Ophthalmol* 117:663-666, 1994.
20. Culbertson WW, Blumenkranz MS, Pepose JS et al: Varicella zoster virus is a cause of the acute retinal necrosis syndrome, *Ophthalmology* 93:559-569, 1986.
21. Matsuo T, Date S, Tsuji T et al: Immune complex containing herpes virus antigen in a patient with acute retinal necrosis, *Am J Ophthalmol* 101:368-371, 1986.
22. Sarkies M, Gregor Z, Forsey T et al: Antibodies to herpes simplex type I in intraocular fluids of patients with acute retinal necrosis, *Br J Ophthalmol* 70:81-84, 1986.
23. Lewis ML, Culbertson WW, Post JD et al: Herpes

simplex virus type I: a cause of the ARN syndrome, *Ophthalmology* 93:875-878, 1989.
24. Margolis T, Irvine AR, Hoyt WF et al: Acute retinal necrosis syndrome presenting with papillitis and arcuate neuroretinitis, *Ophthalmology* 95:937-940, 1988.
25. Rugger-Brandle E, Roux L, Leuenberger PM: Bilateral ARM: identification of the presumed infectious agent, *Ophthalmology* 91:1648-1658, 1984.
26. Whittum JW, McCulley JP, Niederkorn JT et al: Ocular disease induced in mice by anterior chamber inoculation of herpes simplex virus, *Invest Ophthalmol Vis Sci* 25:1065-1073, 1984.
27. Holland GN, Cornell PJ, Park MS et al: An association between acute retinal necrosis syndrome and HLA-DQw7 and phenotype Bw62, DR4, *Am J Ophthalmol* 108:370-374, 1989.
28. Palay DA, Sternberg P, Davis J et al: Decrease in the risk of bilateral ARN by cyclovir therapy, *Am J Ophthalmol* 112:250-255, 1991.
29. Matsuo T, Nakayama T, Koyama T et al: A proposed mild type of ARM syndrome, *Am J Ophthalmol* 112:119-131, 1988.
30. Ando F, Kato M, Goto S et al: Platelet function in bilateral ARN, *Am J Ophthalmol* 96:27-32, 1983.
31. Sternberg P, Han DP, Yeo JH et al: Photocoagulation to prevent retinal detachment in ARN, *Ophthalmology* 95:1389-1393, 1988.
32. Blumenkranz MS, Clarkson J, Culbertson WW et al: Visual results and complications after retinal reattachment in the ARN syndrome: the influence of operative technique, *Retina* 9:170-174, 1989.
33. Blumenkranz MS, Clarkson J, Culbertson WW et al: Vitrectomy for retinal detachment associated with ARN, *Am J Ophthalmol* 106:426-429, 1988.
34. Engstrom RE, Jr, Holland GN, Margolis TP et al: The progressive outer retinal necrosis syndrome: a variant of necrotizing herpetic retinopathy in patients with AIDS, *Ophthalmology* 101:1488-1502, 1994.
35. Forster DJ, Dugel PU, Frangieh GT et al: Rapidly progressive outer retinal necrosis in the acquired immunodeficiency syndrome, *Am J Ophthalmol* 110: 341-348, 1990.
36. Margolis TP, Iowder CY, Holland GN et al: Varicella-zoster virus retinitis in patients with acquired immunodeficiency syndrome, *Am J Ophthalmol* 112:119-131, 1991.

# CHAPTER 13

# Other Viral Diseases

## HERPES SIMPLEX VIRUS INFECTION

Although many viruses can induce intraocular inflammation, herpes simplex keratitis is probably the most common ocular disease associated with uveitis. Patients with stromal keratitis often have a concurrent anterior uveitis.[1] Although in some patients this uveitis develops during the initial onset of epithelial disease, most patients get uveitis with stromal involvement. Recurrent episodes are common and can severely damage the eye. Anterior uveitis may also occur in patients with a history of previous epithelial herpetic infection without currently active corneal disease. Herpetic keratouveitis manifests as a red, photophobic, and often very painful eye with decreased vision.[1] Secondary glaucoma frequently accompanies severe inflammatory episodes.

The diagnosis of herpes simplex keratouveitis is most easily made in patients with a known history of herpes simplex keratitis confirmed by typical dendritic epithelial defects or stromal disease confirmed by culture data. The disease should also be suspected in patients with a significant corneal opacity accompanied by synechiae and anterior chamber cells. Keratic precipitates in the area of corneal disease, hypopyon, and hyphema may be seen in some patients. In some cases the corneal disease may obscure the examination of the anterior chamber. Bacterial keratitis must be ruled out, as well as the possibility of secondary bacterial infection.

It remains unclear whether the uveitis associated with herpes simplex keratitis is a secondary inflammatory response to the corneal disease or whether it is induced by invasion of virus into the anterior uvea. Nevertheless, herpes simplex virus has rarely been isolated from the aqueous humor in patients with the disorder.[1] In experimentally induced herpes simplex uveitis, the combination of sensitized T lymphocytes, herpes-specific antibody, and herpes simplex antigen is required to produce inflammation.[2] If this situation applies to human disease, therapy that inhibits the cellular arm of the immune system could control the inflammation but enhance viral replication.

### Treatment

Herpes simplex keratitis is treated with topical antiviral therapy such as trifluridine solution (Viroptic) every 2 hours or vidarabine ointment (Vira-A) every 3 hours. Cycloplegic agents are also employed to reduce pain and prevent synechiae. In addition, topical corticosteroids should be used in cases of associated uveitis but their use is sometimes delayed until the corneal epithelial disease heals. In a recent controlled trial of topical corticosteroids for herpes simplex stromal keratitis, Wilhelmus and colleagues[3] showed that the use of prednisolone phosphate was significantly better than placebo in reducing persistence or progression of stromal keratitis, as well as the time to resolution of uveitis. In this study both groups received topical trifluridine. Although some episodes may resolve without therapy, inflammation may lead to severe ocular damage. Acyclovir, 400 mg orally 5 times a day, is now used for the treatment of herpetic keratouveitis, and long-term maintenance therapy may be required in severe cases. Nevertheless, it should be noted that Barron and colleagues[4] recently found no statistically or clinically significant beneficial effect of oral acyclovir in treating the stromal keratitis caused by herpes simplex virus in patients receiving concomitant topical corticosteroids and trifluridine with regard to time to treatment failure, proportion of resolution, or 6-month best-corrected visual acuity. However, visual acuity did improve over 6 months in more patients in the acyclovir group than in the placebo group. Secondary glaucoma is associated with herpetic keratouveitis and may be difficult to control, especially in cases with rubeosis.

Herpes simplex retinitis is clearly caused by direct infection of the retina by the virus. As already stated, some cases of ARN may be caused by herpes simplex infection. In addition, herpes simplex retinitis can occur in congenital herpes simplex infection associated with herpes encephalitis.[5] This infection is usually caused by herpes simplex type 2 and may be acquired in utero rather than during birth. Many congenital cases of herpes simplex retinitis have corneal and anterior chamber involvement as well, obscuring a clear view of the retina. When retinal lesions are seen clinically or pathologically, they appear as large, white retinal infiltrates associated with vitritis and retinal vascular sheathing. After the lesions heal, there are large areas of atrophic and scarred retina. Frequently the systemic infection with herpes simplex is overwhelming and fatal.

Herpes simplex retinitis has also been reported in patients who have undergone chemotherapeutic immunosuppression and again this ocular condition is often accompanied by a viral encephalitis. Large areas of white retinitis with retinal necrosis result from the viral infection. The disorder may also occur in patients without immunosupression, and diagnosis in some cases has been made after chorioretinal biopsy.[6] Some cases appear to respond to treatment with acyclovir.

## HERPES ZOSTER VIRUS INFECTION

Uveitis associated with herpes zoster infection often occurs with herpes zoster ophthalmicus. Ocular involvement is noted in two thirds of patients with herpes zoster involving the ophthalmic division of the trigeminal nerve.[7] The varicella-zoster virus (VZV) is a DNA herpes class virus and remains latent in the ganglia after chickenpox. Although reactivation occurs frequently in elderly patients, reactivation may occur in young and healthy persons with no known immunosuppression. Cutaneous herpes zoster has been associated with defects in cellular immunity, and this disorder has been frequently seen with HIV infection.

Anterior uveitis can accompany herpes zoster ophthalmicus and probably results from vascular occlusion and secondary ischemia. Intraocular inflammation occurs in one third to one half of the cases.[7,8] A severe glaucoma often arises in patients with severe inflammatory disease, and corneal disease manifested by dendritic keratitis, stromal keratitis, or exposure keratitis is a common finding. Large keratic precipitates and posterior synechiae accompany the anterior uveitis. Although the anterior uveitis may appear with the initial cutaneous lesions, it often develops 1 to 2 weeks after the onset of dermatologic disease. In a small number of patients, scleritis may be seen. The iris should be closely examined because it may be the key to correct diagnosis. Sector and patchy iris atrophy consistent with ischemic damage is characteristic of the disorder. Hyphema may occur, and some eyes develop phthisis because of severe ischemic destruction of the iris and ciliary body. Histologic study in severe cases reveals vascular inflammation and a granulomatous cellular infiltrate in the uvea.[9] Occasionally a retinal vascular occlusive disease or severe choroiditis with associated vitreal inflammation can be seen.

### Treatment

Treatment with oral acyclovir early in the course of herpes zoster infection, when the cutaneous lesions are still active, appears to reduce viral proliferation and the complications of the infection, including anterior uveitis.[10–12] In contrast, acyclovir appears to have little effect on the development of postherpetic neuralgia. In addition, several weeks into the course of the disease, the anterior uveitis is not caused by active viral replication but by ischemia. Therefore antiviral therapy appears to be no longer useful. The anterior uveitis and glaucoma may persist for weeks to months and must be treated with topical corticosteroids, cycloplegics, and appropriate glaucoma therapy. It is not clear whether the prolonged inflammatory course is due solely to the residual ischemia or whether an immunologic response against retained viral antigen in the ocular tissue is also promoting persistent inflammation.

Although oral corticosteroids are sometimes necessary to treat postherpetic neuralgia, they should be used cautiously in the acute phase of ophthalmic zoster infection because of reports of associated ipsilateral cerebrovascular occlusion with contralateral hemiparesis.[7] Systemic corticosteroids should also be cautiously in patients with herpes zoster infection associated with AIDS, because these agents may cause increased immunosuppression. A new topical inhibitor of substance P, capsaicin (Zostrix), may be effective in preventing postherpetic neuralgia of the skin, but a form for ocular use is not available.

Therapy requires a commitment to long-term management because even after the acute inflammation is quieted, residual damage that limits acuity may be surgically repaired. Many patients are left with severe visual loss. A combination of dry eye, corneal disease, cataract, and posterior synechiae contributes to visual loss and often precludes a thorough evaluation of the posterior segment of the eye. Because the optic nerve and retina may also be involved in the disease process, it is often difficult to determine the exact cause of visual loss in any given patient. Nevertheless, it is important to try to ensure that the retina and optic nerve are not severely damaged before surgery for cataract, corneal disease, or glaucoma is performed.

## OTHER VIRAL INFECTIONS

A number of other viral infections are associated with a transient mild anterior uveitis during the acute stages of infection. These include measles (rubeola), mumps, influenza, and infectious mononucleosis. The anterior uveitis rarely is accompanied by symptoms and is often undiagnosed because these patients do not undergo an ophthalmologic examination in the first week or two after the onset of these viral diseases. Retinitis and choroiditis caused by German measles (rubella) is rarely seen in the active stages of disease because it is a congenital infection. One other manifestation of measles virus infection is the rare, late presentation of subacute sclerosing panencephalitis. In addition to the progressive, fatal CNS disease characterized by dementia, ataxia, and myoclonus, an associated necrotizing retinitis involving the macula has developed in some patients.[13] Lesions have occasionally been mistaken for Vogt-Koyanagi-Harada disease, toxoplasmosis, or juvenile macular degeneration.

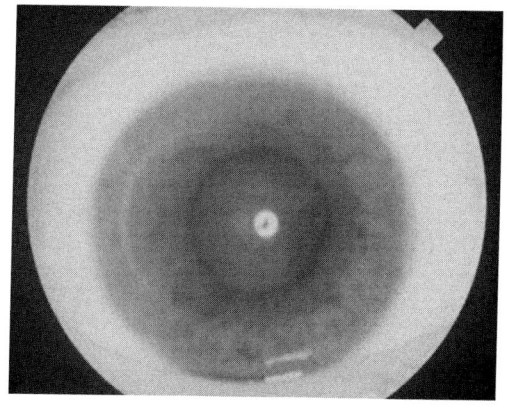

**Fig. 13-1.** Twelve-year-old girl with herpes simplex virus keratitis complicated by anterior uveitis, disciform stromal keratitis, and formation of Wesseley immune ring. (Courtesy Roger George, M.D.) (See Color Plate 29.)

### Case 13-1

A 12-year-old girl with dendritic keratitis was diagnosed with herpes simplex virus keratitis and was treated with topical trifluridine with resolution of the keratitis. Over the course of the next year she had several recurrences of the dendritic keratitis but later developed a disciform stromal keratitis with an associated anterior uveitis. She was then treated with topical trifluridine and topical corticosteroids. On attempts to taper the topical corticosteroids, there was an exacerbation of the stromal keratitis and anterior uveitis with formation of a Wesseley immune ring (Fig. 13-1). Her course was complicated by cataract and glaucoma and has required long-term therapy with topical trifluridine, corticosteroids, and betaxolol.

## REFERENCES

1. O'Connor GR: Recurrent herpes simplex uveitis in humans, *Surv Ophthalmol* 21:165-170, 1976.
2. Oh JO, Minasi P: Role of lymphocyte and antibody in the pathogenesis of immune-mediated herpetic uveitis, *Curr Eye Res* 4:685-691, 1985.
3. Wilhelmus KR, Gee L, Hauck WW et al: Herpetic eye disease study: a controlled trial of topical corticosteroids for herpes simplex stromal keratitis, *Ophthalmology* 101:1883-1896, 1994.
4. Barron BA, Gee L, Hauck WW et al: Herpetic eye disease study: a controlled trial of oral acyclovir for herpes simplex stromal keratitis, *Ophthalmology* 101: 1871-1882, 1994.

5. Reynolds JD, Griebel M, Mallory S et al: Congenital herpes simplex retinitis, *Am J Ophthalmol* 102:33-36, 1986.
6. Grutzmacher RD, Henderson D, McDonald PJ et al: Herpes simplex chorioretinitis in a healthy adult, *Am J Ophthalmol* 96:788-796, 1983.
7. Womack LW, Liesegang TJ: Complications of herpes zoster ophthalmicus, *Arch Ophthalmol* 101:42-45, 1983.
8. Cobo M, Foulks GN, Liesegang T et al: Observations on the natural history of herpes zoster ophthalmicus, *Curr Eye Res* 6:195-199, 1987.
9. Hedges TR, Albert DM: The progression of the ocular abnormalities of herpes zoster: histopathologic observations of nine cases, *Ophthalmology* 89:165-177, 1982.
10. Balfour HH Jr: Acyclovir therapy for herpes zoster: advantages and adverse effects, *JAMA* 255:387-388, 1986.
11. Balfour HH Jr, Bean B, Laskin OL et al: Acyclovir halts progression of herpes zoster in immunocompromised patients, *N Engl J Med* 308:1448-1452, 1983.
12. Cobo LM, Foulks GN, Liesegang TJ et al: Oral acyclovir in the treatment of acute herpes zoster ophthalmicus, *Ophthalmology* 93:763-770, 1986.
13. Otradovec J: Chorioretinitis centralis bei leucoencephalitis subacuta sclerotisans, *Van Bogaert Ophthalmol* 146:65-73, 1963.

# CHAPTER 14

# Ocular Toxoplasmosis

Toxoplasmosis is a common disease in both mammals and birds. The disease is caused by the obligate intracellular protozoan *Toxoplasma gondii*. It is thought that this organism infects at least 500 million persons worldwide, and at least 50% of the adult population in the United States has the chronic symptomless form of the disease.[1] It can cause a passing flulike condition that has little consequence, but it can also cause lymphadenopathy, serious and sometimes fatal disease in immunocompromised hosts, spontaneous abortions, and congenital disease. For the ophthalmologist it is one of the most frequently encountered posterior uveitides, classically producing a necrotic retinitis. It is also one of the few uveitides in which we can potentially make a definitive diagnosis. In the past few years our understanding of the organism and its interrelationship with its host has brought into question several concepts that were readily accepted in ophthalmology practice.

## ORGANISM

In 1908, *T. gondii* was first found in the brain of the North African rodent, the gondii, by Nicolle and Manceaux[2] and by Splendore[3] in a rabbit in Brazil. Janku[4] first described the postmortem findings in a child who had died of disseminated toxoplasmosis. He noted what were probably *Toxoplasma* organisms in the eye, but inoculation of animals with infected tissue did not induce disease. The transmission of the organism to animals via inoculation of infected human tissue was accomplished by Wolf and coworkers.[5]

*T. gondii* is a "cosmopolitan" parasite, being found all over the world. Members of the cat family are the definitive host. Oocysts of *Toxoplasma* are 10 to 12 μm and oval-shaped. They are found uniquely in the intestinal mucosa of cats. Once they are released, they can be spread to human beings or other

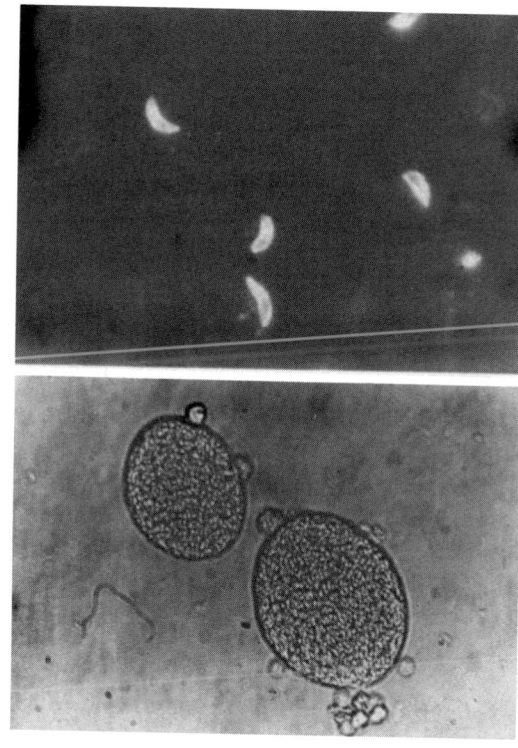

A

B

**Fig. 14-1. A,** Tachyzoites in culture stained with immunofluorescent dye. **B,** *Toxoplasma* cysts containing large numbers of tachyzoites. (Courtesy Leon Jacobs, M.D.)

animals through a variety of vectors. Although invariably thought to be ingested, the organism may also enter the host through other mucosal surfaces.[6] Humans can also be infected secondarily by ingesting meat (pork and lamb particularly, as well as chicken in endemic areas, but probably not beef) contaminated with *Toxoplasma* cysts. The two forms of the organism that can be found in humans are cysts and tachyzoites (Fig. 14-1). The cysts are up to 200 μm in diameter, contain hundreds to thousands of organisms, and have a propensity for cardiac tissue, muscle, and neural tissue, including the retina. The cyst structure is complex and can include elements from the host. It can remain intact outside of a host in soil for at least a year. It is not totally clear what all the factors are that cause ultimate rupture of the cyst and the release of tachyzoites. The tachyzoite is oval or arc-shaped and about 6 to 7 μm in length. It is an obligate intracellular organism, actively proliferates, and is the cause of the acute disease. The *Toxoplasma* organism's entry into and residence within the cell of the host is clearly a complex dynamic, and much is still not known. Joiner[7] describes that the organism forms a parasitophorous vacuole that surrounds the parasite and that lacks plasma membrane markers from the host. It will not fuse with other compartments in the cell,and it is sheltered from all cellular traffic.

Many of the antigens of the organism have been identified (Fig. 14-2). Perhaps the most studied of the antigens is that of p30. This major surface antigen has a molecular weight between 27 and 30 kd. It is serologically useful in the diagnosis of infection[8] and may play a role in the parasite's ability to invade a cell.[9] In animal models, immunization with this antigen or adoptive transfer of immune cells recognizing this antigen will confer a degree of protection against active infection. The p30 gene sequence has been deduced,[10] and its mRNA appears to be 1500 nucleotides in length.

A second antigen that has been characterized is the p22 antigen. This cell-surface antigen (Mol. wt. 22 kd) can participate in antibody-dependent, complement-mediated lysis of the tachyzoite.[11] It appears to be part of a complex

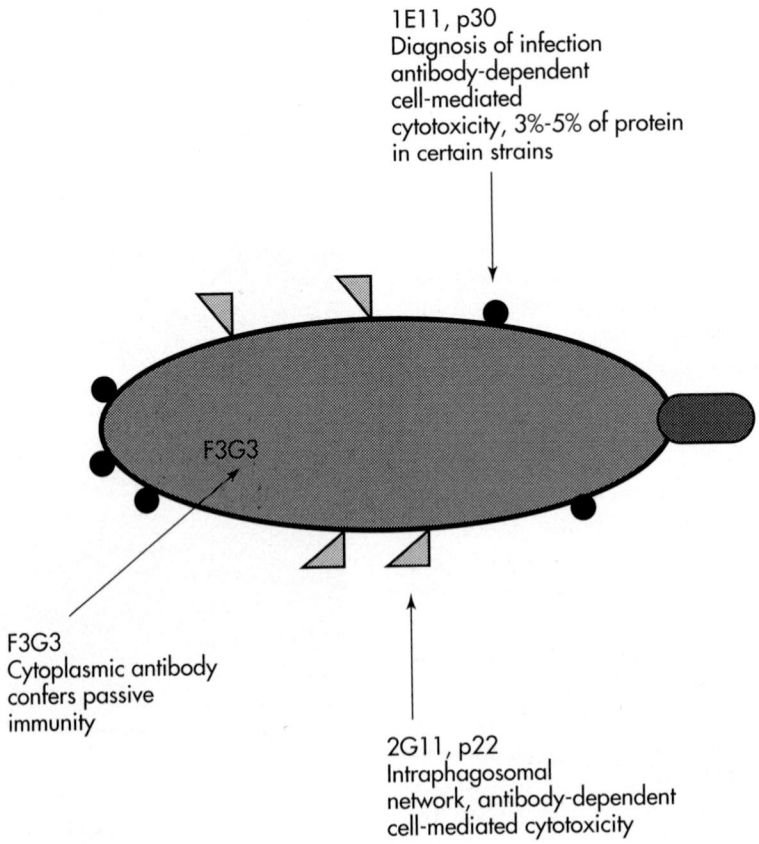


**Fig. 14-2.** Cartoon showing anatomic areas from which purified *Toxoplasma* antigens have been isolated.

phagosomal reticular network.[12] A third antigen that has been studied is known as the *F3G3 antigen.* This 58 kd antigen is cytoplasmic and is not expressed on the cell surface. Passive transfer of antibody that reacts to this antigen has been successful in protecting animals from a lethal challenge of the *Toxoplasma* organism.[13] The study of excreted/secreted antigens of toxoplasmosis continues[14] because it has been demonstrated that 90% of the circulating antigens detected during active infection are those that are actively excreted.[15] These antigens could be used as a basis for vaccine development in that immunization against these antigens might abrogate rapid entry of the tachyzoite into the cell.

## CLINICAL MANIFESTATIONS

### Systemic

The acquired disease in the nonimmunocompromised adult leads to lymphadenopathy in 90% of the cases, with fever, malaise, and sore throat sometimes occurring. More severe disease can occur, affecting muscle, skin, brain, heart, and kidney, as well as other organs. Death due to toxoplasmosis rarely occurs in the immunocompetent person. However, the disease in the immunocompromised patient can be a fulminant central nervous system disease that rapidly leads to death.

### Ocular

The acquired disease in the immunocompetent person has been thought to cause ocular disease only rarely. Perkins,[16] in reviewing the literature, found that uveitis was described in 52 of 1669 cases (3.1%) of acquired toxoplasmosis reported. The uveitis was most commonly seen in cases of toxoplasmic encephalitis.[16] In his treatise *Uveitis and Toxoplasmosis,*[17] Perkins states, "It is probable that the vast majority of cases of toxoplasmic uveitis in adults and children are recurrences of a congenital infection." It has been therefore assumed that acquired disease rarely manifests as purely an ocular disease.

The acquisition of the disease during pregnancy is the period of most concern. In the United States about 2 to 6/1000 woman acquire the infection while pregnant,[1] with about a 40% risk of transmitting the infection to the fetus. The congenital disease can lead to a wide range of symptoms, but most important to this discussion is that most cases of ocular toxoplasmosis are conjectured to be congenital, with late activation. In a European study reported by Koppe and Kloosterman,[18] 5% of the infants infected will either die or become severely affected by the disease. Further, about 70% of infants with congenital infections will show chorioretinal scars compatible with toxoplasmosis after a follow-up of 16 years, with 1% to 2% suffering severe visual impairment because of this infection. However, reports support the notion that acquired infection may lead to ocular disease. Wilson and Teutsch[19] reported that in following up the results of an outbreak of systemic toxoplasmosis that occurred in Atlanta, Georgia, in October 1977, one patient of the original group who became ill or had serologic evidence of acute infection showed evidence of ocular disease.

A large atrophic scar, frequently in the macula—a result of congenital toxoplasmosis—usually is seen (Fig. 14-3). Although such lesions help in diagnosing an old problem, they do not present the ophthalmologist with a therapeutic problem. Rather it is the reactivation or the recent acquisition of toxoplasmosis that poses the problem. In these cases, ocular toxoplasmosis manifests as a focal retinitis. The active lesion can vary greatly in size, but it is usually oval or circular and rarely bullous. Frequently, reactivation sites will be "satellite" lesions, next to old atrophic lesions, indicative of previous toxoplasmic infections. The retina during the acute stage appears thickened rather than transparent and is cream-colored (Fig. 14-4). Cells are found in the vitreous, particularly overlying the active lesion. Some eyes may have one or two small, old lesions, whereas others may have many, some of them very large, involving several clock hours of peripheral retina. In some large and particularly recalcitrant lesions, the vitreal haze and cellular reaction can be so profound as to be the cause of visual decrease. In the surrounds of the area of active retinitis, one may see hemorrhage, as well as sheathing of the retinal blood vessels. Fluorescein angiography of the active lesion demonstrates early blockage with subsequent leakage of the lesion (Fig. 14-5).

Because the *Toxoplasma* organism has a propensity for neural tissue, it is important to keep in mind that the lesion classically begins in the retina, and only with ongoing inflammation will it involve not only multiple layers of the retina but also the choroid. Cells in the anterior chamber may also be noted and may appear to be either a granulomatous or nongranulomatous uveitis. In the immunocompetent host, although evidence of old toxoplasmic activity may be present, the disease usually activates only in one eye at a time. With continuing inflammatory disease, the lesion and overlying vitreous will undergo several changes. The vitreous may contract, and a posterior vitreal detachment is not uncommon. Further vitreal condensation leads to a "scaffolding" of vitreal strands (Fig. 14-6). Roizenblatt and coauthors[20] refer to the development of vitreous cylinders in toxoplasmosis, a result of condensation of

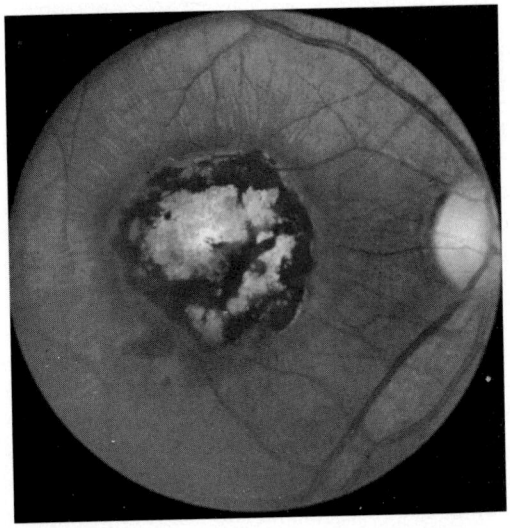

**Fig. 14-3.** Large macular atrophic scar due to congenital toxoplasmosis.

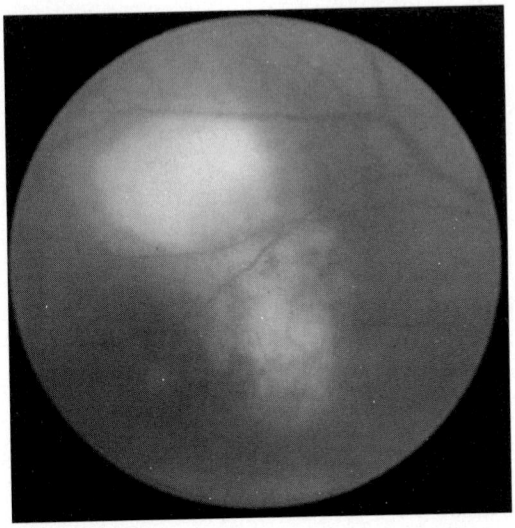

**Fig. 14-4.** Large active toxoplasmic infection in retina; seen as "satellite" to old healed atrophic lesion.

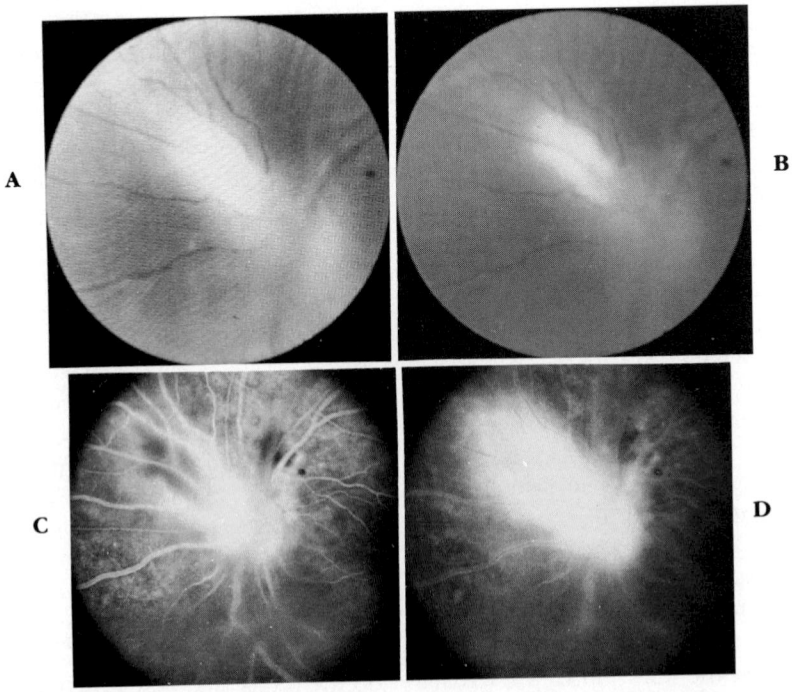


**Fig. 14-5. A,** Fluorescein angiogram showing leakage around borders of macular lesion of toxoplasmosis. Note staining of retinal vein below lesion. **B,** Large toxoplasmosis lesion encroaching on optic disc. **C** and **D,** Fluorescein angiogram of lesion showing hyperfluorescence peripherally with later photograph showing leakage of dye from both lesion and disc. (**A,** Courtesy J.D.M. Gass, M.D.)

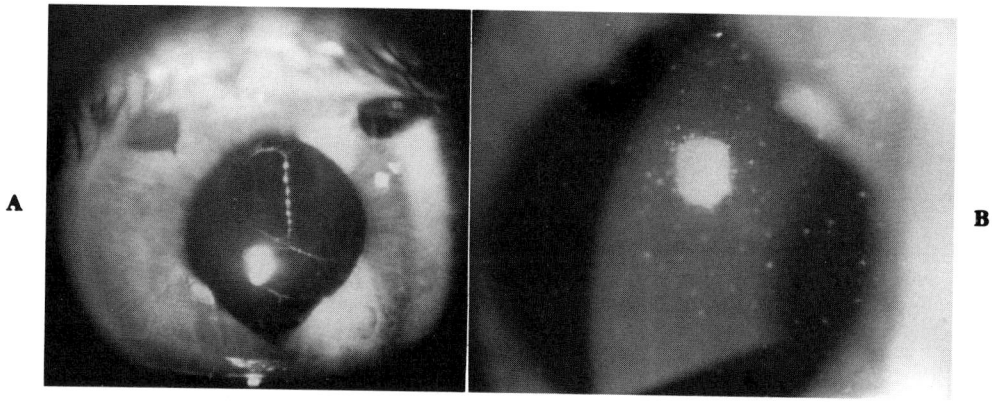


**Fig. 14-6. A,** "Scaffolding" seen in vitreous of patient with severe recurrent ocular toxoplasmosis. **B,** Keratic precipitates on cornea of same eye during inflammatory episode.

the collagen fibers. As the lesion becomes less acute, the area of retinal involvement takes on a less bright-yellow appearance, ultimately becoming atrophic, often with pigment heaping around its edges. Pigment clumping, however, does not surround all old lesions and should not be used as a diagnostic sign. The associated retinal disturbance will also begin to clear. All patients will have visual field defects that correspond to the interruption of the retinal nerve fiber layer.[21]

**Decreased vision.** The vision of the patient with toxoplasmosis is decreased for several reasons. As already mentioned, the vitreal inflammation by itself may be so great as to significantly decrease vision. As well, the lesion may be situated in the posterior pole (although not in the fovea per se), with the edema and probable inflammatory by-products of the reactions affecting central vision; however, the fovea may be relatively far from the center of the retinitis. This may be similar to the phenomenon that is seen in pars planitis (see Chapter 20). Another cause of decreased vision is infection involving the macula. Once the fovea is involved in the actual infection itself, the potential for a significant return of good vision is poor, and all efforts must be made to prevent this from occurring. Schlaegel and Weber[22] noted that in 60 attacks of ocular toxoplasmosis, 7 (12%) had active retinitis within 5 degrees of the umbo, and another 7 (12%) demonstrated some evidence of mild macular edema.

Ocular toxoplasmosis has been noted to present in a variety of ways besides the classic manifestation already described. Friedmann and Knox[23] and more recently Doft and Gass[24] observed a subset of ocular toxoplasmosis that is characterized by gray-white fine punctate lesions of the deep retina and retinal pigment epithelium and, initially, little or no overlying vitreal activity (Fig. 14-7). The resolution of these lesions may leave a typical toxoplasmosis scar. Another important presentation is that of papillitis. These patients may have severe papillitis, vitreal inflammation, and sector-nerve, fiber-bundle defects, with no apparent retinal foci, as was described by Folk and Lobes.[25] Other presentations that we are aware of are bullouslike inflammatory lesions in the midperiphery of the retina (Fig. 14-8), a wide ringlike lesion near the extreme periphery of the retina that resembles a severe uniocular pars planitis, and a scleritis due to the severe retinal inflammation caused by the *Toxoplasma* infection. Numerous anecdotal reports concerning various presentations can be found in the literature. Although some may be without foundation, they stress that one should suspect this disorder in a variety of clinical situations. Friedmann and Knox[23] noted that the 63 patients whose cases they reviewed averaged 2.7 episodes.

**Loss of vision.** The most important sequela of ocular toxoplasmosis can be loss of vision due to direct involvement of the fovea by the infection. However, choroidal neovascularization can also occur as a late complication of the disease.[26,27] Skorska and coworkers[27] found that subretinal neovascular lesions were present in 7 of 36 cases studied. The new vessels were located either directly on the border of the scar or at a distance, with feeder vessels arising from the scar (Fig. 14-9). Retinochoroidal anastomoses have also been observed to occur in toxoplasmosis, with one study placing the incidence at 2.7%[28] (Fig.

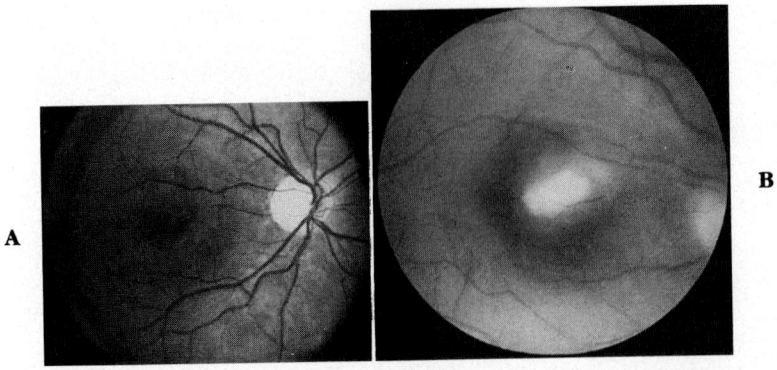


**Fig. 14-7.** Punctate inner retinal layer toxoplasmosis. **A,** Lesion begins as subtle alteration in normal macular pattern. **B,** In follow-up photograph lesion takes on appearance of more classic type of toxoplasmic infection. (Courtesy J.D.M. Gass, M.D.)

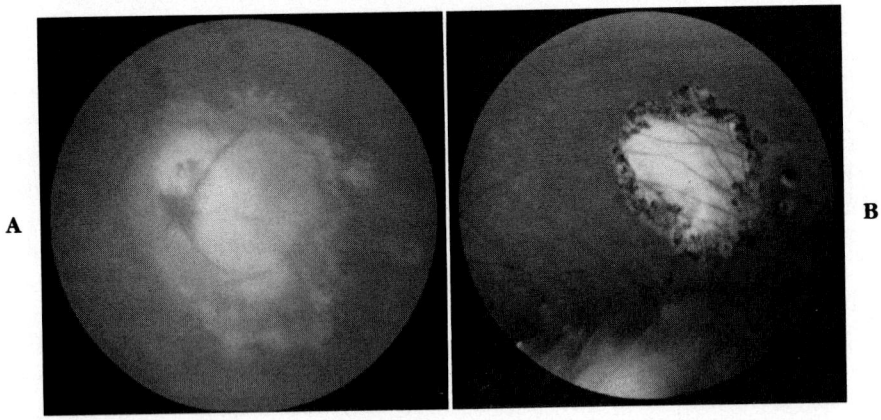


**Fig. 14-8. A,** Large bullous lesion due to toxoplasmosis, with titer of 1:125. **B,** Lesion involuted only after anti-*Toxoplasma* medication.

14-10). Other vascular complications have been reported. Rose[29] reported a case of ocular toxoplasmosis with a retinal vein occlusion, papillitis, and florid disc neovascularization. Pakalin and Arnaud[30] observed a case that manifested with an arteriolar branch occlusion at a site passing through an area of necrosis. They emphasize the need to include toxoplasmosis in the differential diagnosis of even arterial inflammatory phenomena, something not usually done.

A curious association between Fuch's heterochromia and ocular toxoplasmosis was initially made by Toledo de Abreu and coworkers.[31] They studied 13 patients with Fuchs's syndrome who had focal necrotizing chorioretinal toxoplasmic lesions, none of whom had ciliary injection or posterior synechiae but most had keratitic precipitates (KP), anterior chamber reactions, and cataracts. Six of the 13 had iris transillumination. La Hey and colleagues[32] evaluated this possible association in a series of 88 patients with Fuchs's heterochromia, comparing them with control subjects and other patients with uveitis. Although nine (10.2%) of these patients with Fuchs's syndrome had scars compatible with toxoplasmosis, the authors were unable to establish a special relationship between the two entities. Others have confirmed these observations[33] (see Chapter 19). Schwab,[34] in an interesting review, also looked for a relationship between toxoplasmosis and Fuchs's heterochromic iridocyclitis. In his review he found that 13 of the 25 patients with Fuchs's heterochromic iridocyclitis had scars typical of toxoplasmosis and serologic evidence of the organism. This result was compared with the 590 patients seen in the retina clinic at West Virginia University, with only 24 or 4% having retinal lesions typical of toxoplasmosis. Schwab

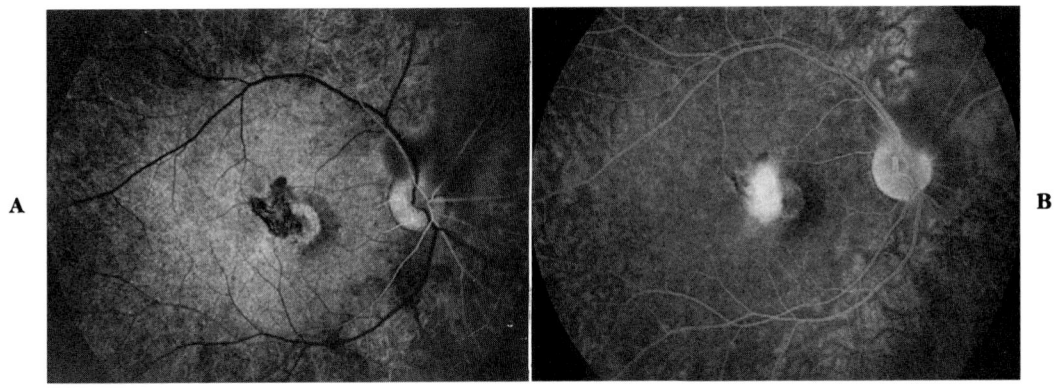


**Fig. 14-9.** Subretinal neovascularization 8 months after acute attack of ocular toxoplasmosis. **A,** Nasal portion of lesion that stains corresponds to area of old scarred lesion. In late-stage angiogram **(B)** nasal hyperfluorescence has not increased in size; however, temporal subretinal neovascular lesion can be noted. (Courtesy Prof. G. Coscas. Reproduced with permission by the *French Ophthalmological Journal,* 7:211-218, 1984.)

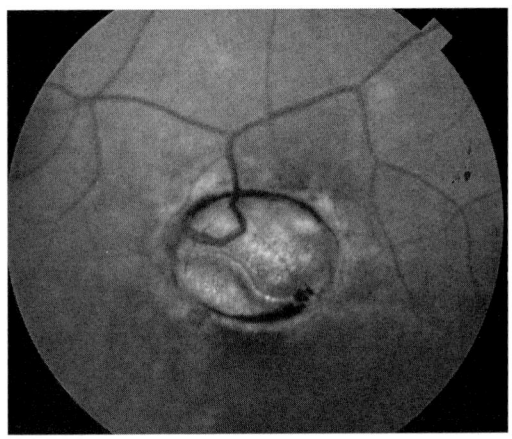

**Fig. 14-10.** Fundus photograph of eye with congenital toxoplasmosis, with retinochoroidal shunt. (Courtesy J. Melamed, M.D., Porto Alegre, Brazil.) (See Color Plate 30.)

concluded that a causal relationship between the two entities appears to exist, at least for a subgroup of patients with Fuchs's hetero chromia.

**Effects in immunocompromised host.** A special word seems appropriate for ocular toxoplasmosis in the immunocompromised host, particularly the patient with the acquired immunodeficiency syndrome (AIDS) (see Chapter 11). In these patients the development of ocular toxoplasmosis does not meet the criteria for an opportunistic infection but can indicate to the clinician that a change in the patient's immune state has occurred. Indeed we have seen active ocular toxoplasmosis in a patient with the AIDS-related complex in whom the full-blown picture of AIDS soon developed. In the AIDS patient the degree of inflammatory disease associated with a toxoplasmic retinitis is usually far greater than that seen with cytomegalovirus (CMV) retinitis, perhaps indicating that reactivation (or acquisition) of the disease occurs earlier in the AIDS patient's course than in CMV retinitis, when the immune repertoire is still capable of mustering a significant inflammatory response. In the United States, toxoplasmic retinitis is still a relatively uncommon disorder in AIDS patients. Often, in toxoplasmic retinitis, numerous lesions will appear to be active at the same time, a most unusual finding in the immunocompetent patient.

The diagnosis of ocular toxoplasmosis in an AIDS patient should initiate an evaluation of possible central nervous system (CNS) disease as well. CNS toxoplasmosis has become a frequently seen problem in this patient population. The reason for the CNS and the eye incidence disparity is not known. The therapeutic management of these ocular lesions can be most difficult. In spite of therapy severe disease can progress. Moorthy and colleagues[35] reported two patients in whom a severe necrotizing retinitis was seen, with one progressing to a panophthalmitis and orbital cellulitis in spite of sulfadiazine, pyrimethamine, and folinic acid therapy. Whether the ocular manifestations of this disease represent reactivation or acquired disease is not known. One could conjecture that both routes are possible. Gagliuso and coworkers[36] offer the observation that most ocular lesions in AIDS patients are unassociated with a preexisting retinochoroidal scar and therefore would suggest acquired disease. This may be, but it is possible that cysts in the retina may remain dormant and become activated only in the immunosuppressed state. As well, it is also possible that small lesions indicative of previous disease are simply engulfed in the large retinal necrotic lesion present in the AIDS patient.

The patient who has undergone iatrogenic immunosuppression is at high risk of experiencing reactivation of ocular toxoplasmosis. As with AIDS, if the immunosuppression cannot be reversed, serious consequences may ensue, as reported by Yeo and colleagues.[37] Singer and coworkers[38] reported the case of ocular toxoplasmic retinochoroiditis occurring after liver transplantation. Because of the difficulty in diagnosing the disorder, the eye was ultimately enucleated. The authors emphasize the fulminant nature of the disease, suggestive far more of the type of ocular disease seen in patients with AIDS.

• • •

In summary, the diagnosis of ocular toxoplasmosis is primarily a clinical one. The typical lesions as described constitute the most important factor in our decision making. The one additional supportive test we believe very important is a positive toxoplasmosis titer at any dilution (see later discussion). When the presentation is highly unusual, the diagnosis rests on a combination of multiple factors. In these cases, toxoplasmosis could be confused with the ocular histoplasmosis syndrome, although vitreal cells are not present in this latter entity and the peripapillary changes are rarely evident in toxoplasmosis (see Chapter 15). The deep retinal presentation of toxoplasmosis may be confused with the white-dot syndromes, such as an unusual case of acute posterior multifocal placoid pigment epitheliopathy (see Chapter 28). In the immunocompromised host, a single toxoplasmosis lesion early on may be confused with CMV retinitis. One possible way to help in discriminating between the two entities is through fluorescein angiography. In an active lesion of toxoplasmosis, the central area will block fluorescein early and stain late, because the central part of the lesion is where the greatest inflammatory response is taking place. This is in contradistinction to CMV retinitis, in which the central area will be atrophic and more readily hyperfluorescent early on in the angiogram (Phuc LeHoang, M.D., personal communication, 1989).

## HISTOPATHOLOGY AND IMMUNE FACTORS

In ocular toxoplasmosis, cysts and tachyzoites can be found in the retina (Fig. 14-11). The *Toxoplasma* organism most frequently is seen in the superficial portions of the retina. The lesion induced is a necrotic one, destroying the architecture of the retina. In many cases the underlying structures are destroyed as well, so that the disease at this point can certainly be classified as a chorioretinitis. Clinically, this destruction will permit the examiner to see underlying sclera quite clearly. Dutton and coworkers[39,40] were able to study these alterations more carefully using a congenital murine model of toxoplasmic retinochoroiditis. They noted that the inflammation ranged from a low-grade mononuclear infiltrate to total destruction of the outer retina, the retinal pigment epithelium, and choroid. Of great interest was that photoreceptor outer segments were phagocytosed by macrophages, whereas the *Toxoplasma* cysts did not appear to be the center of the inflammatory attack. Because of the selective photoreceptor destruction, one can speculate that autoimmune mechanisms may be important in the tissue destruction seen (see discussion of autoimmunity in Chapter 2). Indeed, when we had the opportunity to evaluate this question, we found that 16 of 40 patients with (40%) ocular toxoplasmosis demonstrated an in vitro proliferative response to the retinal S-antigen.[41] This finding could indicate that an autoimmune component to the

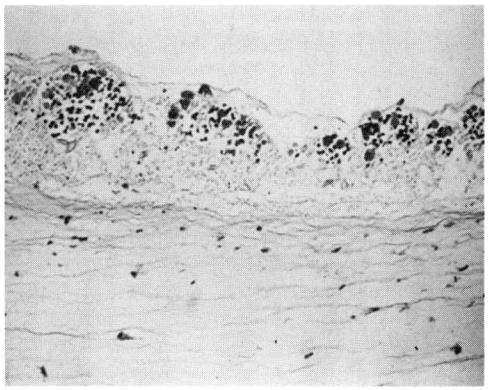

**Fig. 14-11.** Photomicrograph showing toxoplasmic cysts in retina. Cysts are larger circular structures, located mainly in or close to the nerve fiber layer. (Courtesy D. Cogan, M.D.)

inflammatory disease seen is presumably initiated with destruction of the retina by a parasite and subsequent sensitization to the uveitogenic antigen. We also found that proliferative responses to the p22 antigen approached those seen to crude toxoplasmosis antigen, whereas the response to the p30 membrane antigen was considerably less striking.

### Immune response

The host's immune response is exceptionally important in the ultimate expression of toxoplasmosis. In animal models, resistance, as measured by survival after challenge with the organism, has been reported to be regulated by at least five genes,[42] one of which is within the region of the H-2 antigen (the equivalent of the major histocompatibility complex [MHC] in human beings).[43] Brown and McLeod[44] have found that class I MHC genes, as well as the CD8 positive fraction of T cells, determine the cyst number in *Toxoplasma* infection. Others have looked at the effect of cytokines on the multiplication of the *Toxoplasma* organism. Interferon (IFN)–γ, as well as tumor necrosis factor (TNF) – α and transforming growth factor (TGF)–β all appear to play a role in inhibiting multiplication.[45] Gazzinelli and colleagues[46] reported that a reactivation of *T. gondii,* at least in the experimental mouse model, is due to a down-regulation of IFN-γ and TNF-α, which leads to decreased macrophage (with a decrease in inducible nitric oxide synthase and macrophage activation gene 1) and glial activation, a release of parasite growth, and tissue damage. Beaman and colleagues[47] reported that interleukin (IL)-6 enhanced intracellular reproduction of *T. gondii* and actually reversed the effect of IFN-γ–mediated killing. This is of particular note in light of the fact that the retinal pigment epithelium (RPE) produces large amounts of IL-6. It has also been suggested that $CD8^+$ T cells directed against the *Toxoplasma* organism appear during the acute phase of the disease, whereas $CD4^+$–parasite specific T cells appear with chronicity of the disease.[48] Denkers and colleagues[49] reported that *Toxoplasma* possesses a superantigen that expands murine Vβ5-expressing cells, most of which were $CD8^+$. It may be that this superantigen-driven expansion of predominantly IFN-γ–secreting $CD8^+$ cells is in part why this early immune response is seen. Curiel and coworkers[50] recently reported the cloning of human $CD3^+$, $CD4^+$ T cells that lysed autologous target cells that had been pulsed with *Toxoplasma* antigen or infected with live tachyzoites. These results suggest that specific immunotherapy through the development of vaccine may be possible.

Although antibodies are usually readily made, it is the cellular component of the immune system that must be intact for a resolution of the disease process. However, antibody production may play an important role in establishing a state of premunition (infection immunity) in *Toxoplasma* infection.[51] In an attempt to evaluate why newborn infants seem to have difficulty in clearing the *Toxoplasma* infection, Wilson and Haas[52] evaluated the cellular defenses against *T. gondii* in newborns. They noted that newborn and adult macrophages killed the organism equally as well, but supernatants from cord blood–derived concanavalin A–stimulated mononuclear cells less effectively activated macrophages as compared with supernatants produced from adult blood cells. This difference appeared to lie in the $CD4^+$ fraction of T cells. The cord blood appeared to produce fewer lymphokines capable of activating macrophages, including IFN-γ. The authors did not believe that enhanced generation of reactive oxygen intermediates was important in explaining the differences between the adult and newborn responses, although recent notions would suggest that nitrous oxide and its effects in macrophages may indeed play a very important role. Of interest is that the organism replicates in the macrophage, and this decreased killing in the newborn may then lead to greater susceptibility.

### Inflammatory response

What then is the cause of the focal, retinal, inflammatory response? The data to date still support the notion that it is the release of actively proliferating tachyzoites, often from a long-dormant cyst. However, immune studies with patients with ocular toxoplasmosis suggest that other factors are involved. Wyler and coworkers[53] noted that lymphocytes from patients with ocular toxoplasmosis demonstrated in vitro responses not only to *Toxoplasma* antigens but also to a crude retinal preparation. As already mentioned, our patients with toxoplasmosis have demonstrated in vitro cellular responses to the retinal S-antigen, a purified antigen from the photoreceptor region, and the site of the most intense inflammatory response in Dutton and colleagues' murine model for toxoplasmosis.[40] In addition, Abrahams and Gregerson[54] also have detected circulating antibodies to various retinal antigens in patients with toxoplasmosis. These observations raise the provocative argument that the inflammatory disease we see is at least in part, or at times, autoimmune driven. We know that the *Toxoplasma* cyst may include tissue from the host, and perhaps S-antigen is sequestered there until the cyst breaks open. Alternatively, the initial destruction caused by the proliferating organism releases immunogenic antigens to the general circulation, thereby causing sensitization. This then results in a secondary autoimmune response, which then can prolong the initial response or become the center of a recurrent inflammatory episode sometime in the future.

The mechanism for the anterior uveitis and the Fuchs's-like syndrome seen in conjunction with the retinitis of ocular toxoplasmosis still is conjectural. In a rabbit model of experimental ocular toxoplasmosis, toxoplasmic antigen has been found in the vitreous.[55] In a feline model of ocular toxoplasmosis in which chorioretinal lesions form after injection of organisms into the carotid, an anterior uveitis can be seen in some of the animals.[56] It may be in that in the human situation the antigen is also found in the anterior chamber, producing an inflammatory response there; alternatively, immune complexes formed more posteriorly in the eye may fix to the tissue in the anterior chamber, including the iris, giving the clinical findings described. However, an intact *Toxoplasma* organism has been found in only one immunocompromised person with AIDS.[57] Greven and Teot[58] reported recovering encysted bradyzoites from the cytospin of a vitrectomy specimen obtained in the course of a retinal detachment repair, which helped confirm the clinical impression and led to the initiation of therapy.

### Methods of diagnosis

Serologic evidence of the *Toxoplasma* organism is of immense importance in helping the clinician make the diagnosis. We would accept positivity even in undiluted serum, although admittedly this can be problematic because the incidence of false-positive results is high. The presence of IgM titers to the organism suggests a recently acquired infection. Observations by Rubens Belfort in Brazil (personal communication, 1993) suggest that at least in some cases the IgM peak may be highly ephemeral and thus easily missed. The type of serologic testing that is the most reliable is still debatable, although the enzyme-linked immunosorbent assay (ELISA) technique has been recommended by many. Weiss and colleagues[59] reported their experience comparing the immunofluorescence antibody test, the Sabin-Feldman dye test, and the ELISA. They found that in three cases the immunofluorescence test result was negative (titer less than 1:16) whereas the Sabin-Feldman test result was positive for the three, as was the ELISA in the one patient tested. These data suggest performing the Sabin-Feldman test or ELISA antibody tests before excluding the diagnosis of ocular toxoplasmosis on the basis of a negative antibody test result.[59]

The diagnosis of this disease by serologic means alone is not yet feasible, as underlined by a study performed by Rothova and coworkers.[60] They noted that even though 100% of their patients with clinically apparent ocular toxoplasmosis revealed IgG antibody positivity, 58% of the control subjects also showed positive results. Although 7 of 25 (28%) patients with toxoplasmosis had detectable circulating immune complexes with IgG and *Toxoplasma* antigen, 2 of 12 (16%) control subjects did as well. In reviewing normal control subjects and patients with suspected ocular toxoplasmosis, Phaik and coworkers[61] estimated that at least 77% of those with ocular toxoplasmosis had serotiters equal to or greater than 1:256, somewhat higher than that found in control subjects. Nonetheless, we believe that the diagnosis is very much a clinical one, with serologic findings supportive but not definitive.

The serologic examination of the aqueous is a technique reported by Desmonts.[62] In this classic paper, Desmonts postulated that in patients with purely an ocular recurrence of toxoplasmosis, local antibody formation against the organism will occur and therefore the local titer will be greater than that found in the circulation. His impressive demonstration of this phenomenon and the calculation of the "C" value is one that the ophthalmologist should be aware of (see Chapter 6). This technique is not one that is widely used in the United States, although our European colleagues find it of value.[63] Although in most cases we have seen, the clinical appearance of the disease is straightforward, this added technique can be helpful in the evaluation of patients who present real diagnostic dilemmas (see Case 14-4). For example, consider the patient with an underlying malignant process, such as a lymphoma or leukemia, who manifests a focal inflammatory process in the retina, with overlying vitreal activity. Is this lesion a localized form of the neoplasm or rather an activation of toxoplasmosis because of a change in his or her immune status? The evaluation of the aqueous for anti-*Toxoplasma* antibodies may not be a perfect technique but could provide the clinician with important information. Turunen and colleagues[64] emphasized the reliability of this test and found that in both the patients with toxoplasmosis and control subjects, intraocular anti–mumps antibody formation was within the normal range, suggesting that the response may be specific. We are not as convinced that this is necessarily the case, but no more perfect method of evaluation exists.

**Pregnancy.** In pregnant women, testing is routinely performed for toxoplasmosis. It is generally believed that if the mother has anti-*Toxoplasma* antibodies before the beginning of the pregnancy, then the fetus is protected. If the disease is contracted during pregnancy, the highest number of children born with symptoms of *Toxoplasma* infection are those contracting the disease in the third trimester of the pregnancy. It is believed that if one child is born with signs of ocular toxoplasmosis, then succeeding siblings will be protected. Anecdotal reports have appeared to possibly disprove this concept, but most have had extenuating circumstances that could explain the unusual findings without disproving the concept that if one child is born with toxoplasmosis, the siblings that follow will not.

### Newer methods

Newer methods for diagnosis of toxoplasmosis have been developed. Western blot analysis has been used to identify cytoplasmic and membrane antigens of *T. gondii*.[65] Using recently identified genes believed to be specific to this organism as a template and by means of the polymerase chain reaction (PCR), one can search for toxoplasmic DNA, even when it is present in minute quantities. PCR will permit amplification of these DNA fragments adequate to allow detection on standard laboratory techniques, such as Southern blot analysis. Two genes to date have been used. The gene for the p30 antigen is one of the major surface proteins of the organism.[8-10] The B1 gene,[66] which contains an intron but does not encode for a known protein, has been shown to be in the genome of many *Toxoplasma* strains, but not in the mammalian genome. The PCR technique has been applied to deparaffinized ocular sections of two cases. Although cysts could be identified by use of standard microscopic examination in one eye, PCR permitted the identification of the parasite in both cases.[67] This study demonstrates the feasibility of this method even when paraffin slides are used. By means of this method, DNA from toxoplasmosis was identified in the aqueous of three patients with ocular toxoplasmosis.[68] The positive PCR response in these three patients was not related to the "C" coefficient, the analysis used to determine local production of specific antibody.

Another approach to diagnosis has been to develop in vivo tests. One method shown to work in rabbits has been the use of in vivo immunofluorescence. Scheiffarth and associates[69] tagged specific antitoxoplasmosis antibodies with fluorescein, injected them intravenously, and found that an experimentally induced chorioretinitis would stain with this technique. Much work is still needed to bring this technique to the human form of the disease.

### Congenital versus acquired disease

As discussed earlier, it was formerly an established "given" in ophthalmology that most, if not all, of the ocular lesions ascribed to toxoplasmosis were due to a congenitally acquired infection. The classic concepts were that subclinical infection would occur in most cases, resulting in overt clinical symptoms years later, when the patient was a young adult. A corollary to this concept of congenital disease was that a mother, if infected before becoming pregnant, would not transmit the disease to her child. If she did become infected during pregnancy, then she would transmit the disease only to that one offspring; afterward she would be immunized and therefore any other children would be protected.

These ophthalmic "givens" have been seriously questioned by the seminal observations of a family of ophthalmologists, the Silveiras, of Erechim, a small city located in the most southern state (Rio Grande do Sul) of Brazil. These physicians had noted a very high rate of toxoplasmosis in the population of this region. In a survey of 100 normal children, they found that 98% of them between the ages of 10 and 15 years had antibodies to toxoplasmosis. On the basis of their observations, it was calculated that the frequency of retinal scars in the population of this area was 40:200 as compared with 1:200 in the United States and 6:200 in São Paulo, Brazil. In a search for an explanation of this very high rate, it was noted that the residents of this region prepare sausage made of raw or poorly cooked pork. The preparation of the sausage is a family endeavor requiring much tasting to ensure proper preparation. This custom could explain in part the high rate of the disease.

Other observations about ocular toxoplasmosis in this region were most provocative. Ocular toxoplasmosis was observed in families in which the mother and several children (nontwins) had retinal lesions typical of toxoplasmosis; indeed, even three generations in one family were seen.[70] The finding of toxoplasmic cysts, which provided a definitive diagnosis of this disorder, occurred in two siblings, each of whom required enucleation of an eye for intractable pain. Such findings could be better explained if the disease were acquired rather than congenital. Indeed, a rather typical systemic manifestation of this disease seen by one of us (R.B.N.) when visiting Erechim was a febrile child with rather marked lymphadenopathy. These children either have a necrotizing retinal lesion at the same time or will return some months later with one. Other studies showed that IgM antibodies could be found in patients, but the antibody titers do not stay elevated above baseline for very long.

To corroborate these earlier observations, a household survey was undertaken in the Erechim region. Of the 1,042 persons examined, 184 (17.7%) were found to have ocular toxoplasmosis. On the basis of these observations, the prevalence of ocular toxoplasmosis was calculated to be 30 times higher than estimates for this disease in other parts of the world.[71] Of interest as well was the finding that only 0.9% of young children tested had antibodies to *T. gondii,* further suggesting that the ocular disease seen was due to postnatal infection rather than to a congenital cause.

A prospective study investigating the incidence of congenital toxoplasmosis in this region was then undertaken.[72] During a 5-month period, serum was obtained from 283 of 599 newborns and 190 infants younger than 1 year of age. The study showed that 2.1% of the newborns and 0.5% of the infants had evidence of circulating antibodies to the *Toxoplasma* organism. For 21% of adults of this region of Brazil to have ocular toxoplasmosis due to a congenital infection, then more than 20% of the mothers would have to be infected during pregnancy. Indeed, only 0.5% to 0.6% of the cord blood tested revealed antitoxoplasmosis antibodies.

These studies clearly demonstrate that acquired disease is a major mode of transmission of this parasite that leads to the ocular form of the disease—at least for a corner of southern Brazil.[73] But do these observations have any relevance to the disease outside of Brazil? We do not know, of course, and the answer may be quite complex in Brazil as well, because a recent survey within Rio Grande do Sul showed a marked difference in the prevalence rates between the region of Erechim as compared with the southern portion of the state.[74] However, these provocative observations lead to the speculation that these findings may be relevant to the North America population as well. Sibley and Boothroyd[75] have reported that all virulent strains are derived from a single clonal lineage. If this is true, then we can logically assume that similar mechanisms are at play elsewhere and that acquired disease may be an important mode of transmission.

## THERAPY

An initial decision must be made if indeed the *Toxoplasma*-induced lesion needs to be treated at all. We know that in the immunocompetent person the disease is ultimately self-limited. For us, the decision to treat generally would be based on the following criteria:

- A lesion within the temporal arcade
- A lesion abutting the optic nerve or threatening a large retinal vessel
- A lesion that has induced a large degree of hemorrhage
- A lesion that has induced enough of a vitreal inflammatory response so that the vision has dropped below 20/40 in a previously 20/20 eye or at least has sustained a two-line drop from the visual acuity before the acute infection

A relative indication would be the case of multiple recurrences that develop marked vitreal condensation. Here one might be concerned about the continuation of this process leading to retinal detachment.

As the first drug combination for the treatment of ocular toxoplasmosis, we still use sulfadiazine (1 g orally four times daily) and pyrimethamine (50-mg loading dose, then 25 mg orally twice daily), always given concomitantly with folinic acid, 3 to 5 mg three times a week. A baseline platelet count followed by weekly counts are obtained for the duration of the folinic acid therapy, which we continue for 1 week after stopping the pyrimethamine. We generally treat immunocompetent patients for 3 to 4 weeks with this regimen. We judiciously add prednisone to the regimen if the lesion is in the posterior pole or threatening the optic nerve head. Generally we use 20 to 40 mg/day of prednisone in the adult patient, beginning 12 to 24 hours after initiating the specific antimicrobial therapy. If the macula or optic nerve is threatened, we do not hesitate seeing the patient frequently, trying to taper the prednisone in such a way that it is stopped before the anti-*Toxoplasma* therapy is discontinued. It is important to stress that immunosuppressive therapy (prednisone) should never be employed alone, only under the therapeutic cover of the specific antimicrobial therapy, nor do we give it at higher doses for any prolonged period of time. Periocular injections of corticosteroids are not to be used. Sabates and coworkers[76] reported the cases of seven patients in whom the disease was particularly destructive and disseminated, and all were initially treated with corticosteroids alone. Cytotoxic agents do not have a role in the treatment of this infection.

Clindamycin (150-300 mg orally three or four times daily) combined with sulfadiazine has also been shown to be effective in treating this disorder.[77,78] Because the two agents affect unrelated pathways, it may be that the combination could have synergistic effects although not perhaps as effective as the combination of pyrimethamine and sulfadiazine.[79] Although it is a useful approach, the potential for diarrhea and the serious complications of pseudomembranous colitis at worst is problematic. In one study[80] 15 of 90 patients treated with clindamycin combined with fluorocortolon had side effects of treatment, including diarrhea, allergic exanthem, mild lymphopenia, hepatoxicity, and gastrointestinal bleeding. The drug was withdrawn in eight patients. Clindamycin has also been given in 50-mg subconjunctival injections, with positive clinical results observed.[81] No randomized study has evaluated the question as to which therapeutic combination is more effective in treating the acute disease and preventing recurrences. It had been thought that clindamycin may prevent recurrences, but this has not been the case.[82]

A trimethoprim-sulfamethoxazole combination has been used by some clinicians. In principle this combination would inhibit the synthesis of tetrahydrofolic acid, as does pyrimethamine. This combination of trimethoprim-sulfamethoxazole was evaluated in the treatment of toxoplasmosis by Opremcak and colleagues.[83] They found that in 16 patients studied all had resolution of their active retinochoroiditis and an improvement in vision. Two had drug allergies.

A drug that has been used recently with initially positive results in the treatment of toxoplasmosis is atovaquone (Mepron). Of great potential interest is its ability to kill *Toxoplasma* cysts in vitro.[84] If true in vivo, it is conceivable that one therapeutic course with this agent could prevent recurrences, assuming adequate levels of the drug were available to completely sterilize the infection. Atovaquone is a quinolone derivative first developed because of its antimalarial properties. It has been used most extensively in the treatment of CNS toxoplasmosis with reasonably good results.[85] We have reported its use in the treatment of ocular toxoplasmosis in an AIDS patient unable to continue more standard therapy, and with a very good therapeutic response.[86] A new formulation is presently being used in a study evaluating its use in the treatment of ocular toxoplasmosis in AIDS patients in Brazil. It is hoped that this will enhance absorption of the drug and therefore permit high enough levels that will kill the cyst of the parasite.

It should be noted that no randomized masked trial has been performed to definitively demonstrate the therapeutic activity of any of the drugs presently used for the treatment of ocular toxoplasmosis. However, empiric observations in the immunoincompetent host (e.g., with AIDS) has shown that the disease will be arrested only with therapy and will activate once the therapy has been stopped. However, in the immunocompetent host, the observations of Rothova and colleagues[87] provided thought-provoking data. In a multicenter study that was neither randomized nor masked, 149 patients with ocular toxoplasmosis were placed into one of three therapeutic regimens, whereas those with peripheral lesions were not treated. The authors found no difference in the duration of inflammatory activity between the treated and untreated patients. They did find a reduction in the size of the retinal inflammatory lesion in 49% of patients receiving pyrimethamine versus 20% of the untreated group ($p < .01$).

## Additional therapeutic approaches

Cryotherapy of peripheral lesions that cause enough vitreal inflammatory activity to affect the vision can also be considered. Excessive cryotherapy applied to these "hot" eyes could potentially induce unwanted and excessive vitreous condensation and membrane formation, ultimately pulling on the retina and causing a retinal detachment. Photocoagulation has also been advocated by some as a means to treat the disease. Ghartey and Brockhurst[88] described their experience in treating five eyes with toxoplasmic lesions unresponsive to antimicrobial therapy and corticosteroids. Photocoagulation treatment was thought to benefit four eyes, with healing of the lesion after a few weeks. Others have suggested that such treatment could reactivate dormant cysts, leading to a renewal of ocular disease.

Vitrectomy and lensectomy can be performed on these eyes to remove vitreous and lens opacities that affect vision.[89] Significant vitreous condensations can form in eyes having a history of multiple episodes of inflammation due to toxoplasmosis. In patients with toxoplasmosis who are undergoing vitrectomy, we usually begin antimicrobial therapy before surgery and continue postoperatively. The rationale for this approach is the concern that the nonspecific inflammation induced by the vitrectomy might initiate an inflammatory episode of toxoplasmosis. We would not use periocular steroid after the procedure but will give steroids by mouth if it is indicated.

### Case 14-1

A 28-year-old white man was first seen at the National Eye Institute in March 1981. He was complaining of a decrease in vision with floaters in the left eye for over a week's time. The vision in his right eye was 20/20, and in the left, 20/25. The anterior chambers were quiet. There was 1+ haze in the vitreous of the right eye, with a white retinal lesion, 1½ disc diameters, encompassing the vessels of the superior temporal arcade and extending into the posterior pole. The more peripheral portion of the lesion seemed old—that is, less white and raised, with some pigment surrounding the edges—whereas the more active area seemed pointed toward the macula. The left eye also had an old inactive scar in the periphery of the superior portion of the retina. The clinical impression was that of ocular toxoplasmosis. The toxoplasmosis titer was positive at 1:128. The decision was made not to treat the patient.

The patient returned 1 week later with the same visual acuity. However, the lesion had progressed toward the macula. A decision was then made to initiate antitoxoplasmosis therapy: clindamycin 300 mg by mouth four times daily and sulfadiazine 0.5 g by mouth four times daily. No steroid was given. The patient was followed up weekly, and after 3 weeks of the therapy, the disease involuted. Therapy was stopped after 4 weeks. By late April 1981, the patient's visual acuity was 20/15 OU, and the lesion in the right eye was quiet. He had no problems until August 1985, when he noted an increase in floaters in the right eye. An examination at that time showed that there was a small area of active retinitis on the peripheral portion of the old lesion, on the side not facing the macula. It was elected not treat the patient, and lesion has regressed. He has been free of recurrence to date.

**Comment 14-1** We elected to treat the patient in spite of good vision only after following the clinical course and noting its progression toward the macula. It did not seem reasonable to wait any longer. He has continued to have recurrences, even after clindamycin therapy, and he needs to be seen regularly. In passing, it can be argued that a patient presenting today with his or her first attack of ocular toxoplasmosis deserves to be screened for HIV.

### Case 14-2

This 43-year-old white man has congenital toxoplasmosis. He has never had good vision in the left eye because of a large atrophic scar in the macula. The right eye has multiple lesions, all compatible with the diagnosis of ocular toxoplasmosis. In the right eye there is a lesion that encroaches onto the temporal side of the fovea, but his visual acuity was 20/25 in that eye when he was first seen at the National Eye Institute in 1977. In 1979 he complained of a "haziness" to his vision in the right eye. Examination of the parafoveal lesion could not detect an area of activity. In spite of this, he was begun on clindamycin, sulfadiazine, pyrimethamine (Daraprim), folinic acid, and prednisone.

The haziness disappeared over the course of the 3-week therapy period. During the ensuing years, his vision in the right eye has varied from 20/25 to 20/32. He has had one episode every 12 to 18 months when he feels there is a change in the quality of his vision. Examination of serial retinal photographs shows greater pigment around the atrophic scars, but rarely evidence of activity.

**Comment 14-2** The lack of observable activity on the edge of the old lesion abutting the fovea has not dissuaded us from treating him each time he complains of a change in his vision. A small nidus of infection, enough to alter his vision but not enough for the observer to note, could very well be there. This patient always maintains a supply of his medication and begins the antimicrobial therapy (sulfadiazine and clindamycin) immediately in symptoms. He is seen within 24 hours and then pyrimethamine (after a baseline platelet count), folinic acid, and steroid are begun.

### Case 14-3

This 36-year-old white man with AIDS-related complex had chronic granulomatous skin disease, chronic hepatitis, thrombocytopenia, and evidence of exposure to both the HIV and human T-cell leukemia/lymphoma–1 (HTLV1) virus. We first saw the patient in November 1984. He had had uveitis in the right eye for several months. He had also developed a cataract in the left. He had active toxoplasmic retinitis in the right eye and an old pigmented lesion in the left, also compatible with ocular toxoplasmosis. The left eye as well had a dense cataract. He was treated with clindamycin and sulfadiazine, with resolution of his inflammation after a 6-week course of sulfadiazine. The clindamycin was stopped after 3 weeks because of severe gastrointestinal problems, and pyrimethamine with folinic acid was begun for the next 3 weeks. A CT scan of the head showed no evidence of cerebral toxoplasmosis. Under this therapeutic cover the patient underwent cataract surgery, with a good visual result.

The patient continued to have recurrences of his ocular toxoplasmosis as soon as the specific antimicrobial therapy was discontinued. It was therefore decided to maintain long-term sulfadiazine therapy, but this needed to be stopped because of hives. Pyrimethamine was then used. In August 1985 the cataract in the right eye has significantly reduced his vision and made it difficult to maintain close follow-up of his retinitis. There now were cotton-wool spots in both eyes and cells in the left, but the lesion in the right eye seemed to be stable. He therefore underwent lensectomy and vitrectomy in the right eye. HIV was cultured out of the vitreous specimen, his Witmer quotient was markedly elevated, supporting the preoperative diagnosis, and after surgery his right eye (OD) revealed 4+ cells and 3+ haze. This responded only to the addition of sulfadiazine.

**Comment 14-3** This man's ocular course underscores the rapidity of changes and the difficulty in treating them in the immunosuppressed host. The presence of HIV in the vitreous, in addition to his history of chronic hepatitis, emphasizes the great care needed in handling these samples. Further, without an intact cell-mediated immune arm, the disease simply recurred once therapy was discontinued. The only therapeutic option was to "juggle" the available therapeutic agents. He ultimately succumbed to his underlying disease.

### Case 14-4

A 67-year-old white man from Latin America underwent triple coronary artery bypass surgery in his home country. This surgery was complicated by renal failure and the need for acute hemodialysis and transfusions. He subsequently regained renal function, and he returned to his normal routine. Three months later he noted decreased OD visual acuity, followed a week later in the left eye (OS). He had cells in the anterior chamber and in the vitreous. There were deep retinal or subretinal whitish-yellow lesions in both eyes. Findings of a work-up for a blood-borne infectious agent were negative, as were results of a computed tomography (CT) scan of the head and a lumbar puncture. The clinical diagnosis was intraocular lymphoma. An OD vitrectomy showed no malignant cells. However, the suspicion remained high, and an OS vitrectomy and retinal biopsy were performed. Both were negative for a malignant process, and results of a CT scan of the abdomen and chest, as well as bone marrow biopsy, were all normal. Findings of the retinal biopsy showed a large number of mature plasma cells.

The patient was sent to the National Institutes of Health (NIH) for further evaluation. Results of his physical examination were normal. A magnetic resonance image (MRI) showed a few small areas of ischemia consistent with involutional change. The erythrocyte sedimentation rate (ESR) was 34 mm in 1 hour; there were no antibodies to hepatitis B, and, liver and thyroid test results were normal. Chest x-ray films showed no active disease. A repeat OS vitrectomy showed T cells and macrophages but no malignant cells; viral cultures for zoster, varicella, and CMV were negative but showed herpes simplex 1 and 2 antibodies that were higher in the cerebrospinal fluid (CSF). The patient's toxoplasmosis titer (IgG) was elevated at 1 : 1000. Analysis for Lyme and *Leptospira* organisms revealed seronegativity. The patient was begun on oral prednisone therapy and within 1 week new lesions developed in the fundus.

After being seen by infectious disease specialists, he was empirically begun on a regimen of pyrimethamine, sulfadiazine, and ganciclovir. Rhegmatogenous retinal detachment developed, and during surgery the subretinal fluid was sent for toxoplasmosis titers and for culture. The "C" quotient for both vitreous and subretinal fluid was 300 when compared with the serum. The ganciclovir was stopped, and the patient's inflammation cleared on the antitoxoplasmosis medication.

**Comment 14-4** Although we evaluated the patient for toxoplasmosis, we did not consider this diagnosis as a high possibility. We would assume that the patient was infected via one of the transfusions he received after his coronary surgery. The C coefficient was most helpful in this case.

## REFERENCES


1. Krick JA, Remington JS: Current concepts in parasitology: toxoplasmosis in the adult—an overview, *N Engl J Med* 298:550-553, 1978.
2. Nicolle C, Manceaux L: Sur une infection à corps de Leishman (ou organismes voisins) due *Gondii, Compt Rend Acad Sci* 147:763-766, 1908.
3. Splendore A: Un nuovo protozoa parassita dei conigli: incontrato nell lesioni anatomiche d'une malattia che ricorda in molti punti il kala-azar dell'uomo, *Rev Soc Sci Saõ Paulo* 3:109-112, 1908.
4. Janku J: Pathogenesis and pathologic anatomy of coloboma of macula lutea in eye of normal dimensions, and in microphthalmic eye, with parasites in retina, *Cas Lék Cesk* 62:1021-1027, 1054-1059, 1111-1115, 1138-1143, 1923.
5. Wolf A, Cowen D, Paige B: Human toxoplasmosis: occurrence in infants as an encephalomyelitis: verification by transmission to animals, *Science* 89:226-227, 1939.
6. O'Connor GR: The mucosae as possible sites of entrance for *Toxoplasma gondii.* In O'Connor GR, editor: *Immunologic diseases of the mucous membranes,* New York, 1980, Masson.
7. Joiner KA: Cell entry by *Toxoplasma gondii:* all paths do not lead to success, *Res Immunol* 144(1):34-38, 1993.
8. Santoro F, Afchain D, Pierce R et al: Serodiagnosis of *Toxoplasma* infection using a purified parasite protein (P30), *Clin Exp Immunol* 62:262-269, 1985.
9. Kasper LH, Khan IA: Role of P30 in host immunity and pathogenesis of *T. gondii* infection, *Res Immunol* 144(1):45-48, 1993.
10. Burg JL, Perelman D, Kasper LH et al: Molecular analysis of the gene coding the major surface antigen of *Toxoplasma gondii, J Immunol* 141:3584-3591, 1988.
11. Kasper LH, Crabb JH, Pfefferkorn ER: Isolation and characterization of a monoclonal antibody-resistant antigenic mutant of *Toxoplasma gondii, J Immunol* 129:1694-1699, 1982.
12. Sibley LD, Krahenbuhl JL, Adams GM et al: *Toxoplasma* modifies macrophage phagosomes by secretion of a vesicular network rich in surface proteins, *J Cell Biol* 103:867-874, 1986.
13. Sharma SD, Araujo FG, Remington JS: *Toxoplasma* antigen isolated by affinity chromatography with monoclonal antibody protects mice against lethal infection with *Toxoplasma gondii, J Immunol* 133: 2818-2820, 1984.
14. Cesbron-Delauw MF, Capron A: Excreted/secreted antigens of *Toxoplasma gondii*—their origin and role in the host-parasite interaction, *Res Immunol* 144(1): 41-44, 1993.
15. Hughes HPA, Van Knapen F: Characterization of a secretory antigen from *Toxoplasma gondii* and its role in circulating antigen production, *Int J Parasitol* 12:433-437, 1982.
16. Perkins ES: Ocular toxoplasmosis, *Br J Ophthalmol* 57:1-17, 1973.
17. Perkins ES: *Uveitis and toxoplasmosis,* Boston, 1961, Little, Brown & Co.
18. Koppe JG, Kloosterman GJ: Congenital toxoplasmosis: long-term follow up, *Padiatr Padol* 17:171-179, 1982.
19. Wilson LA, Teutsch SM: Acquired toxoplasmosis, *Ophthalmology* 89:1299-1302, 1982.
20. Roizenblatt J, Grant S, Foos RY: Vitreous cylinders, *Arch Ophthalmol* 98:734-739, 1980.

21. Benson WE: Ocular toxoplasmosis and visual field defects, *Am J Ophthalmol* 90:25-29, 1980.
22. Schlaegel TF Jr, Weber JC: The macula in ocular toxoplasmosis, *Arch Ophthalmol* 102:697-698, 1984.
23. Friedmann CT, Knox DL: Variations in recurrent active toxoplasmic retinochoroiditis, *Arch Ophthalmol* 81: 481-493, 1969.
24. Doft BH, Gass JD: Outer retinal layer toxoplasmosis, *Graefes Arch Clin Exp Ophthalmol* 224:78-82, 1986.
25. Folk JC, Lobes LA: Presumed toxoplasmic papillitis, *Ophthalmology* 91:64-67, 1984.
26. Fine SL, Owens SL, Haller JA et al: Choroidal neovascularization as a late complication of ocular toxoplasmosis, *Am J Ophthalmol* 91:318-322, 1981.
27. Skorska I, Soubrane G, Coscas G: Toxoplasmic choroiditis and subretinal neovessels, *J Fr Ophtalmol* 7:211-218, 1984.
28. Potter JW: Vascular anastomoses in ocular toxoplasmosis, *J Am Optom Assoc* 53:549-552, 1982.
29. Rose GE: Papillitis, retinal neovascularization and recurrent retinal vein occlusion in *Toxoplasma* retinochoroiditis: a case report with uncommon clinical signs, *Aust N Z J Ophthalmol* 19:155-157, 1991.
30. Pakalin S, Arnaud B: Arterial occlusion associated with toxoplasmic chorioretinitis, *J Fr Ophtalmol* 13:554-556, 1990.
31. Toledo de Abreu M, Belfort R Jr, Hirata PS: Fuchs' heterochromic cyclitis and ocular toxoplasmosis, *Am J Ophthalmol* 93:739-744, 1982.
32. La Hey E, Rothova A, Baarsma GS et al: Fuchs' heterochromia iridocyclitis is not associated with ocular toxoplasmosis, *Arch Ophthalmol* 110:806-811, 1992.
33. Saraux H, Laroche L, Le Hoang P: Secondary Fuchs' heterochromic cyclitis: a new approach to an old disease, *Ophthalmologica* 190:193-198, 1985.
34. Schwab IR: The epidemiologic association of Fuchs' heterochromic iridocyclitis and ocular toxoplasmosis, *Am J Ophthalmol* 111:356-362, 1991.
35. Moorthy RS, Smith RE, Rao NA: Progressive ocular toxoplasmosis in patients with acquired immunodeficiency syndrome, *Am J Ophthalmol* 115:742-747, 1993.
36. Gagliuso DJ, Teich SA, Friedman AH et al: Ocular toxoplasmosis in AIDS patients, *Trans Am Ophthalmol Soc* 88:63-86, 1990.
37. Yeo JH, Jakobiec FA, Iwamoto T et al: Opportunistic toxoplasmic retinochoroiditis following chemotherapy for systemic lymphoma: a light and electron microscopic study, *Ophthalmology* 90:885-898, 1983.
38. Singer MA, Hagler WS, Grossniklaus HE: *Toxoplasma gondii* retinochoroiditis after liver transplantation, *Retina* 13:40-45, 1993.
39. Dutton GN, Hay J, Hair DM et al: Clinicopathological features of a congenital murine model of ocular toxoplasmosis, *Graefes Arch Clin Exp Ophthalmol* 224:256-264, 1986.
40. Dutton GN, McMenamin PG, Hay J et al: The ultrastructural pathology of congenital murine toxoplasmic retinochoroiditis. II. The morphology of the inflammatory changes, *Exp Eye Res* 43:545-560, 1986.
41. Nussenblatt RB, Mittal KK, Fuhrman S et al: Lymphocyte proliferative responses of patients with ocular toxoplasmosis to parasite and retinal antigens, *Am J Ophthalmol* 107:632-641, 1989.
42. McLeod R, Skamene E, Brown C et al: Genetic regulation of early survival and cyst number after peroral *Toxoplasma gondii* infection of AXB/BXA recombinant inbred and B10 congenic mice, *J Immunol* 142:3247-3255, 1989.
43. McLeod R, Brown C, Mack D: Immunogenetics influence outcome of *Toxoplasma gondii* infection, *Res Immunol* 144(1):61-65, 1993.
44. Brown CR, McLeod R: Class I MHC genes and CD8+ T cells determine cyst number in *Toxoplasma* infection, *J Immunol* 145:3438-3441, 1990.
45. Chao CC, Hu S, Gekker G et al: Effects of cytokines on multiplication of *Toxoplasma gondii* in microglial cells, *J Immunol* 150:3404-3410, 1993.
46. Gazzinelli RT, Eltoum I, Wynn TA et al: Acute cerebral toxoplasmosis is induced by in vivo neutralization of TNF-alpha and correlates with the down-regulated expression of inducible nitric oxide synthase and other markers of macrophage activation, *J Immunol* 151:3672-3681, 1993.
47. Beaman MH, Hunter CA, Remington JS: Enhancement of intracellular replication of *Toxoplasma gondii* by IL-6, *J Immunol* 153:4583-4587, 1994.
48. Hérion P, Saavedra R: Human T-cell clones as tools for the characterization of the cell-mediated immune response to *Toxoplasma gondii, Res Immunol* 144(1): 48-51, 1993.
49. Denkers EY, Caspar P, Sher A: *Toxoplasma gondii* possesses a superantigen activity that selectively expands murine T cell receptor Vβ5-bearing CD8+ lymphocytes, *J Exp Med* 180:985-994, 1994.
50. Curiel TJ, Krug ED, Purner MB et al: Cloned human CD4+ cytotoxic T lymphocytes specific for *Toxoplasma gondii* lyse tachyzoite-infected target cells, *J Immunol* 151:2024-2031, 1993.
51. Hafizi A, Modabber FZ: Effect of cyclophosphamide on *Toxoplasma gondii* infection: reversal of the effect by passive immunization, *Clin Exp Immunol* 33:389-394, 1978.
52. Wilson CB, Haas JE: Cellular defenses against *Toxoplasma gondii* in newborns, *J Clin Invest* 73:1606-1616, 1984.
53. Wyler DJ, Blackman JH, Lunde MN: Cellular hypersensitivity to toxoplasmal and retinal antigens in patients with toxoplasmal retinochoroiditis, *Am J Trop Med Hyg* 29:1181-1186, 1980.
54. Abrahams IW, Gregerson DS: Longitudinal study of serum antibody responses to retinal antigens in acute ocular toxoplasmosis, *Am J Ophthalmol* 93:224-231, 1982.
55. Rollins DF, Tabbara KF, O'Connor GR et al: Detection of toxoplasmal antigen and antibody in ocular fluids in experimental ocular toxoplasmosis, *Arch Ophthalmol* 101:455-457, 1983.
56. Davidson MG, Lappin MR, English RV et al: A Feline model of ocular toxoplasmosis, *Invest Ophthalmol Vis Sci* 34:3653-3660, 1993.
57. Rehder JR, Burnier MB Jr, Pavesio CE et al: Acute unilateral toxoplasmic iridocyclitis in an AIDS patient, *Am J Ophthalmol* 106:740-741, 1988.
58. Greven CM, Teot LA: Cytologic identification of *Toxoplasma gondii* from vitreous fluid, *Arch Ophthalmol* 112:1086-1088, 1994.
59. Weiss MJ, Velazquez N, Hofeldt AJ: Serologic tests in the diagnosis of presumed toxoplasmic retinochoroiditis, *Am J Ophthalmol* 109:407-411, 1990.

60. Rothova A, van Knapen F, Baarsma GS et al: Serology in ocular toxoplasmosis, *Br J Ophthalmol* 70:615-622, 1986.
61. Phaik CS, Seah S, Guan OS et al: Anti-*Toxoplasma* serotitres in ocular toxoplasmosis, *Eye* 5(pt 5):636-639, 1991.
62. Desmonts G: Definitive serological diagnosis of ocular toxoplasmosis, *Arch Ophthalmol* 76:839-853, 1966.
63. Goichot EL, Bloch-Michel E: Intérêt de l'étude détaillée de la sérologie quantitative de l'humeur aqueuse pour le diagnostic de la toxoplasmose ocualaire: a propos de 180 cas, *J Fr Ophtalmol* 3:21-26, 1980.
64. Turunen HJ, Leinikki PO, Saari KM: Demonstration of intraocular synthesis of immunoglobulin G *Toxoplasma* antibodies for specific diagnosis of toxoplasmic chorioretinitis by enzyme immunoassay, *J Clin Microbiol* 17:988-992, 1983.
65. Ware PL, Kasper LH: Strain-specific antigens of *Toxoplasma gondii, Infect Immun* 55:778-783, 1987.
66. Boothroyd JC, Burg JL, Nagel S et al: Antigen and tubulin genes of *Toxoplasma gondii.* In Agabian N, Goodman H, Nogueria N, editors: *Molecular strategies of parasitic invasion,* New York, 1987, AR Liss.
67. Brézin AP, Egwuagu CE, Burner M Jr et al: Identification of *Toxoplasma gondii* in paraffin-embedded sections by the polymerase chain reaction, *Am J Ophthalmol* 110:599-604, 1990.
68. Brézin AP, Eqwuagu CE, Silveira C et al: Analysis of aqueous humor in ocular toxoplasmosis, *N Engl J Med* 324:699, 1991.
69. Scheiffarth OF, Zrenner E, Disko R et al: Intraocular in vivo immunofluorescence, *Invest Ophthalmol Vis Sci* 31:272-276, 1990.
70. Silveira C, Belfort R Jr, Burnier M et al: Acquired toxoplasmosis infection as the cause of toxoplasmic retinochoroiditis in families, *Am J Ophthalmol* 106: 362-364, 1988.
71. Glasner PD, Silveira C, Kruszon-Moran D et al: An unusually high prevalence of ocular toxoplasmosis in southern Brazil, *Am J Ophthalmol* 114:136-144, 1992.
72. Glasner PD, Silveira CM, Camargo ME et al: Low frequency of congenital *Toxoplasma gondii* (TG) infection in the Erechim region of Rio Grande do Sul, Brazil, *Ophthalmology (suppl)* 99:150, 1992.
73. Nussenblatt RB, Belfort R Jr: Ocular toxoplasmosis: an old disease revisited, *JAMA* 271:304-307, 1994.
74. Melamed J, Sebben JC, Maestri M et al: Epidemiology of ocular toxoplasmosis in Rio Grande do Sul, Brazil. In Dernouchamps JP, Verougstraete C, Caspers-Velu L, editors: *Recent advances in uveitis: Proceedings of the Third International Symposium on Uveitis, Brussels, Belgium,* Amsterdam, 1993, Kugler.
75. Sibley LD, Boothroyd JC: Virulent strains of *Toxoplasma gondii* comprise a single clonal lineage, *Nature* 359:82-85, 1992.
76. Sabates R, Pruett RC, Brockhurst RJ: Fulminary ocular toxoplasmosis, *Am J Ophthalmol* 92:497-503, 1981.
77. Tabbara KF, O'Connor GR: Treatment of ocular toxoplasmosis with clindamycin and sulfadiazine, *Ophthalmology* 87:129-134, 1980.
78. Lakhanpal V, Schocket SS, Nirankari VS: Clindamycin in the treatment of toxoplasmic retinochoroiditis, *Am J Ophthalmol* 95:605-613, 1983.
79. Thiermann E, Apt W, Atias A et al: Comparative study of some combined treatment regimens in acute toxoplasmosis in mice, *Am J Trop Med Hyg* 27:747-750, 1978.
80. Mittelviefhaus H: Clindamycin therapy of suspected toxoplasmosis retinochoroiditis, *Klin Monatsbl Augenheilkd* 200:123-127, 1992.
81. Ferguson JG Jr: Clindamycin therapy for toxoplasmosis, *Ann Ophthalmol* 13:95-100, 1981.
82. Belfort R Jr: Personal communication, 1992.
83. Opremcak EM, Scales DK, Sharpe MR: Trimethoprim-sulfamethoxazole therapy for ocular toxoplasmosis, *Ophthalmology* 99:920-925, 1992.
84. Araujo FG, Huskinson J, Remington JS: Remarkable in vitro and in vivo activities of the hydroxynaphthoquinone 566C80 against tachyzoites and tissue cysts of *Toxoplasma gondii, Antimicrob Agents Chemother* 35:293-299, 1991.
85. Lane HC, Laughon BE, Falloon J et al: NIH conference: recent advances in the management of AIDS-related opportunistic infections, *Ann Intern Med* 120:945-955, 1994.
86. Lopez JS, de Smet MD, Masur H et al: Orally administered 566C80 for treatment of ocular toxoplasmosis in a patient with the acquired immunodeficiency syndrome, *Am J Ophthalmol* 113:331-333, 1992.
87. Rothova A, Meenken C, Buitenhuis HJ et al: Therapy for ocular toxoplasmosis, *Am J Ophthalmol* 115:517-523, 1993.
88. Ghartey KN, Brockhurst RJ: Photocoagulation of active toxoplasmic retinochoroiditis, *Am J Ophthalmol* 89: 858-864, 1980.
89. Fitzgerald CR: Pars plana vitrectomy for vitreous opacity secondary to presumed toxoplasmosis, *Arch Ophthalmol* 98:321-323, 1980.

# CHAPTER 15

# Ocular Histoplasmosis

Ocular histoplasmosis is the only syndrome in the spectrum of ocular inflammation in which "presumed" has appeared in its name. Epidemiologic evidence supports the concept that an invading organism is the cause of this ocular disease. However, accruing evidence supports the notion that there is a complex interaction between the exogenous pathogen and the immune response. As well, the recent advances in submacular surgery have provided sufferers with this entity a possible, yet to be fully proved, alternative therapeutic approach to consider besides medical and laser therapy or simply observation.

## SYSTEMIC FINDINGS

*Histoplasma capsulatum,* a fungus found worldwide in valleys with rivers, is endemic to the midwestern United States. Found in the soil, it is readily inhaled and phagocytosed. Although the disease may start in the lungs, it can spread to the liver and spleen, leaving small calcified lesions that can be seen on x-ray examination. The disease can take three major forms: (1) a nonfatal acute pneumonitis with fever, (2) an acute progressive form that can be fatal in 1 to 2 months, and (3) a chronic form similar to tuberculosis.[1] These disease presentations rarely have ocular manifestations. The ocular histoplasmosis syndrome is rather a distinct entity found almost exclusively in the United States, and it usually occurs in symptom-free persons living in endemic regions.

## OCULAR APPEARANCE

Probably Reid and coworkers[2] described the first ocular case that we now recognize as the ocular histoplasmosis syndrome, but Woods and Wahlen[3] were the first to describe the ocular syndrome in full detail. They believed that *H. capsulatum* might be the cause for both the typical atrophic spots in the retinal periphery and the disciform changes in the macula. Although the disorder is found most commonly in the midwestern United States, particularly in the Ohio-Mississippi valleys, it also appears in the middle Atlantic states such as Maryland. In these areas, skin tests for histoplasmosis show positive results in a high percentage of the population, indicating systemic sensitization by the immune system. The ocular histoplasmosis syndrome is a rare disease in other parts of the world, even in areas endemic for histoplasmosis.[4] There are reports of cases that meet the criteria for the diagnosis; however, test results are negative for evidence of histoplasmosis infection and sensitization.[5,6]

Studies in the United States have suggested that typical findings of ocular histoplasmosis will be found in 1.6%[1] to 12.9%[7] of the population in an endemic area. Further, Smith and Ganley[8] determined from the Walkersville, Maryland, study that maculopathy due to ocular histoplasmosis will develop in 1 adult/1000 in an endemic area. The disease appears most commonly in the third to fourth decade of life, with men more likely to have involvement of both maculae.[4] It appears that the disease is considerably less common in African-Americans[9] (see Box 15-1).

*H. capsulatum* causes four major clinical manifestations of the ocular disease: "histo spots," maculopathy, peripapillary pigment changes, and clear vitreous.

### "Histo spots"

A disseminated choroiditis produces the typical histo spots. Numbering on average four to eight per eye, these choroidal scars are circular, depigmented, atrophic; have a disc diameter (DD) 0.2 to 0.7; and may have a pigment clump centrally[10] (Fig. 15-1). The peripheral lesions are not thought significant in terms of the prognosis for the maintenance of good visual acuity. In a small number of patients, these lesions occur in the equatorial ocular region as streaks running parallel to the ora serrata. They can become larger or smaller, and they may disappear.

**Box 15-1**
**Characteristics of ocular histoplasmosis syndrome**

Resident of histoplasmosis belt of the United States
White, 20-50 years of age
Multiple choroidal spots ("histo" spots)
Peripapillary changes
Disciform scar
No vitreous inflammatory disease
HLA-B7 positivity (macular disease)

### Maculopathy

Maculopathy results in a macular lesion that is sight-threatening, causing sudden, abrupt change in vision. During the initial stage, the choroid may take on a ground-glass appearance and push the retina upward. In the macula, a retinal pigment epithelial detachment can occur, and in 7% of patients, a central serous choroidopathy is seen.[11] In a large number of patients (63%), the lesion is hemorrhagic[11] and in rare instances causes vitreous hemorrhage.[12] Intervals between macular attacks may vary from 1 month to years, leading to a disciform scar (Fig. 15-2). Schlaegel[4] informed his patients that if there were histo scars in a macula, then there was a 1:4 chance of recurrence in the macula over the ensuing 3 years. However, if no scars are noted, then the chances for ocular problems are about 1:50. About 60% of

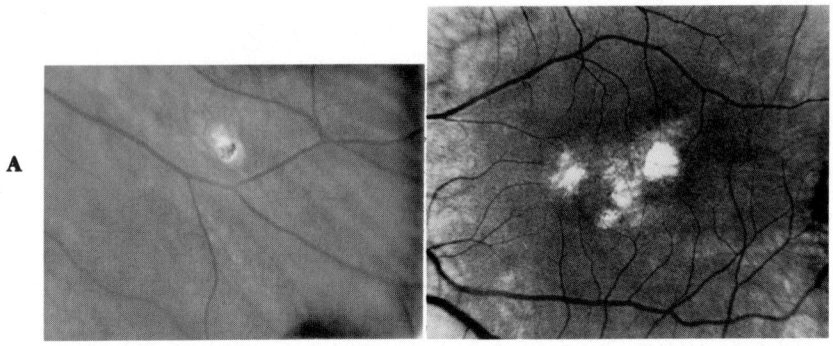


**Fig. 15-1. A,** Peripheral "histo" lesion. These lesions are round and deep to retina. Media has no cells. **B,** Similar lesions in macula.

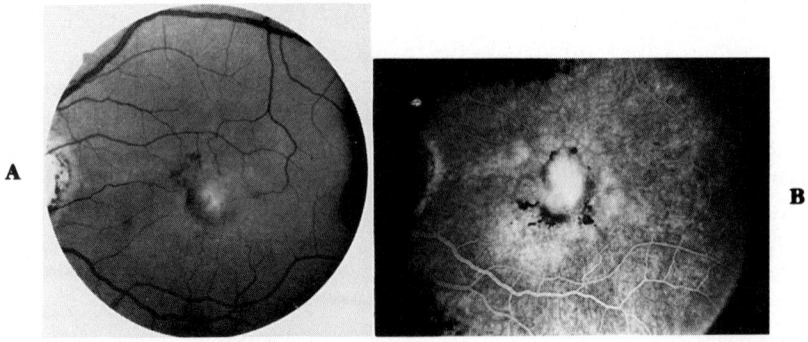


**Fig. 15-2. A,** Patient with macular disciform lesion due to multiple recurrences of presumed ocular histoplasmosis. **B,** Late-stage fluorescein angiogram showing subretinal alterations.

the time this process leads to severe visual impairment, and only 10% to 15% will maintain 20/20 vision in the affected eye after a 2-year period. The development of a disciform lesion in the second eye depends on whether there are old atrophic histo scars in the macular region, because these lesions appear to arise at the edges of old lesions.[9] At times these membranes can be difficult to diagnose because of the absence of hemorrhage or pigmentation.[13] Rarely, subretinal neovascularization leading to a disciform scar can appear in the absence of previous pigmentary changes, usually denoting a nidus of activity,[14] supporting the concept that there are invisible foci of choroidal inflammation in this disorder.[15]

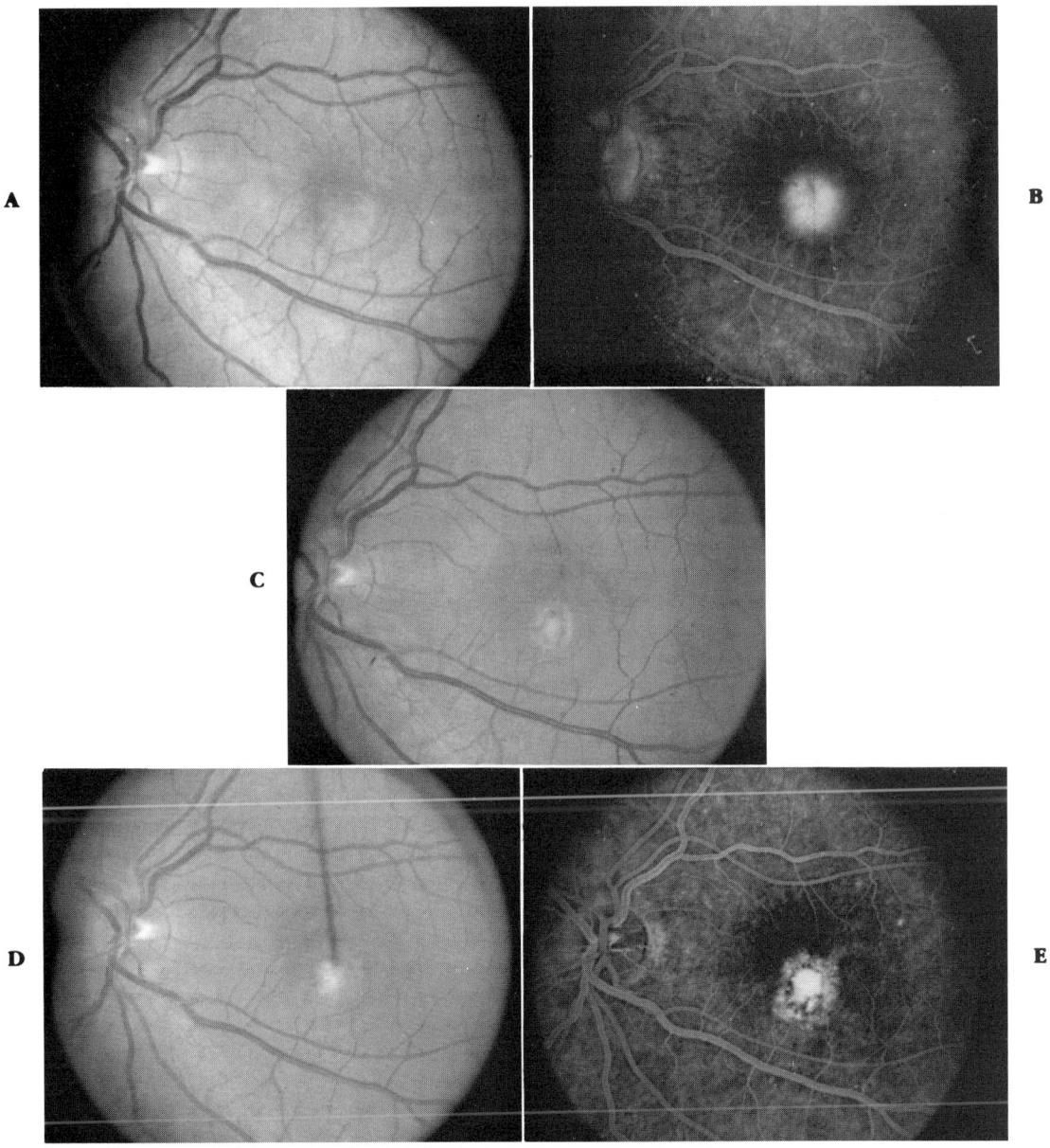


**Fig. 15-3.** Fundus photographs and angiograms of 30-year-old patient who reported metamorphopsia for several weeks in left eye. Visual acuity was 20/40, with 20/20 vision in right eye. **A** shows raised macular lesion. Angiogram **(B)** shows hyperfluorescence compatible with subfoveal neovascularization. Vision in left eye decreased to 20/100 at 3 months and was 20/80 at 6 months. However, pigmented ring around lesion **(C)** was noted. By 24 months, vision had returned to 20/20, with atrophic lesion in macula present **(D),** with staining but not leakage noted on angiogram **(E).** (Courtesy Peter A. Campochiaro, M.D.) (See Color Plate 31.)

A point of great interest is the natural history of disciform lesions due to ocular histoplasmosis, particularly in light of new surgical techniques (see later discussion). In ocular histoplasmosis, a spontaneous improvement of visual acuity is possible in patients with disciform changes due to this disorder. Jost and coworkers[16] found that 10 of 700 patients with ocular histoplasmosis had a spontaneous improvement. In a report by Kleiner and colleagues,[17] the visual outcome of 74 eyes having ocular histoplasmosis and active subretinal neovascular membranes was studied. The authors found, in a follow-up period that ranged from 12 to 109 months (median, 36.5 months), that 14% of eyes retained a visual acuity of 20/40 or better. Some of the factors associated with the retention of good vision were the patient's age (younger than 30 years old), the small size of the membrane, and an absence of visual loss due to ocular histoplasmosis in the other eye. Campochiaro and colleagues[18] reported on the cases of five patients who maintained or spontaneously regained good visual acuity in the presence of a subfoveal neovascular membrane. They believed that a typical pattern emerged for all of these patients when the sequential photographs and angiograms were studied. A pigmented ring forms around the membrane, and the membrane begins to change character on the angiogram, going from one that leaks fluorescein to one that stains but does not leak. With time, there is resorption of subretinal fluid, with limitation of the hemorrhage and fibrosis (Fig. 15-3).

### Peripapillary pigment changes

Peripapillary pigment changes occur, presumably due to an underlying choroiditis. These changes are important because they can help the ophthalmologist diagnose the disease. A line of pigment is seen bordering the disc inside a depigmented area. Sometimes these lesions appear to be nodular and can harbor subretinal nets with resultant hemorrhagic episodes.

### Clear vitreous

A clear vitreous is an important part of the clinical appearance of ocular histoplasmosis. The presence of cells must make the observer reconsider the diagnosis.

The differential diagnosis of this condition includes many granulomatous lesions that appear deep to the retina, including tuberculosis, coccidioidomycosis, cryptococcosis, and sarcoidosis. The pseudohistoplasmosis entity reported by Nozik and Dorsch[19] has lesions in the posterior segment highly suggestive of ocular histoplasmosis (see Chapter 28). Deutsch and Tessler[20] found that sarcoidosis could be identified as the underlying cause of the histoplasmosis-like profile in many of the patients they observed. All these entities should have obvious inflammatory activity in the vitreous, unlike the ocular histoplasmosis syndrome. Some noninflammatory conditions that simulate this condition include myopic degeneration, drusen of the optic disc, and angioid streaks. It is important to keep in mind that if vitreal cells are present, then the diagnosis of presumed ocular histoplasmosis must be reconsidered.

## ETIOLOGY AND IMMUNOLOGY

Few clinically relevant tests are required to corroborate the clinical impression of ocular histoplasmosis. A skin test using histoplasmin antigen is most helpful, with this reactivity usually appearing early after exposure and persisting a lifetime. However, there is a risk that ocular lesions may reactivate with this test, so that it is best not undertaken in those patients with macular disease. One can argue that because "invisible" lesions may be present in the macula, the test may pose a risk to all patients. This test is therefore not often performed. The complement-fixation test for circulating antibodies is not a particularly effective way to evaluate exposure, with Schlaegel[4] finding seropositivity in only one third of typical cases. A chest x-ray film to detect any calcification can help establish whether the patient has been previously exposed to this pathogen.

The exact role that *H. capsulatum* plays in ocular histoplasmosis still remains to be elucidated. *Histoplasma* organisms have been found in the eyes of patients who have been immunosuppressed.[21] Indeed, in one report of a patient with a 12-year history of relapsing disseminated histoplasmosis, the ocular lesion manifested was that of an endophthalmitis rather than the typical findings of the ocular histoplasmosis syndrome.[22] Specht and colleagues[23] reported the ocular findings in an AIDS patient who had disseminated histoplasmosis. Creamy white intraretinal and subretinal lesions were noted, and postmortem examination of the globe showed the presence of *Histoplasma* yeast cells in the area of the retinitis, as well as in optic nerve. Pulido and coworkers[24] reported a case of exogenous postoperative *Histoplasma* endophthalmitis. The enucleated specimen of this 60-year-old man (after intraocular lens [IOL] surgery) showed *Histoplasma* organisms but seronegativity and an absence of systemic infection. However, other histopathologic correlations in which the presence of *Histoplasma* antigen has been suspected have occurred in cases thought to be compatible with the ocular histoplasmosis syndrome.[25–27]

Histoplasmosis has been seen to occur naturally in both cats and dogs, inducing a choroiditis and retinitis, respectively.[28] Intracarotid inoculation of nonhuman primates with live *H. capsulatum* showed that acute lesions took on several clinical features seen in human beings, including chorioretinal scarring and retinal pigment epithelial defects, as well as "disappearing" lesions. However, organisms were not demonstrated by culture or special stains in lesions present for longer than 6 weeks.[29] Subretinal neovascularization was observed in one eye of a nonhuman primate 1 year after injection with the organism.[30] Of interest was the failure of fluorescein angiography to demonstrate the presence of this abnormality, presumably due to the presence of tight junctions and therefore no leakage.

Anderson and colleagues[31] have characterized the lesions of histoplasmic choroiditis in the nonhuman primate with the use of antihuman monoclonal antibodies. They found variability in the cellular components of typical histo spots, even in the same eye. Of interest was a chronic lesion with a B-cell focus with high numbers of mature B cells and helper/inducer T cells.

Immunologic monitoring has not been exceptionally helpful in understanding the basic mechanisms of this disease. Check and colleagues[32] believed that in vitro lymphocyte proliferation assays with *Histoplasma* organisms seemed to correlate with the severity of disease. Brahmi and coworkers[33] found similar lymphocyte transformation responses in both patients with presumed ocular disease and with acute histoplasmosis syndrome, whereas other parameters, such as natural killer cell activity and helper/suppressor ratios, were different between these groups.

With use of HLA typing, a potential immunogenetic predisposition to the development of the macular lesions appears to have been identified. Godfrey and coworkers[34] and Braley and colleagues[35] found an association between HLA-B7 and the macular lesions of this syndrome, giving a calculated relative risk of 11.8. This association has not been noted with those patients manifesting only peripheral retinal lesions. Spaide and colleagues[36] found an absence of HLA-DR2 in 17 patients with multifocal choroiditis and panuveitis, whereas this antigen was found in 17 patients with subretinal neovascularization associated with the ocular histoplasmosis syndrome. The authors believe that these data suggest that in spite of the ocular fundus similarities of these two entities, the disorders appear to have differing genetic dispositions.

Many questions remain concerning the underlying mechanism of this entity. Many years ago, Dr. Richard O'Connor, who at that time was the at the University of California, San Francisco, studied patients in whom typical lesions of ocular histoplasmosis developed several decades after leaving an endemic area. Several explanations can be given. It may be that genetically prone persons are unable to clear the organism and that they continuously "shed" antigen from a site, such as the spleen. Once it has lodged in the eye, the low-grade inflammatory response in the choroid occurs again. Another possibility is that molecular mimicry may be the reason for repeated attacks (see Chapter 2). A third possibility is that in genetically prone persons the fungal antigen acts as an adjuvant to induce an inflammatory response wherever it lodges, for example, the choroid (Fig. 15-4).

## THERAPY

Amphotericin B has no role to play in the treatment of ocular histoplasmosis. It not only is ineffective but exposes the patient to a medication with serious secondary effects. Until recently the two major forms of therapy were those of corticosteroids and laser photocoagulation, but a third approach has most provocative implications (to be discussed). Corticosteroids can be given for the acute macular lesion that causes a sudden drop in visual acuity or in preparation for laser therapy. Patients with macular lesions, particularly those with one eye already visually handicapped because of the disease, may consider carrying prednisone with them and checking themselves daily for any changes in vision or distortions that occur as noted on an Amsler grid. Short-term corticosteroid therapy should be

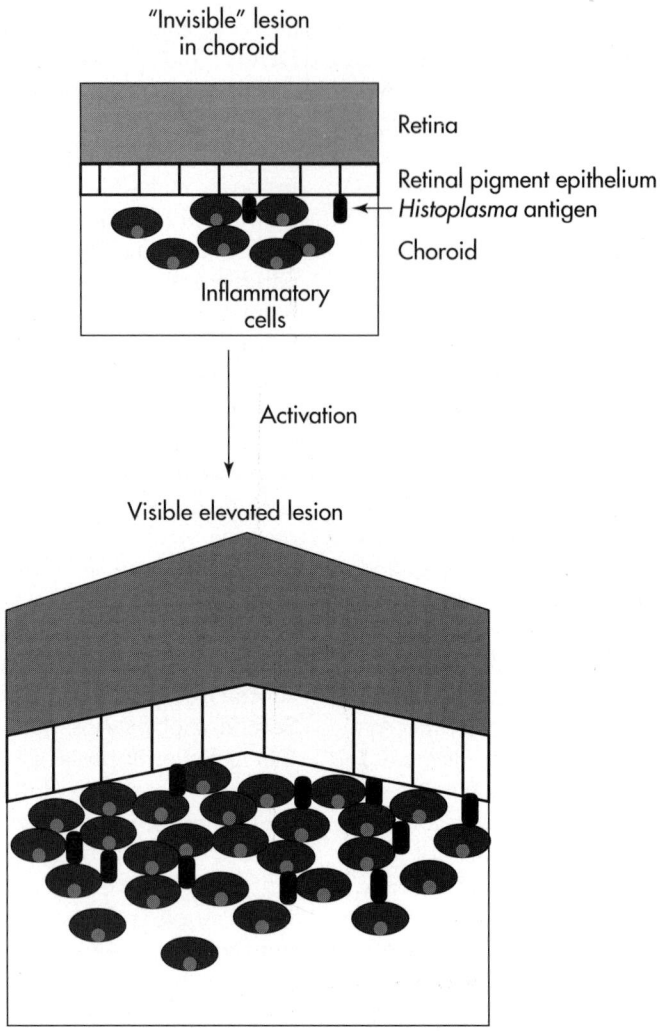


**Fig. 15-4.** Scheme showing presence of "invisible" lesions in choroid. *Histoplasma* antigen may be present, inducing a minimal inflammatory response, and therefore is not seen. If more antigen is released from distant site and lodges in same area, or if *Histoplasma* antigen already there acts as adjuvant, more pronounced inflammatory response will occur, which now can be visualized as "active" lesion.

given in high doses (60 mg daily, 50-120 mg every other day) to effect a change. The chronicity of the disorder (at least 2 years) suggests that a long-term therapeutic commitment must be made by the patient and the physician. The final visual outcome when subretinal neovascular nets encroach the foveal and juxtafoveal region is not affected by corticosteroid therapy[37]; with a follow-up of 39 months on the average, 81% of eyes had visual acuities worse than 6/12, and almost 70% of these were 6/60 or worse using this form of therapy.

Maumenee first suggested the use of laser photocoagulation to treat the ocular histoplasmosis syndrome.[4] The results of a randomized clinical trial evaluating the effectiveness of argon laser photocoagulation for choroidal neovascular membranes have shown this approach to be the treatment of choice until now.[38] After an 18-month follow-up, 34% (39/114) of untreated eyes versus 9.4% (11/117) of treated eyes had lost six lines or more of visual acuity from baseline. In 1991 the Macular Photocoagulation Study Group[39] published their 5-year results of three randomized studies using argon laser photocoagulation in the treatment of extrafoveal choroidal neovascularization due to various disorders, including ocular histoplasmosis. In these studies, untreated eyes with extrafoveal choroidal neovascularization due to ocular histoplasmosis had a 3.6 times greater risk of losing six or more lines of visual acuity than laser-treated eyes. However, recurrent neovascularization was noted in 26% of the treated eyes. The Canadian Ophthalmology Study Group,[40] in a multicenter, randomized, controlled clinical trial, found that krypton red laser photocoagulation was not better for well-defined extrafoveal nets than was argon green laser.

A recent pilot study was reported in which laser therapy was directed to treating subfoveal neovascular nets.[41] Only a total of 25 patients were enrolled, and there was a fairly short follow-up period. The observers could not conclude whether the approach was useful or not, but a marked decrease in vision did not appear to occur in the group treated with laser photocoagulation, nor was there a striking increase either. One interesting aspect of this report was the difficulty in recruiting patients; the authors hypothesized that most patients' nets begin outside the fovea and therefore are treated before reaching the more advanced stage.

Recurrence of subretinal neovascular nets is problematic. Green[42] has reported a clinicopathologic study of treated choroidal neovascular membranes. He noted that recurrences of choroidal neovascularization, some contiguous and some not contiguous to treated areas, occurred in 9 of 12 lesions in the 10 eyes he studied. It is interesting to note that the scar induced by laser photocoagulation resembled that of the naturally occurring scar, portions of which consisted of hyperplastic retinal pigment epithelium.

### Subretinal surgery

The removal of choroidal neovascular nets by means of subretinal surgery techniques has especially provocative implications. Although subretinal surgery reports appeared in the 1980s,[43,44] this type of surgery did not really develop until the 1990s, with the advent of new instruments and indications. Choroidal neovascularization due to ocular histoplasmosis has been one disease in which this approach has been explored in some depth (see Chapter 9). An initial paper by Thomas and Kaplan[45] reported on two patients with subfoveal neovascularization due to the ocular histoplasmosis syndrome whose visual acuities were 20/400. After surgery the visual acuity returned to 20/20 in one patient and 20/40 in the other, with a short follow-up time. Subsequent reports have put the technique in perspective, albeit not definitively. Berger and Kaplan[46] reported that 8 of 15 patients with subfoveal choroidal neovascularization due to ocular histoplasmosis had an improvement of two lines or better after subretinal surgery and removal of the membrane. They noted an improvement in vision even after 6 months of decreased vision. Recurrent neovascularization occurred in 2 of the 15 eyes. Thomas and coworkers[47] performed two types of procedures on patients with histoplasmosis who had subfoveal nets. After performing a vitrectomy, the authors either disconnected the choroidal circulation or extracted the net through their retinotomy site. Of 16 eyes that had membranes removed 6 improved by at least two Snellen lines, whereas none of the 4 patients who had the membranes' choroidal circulation disconnected showed such improvement.

Although these observations are encouraging, there are several points to keep in mind. The first is that all who have reported on this procedure stress the importance of choosing the prospective patient very carefully. This brings into question the applicability of this procedure for most patients. Certainly the initial reports concerning this procedure—when applied to patients with age-related maculopathy—have not been especially impressive. Those patients may need much more than "simply" removing a subretinal net, that is, the replacement of their nonfunctioning or barely functioning retinal pigment epithelial cells. Another point to consider is the possible recurrence rate after surgery and whether it is substantially different from present therapeutic modalities. Finally, a confounding point is the spontaneous regression of some of these nets in patients with this ocular histoplasmosis, particularly in those patients who are young and would be particularly good candidates for surgery. This approach holds promise for the future and is cause for guarded optimism.

### REFERENCES

1. Asbury T: The status of presumed ocular histoplasmosis: including a report of a survey, *Trans Am Ophthalmol Soc* 64:371-400, 1966.
2. Reid JD, Scherer JH, Herbut PA et al: Systemic histoplasmosis diagnosed before death and produced experimentally in guinea pigs, *J Lab Clin Med* 27:419-434, 1942.
3. Woods AC, Wahlen HE: The probable role of benign histoplasmosis in the etiology of granulomatous uveitis, *Am J Ophthalmol* 49:205-220, 1960.

4. Schlaegel TF Jr: *Ocular histoplasmosis,* New York, 1977, Grune & Stratton.
5. Saraux H, Pelosse B, Guigui A: Multifocal inner choroiditis: pseudohistoplasmosis—the European form of the presumed American histoplasmosis, *J Fr Ophthalmol* 9:645-651, 1986.
6. Braunstein RA, Rosen DA, Bird AC: Ocular histoplasmosis syndrome in the United Kingdom, *Br J Ophthalmol* 58:893-898, 1974.
7. Davidorf FH, Anderson JD: Ocular lesions in the Earth Day 1970 histoplasmosis epidemic, *Int Ophthalmol Clin* 15(3):51-60, 1975.
8. Smith RE, Ganley JP: An epidemiologic study of presumed ocular histoplasmosis, *Trans Am Acad Ophthalmol Otolaryngol* 75:994-1005, 1971.
9. Gass JDM, Wilkinson CP: Follow-up study of presumed ocular histoplasmosis, *Trans Am Acad Ophthalmol Otolaryngol* 76:672-694, 1972.
10. Smith RE, Ganley JP, Knox DL: Presumed ocular histoplasmosis. II. Patterns of peripheral and peripapillary scarring in persons with nonmacular disease, *Arch Ophthalmol* 87:251-257, 1972.
11. Walma D, Schlaegel TF Jr: Presumed histoplasmic choroiditis, *Am J Ophthalmol* 57:107-110, 1964.
12. Kranias G: Vitreous hemorrhage secondary to presumed ocular histoplasmosis syndrome, *Ann Ophthalmol* 17:295-298, 1985.
13. Rivers MB, Pulido JS, Folk JC: Ill-defined choroidal neovascularization within ocular histoplasmosis scars, *Retina* 12:90-95, 1992.
14. Ryan SJ Jr: De novo subretinal neovascularization in the histoplasmosis syndrome, *Arch Ophthalmol* 94:321-327, 1976.
15. Schlaegel TF Jr: The concept of invisible choroiditis in the ocular histoplasmosis syndrome, *Int Ophthalmol Clin* 23:55-63, 1983.
16. Jost BF, Olk RJ, Burgess DB: Factors related to spontaneous visual recovery in the ocular histoplasmosis syndrome, *Retina* 7:1-8, 1987.
17. Kleiner RC, Ratner CM, Enger C et al: Subfoveal neovascularization in the ocular histoplasmosis syndrome: a natural history study, *Retina* 8:225-227, 1988.
18. Campochiaro PA, Morgan KM, Conway BP et al: Spontaneous involution of subfoveal neovascularization, *Am J Ophthalmol* 109:668-675, 1990.
19. Nozik RA, Dorsch W: A new chorioretinopathy associated with anterior uveitis, *Am J Ophthalmol* 76:758-762, 1973.
20. Deutsch TA, Tessler HH: Inflammatory pseudohistoplasmosis, *Ann Ophthalmol* 17:461-465, 1985.
21. Scholz R, Green WR, Kutys R et al: *Histoplasma capsulatum* in the eye, *Ophthalmology* 91:1100-1104, 1984.
22. Goldstein BG, Buettner H: Histoplasmic endophthalmitis: a clinicopathologic correlation, *Arch Ophthalmol* 101:774-777, 1983.
23. Specht CS, Mitchell KT, Bauman AE et al: Ocular histoplasmosis with retinitis in a patient with acquired immune deficiency syndrome, *Ophthalmology* 98: 1356-1359, 1991.
24. Pulido JS, Folberg R, Carter KD et al: *Histoplasma capsulatum* endophthalmitis after cataract extraction, *Ophthalmology* 97:217-220, 1990.
25. Khalil MK: Histopathology of presumed ocular histoplasmosis, *Am J Ophthalmol* 94:369-376, 1982.
26. Ryan SJ: Histopathological correlates of presumed ocular histoplasmosis, *Int Ophthalmol Clin* 15(3):125-137, 1975.
27. Maumenee AE: Clinical entities in "uveitis": an approach to the study of intraocular inflammation, *Am J Ophthalmol* 69:1-27, 1970.
28. Gwin RM, Makley TA Jr, Wyman M et al: Multifocal ocular histoplasmosis in a dog and cat, *J Am Vet Med Assoc* 176:638-642, 1980.
29. Smith RE, Dunn S, Jester JV: Natural history of experimental histoplasmic choroiditis in the primate, *Invest Ophthalmol Vis Sci* 25:810-819, 1984.
30. Jester JV, Smith RE: Subretinal neovascularization after experimental ocular histoplasmosis in a subhuman primate, *Am J Ophthalmol* 100:252-258, 1985.
31. Anderson A, Clifford W, Palvolgyi I et al: Immunopathology of chronic experimental histoplasmic choroiditis in the primate, *Invest Ophthalmol Vis Sci* 33:1637-1641, 1992.
32. Check IJ, Diddie KR, Jay WM et al: Lymphocyte stimulation by yeast phase *Histoplasma capsulatum* in presumed ocular histoplasmosis syndrome, *Am J Ophthalmol* 87:311-316, 1979.
33. Brahmi Z, Wheat J, Rubin RH et al: Humoral and cellular immune response in ocular histoplasmosis, *Ann Ophthalmol* 17:440-444, 1985.
34. Godfrey WA, Sabates R, Cross DE: Association of presumed ocular histoplasmosis with HLA-B7, *Am J Ophthalmol* 85:854-858, 1978.
35. Braley RE, Meredith TA, Aaberg TM et al: The prevalence of HLA-B7 in presumed ocular histoplasmosis, *Am J Ophthalmol* 85:859-861, 1978.
36. Spaide RF, Skerry JE, Yannuzzi LA et al: Lack of HLA-DR2 specificity in multifocal choroiditis and panuveitis, *Br J Ophthalmol* 74:536-537, 1990.
37. Olk RJ, Burgess DB, McCormick PA: Subfoveal and juxtafoveal subretinal neovascularization in the presumed ocular histoplasmosis syndrome, *Ophthalmology* 91:1592-1602, 1984.
38. Ocular Histoplasmosis Study: Argon laser photocoagulation for ocular histoplasmosis: results of a randomized clinical trial, *Arch Ophthalmol* 101:1347-1357, 1983.
39. Macular Photocoagulation Study Group: Argon laser photocoagulation for neovascular maculopathy: five-year results from randomized clinical trials, *Arch Ophthalmol* 109:1109-1114, 1991.
40. Canadian Ophthalmology Study Group: Argon green vs krypton red laser photocoagulation for extrafoveal choroidal neovascularization, *Arch Ophthalmol* 112: 1166-1173, 1994.
41. Fine SL, Wood WJ, Isernhagen RD et al: Laser treatment for subfoveal neovascular membranes in ocular histoplasmosis syndrome: results of a pilot randomized clinical trial, *Arch Ophthalmol* 111:19-20, 1993.
42. Green WR: Clinicopathologic studies of treated choroidal neovascular membranes: a review and report of two cases, *Retina* 11:328-356, 1991.
43. Machemer R: Surgical approaches to subretinal strands, *Am J Ophthalmol* 90(1):81-85, 1980.

44. de Juan E Jr, Machemer R: Vitreous surgery for hemorrhagic and fibrous complications of age-related macular degeneration, *Am J Ophthalmol* 105(1):25-29, 1988.
45. Thomas MA, Kaplan HJ: Surgical removal of subfoveal neovascularization in the presumed ocular histoplasmosis syndrome, *Am J Ophthalmol* 111:1-7, 1991.
46. Berger AS, Kaplan HJ: Clinical experience with the surgical removal of subfoveal neovascular membranes: short-term postoperative results, *Ophthalmology* 99: 969-975, 1992.
47. Thomas MA, Grand MG, Williams DF et al: Surgical management of subfoveal choroidal neovascularization, *Ophthalmology* 99:952-968, 1992.

# CHAPTER 16

# Toxocara Canis

Nematode infections of the eye have been noted for some time; Calhoun[1] in 1937 observed a larva in the anterior chamber of an 8-year-old boy that ultimately was resorbed. By its description, it was thought to be an ascarid. In 1950, Wilder[2] reported 24 cases in which eyes enucleated for suspected retinoblastoma were found to have nematodes. Four of these cases were later determined by Nichols[3] to be caused by *Toxocara canis.* Over the years, this entity has been recognized as a disorder with potentially serious consequences for vision.

*Toxocara canis* is an ascarid that can only complete its life cycle in the dog. An adult dog can acquire the infection by ingesting eggs with stage I encapsulated larvae that are found in the soil, by ingesting second stage larvae from infected meat (mice, rabbits, etc.), or by ingesting advanced stage larvae from the feces of prenatally infected pups.[4] In some parts of the United States, toxocariasis is found in 100% of puppies under 6 months of age.[5] Eggs in the intestine will ultimately hatch, and the larvae will migrate out of the intestine to all parts of the body. Most will encyst as stage II larvae and not develop further. However, pregnancy will reactivate some of these dormant larvae, allowing them to reenter the bloodstream and pass through the placenta to infest the growing pups. At birth, the larvae will migrate to the lungs and become stage III larvae. These can be coughed up and then swallowed, whereupon these larvae go on to a stage IV larvae and ultimately to the adult worm. These adult worms will lay massive numbers of eggs that pass out of the host in the feces. Human beings enter the pathway when they ingest soil, food, or other materials contaminated with these eggs. A survey of sandpits in parks in Japan showed that *Toxocara* eggs could be found in 12 of 13 surveyed. The eggs were present on the surface and in the depths of the sand.[6] Once in the human intestine, the stage II larvae will leave the intestine and enter the bloodstream, migrating throughout the body until the vascular lumen becomes small enough to block its progress. At this point the larva bores into the tissue and encysts. In addition to the eye, such cysts are frequently found in the brain, liver, and lungs. Because the larvae cannot migrate out of the human lungs, the life cycle ends at the stage II larval state, and *Toxocara* eggs will not be found in the feces of infected persons.

The encysted larvae may stay dormant without causing any clinically overt symptoms although they are present in large numbers. However, one encysted larva in the eye can lead to serious visual disturbance. An acute systemic disease (visceral larval migrans, VLM) is due to the migration of the stage II larva of the *Toxocara canis.* This is associated with fever, pulmonary symptoms such as a dry hacking cough or asthma-like attacks, splenomegaly and hepatomegaly, skin lesions, neurologic symptoms such as convulsions, and a meningitic picture.

*Toxocara canis* is an ubiquitous parasite found worldwide. The incidence of infected puppies has been estimated to vary from 33% in London to 98% in Columbus, Ohio, to 100% in Brisbane, Australia.[7] In one case control study that compared 24 age- and sex-matched patients with VLM and controls, 23 of the patients with VLM had had dogs in their homes some time before their illness, and an association with puppies in households of patients with VLM within 1 year of onset was statistically significant.[8]

## OCULAR MANIFESTATIONS

This disorder is typically found in children; the average age is estimated as 7.5 years with a range from 2 to 31 years,[9] and 80% of the cases are below the age of 16.[10] Though certainly exceptions have been reported, this tends to be an uniocular disorder.

Several "typical" ocular presentations have been recognized. Probably the most common presentation is that of a granuloma either in the posterior pole or in the periphery. This is presumed to arise after a stage II larva has been lodged in the choroid and becomes encysted.[11] The lesion itself will be raised and whitish in color with a width of 3/4 to 2 or 3 disc diameters (Fig. 16-1). This diagnosis must also be considered in the differential diagnosis of leukokoria because the lesion may attain a very large size and encompass a large portion of the vitreal cavity and look suspiciously like a retinoblastoma. The disorder is frequently associated with a massive vitritis, probably the result of the release of highly immunogenic antigens from a dead worm.

Live larvae have been observed in the retinal vessels.[12] Another recognized presentation of this entity is a peripheral retinitis, which is thought to be the result of a lodging of a larva in the peripheral retinal vasculature. An hypopyon uveitis can be seen with any of these posterior pole manifestations.

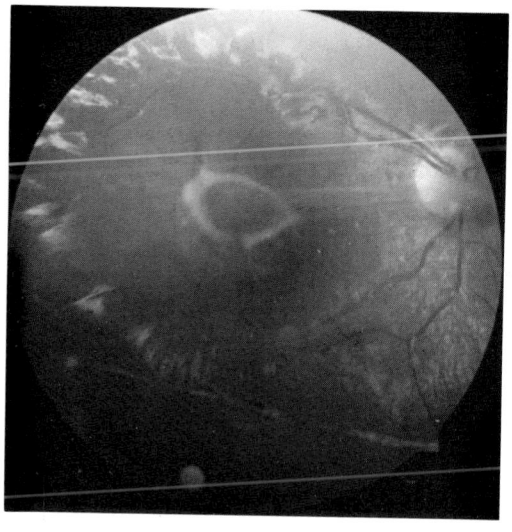

**Fig. 16-1.** *Toxocara* lesion in macula of 6-year-old girl. Choroidal lesion is raised, also pushing overlying retina upward; note epiretinal changes.

Less common presentations of *Toxocara canis* in the eye include optic nerve disease[13,14]; Brown and Tasman[15] reported an 11-year-old child with a presumed toxocaral neuroretinitis associated with a branch retinal artery obstruction. Karel and colleagues[16] reported a case in which the *Toxocara* larva observed in a choroidal granuloma migrated into the lens through the posterior capsule. Five cases of ocular toxocariasis in adults were reported by Steahly and Mader,[17] all with presentations similar to those seen in children.

As mentioned above, the most important alternative diagnosis to consider is that of retinoblastoma. Shields[18] has written that *T. canis* endophthalmitis is the most common entity confused with retinoblastoma. Further, presumed ocular toxocariasis accounted for 26% of the pseudoretinoblastomas seen at the Oncology Service of the Wills Eye Hospital, Philadelphia, Penn. Children with retinoblastoma usually are younger than those with ocular toxocariasis, the vitreous is usually clear, and there may be a familial history of the disorder. Ultrasound,[19] x-ray, or other imaging methods will frequently help distinguish this entity from retinoblastoma because calcification is found frequently in retinoblastoma, though this has been reported in some cases of toxocariasis.[20] With the use of a standardized echographic approach, Wan and colleagues[21] studied the eyes of 11 toxocariasis patients. In 10 of these patients, the following characteristics were found: (1) a solid highly reflective mass, (2) vitreous bands or membranes that extend from the mass to the posterior pole, and (3) a traction retinal detachment or fold from the mass to the posterior pole.

The lactate dehydrogenase aqueous to serum ratio is greater than one in retinoblastoma patients, and the phosphoglucose-isomerase ratio should be greater than two in eyes with retinoblastoma. Other diagnoses to consider include toxoplasmosis, primary hyperplastic primary vitreous, Coats' disease, focal choroiditis of other cause, such as sarcoid, and retrolental fibroplasia.

## HISTOPATHOLOGY AND IMMUNE FACTORS

The immune reaction to the *Toxocara* organism is similar to that seen for other parasites of this type. A profound eosinophilic response is initially noted histologically. Later on, the immune response will change to include macrophages, lymphocytes, and epithelioid cells. A large granulomatous response to the organism is not unusual (Fig. 16-1). In late lesions, scarring may be prominent. The inflammatory response may be quite profound and cause more destruction than the offending organism. Therefore a careful search of the lesion is needed sometimes to discover the parasite. In addition, in severe inflammatory reactions the organism may be essentially destroyed, and therefore the diagnosis can only be suspected on the basis of the massive inflammatory response. Recent in vitro work by Del Prete and colleagues[22] isolated clones of T cells from patients with the use of the *Toxocara canis* excretory/secretory antigen. They found that these clones secreted IL-4 and IL-5 but no or minimal amounts of IL-2 and IFN-γ, the reverse of what was seen from clones that were specific to the purified protein derivative of *Mycobacterium tuberculosis.*

An eosinophilic amorphous material called the Splendore-Hoeppli phenomenon can be seen in the organs of children with VLM. This reaction is not specific to the *Toxocara* organism but rather is seen for several parasites that probably initiate a similar type of eosinophilic response. Experimentally induced disease will produce a marked eosinophilic response and an histologic picture not unlike that seen in human beings.[23] Further, Rockey and colleagues[24] have noted that eosinophils adhere firmly to the larval sheath. But the parasite is able to partially evade eosinophils in culture by shedding its sheath. This in vitro observation would support the notion that the larval sheath could act as an antigenic stimulus without the presence of the parasite itself.

Carter[25] used $S^{35}$-labeled *Toxocara canis* to determine larval numbers in various tissues. It was found that although initially the larvae congregated in the liver, by day 14 postinfection the majority of the isotope was found in the brain. Cuellar and colleagues[26] reported that immune complexes may be a good technique for monitoring treatment efficiency because they fell quickly and remained low with therapy. In yet another animal model with Swiss mice,[27] the administration of cyclosporine was tested. Of interest was that the medication increased susceptibility of the mice to the *Toxocara* larvae, but the antiparasitic effect of the medication was great, leading to a diminution in the number of living *Toxocara canis* larvae.

Laboratory tests can be important in the diagnosis of *Toxocara canis* infection. Children with VLM will have an eosinophilia and hyperglobulinemia.[18] No eggs will be found in the stool because the eggs' life cycle in human beings would not reach this stage. Children with this condition tend to be 2 to 4 years of age. Those with ocular toxocariasis are generally older (7 years and older), and they may or may not have a history of VLM. Further, because there is no acute systemic illness, elevated immune parameters are rarely present.

### Enzyme-linked immunoabsorbent assay

Many of the older methods used to evaluate antibody responses to the *Toxocara* organism were not specific, cross reacting with other ascarids. The enzyme-linked immunoabsorbent assay (ELISA) is to date the most reliable and readily available test for the evaluation of antibodies directed against this organism. This test has used at least two *Toxocara*-derived antigens, that from the embryonated egg and the excretory-secretory or exoantigen. A report[28] would suggest that the exoantigen may be somewhat better at giving consistent findings. Gillespie and colleagues[29] found that a two-site antigen capture ELISA that detects a carbohydrate epitope on the excretory-secretory antigens of *Toxocara* was reasonably efficient (in 50% of cases) in detecting antibodies in patients with acute toxocariasis but was not effective in detecting antibodies in those with inactive or ocular disease. One ELISA kit evaluated[30] had a calculated diagnostic sensitivity of 91%, but 14% of serum samples had false positives because of cross-reactions with other protozoan or helminthic infections.

A titer of 1:8 in the serum is usually taken as evidence of a positive test for ocular toxocariasis (Table 16-1). As with all tests, this is not foolproof. Albert and Marcus[31] reported a case of a 4-year-old boy with a serum ELISA of 1:4; examination of the enucleated eye revealed a second stage larva of *Toxocara.* Kieler[32] reported the case of a 5-year-old with an ELISA titer of 1:2 and the *Toxocara* parasite present in an eosinophilic granuloma in the vitreous cavity, whereas Sharkey and McKay[33] reported a case with a repeatedly negative ELISA test.

Magnaval and colleagues[34] tested the value of Western blotting techniques as compared with

**Table 16-1.** Sensitivity and specificity of ELISA for diagnosis of ocular *Toxocara canis*

| Cutoff titer of positive test | Sensitivity (%) | Specificity (%) |
|---|---|---|
| 1:2 | 95 | 72 |
| 1:4 | 93 | 86 |
| 1:8 | 90 | 91 |
| 1:16 | 85 | 94 |
| 1:32 | 73 | 95 |
| 1:64 | 51 | 97 |
| 1:128 | 24 | 99 |
| 1:256 | 15 | 100 |
| 1:512 | 5 | 100 |

From Hagler WS et al.: Results of surgery for ocular *Toxocara canis, Ophthalmology* 88:1081-1086, 1981.

the standard ELISA. With the use of the same excretory/secretory antigens for both, the Western blotting technique correlated well with the ELISA technique. One advantage of the Western blotting technique was that banding patterns were such as to avoid problems of cross-reactivity with sera infected with other helminths.

The study of the aqueous or vitreous for local production of specific antibody or its cellular components has been done. Felberg and colleagues[35] found higher anti-*Toxocara* titers in the aqueous of ocular toxocariasis patients when compared with the serum, which suggests that local production of the antibody was taking place. The cytology of the aspirate in ocular toxocariasis should demonstrate eosinophils and not lymphocytes as in other types of uveitides. Further, one may see tumor cells in the aspirate from an eye with retinoblastoma.

## TREATMENT

Several treatment approaches have been suggested for this disorder, which perhaps suggests that the results for each therapy remain unclear or unsatisfactory. The medical therapy for *Toxocara canis* centers around two very different approaches. The first is the treatment of the patient with antihelminthics, such as thiabendazole or diethylcarbamazine, and the second with prednisone to decrease the secondary inflammatory response. Rubin and colleagues[12] reported the use of systemic prednisone (40 mg per day) with thiabendazole (2 g daily for 5 days) with disappearance of the active larva 24 hours after the initiation of therapy, but with no change in the pre- and postvisual acuity. Wilkinson and Welch[36] reported that thiabendazole and prednisone given to different patients were not successful in treating the disorder.

It is clear that the live larva may not induce a significant inflammatory response but that on death the inflammation may be considerable with serious sequelae to the eye. It is not clear how helpful the addition of antihelminthics are in the published studies because most successful cases received corticosteroids simultaneously. The use of corticosteroids seems justified in the light of severe intraocular infection, whereas the treatment of patients with antihelminthics (thiabendazole), if used, should be accompanied by steroids, and the patients need to be followed up by either a pediatrician or internist. Dinning and colleagues[37] proposed the use of a three-step approach for the ocular manifestations of toxocariasis. Initially, local, periocular, and systemic steroids combined with surgery if appropriate is suggested. If this approach is not successful, thiabendazole (50 mg/kg/day) should be considered. Finally, if the eye disease is associated with visceral larva migrans or a high antibody titer, local and systemic steroids combined with thiabendazole may be used.

Vitreous surgery has also been suggested as an effective method by which the secondary effects of *Toxocara canis* can be managed. Hagler and colleagues[38] operated on 17 patients with retinal complications of this disorder; three of these had active infection at the time of surgery. They were able to reattach the retina in 12 of these cases, and in 15 patients a stabilization or improvement of visual acuity was obtained. Belmont and colleagues[39] also reported a favorable outcome in patients with ocular toxocariasis who undergo pars plana vitrectomy. Gonvers and colleagues[40] reported the case of a 30-year-old patient with a traction detachment as a result of an inflammatory granuloma. The granuloma was removed in toto demonstrating a typical toxocariasis lesion. Results of the ELISA performed on the vitreous sample were strongly positive (Fig. 16-2). Maguire and colleagues[41] performed a vitrectomy for vitreopapillary traction and extracted from the eye an intact *Toxocara canis* organism. If the larva is visible and is at least 3 mm from the foveola, photocoagulation can be attempted to kill the organism.[18] This may induce inflammation that will require prednisone therapy.

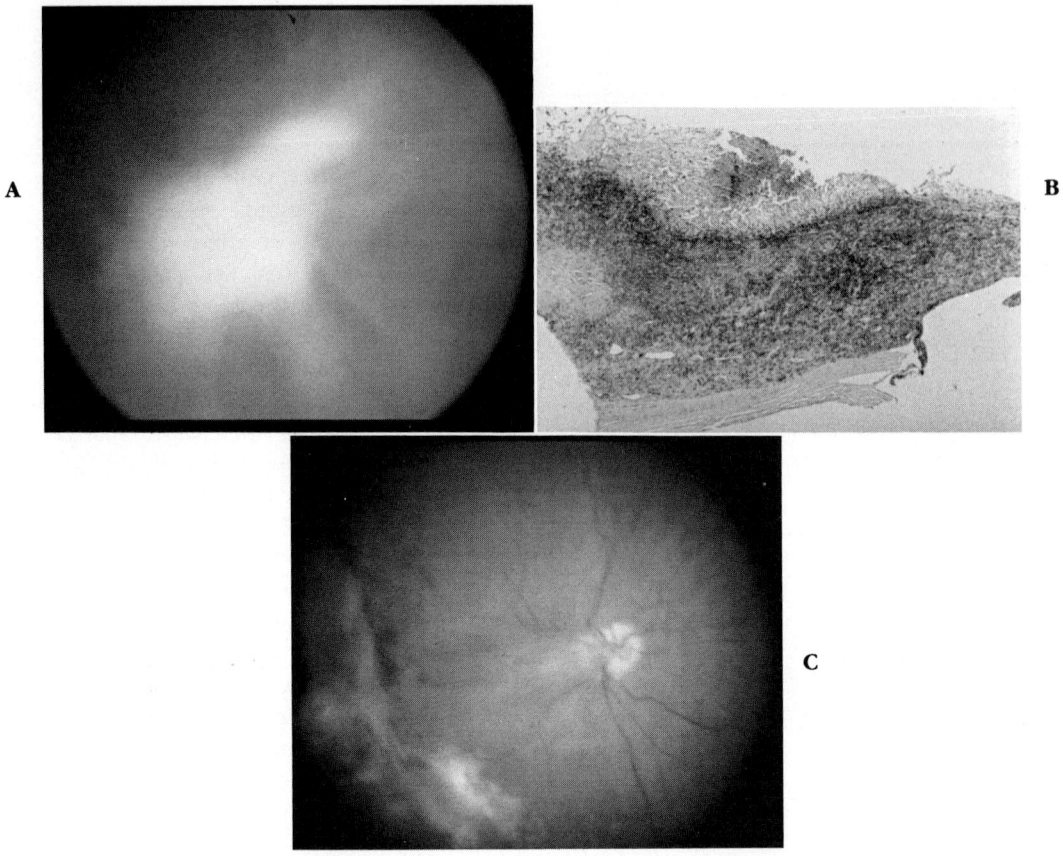


**Fig. 16-2. A,** Posterior traction detachment caused by large granuloma. After pars plana vitrectomy, lesion was removed in toto through retinotomy site. **B,** Histologic findings of lesion were characteristic of toxocariasis lesion. Result of ELISA for *Toxocara canis* found vitreous sample markedly positive. **C,** Posterior pole after surgery. Vision improved from hand motion (HM) to 15/200. (Courtesy Prof. M. Gonvers, Lausanne, Switzerland.) (See Color Plate 32.)

### Case 16-1

A 5-year-old boy was referred for examination after having failed a routine eye-screening examination in his pediatrician's office. According to his parents, he had no visual complaints and his behavior appeared normal. Both a physical examination performed by the pediatrician and a complete blood cell count with a differential were normal. Although the family had no pets, several neighbors owned dogs. The visual acuity was 20/400 OD, 20/20 OS. There was a small angle exotropia. The anterior segment was quiet. The intraocular pressure was normal. The lens was clear. The vitreous in the right eye had 1+ cell with trace haze. The vitreous of the left eye was quiet. In the macula of the right eye, there was a gray-white subretinal granulomatous macular lesion, preretinal gliosis extending from the disk to the macula associated with retinal wrinkling. The left eye was normal. Result of the ELISA for *Toxocara canis* was positive at 1:64, and the diagnosis of ocular *Toxocara canis* was made. The child was started on a course of systemic corticosteroids, but there was no improvement of visual acuity in that eye, and the therapy was stopped. The posterior segment has remained unchanged for over 3 years.

## REFERENCES

1. Calhoun FP: Intraocular invasion by the larva of the ascaris, *Arch Ophthalmol* 18:963-970, 1937.
2. Wilder HC: Nematode endophthalmitis, *Trans Am Acad Ophthalmol Otolaryngol* 55:99-109, 1950.
3. Nichols RL: The etiology of visceral larava migrans. I. Diagnostic morphology of infective second stage *Toxocara* larvae, *J Parasitol* 42:349-362, 1956.
4. Molk R: Ocular toxocariasis: a review of the literature, *Ann Ophthalmol* 15:216-231, 1983.
5. Kazacos KR: Visceral and ocular larva migrans, *Semin Vet Med Surg (small animal)* 6:227-235, 1991.
6. Uga S: Prevalence of *Toxocara* eggs and number of faecal deposits from dogs and cats in sandpits of public parks in Japan, *J Helminthol* 67:78-82, 1993.

7. Mok CH: Visceral larva migrans, *Clin Pediatr* 7:565-573, 1968.
8. Schantz PM, Weis PE, Pollard ZF, White MC: Risk factors for toxocaral ocular larva migrans: a case-control study, *Am J Public Health* 12:1269-1272, 1980.
9. Brown DH: Ocular *Toxocara canis*. II. clinical review, *J Pediatr Ophthalmol* 7:182-191, 1970.
10. Diallo JS: Syndromes de larva migrans. In *Manifestations opthalmologiques des parasitoses,* Paris, 1985, Masson, 155-161.
11. Upadhyay MP, Rai NC: Toxocara granuloma of the retina, *Jap J Ophthalmol* 24:278-281, 1980.
12. Rubin ML, Kaufman HE, Tierney JP, Lucas HC: An intraretinal nematode, *Trans Am Acad Ophthalmol Otolaryngol* 72:855-866, 1968.
13. Bird AC, Smith JL, Curtin VT: Nematode optic neuritis, *Am J Ophthalmol* 69:72-77, 1964.
14. Cox TA, Haskins GE, Gangitano JL et al: Bilateral toxocara optic neuropathy, *J Clin Neuro Ophthalmol* 3:267-274, 1983.
15. Brown GC, Tasman WS: Retinal arterial obstruction in association with presumed *Toxocara canis* neuroretinitis, *Ann Ophthalmol* 13:1385-1387, 1981.
16. Karel I, Peleska M, Uhlikova M et al: Larval migrans lentis, *Ophthalmologica* 174:14-19, 1977.
17. Steahly LP, Mader T: Acute ocular toxocariasis in adults, *J Ocul Ther Surg* 4:93-99, 1985.
18. Shields JA: Ocular toxocariasis: a review, *Surv Ophthalmol* 28:361-381, 1984.
19. Kennedy JJ, Defeo E: Ocular toxocariasis demonstrated by ultrasound, *Ann Ophthalmol* 13:1357-1358, 1981.
20. Howard GM, Ellsworth RM: Differential diagnosis of retinoblastoma, *Am J Ophthalmol* 60:610-616, 1965.
21. Wan WL, Cano MR, Pince KJ et al: Echographic characteristics of ocular toxocariasis, *Ophthalmology* 98:28-32, 1991.
22. Del Prete GF, De Carli M, Mastromauro C et al: Purified protein derivative of *Mycobacterium tuberculosis* and excretory-secretory antigen(s) of *Toxocara canis* expand in vitro human T cells with stable and opposite (type 1 T helper or type 2 T helper) profile of cytokine production, *J Clin Invest* 88:346-350, 1991.
23. Rockey JH, Donnelly JJ, Stromberg BE et al: Immunopathology of *Toxocara canis* and *Ascaris suum* infections of the eye: the role of the eosinophil, *Invest Ophthalmol Visual Sci* 18:1172-1184, 1979.
24. Rockey JH, John T, Donnelly JJ et al: In vitro interaction of eosinophils from ascarid-infected eyes with *Ascaris suum* and *Toxocara canis* larvae, *Invest Ophthalmol Visual Sci* 24:1346-1357, 1983.
25. Carter KC: The use of 35S-labelled *Toxocara canis* to determine larval numbers in tissues, *J Helminthol* 66:279-287, 1992.
26. Cuellar C, Fenoy S, Aguila C et al: Evaluation of chemotherapy in experimental toxocariasis by determination of specific immune complexes, *J Helminthol* 64:279-289, 1990.
27. el-Ganayni GA, Handousa AE: The effect of cyclosporin A (CSA) on murine visceral toxocariasis canis, *J Egypt Soc Parasitol* 22:487-494, 1992.
28. Glickman LT, Grieve RB, Lauria SS et al: Serodiagnosis of ocular toxocariasis: a comparison of two antigens, *J Clin Pathol* 38:103-107, 1985.
29. Gillespie SH, Bidwell D, Voller A et al: Diagnosis of human toxocariasis by antigen capture enzyme linked immunosorbent assay, *J Clin Pathol* 46:551-554, 1993.
30. Jacquier P, Gottstein B, Stingelin Y et al: Immunodiagnosis of toxocariasis in humans: evaluation of a new enzyme-linked immunosorbent assay kit, *J Clin Microbiol* 29:1831-1835, 1991.
31. Albert DM, Marcus LC: Ocular toxocariasis presenting as leukocoria in a patient with low ELISA titer to *Toxocara canis, Ophthalmology* 88:1302-1306, 1981.
32. Kieler RA: *Toxocara canis* endophthalmitis with low ELISA titer, *Ann Ophthalmol* 15:447-449, 1983.
33. Sharkey JA, McKay PS: Ocular toxocariasis in a patient with repeatedly negative ELISA titre to *Toxocara canis, Br J Ophthalmol* 77:253-254, 1993.
34. Magnaval JF, Fabre R, Maurieres P et al: Application of the western blotting procedure for the immunodiagnosis of human toxocariasis, *Parasitol Res* 77:697-702, 1991.
35. Felberg NT, Shields JA, Federman JL: Antibody to *Toxocara canis* in the aqueous humor, *Arch Ophthalmol* 99:1563-1564, 1981.
36. Wilkinson CP, Welch RB: Intraocular toxocara, *Am J Ophthalmol* 71:921-930, 1971.
37. Dinning WJ, Gillespie SH, Cooling RJ et al: Toxocariasis: a practical approach to management of ocular disease, *Eye* 2:580-582, 1988.
38. Hagler WS, Pollard ZF, Jarrett WH et al: Results of surgery for ocular *Toxocara canis, Ophthalmology* 88:1081-1086, 1981.
39. Belmont JB, Irvine A, Benson W et al: Vitrectomy in ocular toxocariasis, *Arch Ophthalmol* 100:1912-1915, 1982.
40. Gonvers M, Mermoud A, Uffer S et al: Ocular *Toxocara canis* in a 30-year-old adult, *Klin Monatsbl Augenheilkd* 200(5):522-524, 1992.
41. Maguire AM, Green WR, Michels RG et al: Recovery of intraocular *Toxocara canis* by pars plana vitrectomy, *Ophthalmology* 97:675-680, 1990.

# CHAPTER 17

# Onchocerciasis and Other Parasitic Diseases

## ONCHOCERCIASIS

### Clinical appearance

Onchocerciasis or river blindness is a disease that affects about 18 to 20 million people in the world with some 10% considered visually handicapped as a direct result of the disorder.[1,2] In developing countries, blindness occurs at 10 times the rate reported in the industrialized world.[3] Ocular onchocerciasis has been declared one of the five major preventable causes of blindness by the World Health Organization (the others include cataract, trachoma, and xerophthalmia). The disease is caused by the tissue-dwelling parasite, the nematode *Onchocerca volvulus.* It is spread by the black flies of the *Simulium* species and is found in a broad belt across western and central Africa, as well as in Central America with small pockets in northern South America and the Arabian peninsula. The blackfly needs rapid running water to propagate, and therefore the endemic areas are usually the most fertile, which makes this disease of extraordinary import for the Third World countries affected.

The infected blackfly bites human beings, thereby introducing the infection. Polymerase chain reaction–mediated amplification methods and immunoblotting of the silk proteins permit the identification of sibling species of biting adult females.[4] Adult worms will ultimately develop and form into nodules found throughout the body often subcutaneously. The adult worms will lead to the production of the microfilariae that are released in extraordinary numbers. The diagnosis of the disease and the determination of the infestation rate is made by skin snips and counting the number of microfilariae found. The microfilariae are the major cause of most of the ocular disease. Table 17-1 describes other ocular manifestations involved in parasitic infections of the eye.

A major complication of onchocerca infestation is corneal disease. Microfilarial infestation in the cornea is related to visual loss over time,[5] and a large number of microfilariae in the anterior segment is related to irreversible visual loss.[6] In the cornea there is a punctate keratitis; there is the presence of "snowflake" opacities in the cornea associated with a fairly mild infestation. With a more intense infestation and time, there is a sclerosing keratitis and loss of vision (Figs. 17-1 and 17-2).

An iridocyclitis can be seen in conjunction with other aspects of the disease, though the intensity of the reaction can vary considerably.[7] In addition to atrophy of the iris, more serious

**Table 17-1.** Parasitic infections of eye

| Ocular manifestation | Disease |
|---|---|
| **ANTERIOR CHAMBER** | |
| Hyphema | *Loa-loa* (Central and West Africa),[76,77] gnathostomiasis (Asia)[78-80] |
| Hypopyon | Amebiasis (worldwide), cysticercosis (Latin America, India), gnathostomiasis, onchocerciasis (Africa, Latin America), toxocariasis |
| Iritis | Amebiasis, angiostrongylodiasis (Pacific),[80] hookworm, ascariasis, schistosomiasis (tropics),[81] caterpillar hairs, cysticercosis, *Giardia,* gnathostomiasis, leishmania (Asia, Latin America), *Loa-loa,* myiasis, onchocerciasis, tapeworm trichinosis, toxocariasis, trypanosomiasis (Africa, Latin America), Bancroft's filariasis (tropics) |
| **VITREOUS** | |
| Hemorrhage | Ascariasis, schistosomiasis, *Loa-loa,* trichinosis |
| Vitritis | Schistosomiasis,[82] caterpillar hairs, cysticercus, gnathostomiasis, onchocerciasis, toxocariasis, trichinosis |
| **CHOROID/RETINA** | |
| Degeneration, exudates, nodules, detachment | Angiostrongyliasis, amebiasis, babesiosis, caterpillar hairs, cysticercus, leishmania, *Loa-loa,* myiasis, onchocerciasis, trichinosis,[83] toxocariasis |
| Hemorrhage | Amebiasis, hookworm, ascariasis, schistosomiasis, cysticercus, giardia, gnathostomiasis, leishmania, linguatulosia, *Loa-loa,* myiasis, malaria, toxocariasis, trichinosis, trypanosomiasis |
| Arteriolar and venule occlusion | Toxocariasis, schistosomiasis, *Loa-loa* |
| Inflammation of RPE and retinal vasculitis | *Wuchereia bancrofti,*[84] onchocerciasis |

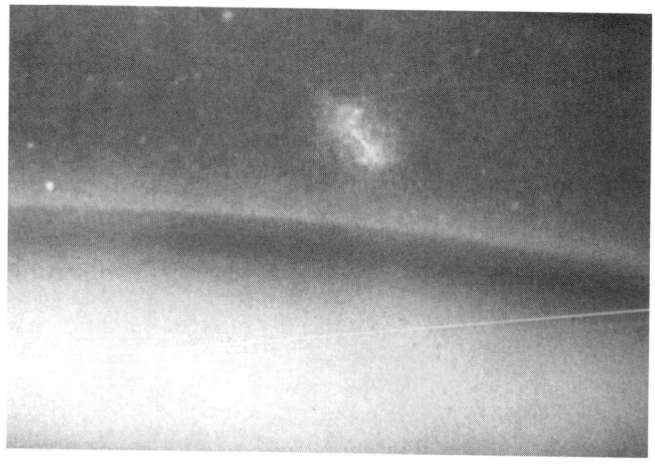

**Fig. 17-1.** Dead microfilaria of *Onchocerca* in cornea inducing localized inflammatory response recognized clinically as snowflake opacity. (Courtesy Hugh Taylor, M.D.)

complications such as secondary glaucoma and secondary cataract can occur. Glaucoma has been recognized as a possibly important cause of irreversible visual loss in these patients.[8] In addition, even without the presence of the inflammatory response, microfilariae can be seen in the anterior chamber. However, the patient needs to be placed in a darkened room with his/her head down between the knees for a few minutes. With the use of a slit lamp the observer will note the presence of the swirling microfilariae in the anterior chamber.

Alterations of the posterior pole have been seen as well, and the degree of visual impair-

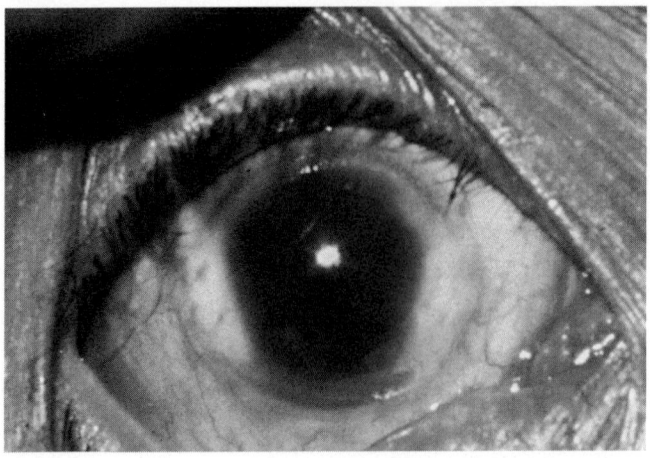

**Fig. 17-2.** Sclerosing keratitis in case of onchocerciasis. (Courtesy Hugh Taylor, M.D.)

ment caused by these changes have probably been underestimated in the past. Large areas of chorioretinitis as well as optic nerve disease leading to atrophy can be seen (Fig. 17-3). Newland and colleagues[9] examined 800 persons in an hyperendemic region of the rain forest in Liberia, West Africa. They found chorioretinal changes in 75% of the people examined; this strongly suggests that the visual impairment in this rain forest region was due largely to chorioretinal disease and not to anterior segment changes.

Relatively few eyes with this condition have been studied histologically. It is thought that the microfilariae may enter through the ciliary vessels, both the short as well as the long.[10,11] Another possibility is the passage of microfilariae through the cerebrospinal fluid into the optic nerve sheath[12] or direct invasion through the sclera through the parasite's release of digestive enzymes.[13]

It should be noted that the ocular disease is thought in most patients to be a result of slow, chronic, and relatively insidious changes. However, acute episodes of glaucoma, uveitis, and optic nerve disease may be an important component to some patients' disease.

Laboratory studies have been attempted to better deduce the mechanism of systemic infestation, and to a lesser degree work has concentrated on ocular disease. The only known natural animal host besides the human being is the gorilla,[14] although the disease has been induced in the chimpanzee[15] and the

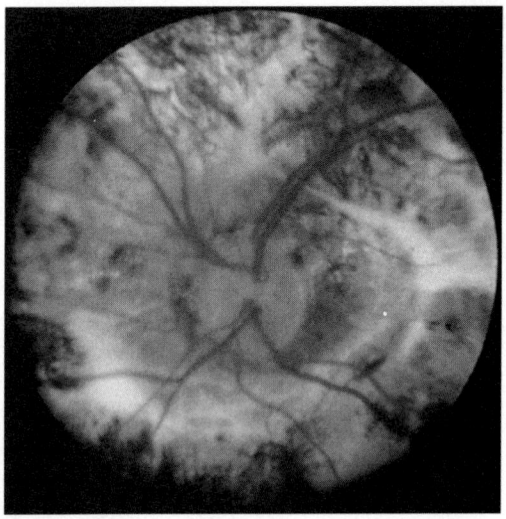

**Fig. 17-3.** Montage of retina of patient with ocular manifestations of onchocerciasis. Extensive chorioretinal al-terations can be seen. This change is underrecognized as cause of visual handicap in this disorder. (Courtesy David Cogan, M.D.)

cynomolgus monkey where *Onchocerca lienalis* was used.[16] Using a rabbit model, Duke and Garner[17] placed *Onchocerca volvulus* into the vitreous or subretinally and observed chorioretinal alterations. The injection of *O. lienalis* subconjunctivally in guinea pigs produced a lesion that resembled that seen in human onchocercal punctate keratitis.[18] A monkey model for this disease that was induced with the injection of 10,000 live *O. volvulus* microfilariae into the vitreous of monkeys has produced posterior segment lesions similar to that seen in the human disease.[19]

### Tests

Laboratory studies would suggest that the parasite induces a complex immune response, perhaps in part autoimmune. IgE production is a prominent feature of onchocerca infestation, and circulating immune complexes that presumably contain parasite antigen can be detected.[20] Cell-mediated responsivity is decreased,[21] a phenomenon noted in other helminth infections. Chan and colleagues[22] examined the ocular fluids and sera from patients with onchocerciasis for the presence of antiretinal autoantibodies. They found that these patients had antibodies directed toward the inner retina (nerve fiber, ganglion cell, and Müller cell) that could not be absorbed with the use of either S-antigen or the interphotoreceptor binding protein. These observations suggested that autoimmune mechanisms may play a role in the retinal degeneration and optic nerve disease seen so frequently in these patients. Van der Lelij and colleagues,[23] in finding high titers of antionchocerca antibodies in the aqueous of onchocerciasis patients with ocular disease, believed that retinal autoimmunity was an improbable factor in the pathogenesis of onchocercal chorioretinopathy.

However, an immunologic cross-reactivity between an antigen of *O. volvulus* and that found in the retinal pigment epithelium was recently identified. Antisera from patients with onchocerciasis will identify a 22,000 Mr antigen from onchocerca, whereas a 44,000 Mr antigen from cultured human retinal pigment epithelium will be immunoprecipitated with the same antiserum.[24] Kläger and colleagues[25] used Western blots and showed that antibody reactions against this antigen were seen in all patients tested with onchocerciasis and posterior pole disease but were not seen in controls. These provocative results would suggest that molecular mimicry plays an important role in the development of at least certain aspects of the ocular complications noted in this disorder. It further strengthens the notion as with ocular toxoplasmosis that our notions of inflammatory systems can no longer be restricted to only one mechanism, but indeed multiple and in some ways intellectually contradictory routes may have been stimulated. Autoantibody responses are not restricted to the eye. Such cross-reactivity has been reported against five major autoantigens, anticalreticulum activity, and the 65-kDa arthritis-associated mycobacterial heat shock protein.[26]

The regulation of IL-5 production in onchocerciasis has recently been evaluated. It has been suggested that in some helminthic infections the production of IL-5 may be associated with an immune or resistant state. It appears that in patients who are "immune" to *Onchocerca,* both IL-2 and IL-5 are produced in significantly higher levels than in those patients with acute infection. Further, IL-2 production is required to induce IL-5.[27]

### Therapy

Therapeutic strategies have been varied. A long-term approach has been an attempt to rid the endemic regions of the vector, the blackfly. This has been successful in a large area of West Africa, but this approach has been expensive and needs constant monitoring to prevent encroachment of blackflies from non-insec-ticide–treated regions. Until recently, three modalities were available to treat the patient. The first was nodulectomy, i.e., removing the adult worms that produce the microfilariae. Nodulectomy was reported by Rodolfo Robles in Central America in 1915 to improve the ophthalmic disease, and this approach has been practiced in Guatemala since 1935. Indeed, though hard evidence concerning its effectiveness is lacking, the rate of blindness in the endemic regions has decreased from 1935 to 1979, during which 1.5 million people have been examined and 257,883 nodules excised.[28] Nodulectomy has not significantly altered the number of microfilariae in skin snips from patients in West Africa.

The second and third modalities available were specific therapies against the *Onchocerca* organism. Specific therapy for the onchocerca organism was for many years limited to diethylcarbamazine citrate (DEC-C) and suramin. DEC-C is microfilaricidal, and with the massive killing of these organisms a severe systemic reaction occurs (Mazzotti reaction). An aggravation of the ocular condition, with limbitis, increase in corneal opacities, and advancement of sclerosing keratitis can also occur. Further,

Bird and colleagues[29] observed that DEC-C administration induced transient pigment epithelial lesions, optic disc leakage, and visual field loss. Its administration sometimes necessitates corticosteroid coverage. Though suramin is more toxic to adult worms than to microfilariae, killing of the microfilariae still leads to secondary reactions. Further, this drug has an intrinsic toxicity that may be fatal. Because of this, suramin is best given in progressive doses over 6 to 8 weeks until a total dosage of 60 to 67 mg/kg is reached. Both of these drugs must be used with great care, and patients should be followed-up closely by physicians with experience in their use.

Other drugs that were evaluated include the benzimidazoles, and a quantification of ocular reactions as a result of the therapy has been published.[30] These compounds have an effect on the embryogenesis of various *Onchocerca* species, thereby sterilizing the adult worms. Testing of these compounds suggested embryogenesis was interrupted in adult worms in the nodules of onchocerca patients 2 months after therapy.[31] However, these drugs are poorly absorbed orally, and standard dosages may not be particularly effective.

A macrofilaricidal agent, ivermectin, has shown enormous potential in the treatment of onchocerciasis. Given as a single oral dose of 150 μmg/kg, it is believed that it will control or curtail the disease if given on a wide scale in endemic areas.[1,3] Ivermectin was compared with DEC-C in a double-masked randomized study in the treatment of the ocular changes caused by onchocerciasis.[32] It was found that although DEC-C caused a marked increase in both living and dead microfilariae in the cornea inducing a limbitis and punctate keratitis, ivermectin did not. Further, ivermectin resulted in a long-term reduction in intraocular microfilariae when given in a single oral dose of 200 μg/kg. Other studies have demonstrated similar results.[33,34] Diallo and colleagues[33] noted that microfilarial densities reached 4% of pretherapy levels 1 year after a single 12 mg dose of ivermectin, but one of 10 ivermectin-treated patients needed systemic steroids to deal with the adverse systemic reactions. In this study, adult worms taken from patients treated with ivermectin were examined; they contained deformed and degenerated intrauterine forms of the microfilariae. In one report preliminary findings in the distribution of ivermectin to 118,925 persons in Nigeria, Ogunba, and Gemade were that the drug was extremely well tolerated; only 0.7% of recipients reported adverse reactions within 3 days of treatment.[35] Whitworth and colleagues[36] reported the results of a randomized double-masked study in Sierra Leone that compared the effects of ivermectin to placebo on ocular disease. They found that the 296 persons who received ivermectin had less anterior segment disease, lower prevalence of microfilariae in the anterior chamber and cornea, and less punctate keratitis and iritis than seen in the 272 patients who received placebo. No difference was found between the two groups when comparing optic atrophy or chorio-retinitis, and the visual acuities in the two groups were not statistically significantly different though the results favored the ivermectin group. Dadzie and colleagues[37] found very low ocular microfilariae loads in 334 patients in Ghana who were treated twice with the medication. Three new cases of blindness did occur in the ivermectin group; these were thought to have occurred in patients with advanced disease. However, one report by Njoo and colleagues[38] is somewhat less heartening. In a considerably smaller study of patients with onchocerciasis from an hyperendemic area with no vector control, 44% of 25 patients who received three doses of ivermectin still had positive skin snips, but the number of adverse reactions did decrease with repeated administration. The study did suggest that therapy alone without vector control may not be the ideal approach in many areas.

Another drug that has received a great deal of interest for the treatment of onchocerciasis is amocarzine. This drug, now being actively tested, was found (at a dose of 3 mg/kg twice daily) to have killed 73% of 1477 female worms at nodulectomy 4 months after treatment. There was as well a marked drop in the microfilarial skin count, and it remained low for at least 6 months.[39]

## GIARDIASIS

*Giardia lamblia* is a flagellated binucleate protozoan about 12 to 14 μm in length. It can be in a motile form (trophozoite) or in a cystic state. Ingestion of contaminated food or drinking water is the usual mode of spread. It has a propensity to inhabit the jejunum of human beings where it will multiply and cause swelling of the microvilli of the intestinal epithelial cells. Gastrointestinal symptoms include epigastric burning, cramps, diarrhea, constipation, and weight loss. Though extraintestinal spread of the organism has not been documented to date, there have been reports of patients with extraintestinal manifestations attributed to *Giardia*.[40,41] These manifestations include nervousness, headache, and emotional instability. To our knowledge, Barraquer[42] was the first to make the association between giardiasis and ocular inflammatory disease, noting choroiditis, hemorrhagic retinopathy, and iridocyclitis. Knox and King[43] reported the finding of *Giardia* in the stool of three patients with retinal arteritis, which was associated with an iridocyclitis in two of them. It was felt that antiparasitic therapy improved their ocular state. The underlying cause of the ocular inflammatory disease is unknown, though the most plausible explanation at this point is that the inflammation results from an hypersensitivity reaction.

The diagnosis is based on finding the organism in the stools, which is not always easy to do. Multiple examinations or even the biopsy of jejunal tissue is needed. The disease is treated with quinaquine hydrochloride (Atabrine) (100 mg) given three times a day for 10 days.

## OPHTHALMOMYIASIS

The term *opthalmomyiasis* refers to the infestation of the eye by the larval forms of flies in the order Diptera. Ophthalmomyiasis externa would indicate infestation of the conjunctiva, whereas interna would mean inside the globe. Usually, these larval forms are obligate tissue parasites that require the host's tissue to complete its developmental cycle. In addition to human beings, the usual hosts for these larvae include cattle, deer, sheep, horses, and reindeer. The larvae may get to the eye via a vector such as the adult fly that carries the larvae or eggs to the region or by touching of the ocular region with hands contaminated with the larvae. Most patients do not give a history of being "bitten." The larva is thought to bore through the coats of the eye until coming to rest within. However, an early report by DeBoe[44] described the emergence of the larva from the optic nerve head into the vitreous. A handful of cases have been described in the literature.

Seventeen cases of ophthalmomyiasis externa were seen by Amr and colleagues[45] in northern Jordan. These were due to the sheep nasal botfly, *Oestrus ovis;* the symptoms were mild to severe conjunctivitis, cellulitis, and lacrimation. Four reported cases were due to *Oestrus ovis* in Kuwait both before and after Operations Desert Shield and Desert Storm.[46] Other species involved include *Cochliomyia hominivorax*.[47]

In cases of ophthalmomyiasis interna, the invading larva may initially cause little or no pain, but discomfort and an intraocular inflammatory reaction can certainly occur,[48] particularly after its death.[49] The characteristic features of ophthalmomyiasis interna include the presence of subretinal tracks[50,51] along with the finding of an encysted larva either subretinally or even free floating in the vitreous. Without finding the maggot in the eye, a definitive diagnosis cannot be made; the maggot is white or semitranslucent, segmented, and tapered at both ends.[50] Vision may be lost because of macular hemorrhage, optic nerve invasion by the maggot, or retinal detachment. Recently, Campbell and colleagues[52] reported that an interesting retinopathy that resembled ophthalmomyiasis interna was seen in 10% of a sample Chamorro population examined on the island of Guam. In addition, this retinopathy was found in 50% of a population with amyotrophic lateral sclerosis/Parkinsonism-dementia complex. Though the retinopathy appears to be similar to the changes seen with parasitic infestation, they were not able to establish a definitive diagnosis in spite of obtaining eyes for histologic study.

The treatment of ophthalmomyiasis must be tailored to the ocular findings. If there is no inflammatory disease and good vision, the ophthalmologist may elect to follow the patient. However, if there is a severe inflammatory reaction, antiinflammatory therapy should be instituted. If the larva can be visualized in the subretinal space, and if the decision is made to treat it, Gass and Lewis[50] have recommended the use of photocoagulation over removal of the organism by sclerotomy. Forman and colleagues[53] described a case of a 16-year-old patient with a subretinal fly larva in which the larva was killed with argon laser therapy. The visual acuity improved from 20/200 to 20/20. Syrdalen and colleagues[54] reported the removal of the reindeer warble fly larva through a pars plana opening after vitrectomy freed the surrounding vitreous attachments. The patient retained good vision.

## CYSTICERCOSIS

Cysticercosis is more common in areas with poor hygiene. It is more common in the first four decades of life and is rare in the United States, but it is commonly seen in Central and South America. This disease is caused by the ingestion of the eggs of *Taenia solium*. The larva migrate to the eye where it encysts (Fig. 17-4). Often the scolex of the larva can be seen moving slowly in the vitreous.[55] An anterior chamber tap will reveal a large number of eosinophils. The presence of the parasite can be disastrous for the eye, particularly if it is located in the subretinal space. Vitrectomy can be used to remove the larva if it is in the vitreous[56] with a potential for good postoperative vision. However, the removal of subretinal lesions may not lead to a good visual outcome.[57] The larva can be removed via a sclerotomy site, and repair of the detachment caused by the presence of the parasite with a scleral buckling procedure can be tried.[56] There are usually no overt systemic findings in this disorder. However, cysticercosis has been identified as the cause of severe medial rectus muscle myositis.[58]

## CATERPILLAR HAIRS

Caterpillar hairs have been known since ancient times to be toxic to human beings. Ocular disease was first associated with the caterpillar in the last century. Several species of caterpillar have hairs that form a row on their dorsal surface and that contain histamine-liberating substances[59] that are released only if the hair is broken. It is theorized that these hairs reach the eye by being airborne or when a person prunes a tree or bush containing these caterpillars. Once the hair reaches the eye, the movement of the globe and lids may force the hair into the eye itself and cause the disease described here. If it stays on the surface of the globe, then a small granulomatous reaction in the conjunctiva will ensue. A caterpillar hair keratitis has also been reported.[60]

The initial entry into the eye may cause an immediate inflammatory reaction with pain, photophobia, and anterior uveitis. Later findings include chorioretinal lesions. According to Raspiller and colleagues,[61] this may occur anywhere from 1½ to 16 years after the initial insult. They stress two characteristics of these chorioretinal lesions. The first is the presence of a track or tracks that represent the migration of the hairs that align in the anteroposterior direction and reflect the hairs' migration from the anterior to the posterior portion of the globe. The second aspect to these lesions is the formation of white nodules or outpouchings along the track (Fig. 17-5).

Treatment for this problem lies in trying to prevent situations in which caterpillar hairs can be released. Certainly if a caterpillar hair can be seen on the ocular surface, one should attempt

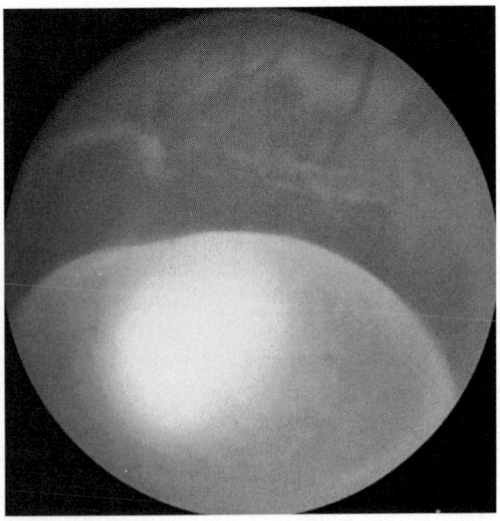

**Fig. 17-4.** *Cysticerca* organism seen through cystic retina. (Courtesy Miguel Burnier, Jr., M.D.)

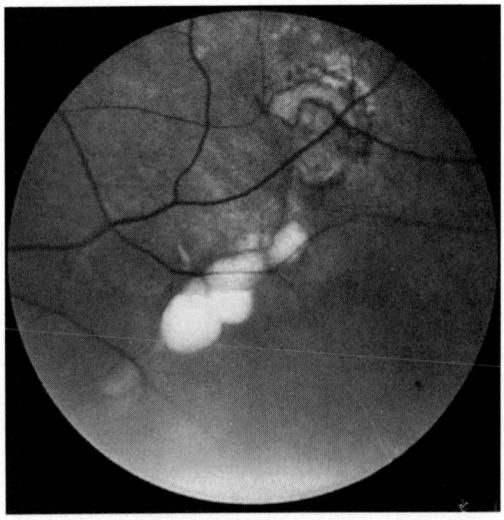

**Fig. 17-5.** Presumed caterpillar hairs causing track anteroposteriorly in temporal retina.

to remove it at the slit lamp. If the hair is noted in the anterior chamber or vitreous, then its surgical removal may be considered. Raspiller and colleagues[61] have suggested placing a barrier of laser photocoagulation in front of the progressing track to prevent it from extending into the macular region. The use of antiinflammatory agents is certainly indicated to reduce the inflammatory response and to make the patient more comfortable.

## AMEBIASIS

It is estimated that 10% of the world population is infested with *Amoeba,* and at least half the population in Central and South America as well as Asia. Most of the symptoms are gastrointestinal. However, intraocular inflammatory disease has on occasion been associated with the parasite. Rodger and colleagues[62] reported that intermediate uveitis was common in patients with amebic dysentery. Several reports have reported that various *Entamoeba*[63] as well as *Acanthamoeba*[64] cause a chorioretinal lesion. The disease is characterized by a subretinal whitish exudative lesion most commonly in the macular region. Associated with this will be hemorrhage as well as disturbances of the retinal pigment epithelium. In cases of dysentery, the ameba can be found in stool samples, but this is not always the case in hepatic amebiasis.

## DIFFUSE UNILATERAL SUBACUTE NEURORETINITIS

Although *Toxocara canis* involvement of the eye has been recognized for a long while, there is certainly the possibility that other heretofore unrecognized nematodes may also cause ocular disease. An example of this is diffuse unilateral subacute neuroretinitis (DUSN). This ocular disease was first described by Gass[65] in 1977 and termed the unilateral wipe-out syndrome. In 1978 he changed the name to DUSN to better describe the syndrome.[66] Later in that year Gass published an article in which he observed a motile subretinal nematode in two patients with DUSN.[67] On further searching of the literature, Gass was able to identify previously reported cases of similar nematodes that produced the same clinical picture as early as 1952.[68] Hence a syndrome of initially unknown cause that was classified only by clinical description was later found to be related to a nematode in the subretinal space. The understanding of the cause thereby suggested possible therapies that were not considered when the disease was thought to be idiopathic.

DUSN begins as scattered recurrent deep gray-white retinal lesions and marked loss of central acuity. There is often moderate vitreal inflammation, but there may be no observable inflammation in some cases. Optic disc swelling may be present. As the disease advances, there is progressive optic atrophy, narrowing of the retinal vessels, pigment epithelial stippling, and further visual field loss. The electroretinogram is significantly decreased. Careful examination with a contact lens may disclose a motile worm moving in the subretinal space. The details about the worm's size will be discussed below. Occasionally the worm may be seen in the vitreous. In some patients subretinal tracks that correspond to previous movement of the worm can be seen. The examination light may cause the worm to move. Granulomatous masses, such as those that are seen in classic *Toxocara canis,* are not observed in DUSN. Fluorescein angiography has demonstrated no fluorescence of the gray-white lesions in the early angiogram stages with late staining of these lesions.[67] Perivascular staining and mottled retinal pigment epithelial window defects are also seen. Before the identification of the worm, several disorders can be considered in the differential diagnosis. These would include acute multifocal posterior placoid epitheliopathy (AMPPE), toxoplasmosis, optic neuritis, as well as posttraumatic retinal and choroidal ischemia.

Because the movement of the worm is thought to cause destruction of the retinal outer segments, visual loss is rarely reversible. An acuity of less than 20/200 is seen in about one half the cases.[67] Occasional patients have retained good vision without treatment. An associated creeping skin eruption suggestive of systemic nematode infection is seen in some patients.

Worms of two sizes have been described in eyes with DUSN.[68] A smaller worm between 400 and 1200 micra was seen in most cases in which the patient lived in the southeast United States. A larger (1500 to 2000 micra) worm has been seen in patients residing in the northern and midwestern states (Fig. 17-6). However, this geographic relationship does not always hold up to careful scrutiny. The worms have been

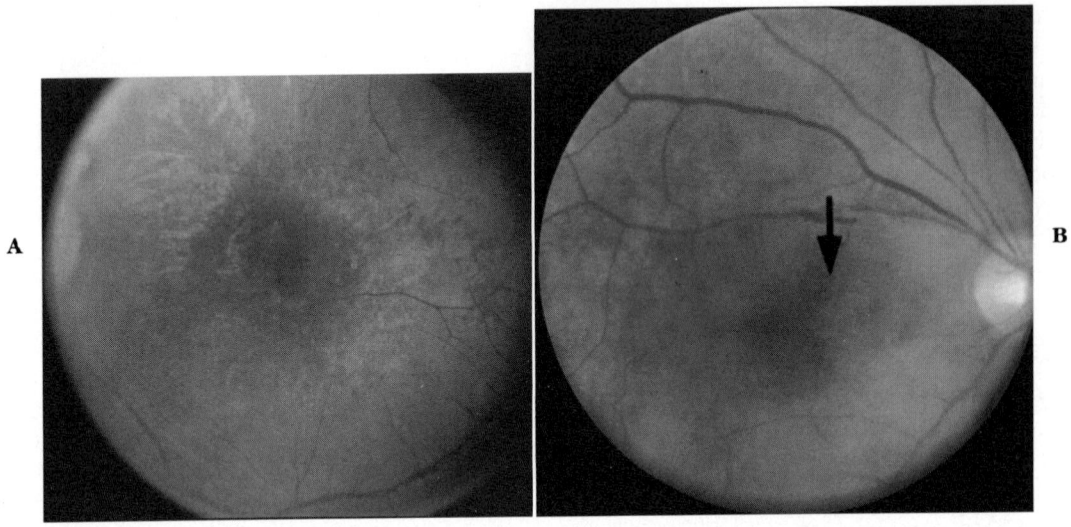


**Fig. 17-6.** Fundus photographs of worms causing DUSN from **A,** southern part of United States and **B,** northern part of United States. (Courtesy J. Donald Gass, M.D.) (See Color Plate 33.)

described as about 1/20 their length in diameter.

Identification of the type of nematode in DUSN is still unsettled. Titers for *Toxocara canis* have been looked for in patients with DUSN and are invariably negative. Eosinophilia is occasionally seen. In 1984 it was suggested that the larger worms in patients living in more northern climates were *Baylisascaris procyonis,* a nematode found in racoons.[69] *Toxocara* rarely exceeds 400 micra in length. Experimental infection of subhuman primates and other experimental animals by *Baylisascaris procyonis* eggs orally has produced a clinical picture that is similar to DUSN.[70] A recently reported case of unilateral DUSN from the western United States implicated *Baylisascaris* as the causative agent as well.[71] However, no patient with DUSN has had the neurologic complications that have been associated with infection by this nematode. It is likely that the clinical picture of DUSN can be produced by a variety of nematodes that find their way by chance to the eye and destroy the retina. These nematodes may include toxocara in some patients in spite of the very low toxocara antibodies that are found because the smaller worms seen in DUSN are of the correct size for toxocara.

Medical therapy with thiabendazole, an antihelminthic agent, or corticosteroids have not been successful in the treatment of DUSN. The worm has been successfully destroyed by photocoagulation.[68,72] In this disease, death of the worm is not associated with an increased inflammatory response. In addition, if the worm can be localized in the periphery of the retina, it can be surrounded by photocoagulation and then excised. Destruction of the worm by photocoagulation appears to halt the progression of DUSN. Although the risk factors for the development of this type of ocular larval migrans are uncertain and the exact type of nematode in each case is still not specified, the recognition of the cause of this disease has led to the beginnings of a logical therapeutic approach.

Although nematodes have been reported in the eye, there are few reports of trematodes. McDonald and colleagues[73] reported two cases of *Alaria mesocercaria,* a trematode, in the eyes of two unrelated Asian men who presumably were exposed while eating poorly cooked frog's legs. They both presented with unilateral disease, choroidal tracks, and other findings similar to that of DUSN. In one case the organism was killed with laser, and in the other case the trematode was removed surgically from the vitreous.

## SEASONAL HYPERACUTE PANUVEITIS

A curious entity has been reported by Upadhyay and colleagues[74] in Nepal. This severe and usually unilateral disease has been noted to occur principally in children. It has occurred in two cycles; the first was recognized soon after the monsoon season of 1975. The disease begins very acutely with a red eye and leukocoria with little pain. There may be a

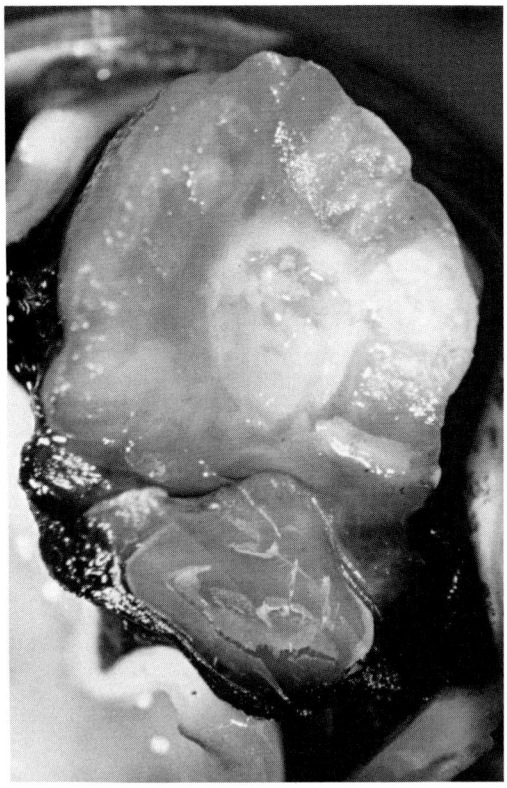

**Fig. 17-7.** Sectioned eye with seasonal hyperacute panuveitis. Eye has intraocular hemorrhage and cataract. Dense white structure in center of vitreous is totally detached retina.

fibrinoid reaction in the anterior chamber and often there is also an hypopyon. This is followed by hypotony and a very sudden drop in vision. Examination of the posterior segment is obscured by the leukocoria. The anterior chamber ultimately becomes flat and the eye becomes phthisical (Fig. 17-7). Therapy to date has not been able to reverse the disease.

Work-up of these children has revealed no systemic abnormalities to date. Circulating immune complexes were not elevated. Evidence of S-antigen sensitization could not be demonstrated.[75] Several children were noted to be exposed to moths, but laboratory experiments attempting to define if antigens from the moth induced uveitis were not successful.[45] Histologic examination reveals a severe inflammatory response with lymphocytes and plasma cells noted and with the retina drawn up into the retrolenticular mass. Eosinophils did not make up a significant proportion of the cell population. Neither worms nor virus particles could be identified. At present the underlying cause of this disorder remains unknown.

## REFERENCES


1. Malatt HR, Taylor HR: Onchocerciasis, *Infect Dis Clin North Am* 6:963-977, 1992.
2. World Health Organization: WHO Onchocerciasis: report of the WHO expert committee on onchocerciasis, WHO technical report series no. 752, Geneva, Switzerland, 1987.
3. Narita AS, Taylor HR: Blindness in the tropics, *Med J Aust* 159:416-420, 1993.
4. Brockhouse CL, Vajime CG, Marin R et al: Molecular identification of onchocerciasis vector sibling species in black flies *(Diptera: Simuliidae), Biochem Biophys Res Commun* 194:628-634, 1993.
5. Anderson J, Fuglsang H, Marshall TF: Effects of diethylcarbamazine on ocular onchocerciasis, *Tropenmed Parasitol* 27:263-275, 1976.
6. Thylefors B, Brinkman UK: The microfilarial load in the anterior segment of the eye: a parameter of intensity of onchocerciasis, *Bull World Health Org* 55:731-737, 1977.
7. Maertens K: Tonography in onchocerciasis, *Bull Soc Panafr Ophthal* 5:23-27, 1982.
8. Thylefors B, Duppenthaler JL: Epidemiological aspects of intraocular pressure in an onchocerciasis endemic area, *Bull World Health Org* 57:963-969, 1979.
9. Newland HS, White AT, Greene BM et al: Ocular manifestations of onchocerciasis in a rain forest area of West Africa, *Br J Ophthalmol* 75:163-169, 1991.
10. Neumann E, Gunders AE: Pathogenesis of the posterior segment lesion of ocular onchocerciasis, *Am J Ophthalmol* 75:82, 1973.
11. Budden FH: The natural history of ocular onchocerciasis over a period of 14-15 years and the effect on this of a single course of suramin, *Trans Roy Soc Trop Med Hyg* 70:484-491, 1976.
12. Duke BOL, Vincelette J, Moore PJ: Microfilariae in the cerebrospinal fluid, and neurological complications during treatment of onchocerciasis with diethylcarbamazine, *Tropenmed Parasitol* 27:123-132, 1976.
13. Tonjum AM, Thylefors B: Aspects of corneal changes in onchocerciasis, *Brit J Ophthalmol* 62:458-461, 1978.
14. Van den Berghe L, Chardome M, Peel E: The filiarial parasites of the eastern gorilla in the Congo, *J Helminthol* 38:349-368, 1964.
15. Duke BOL: Experimental transmission of *Onchocerca volvulus* from man to chimpanzee, *Trans Roy Soc Trop Med Hyg* 56:271, 1962.
16. Donnelly JJ, Taylor HR, Young E et al: Experimental ocular onchocerciasis in Cynomolgus monkeys, *Invest Ophthalmol Vis Sci* 27:492-499, 1986.
17. Duke BOL, Garner A: Fundus lesions in the rabbit eye following inoculation of *Onchocerca volvulus* microfilariae into the posterior segment. II. pathology, *Tropenmed Parasitol* 27:19-29, 1976.
18. Sakla AA, Donnelly JJ, Lok JB et al: Punctate keratitis induced by subconjunctivally injected microfilariae of *Onchocera lienalis, Arch Ophthalmol* 104:894-898, 1986.
19. Semba RD, Donnelly JJ, Young E et al: Experimental ocular onchocerciasis in cynomologous monkeys. IV. chorioretinitis elicited by *Onchocerca volvulus* microfilariae, *Invest Ophthalmol Vis Sci*32:1499-1507, 1991.

20. Somorin AO, Hewer DC, Ajugwo RE: Immunoglobulin in Nigerian onchocerciasis, *Ann J Trop Med Hyg* 26:872-876, 1977.
21. Ngu JL, Blackett K: Immunological studies in onchocerciasis in Cameroon, *Trop Geogr Med* 28:111-120, 1976.
22. Chan CC, Nussenblatt RB, Kim MK et al: Immunopathology of ocular onchocerciasis. II. Anti-retinal autoantibodies in serum and ocular fluids, *Ophthalmology* 94:439-443, 1987.
23. Van der Lelij A, Rothova A, de Vries JP et al: Analysis of aqueous humour in ocular onchocerciasis, *Curr Eye Res* 10:169-176, 1991.
24. Braun G, McKechnie NM, Connor V et al: Immunological cross-reactivity between a cloned antigen of *Onchocerca volvulus* and a component of the retinal pigment epithelium, *J Exp Med* 174:169-177, 1991.
25. Kläger S, Taylor DW, Alexander RA et al: Immunologic cross-reactivity in the pathogenesis of ocular onchocerciasis, *Invest Ophthalmol Vis Sci* 34:2888-2902, 1993.
26. Meilof JF, Van der Lelij A, Rokeach LA et al: Autoimmunity and filariasis: autoantibodies against cytoplasmic cellular proteins in sera of patients with onchocerciasis, *J Immunol* 151:5800-5809, 1993.
27. Steel C, Nutman TB: Regulation of IL-5 in Onchocerciasis: a critical role for IL-2, *J Immunol* 150:5511-5518, 1993.
28. UNDP/World Bank/WHO special programme for research and training in tropical diseases: The pathogenesis and treatment of ocular onchocerciasis: report of the eighth meeting on the scientific working group on filariasis in collaboration with the programme for the prevention of blindness, Geneva, Switzerland, October 20-22, 1982.
29. Bird AC, El Sheikh H, Anderson J et al: Changes in visual function and in the posterior segment of the eye during treatment of onchocerciasis with diethylcarbamazine citrate, *Brit J Ophthalmol* 64:191-200, 1980.
30. Hero M, Bird AC, Awadzi K: Quantification of the ocular reactions to microfilaricides in the chemotherapy of onchocerciasis, *Eye* 6(Part 1):93-96, 1992.
31. Rivas-Alcala AR, Greene BM, Taylor HR et al: Chemotherapy of onchocerciasis: a controlled comparison of mebendazole, levamisole, and diethylcarbamazine, *Lancet* 2:485-492, 1981.
32. Taylor HR, Murphy RP, Newland HS et al: Treatment of onchocerciasis: the ocular effects of ivermectin and diethylcarbamazine, *Arch Ophthalmol* 104:863-870, 1986.
33. Diallo S, Aziz MA, Lariviere M et al: A double-blind comparison of the efficacy and safety of ivermectin and diethylcarbamazine in a placebo-controlled study of Senegalese patients with onchocerciasis, *Trans R Soc Trop Med Hyg* 80:927-934, 1986.
34. Dadzie KY, Bird AC, Awadzi K et al: Ocular findings in a double-blind study of ivermectin versus diethylcarbazine versus placebo in the treatment of onchocerciasis, *Br J Ophthalmol* 71:78-85, 1987.
35. Ogunba EO, Gemade EI: Preliminary observations on the distribution of ivermectin in Nigeria for control of river blindness, *Ann Trop Med Parasitol* 86:649-655, 1992.
36. Whitworth JA, Gilbert CE, Mabey DM et al: Effects of repeated doses of ivermectin on ocular onchocerciasis: community-based trial in Sierra Leone, *Lancet* 338: 1100-1103, 1991.
37. Dadzie KY, Remme J, De Sole G: Changes in ocular onchocerciasis after two rounds of community-based ivermectin treatment in a holoendemic onchocerciasis focus, *Trans R Soc Trop Med Hyg* 85:267-271, 1991.
38. Njoo FL, Stilma JS, van der Lelij A: Effects of repeated ivermectin treatment in onchocerciasis, *Doc Ophthalmol* 79:261-267, 1992.
39. Poltera AA, Zea-Flores G, Guderian R et al: Onchocercacidal effects of amocarzine (CGP 6140) in Latin America, *Lancet* 337:583-584, 1991.
40. Welch PB: Giardiasis with unusual clinical findings: preliminary report, *Am J Digest Dis* 10:52-55, 1943.
41. Webster BH: Human infection with Giardia lamblia: an analysis of 32 cases, *Am J Digest Dis (New Series)* 3:64-71, 1958.
42. Barraquer I: Sur la coincidence de la lambliase et de certaines lésions du fond de l'oeil, *Bull Soc Pathol Exot (Paris)* 31:55-58, 1938.
43. Knox DL, King J Jr: Retinal arteritis, iridocyclitis, and giardiasis, *Ophthalmology* 89:1303-1308, 1982.
44. DeBoe MP: Dipterous larva passing from the optic nerve into the vitreous chamber, *Arch Ophthalmol* 10:824-825, 1933.
45. Amr ZS, Amr BS, Abo-Shehada MN: Ophthalmomyiasis externa caused by *Oestrus ovis* L. in the Ajloun area of northern Jordan, *Ann Trop Med Parasitol* 87:259-262, 1993.
46. Hira PR, Hajj B, al-Ali F, Hall MJ: Ophthalmomyiasis in Kuwait: first report of *Oestrus ovis* before and after the Gulf conflict, *J Trop Med Hyg* 96:241-244, 1993.
47. Chodosh J, Clarridge J: Ophthalmomyiasis: a review with special reference to Cochliomyia hominivorax, *Clin Infect Dis* 14:444-449, 1992.
48. Dixon JM, Winkler CH, Nelson JH: Ophthalmomyasis interna caused by *Cuterebra* larva, *Trans Am Ophthalmol Soc* 67:110-115, 1969.
49. Godde-Jolly D, Brumpt ML, Stofft P: Un cas d'ophtalmomyase "hypoderma boris" de la chambre anterieure, *Bull Soc Ophtal Fr* 2:48-56, 1966.
50. Gass JDM, Lewis RA: Subretinal tracks in ophthalmomyiasis. *Arch Ophthalmol* 94:1500-1505, 1976.
51. Slusher MM, Holland WD, Weaver RG et al: Ophthalmomyiasis interna posterior: subretinal tracks and intraocular larvae, *Arch Ophthalmol* 97:885-887, 1979.
52. Campbell RJ, Steele JC, Cox TA et al: Pathologic findings in the retinal pigment epitheliopathy associated with the amyotrophic lateral sclerosis/Parkinsonism-dementia complex of Guam, *Ophthalmology* 100:37-42, 1993.
53. Forman AR, Cruess AF, Benson WE: Ophthalmomyiasis treated by argon-laser photocoagulation, *Retina* 4:163-165, 1984.
54. Syrdalen P, Nitter T, Mehl R: Ophthalmomyiasis interna posterior: report of case caused by reindeer warble fly larva and review of previous reported cases, *Br J Ophthalmol* 66:589-593, 1982.
55. Meyerson L, Pienaar BT: Intraocular cysticercus, *Br J Ophthalmol* 45:148-153, 1961.
56. Topilow HW, Yimoyines DJ, Young GA et al: Bilateral multifocal intraocular cysticercosis, *Ophthalmology* 88:1166-1172, 1981.
57. Segal P, Mrzyglod S, Dudarewiex JS: Subretinal cysticercosis in the macular region, *Am J Ophthalmol* 57:655-664, 1964.

58. Stewart CR, Salmon JF, Murray ADN et al: Cysticercosis as a cause of severe medial rectus muscle myositis, *Am J Ophthalmol* 116:510-511, 1993.
59. Diallo JS: *Manifestations Ophtalmologiques des parasitoses,* Paris, 1985, Masson.
60. Teske SA, Hirst LW, Gibson BH et al: Caterpillar induced keratitis, *Cornea* 10:317-321, 1991.
61. Raspiller A, Lepori JC, George JL: Choriorétinopathie par migration de poils de chenilles, *Bull Mem Soc Fr Opthalmol* 95:153-156, 1984.
62. Rodger FC, Chir PK, Hosain ATMM: Night blindness in the tropics, *Arch Ophthalmol* 63:927-935, 1960.
63. Braley AE, Hamilton HE: Central serous choroiditis associated with amebiasis, *Arch Ophthalmol* 58:1-14, 1957.
64. Schlaegel TF Jr, Culbertson C: Experimental Hartmanella optic neuritis and uveitis, *Ann Ophthalmol* 4:103-112, 1972.
65. Gass JDM: Some problems in the diagnosis of macular diseases. In *Symposium on Retinal Disease;* Trans of the New Orleans Acad of Ophthalmol, St Louis, 1977, Mosby, 260-274.
66. Gass JDM, Scelfo R: Diffuse unilateral subacute neuroretinitis, *J R Soc Med* 71:95-111, 1978.
67. Gass JDM, Braunstein RA: Further observations concerning the diffuse unilateral subacute neuroretinitis syndrome, *Arch Ophthalmol* 101:1689-1697, 1983.
68. Parson HE: Nematode chorioretinitis: report of a case with photographs of a viable worm, *Arch Ophthalmol* 47:799-800, 1952.
69. Kazacos KR, Vestre WA, Kazacos EA et al: Diffuse unilateral subacute neuroretinitis syndrome: a probable cause, *Arch Ophthalmol* 102:967-968, 1984.
70. Kazacos KR, Raymond LA, Kazacos EA et al: The racoon ascarid: a probable cause of human ocular larva migrans, *Ophthalmology* 92:1735-1744, 1985.
71. Goldberg MA, Kazacos KR, Boyce WM et al: Diffuse unilateral subacute neuroretinitis: morphometric, serologic, and epidemiologic support for Baylisascaris as a causative agent, *Ophthalmology* 100:1695-1701, 1993.
72. Raymond LA, Gutierrez Y, Strong LE et al: Living retinal nematode destroyed by photocoagulation, *Ophthalmology* 85:944-949, 1978.
73. McDonald HR, Kazacos KR, Schatz H et al: Two cases of intraocular infection with *Alaria mesocercaria (Trematoda), Am J Ophthalmol* 117(4):447-55, 1994.
74. Upadhyay MP, Rai NC, Ogg JE et al: Seasonal hyperacute panuveitis of unknown etiology, *Ann Ophthalmol* 16:38-44, 1984.
75. Upadhyay MP, Rai N, Ogg JE et al: Seasonal hyperacute panuveitis. In Saari KM, editor: *Uveitis update,* Amsterdam, 1984, Excerpta Medica, pp 257-262.
76. Botero D, Aguledo LM, Uribe FJ et al: Intraocular filaria, a *Loaina* species, from man in Columbia, *Am J Trop Med Hyg* 33:578-582, 1984.
77. Lee BY, McMillian R: Loa loa: ocular filariasis in an African student in Missouri, *Ann Ophthalmol* 16:456-458, 1984.
78. Tuder RC, Blair E: Gnathostoma spingerum: an unusual cause of ocular nematodiasis in the western hemisphere, *Am J Ophthalmol* 72:185-190, 1971.
79. Bathrick ME, Mango CA, Mueller JF: Intraocular gnathostomiasis, *Ophthalmology* 88:1293-1295, 1981.
80. Singalavanija A, Wangspa S, Teschareon S: Intravitreal angiostrongyliasis, *Aust NZ J Ophthalmol* 14:381-384, 1986.
81. Newton JC, Kanchanaranya C, Previte LR: Intraocular Schistosoma mansoni, *Am J Ophthalmol* 65:774-778, 1968.
82. Vedy J, Carrica A, Rivaud C et al: A propos d'un cas de rétinite chez un bilharzien, *Med Trop* 39:603-609, 1979.
83. Behrens-Baumann W, Freissler G: Retinochoroidopathy in a patient with seropositive trichinosis, *Klin Monatsbl Augenheilkd* 199:114-117, 1991.
84. Gupta A, Agarwal A, Dogra MR: Retinal involvement in Wucheria bancrofti filariasis, *Acta Ophthalmol (Copenh)* 70:832-835, 1992.

# CHAPTER 18

# Postsurgical Uveitis

Intraocular inflammation can occur after any ocular surgical procedure. It is especially important in the postoperative patient, to differentiate infectious causes of uveitis from other causes of intraocular inflammation because bacterial and fungal endophthalmitis require prompt treatment with specific antimicrobial therapy. The major causes of postsurgical uveitis are listed in Box 18-1.

Patients with a preexisting uveitis often have an exacerbation of intraocular inflammation after surgery. The flare-up usually occurs 3 days to a week after the surgery in patients who receive subconjunctival corticosteroids at the end of the surgical procedure. The inflammation may occur earlier in patients who do not receive steroids. Occasionally, the uveitis can be severe enough to be confused with an infectious endophthalmitis, although hypopyon and severe pain are rare in cases of noninfectious postsurgical uveitis. In contrast, low-grade intraocular inflammation is common after many ocular surgeries, especially after cataract extraction. This inflammation appears to be mediated by prostaglandins and can be inhibited by prostaglandin inhibitors.[1] However, some infectious agents such as *Propionibacterium acnes* may produce a low-grade postsurgical endophthalmitis that may take months to develop.

**Box 18-1**
**Causes of postoperative intraocular inflammation**

**DAY 1–DAY 30**

Acute aerobic bacterial endophthalmitis
Sterile endophthalmitis
Increased activity of previous uveitis
Phacogenic (lens-related) uveitis
Toxic reaction to intraocular lens

**DAY 15–2 YEARS**

Fungal endophthalmitis
*Propionibacterium acnes* or other anaerobic endophthalmitis
Low virulence aerobic bacterial endophthalmitis
Phacogenic (lens-related) uveitis
Sympathetic ophthalmia
Toxic reaction to intraocular lens
Iris-ciliary body irritation related to physical contact with intraocular lens
New onset of idiopathic uveitis

## ACUTE BACTERIAL ENDOPHTHALMITIS

Most cases of bacterial endophthalmitis occur after intraocular surgery and are a surgical emergency. Fortunately, postsurgical endophthalmitis is a rare condition that occurs in less than 1% of cases. Allen and Mangiaracine reported 22 cases of endophthalmitis in a series of 20,000 ocular operations (0.11%),[2] and nine cases in a second series of 16,000 operations (0.056%).[3] Wound problems appear to be an important contributing factor in about 25% of endophthalmitis cases,[4] and infectious endophthalmitis may be a more common problem after glaucoma surgery.[5]

The time interval between surgery and the

onset of inflammation is helpful in distinguishing bacterial endophthalmitis from other causes of postoperative inflammation. Most cases of aerobic bacterial infections occur within 3 to 7 days after surgery. Pain and diminished vision are accompanied by conjunctival hyperemia, chemosis, and lid edema. Anterior uveitis with fibrin, hypopyon, and vitritis are also characteristic of a bacterial endophthalmitis. These symptoms and signs should prompt a diagnostic evaluation that includes culture of intraocular fluids usually obtained during vitrectomy surgery. Even in cases of endophthalmitis after anterior segment surgery, cultures of the vitreous more frequently yield positive cultures than those of the aqueous.[6] The most common organisms include *Staphylococcus aureus* and *Staphylococcus epidermidis.*

The management of bacterial endophthalmitis includes vitrectomy, intravitreal, systemic, subconjunctival and topical antibiotics, and corticosteroids.[4,7] However, only 75% of eyes with a clinical picture consistent with bacterial endophthalmitis will have a positive bacterial culture.[4] These cases should, however, initially be treated as bacterial endophthalmitis until they have improved or until other clinical information suggests an alternative diagnosis. Although sterile endophthalmitis can occur in the early postoperative period and may mimic a bacterial infection, the consequences of untreated bacterial endophthalmitis are so severe that cultures and antibiotic therapy should not be delayed.

## CHRONIC BACTERIAL ENDOPHTHALMITIS

Although most cases of postsurgical bacterial endophthalmitis present with the acute onset of severe inflammation and loss of vision and pain, some bacteria can cause a chronic indolent intraocular infection. These organisms are more difficult to culture and grow more slowly. *Propionibacterium acnes* has recently been recognized as an organisms that can cause a chronic postoperative uveitis, especially after cataract extraction with intraocular lens placement.[8–10] The typical patient with *P. acnes* endophthalmitis presents with chronic low-grade anterior segment inflammation that starts from 2 months to 2 years after cataract surgery. Topical corticosteroids often suppress the inflammation early in the course of the disease but do not prevent the protracted low-grade inflammatory response. White

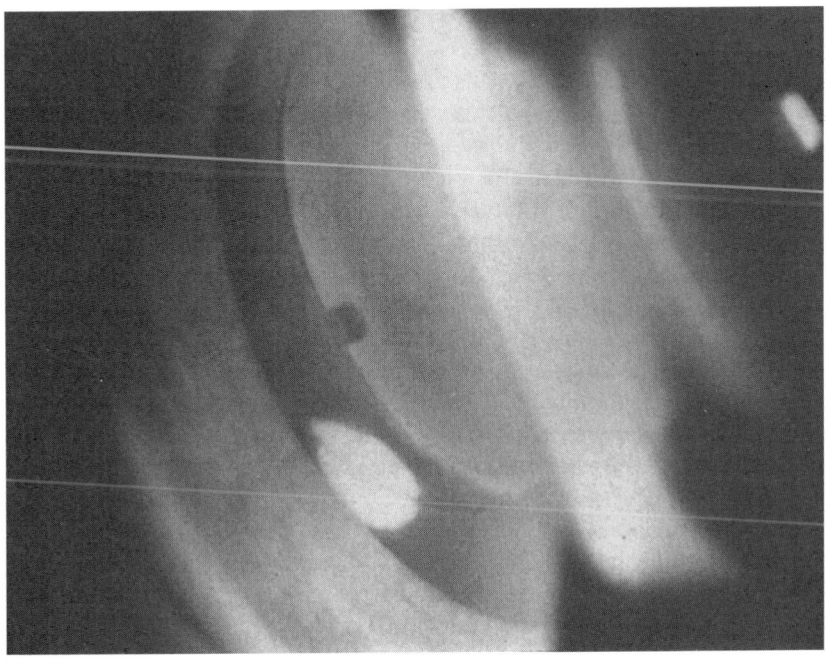

**Fig. 18-1.** Infiltrate on lens haptic in patient with late-onset postoperative endophthalmitis caused by *Propionibacterium acnes.* (Courtesy Robert Martin, M.D.) (See Color Plate 34.)

plaques composed of bacteria are often seen between the intraocular lens and the posterior capsule or on the intraocular lens haptics (Fig. 18-1). The clinical course of *P. acnes* endophthalmitis may resemble that of pseudophakic phacoanaphylaxis,[11,12] and it is not clear whether some of these cases were actually undiagnosed *P. acnes* infection.

We have shown that in addition to the predominance of polymorphonuclear cells, the inflammatory infiltrate in eyes with *P. acnes* endophthalmitis includes a large number of macrophages (10% to 15%).[13] The presence of residual lens material in some cases suggests that lens-induced uveitis may be contributing to the inflammation.[9,12] Others have suggested that *P. acnes* immunopotentiation may be caused by an inhibition of suppressor T cells caused by stimulated macrophages.[14]

Diagnosis of *P. acnes* endophthalmitis is based on culture data. It is important to inform the microbiology laboratory not to discard the cultures after the normal 3 to 4 days. Because the organism is slow growing, cultures should be maintained by the microbiology laboratory for 14 days before they are read as negative. Therapy for *P. acnes* endophthalmitis usually involves a combination of vitrectomy with posterior capsulectomy, intravitreal vancomycin, and systemic cephalosporins. Although the intraocular lens does not need to be removed at the time of initial therapy, recurrent cases are managed with repeat intravitreal antibiotics and removal of residual posterior capsule and the intraocular lens. Despite the delay in diagnosis and therapy of this chronic endophthalmitis, the visual prognosis is usually good. Other organisms including *Propionibacterium granulosum, Achromobacter,* and *Staphylococcus epidermidis* may also cause a chronic bacterial endophthalmitis.[15] However, in addition to these bacteria, fungal endophthalmitis may also cause chronic smoldering postoperative intraocular inflammation.

## FUNGAL ENDOPHTHALMITIS

Fungal endophthalmitis is a relatively rare condition; however, as our diagnostic abilities improve, the incidence of this condition appears to be increasing. Recent studies show that fungus accounts for 8% to 13% of culture positive isolates, and the *Candida* species predominate.[4,6] Fungal infections may not become symptomatic for months after the surgery. They often start with low-grade iridocyclitis or vitritis. Symptoms of blurred vision, redness, and pain gradually increase. Corticosteroid therapy can temporarily ameliorate the symptoms but should be avoided. With time the infection progresses, and "fluff balls" may form in the vitreous in addition to anterior uveitis and vitritis. A discrete fungal mass may be present in the vitreous or anterior chamber in some eyes.[16] The risk factors and ocular characteristics of postsurgical and endogenous fungal infection are listed in Table 18-1.

Untreated fungal endophthalmitis leads to blindness. Even after the correct diagnosis is made, treatment initiated late in the course of the disease may be unsuccessful at restoring vision. In a recent study only 42% of eyes had a visual acuity of 20/400 or better after treat-

**Table 18-1.** Characteristics of fungal infections (postsurgical and endogenous)

| Organism | Risk factors | Ocular characteristics |
|---|---|---|
| *Candida* sp. | IV drug use, chronic IV therapy, surgery | Yellow-white chorioretinal lesions, vitreous fluff balls |
| *Aspergillus* sp. | IV drug use, immunosuppression, surgery | Yellow-white chorioretinal lesions, vitreous fluff balls |
| *Coccidioides immitis* | Southwest USA | Multiple yellow-white chorioretinal lesions, punched-out choroidal lesions; often associated with pulmonary *C. immitis* infection |
| *Cryptococcus neoformans* | Immunosuppression, lymphoma | Small or large yellow-white chorioretinal lesions; often associated with meningitis |
| *Histoplasma capsulatum* | Immunosuppression | Panuveitis with iris involvement |
| *Sporotrichum schenckii* | Horticulturists | Panuveitis |
| *Blastomyces dermatitidis* | Systemic North American blastomycosis | Panuveitis or multiple small chorioretinal lesions |

ment for fungal endophthalmitis.[16] Patients who present early with good acuity (better than 20/60) have a more favorable visual prognosis.[16] Infection with *Acremonium* or *Fusarium* are associated with a poorer prognosis.

The diagnosis of fungal endophthalmitis should be suspected in all cases of postoperative inflammation that occur weeks to months after the surgery. Rarely, fungal infection may occur within a week after the surgical procedure. If fungal infection is suspected, it is helpful to pass part of the vitreous specimen through a millipore filter and to culture the filter as a method of concentrating the organisms. It takes days for the cultures to grow, and *Candida, Fusarium,* and *Aspergillus* are the most common causes of the disorder. The use of Calcofluor or Calcofluor white staining techniques on vitreous samples allows the rapid identification of fungal elements and has improved diagnostic speed and accuracy.[17]

Antifungal therapy combined with vitrectomy and removal of an intraocular lens offer the best chance of a favorable outcome. Some cases have been successfully managed without intraocular lens removal, especially in candida endophthalmitis.[16,18] Amphotericin B is still the mainstay of therapy. Ten micrograms of amphotericin B are instilled into the vitreous; this dose can be repeated once if needed. Intraocular miconazole (25 to 50 μg) can be used in patients not responding to treatment with amphotericin B. Topical and subconjunctival antifungal agents may be used in infections that involve the cornea. Oral flucytosine is useful in candidal infections that are not resistant. Oral ketoconazole may also be beneficial in preventing recurrence, and some experts have suggested this drug as a primary therapy instead of amphotericin B.[16]

## LENS-INDUCED UVEITIS

Phacoanaphylactic (phacoantigenic) uveitis is a granulomatous inflammatory response that is thought to represent an immunologic reaction against lens proteins released after surgical or traumatic disruption of the lens capsule. Phacoanaphylactic uveitis is somewhat of a misnomer because the reaction is not an anaphylactoid or type I hypersensitivity reaction. This form of lens-induced uveitis is differentiated from the nongranulomatous phacogenic (phacotoxic) uveitis, although there is no evidence to support the theory that lens degradation products are directly toxic to the eye.[19,20] It now appears that all these entities may represent varying severity of the same immunologic process that is better termed *lens-induced uveitis.*

Lens-induced uveitis may occur spontaneously in an eye with a hypermature lens or may follow ocular trauma or cataract surgery. A number of researchers have reported a high incidence of lens-induced uveitis after sympathetic ophthalmia.[19,20] However, isolated lens-induced uveitis is usually uniocular occurring in the most recently surgically treated eye; sympathetic ophthalmia is a bilateral disease.[21] The inflammation may occur hours or months after disruption of the lens capsule. Granulomatous keratic precipitates, anterior chamber cells and flare, and occasionally a hypopyon may be seen.

The inflammation can be severe and associated with both anterior uveitis and vitritis. Removal of all residual lens material is usually curative. Response to corticosteroids is poor. If some lens material is mixed with vitreous, a vitrectomy may be indicated. Lens-induced uveitis was rare in the 1960s when intracapsular cataract surgery was performed, but it is much more common with extracapsular cataract extraction. Lens-induced uveitis may be difficult to distinguish clinically from chronic endophthalmitis such as *P. acnes* infection[8,9]; therefore cultures should be obtained in most cases of chronic postoperative intraocular inflammation.

## INFLAMMATION FROM AN INTRAOCULAR LENS

Early intraocular lenses were associated with a variety of toxic reactions caused by problems with lens design material. Cases of intraocular lens-related uveitis included reactions against metal haptics,[22] impurities on the lens from the manufacturer,[23] certain methods of sterilization,[24] and degradation of lens haptics.[25] Although these reactions are usually not immunologically driven, the resultant tissue damage can then lead to prostaglandin and cytokine release and the recruitment of lymphocytes and other inflammatory cells into the eye. This secondary immune-mediated inflammation can often be more damaging than the initial toxic reaction to the intraocular lens. Some old models of anterior chamber intraocular lenses were associated with the development of a syndrome characterized by uveitis, glaucoma, and hyphema (the UGH syndrome).[26] Fortunately, the UGH syndrome is uncommon with current anterior chamber intraocular lenses with flexible haptics.

Intraocular lenses sometimes cause mild inflammation that leads to the accumulation of cellular deposits on the anterior surface of the lens.[27,28] These deposits are often composed of macrophages and giant cells but may be acellular.[28] Membranes are often associated with these intraocular lens deposits. Clearly, most eyes tolerate a posterior chamber intraocular lens with little inflammation.[29] However, some patients have a mild iridocyclitis that can be seen histologically, even if the lens was clinically well tolerated.[30] The safety of intraocular lens placement in patients with chronic uveitis remains debatable and is discussed in greater detail in Chapter 9 on the role of surgery in the uveitis patient.

## LASER-INDUCED UVEITIS

Yttrium-aluminum-garnet (YAG) laser capsulotomy has been associated with low-grade inflammation.[31] The shock wave created by the laser is capable of causing a physical alteration in the blood-ocular barrier. We have observed several cases of patients with a history of ongoing intraocular inflammation in which the YAG laser capsulotomy caused a significant increase in inflammation. Increased topical, periocular, or even systemic corticosteroids may be required at the time of the laser procedure in some patients. We recently diagnosed an unusual case of endophthalmitis that appeared to be induced after a YAG laser iridectomy. The iridectomy was performed in a patient with closed-angle glaucoma with minimal bleeding from an iris vessel. Two days after the procedure the patient developed a hypopyon. The patient was diagnosed as having a sepsis, and the same organism grew from both cultures of the eye and from blood cultures.

### Case 18-1

A 66-year-old woman underwent bilateral extracapsular cataract surgery with posterior chamber intraocular lens implantation. The two surgical procedures were performed 6 weeks apart. After surgery the visual acuity was 20/20 in each eye. Two months after surgery an anterior uveitis developed in the right eye, and white material was noted on the polypropylene lens haptic (Fig. 18-1).

The anterior uveitis initially resolved with topical and periocular corticosteroids. However, the patient had recurrent episodes of uveitis and eventually developed a hypopyon and vitritis. The intraocular lens was removed and replaced with a new intraocular lens. Bacterial and fungal cultures were reported as negative. The intraocular inflammation persisted despite oral corticosteroids. Repeat aqueous and vitreous cultures were obtained and both were positive for *P. acnes* 5 days after inoculation. Cytologic examination of the specimens showed macrophages and neutrophils with few lymphocytes. The patient received intravitreal cephazolin and intravenous cephalexin. Two weeks later there was a moderate amount of persistent inflammation and a second intravitreal injection of cephazolin was given. The inflammation resolved, and the patient's vision improved to 20/20.

## REFERENCES


1. Huang K, Peyman GA, McGetrick J et al: Indomethacin inhibition of prostaglandin mediated inflammation following intraocular surgery, *Invest Ophthalmol Vis Sci* 16:1760-1762, 1977.
2. Allen HF, Mangiaracine AB: A study of 22 infections in 20,000 operations, *Arch Ophthalmol* 72:454-462, 1964.
3. Allen HF, Mangiaracine AB: Bacterial endophthalmitis after cataract extraction. II. Incidence in 36,000 consecutive operations with special reference to preoperative topical antibiotics, *Arch Ophthalmol* 91:3-7, 1974.
4. Driebe WT, Mandelbaum S, Forster RK et al: Pseudophakic endophthalmitis: diagnosis and management, *Ophthalmology* 93:442-448, 1986.
5. Katz LJ, Cantor LB, Spaeth GL: Complications of surgery in glaucoma: early and late bacterial endophthalmitis following glaucoma filtering surgery, *Ophthalmology* 92:959-963, 1985.
6. Forster RK, Zachary IG, Cottingham AJ et al: Further observation on the diagnosis, cause, and treatment of endophthalmitis, *Am J Ophthalmol* 81:52-56, 1976.
7. Weber DJ, Hoffman KL, Thoft RA et al: Endophthalmitis following intraocular lens implantation, *Rev Infect Dis* 8:12-20, 1986.
8. Meisler DM, Palestine AG, Vastine DW et al: Chronic *Propionibacterium endophthalmitis* after extracapsular cataract extraction and intraocular lens implantation, *Am J Ophthalmol* 102:733-739, 1986.
9. Roussel TJ, Culbertson WW, Jaffe NS: Chronic postoperative endophthalmitis associated with *Propionibacterium acnes, Arch Ophthalmol* 105:1199-1120, 1987.
10. Jaffe NS: *Propionibacterium acnes* and endophthalmitis seven months after extracapsular cataract extraction and intraocular lens implantation, *Ophthalmic Surg* 17:791-793, 1986.
11. Apple DJ, Mamalis N, Steinmetz RL et al: Phacoanaphylactic endophthalmitis associated with extracapsular

cataract extraction and posterior chamber intraocular lens, *Arch Ophthalmol* 102:1528-1532, 1984.
12. McMahon MS, Weiss JS, Riedel KG et al: Clinically unsuspected phacoanaphylaxis after extracapsular cataract extraction with intraocular lens, *Br J Ophthalmol* 69:836-840, 1985.
13. Whitcup SM, Belfort R Jr, de Smet MD et al: Immunohistochemistry of the inflammatory response in *Propionibacterium acnes* endophthalmitis, *Arch Ophthalmol* 109:978, 1991.
14. Maguire HC Jr, Cipriano D: Immunopotentiation of cell-mediated hypersensitivity by *Corynebacterium parvum (Propionibacterium acnes), Int Arch Allergy Appl Immun* 70:34-39, 1983.
15. Flicker L, Meredith TA, Wilson LA et al: Chronic bacterial endophthalmitis, *Am J Ophthalmol* 103:745-748, 1987.
16. Pflugfelder SC, Flynn HW Jr, Zwickey TA et al: Exogenous fungal endophthalmitis, *Ophthalmology* 95:19-30, 1988.
17. Sutphin JE, Robinson NM, Wilhelmus KR et al: Improved detection of oculomycoses using induced fluorescence with Cellufluor, *Ophthalmology* 93:416-417, 1986.
18. Gilbert CM, Novak MA: Successful treatment of postoperative *Candida endophthalmitis* in an eye with an intraocular lens implant, *Am J Ophthalmol* 97:593-595, 1984.
19. Blodi FC: Sympathetic uveitis as an allergic phenomena, *Trans Am Acad Ophthalmol Otolaryngol* 63:642-656, 1959.
20. Easom HA, Zimmerman LE: Sympathetic ophthalmia and bilateral phacoanaphylaxis, *Arch Ophthalmol* 72: 9-15, 1964.
21. de Veer JA: Bilateral endophthalmitis phacoanaphylactica, *Arch Ophthalmol* 49:607-614, 1953.
22. Shepard DD: The dangers of metal loop intraocular lenses, *Ophthalmic Surg* 8:93-95, 1977.
23. Meltzer DW: Sterile hypopyon following intraocular lens surgery, *Arch Ophthalmol* 98:100-104, 1980.
24. Stark WJ, Rosenblum P, Maumenee AE et al: Postoperative inflammatory reactions to intraocular lens sterilized with ethylene oxide, *Ophthalmology* 87:385-389, 1980.
25. Krause U, Alanko HI: Dislocated intraocular lens after biodegradation of fixation loops, *Acta Ophthalmol* 64:338-343, 1986.
26. Ellingson FT: The uveitis-glaucoma-hyphema syndrome associated with the Mark VIII anterior chamber lens implant, *J Am Intraocul Implant Soc* 4:50-53, 1978.
27. Eifrig DE: Deposits on the surface of intraocular lenses, *South Med J* 73:6-8, 1980.
28. Wolter JR, Sugar A, Meyer RF: Reactive membranes on posterior chamber lens implants, *Ophthalmic Surg* 16:699-702, 1985.
29. Crawford JB: A histopathologic study of the position of the Shearing intraocular lens in the posterior chamber, *Am J Ophthalmol* 91:458-461, 1981.
30. McDonnell PJ, Green WR, Maumenee AE et al: Pathology of intraocular lenses in 33 eyes examined postmortem, *Ophthalmology* 90:386-403, 1983.
31. Flohr MJ, Robin AL, Kelley JS: Early complications following Q-switched neodymium YAG laser posterior capsulotomy, *Ophthalmology* 92:360-363, 1985.

# PART 5

# NONINFECTIOUS UVEITIC CONDITIONS

# CHAPTER 19

# Anterior Uveitis

## EPIDEMIOLOGY

Anterior uveitis is the most common form of uveitis and accounts for approximately three fourths of cases with an annual incidence rate of about 8 cases per 100,000 population.[1-3] Although anterior uveitis is usually the most easily managed form of uveitis, associated complications such as glaucoma may result in severe visual loss. In addition, many disorders that can cause a panuveitis, such as sarcoidosis, Behçet's disease, and bacterial endophthalmitis, may start as an anterior uveitis.

## CLINICAL DESCRIPTION

Anterior uveitis includes diseases previously categorized as both iritis (inflammation of the iris) and iridocyclitis (inflammation of the iris and ciliary body). Patients with anterior uveitis often complain of redness, pain, and photophobia; some patients are relatively asymptomatic. Tearing may occur, but ocular discharge is rare. Some patients with severe anterior uveitis may also complain of blurred vision. Conjunctival injection is frequently noted on examination. Ciliary flush, conjunctival injection in the perilimbal area, is characteristic of many forms of the disease. Pupillary miosis, posterior synechiae, and dilated iris vessels are common findings in all forms of anterior uveitis. However, sector abnormalities of the iris may suggest herpes zoster ophthalmicus as an underlying cause. The iris may also adhere to the trabecular meshwork forming peripheral anterior synechiae (PAS). These PAS should be looked for on gonioscopy because patients with severe PAS are at risk for secondary glaucoma. In addition, patients with severe posterior synechiae, iris adhesions to the lens, can develop pupillary block and may require prophylactic iridectomy.

The major indicators of anterior uveitis are the presence of cells and flare in the anterior chamber. Anterior chamber inflammation is assessed on slit-lamp biomicroscopy and is detailed in Chapter 4. These cells and flare represent extravasated inflammatory cells and protein as a result of a breakdown of the blood-aqueous barrier. A device has been developed that uses laser photometry to objectively assess anterior chamber cells and flare. Guex-Crosier and colleagues[4] recently used laser flare-cell photometry to demonstrate that blood-aqueous barrier disruption was very pronounced in idiopathic anterior uveitis, acute retinal necrosis, but minimal in patients with toxoplasmosis or Fuchs' heterochromic cyclitis. These authors suggest that laser flare-cell photometry provides a quantitative and sensitive assessment of anterior segment inflammation and may be useful for the management of patients with uveitis.

Fibrin may accumulate in the anterior chamber and may cause the once mobile cells that circulate in the aqueous to become frozen. This plasmoid aqueous is a sign of severe anterior uveitis that requires aggressive therapy. Another sign of severe anterior uveitis is a hypopyon composed of layered leukocytes. A hypopyon can be seen in a number of forms of anterior uveitis, but it is frequently

**Table 19-1.** Syndromes of anterior uveitis

| Disease | Age (yr) | Sex | Ocular redness | HLA-B27 | Systemic findings | Steroid response |
|---|---|---|---|---|---|---|
| Idiopathic | Any | Either | Yes | No | None | Yes |
| HLA-B27, ocular only | 15-40 | M > F | Yes | Yes | None | Yes |
| Ankylosing spondylitis | 15-40 | M > F | Yes | Yes | Spondylitis, sacroliitis | Yes |
| Reiter's syndrome | 15-40 | M > F | Yes | Yes | Arthritis, urethritis, mucocutaneous lesions | Yes |
| Juvenile rheumatoid arthritis | 3-16 | F > M | No | No | Pauciarticular arthritis, ANA* positive, RF† negative | Yes |
| Fuchs' iridocyclitis | Any | Either | No | No | None | Yes/No |
| Posner-Schlossman syndrome | Adult | Either | No | No | None | Yes |
| Schwartz syndrome | Adult | Either | No | No | None | No |
| Ocular ischemia | >50 | Either | Yes | No | Carotid insufficiency | No |
| Kawasaki syndrome | 1-18 | Either | Yes | No | Skin rash, lymphadenopathy, fever, cardiac lesions | Yes |

*ANA, antinuclear antibody.
†RF, rheumatoid factor.

associated with Behçet's disease or infectious endophthalmitis. Recently anterior uveitis, including some cases with hypopyons, has been described in patients with AIDS who are receiving the drug rifabutin as a treatment or prophylaxis for mycobacterial infection.[5-7] Also, hyphema may occur in patients with anterior uveitis, but it usually resolves without permanent damage.[8]

Inflammatory cells may also collect and adhere to the corneal endothelium and form keratic precipitates. The mechanism appears to involve the expression of cell adhesion molecules that are upregulated in the presence of inflammatory cytokines such as IL-1.[9–11] Large greasy-appearing keratic precipitates are suggestive of a granulomatous inflammation and may help in determining the cause of the uveitis (see Chapter 5).

During the acute inflammatory episode, the intraocular pressure is often decreased because of ciliary body shutdown with decreased aqueous production. As the inflammation subsides, however, the intraocular pressure may rapidly increase, especially in cases with severe PAS. In some patients, it is difficult to determine whether the increased intraocular pressure is a result of underlying inflammation or a steroid response to the corticosteroids used to control the disease. In cases of secondary glaucoma caused by active inflammatory disease, increased corticosteroid therapy will lead to a decrease in the intraocular pressure.

Although some of the clinical symptoms and signs of anterior uveitis are specific for certain diseases, most disorders are differentiated by their associated systemic findings. The clinical findings of the common disorders that cause anterior uveitis are summarized in Table 19-1. Some disorders, such as postsurgical inflammation, infectious uveitis, Behçet's disease, sarcoidosis, and the masquerade syndromes, are discussed in separate chapters.

## IDIOPATHIC ANTERIOR UVEITIS

After a thorough medical history and an ocular and general physical examination, almost 50% of patients are found to have an anterior segment inflammation that is not associated with other defined clinical syndromes. This form of anterior uveitis is referred to as idiopathic anterior uveitis. Patients with idiopathic anterior uveitis must not only lack systemic disease associations but also cannot have the HLA-B27 haplotype, which is associated with anterior segment inflammatory disease. In one study, 47% of anterior uveitis patients had HLA-B27–associated anterior uveitis[1]; however, about a quarter of these HLA-B27 positive patients also had underlying systemic disorders including ankylosing spondylitis and Reiter's syndrome. Nevertheless, the diagnosis of idiopathic anterior uveitis depends greatly on the extent of the evaluation for an underlying condition. Many of the cases initially diagnosed as idiopathic anterior uveitis are later diagnosed as a specific disorder.

### Diagnostic workup

A controversial topic in uveitis concerns the diagnostic evaluation of patients with a first episode of anterior uveitis. Some suggest that no evaluation is needed. Others state that a long laundry list of tests should be ordered. As with most things in life, the prudent approach probably lies somewhere in the middle, and as we discussed in Chapter 6; a complete medical history and thorough examination can help you target the workup. Clearly if the patient complains of lower back pain, a diagnosis of ankylosing spondylitis is suggested and the evaluation might consist solely of sacroiliac joint films and HLA-B27 testing. Similarly, a child with anterior uveitis with band keratopathy and a history of arthritis suggests a diagnosis of juvenile rheumatoid arthritis, and a targeted evaluation consisting of an antinuclear antibody (ANA) test and a rheumatoid factor may suffice.

However, when a thorough history and examination fail to suggest specific diagnoses, what tests should be ordered? We tend to do a limited workup of all patients with anterior uveitis even if it is their first episode. If the uveitis is nongranulomatous, we order a fluorescent treponemal antibody absorption test to rule out syphilis, because this test is both highly sensitive and specific for the disease, and because syphilis is treatable and early treatment can prevent long-term complications. Similarly we obtain results of a complete blood cell count and urinalysis to rule out an underlying systemic disorder such as connective tissue disease because the associated renal disease or anemia may be asymptomatic yet warrant therapy. If the inflammation is granulomatous a number of other disorders are suggested (see Chapter 5). In cases of a granulomatous anterior uveitis we will also require a purified protein derivative test, obtain a chest x-ray, and order a serum and urine calcium test and a serum angiotensive-converting enzyme (ACE) level to rule out asymptomatic tuberculosis or sarcoidosis.

### Treatment

Patients with idiopathic anterior uveitis tend to have nongranulomatous inflammation that responds well to topical corticosteroid therapy. Acetate preparations of topical corticosteroids tend to penetrate the cornea better than other preparations especially if the epithelium is intact, and we tend to use prednisolone acetate 1%. To prevent the development of posterior synechiae and to moderate symptoms of pain and photophobia caused by inflammation of the ciliary muscle, mydriasis and cycloplegia are indicated. Scopolamine 0.25% given twice daily is usually sufficient. In resistant cases, periocular injections of corticosteroids may be useful. Systemic corticosteroids are rarely needed.

## HLA-B27–ASSOCIATED ANTERIOR UVEITIS

HLA-B27–associated anterior uveitis appears to be a distinct clinical disorder. This form of the disease has frequent associations with systemic diseases including ankylosing spondylitis, Reiter's syndrome, inflammatory bowel disease, Whipple's disease, and psoriatic arthritis.[12] Nevertheless, as stated earlier, many patients with the HLA-B27 haplotype and anterior uveitis have no associated systemic illness. Patients with HLA-B27–associated anterior uveitis are more often male and tend to develop uveitis at a younger age than patients who are HLA-B27 negative.[3] However, some studies indicate that the long-term visual prognosis is similar between both groups.[3]

Should HLA typing be performed in all patients with anterior uveitis? We obtain HLA typing on patients with their first episode of acute anterior uveitis especially if they have back pain or other systemic symptoms or signs. In addition, if patients develop severe chronic anterior uveitis, we will often HLA type the patient because the finding of the HLA-B27 haplotype often obviates the need for an extensive laboratory evaluation to rule out infectious or other treatable causes of the disease.

The finding of the HLA-B27 haplotype is also of interest as a clue to the possible pathogenesis of the disease. Of particular interest is the potential role of gram-negative bacteria and their interaction with major histocompatibility complex class I antigens in triggering the anterior uveitis.[12,13] Unfortunately, this possible link between microbial antigens, HLA-B27, and anterior uveitis has not lead to improved therapy for the disorder because antimicrobial agents do not have any effect on the course of disease.

Other immunologic studies have been done in an attempt to determine the pathogenesis of anterior uveitis. Increased levels of complement and IgG compatible with breakdown of the blood-aqueous barrier can be detected in the aqueous of patients with anterior uveitis.[14] There is also evidence of complement activation in the aqueous of patients with anterior uveitis, measured by the presence of C3a, C4a, and C5a.[15] Evidence of increased serum fibrin degradation products has suggested a pathogenic role of the clotting pathways.[16] Increased expression of cell adhesion molecules has been associated with the development of intraocular inflammation. Increased expression of ICAM-1 in the irides of uveitis patients has been reported,[17] and expression of cell adhesion molecules in the anterior uvea has been shown to precede the infiltration of inflammatory cells in animal models of acute anterior uveitis.[9,10]

## HLA-B27–ASSOCIATED ANTERIOR UVEITIS WITH SYSTEMIC DISEASE

### Ankylosing spondylitis

Ocular involvement occurs in 25% of patients with ankylosing spondylitis.[18] Both eyes are involved in 80% of patients, but they are rarely simultaneously inflamed. Although the ocular findings associated with ankylosing spondylitis include both iritis and conjunctivitis, the iritis is the more significant manifestation. The disease course is quite variable. Recurrence of the ocular inflammation may occur as frequently as every 2 to 3 weeks. Some patients have fewer than one exacerbation per year. Interestingly, recurrence may be seasonal, although this seasonal variation appears to be more frequent in patients with idiopathic anterior uveitis.[19]

The anterior uveitis associated with ankylosing spondylitis usually has a presentation similar to idiopathic disease, occurring as a unilateral acute iritis with pain, photophobia, and redness (Fig. 19-1, *A*). Patients often complain of the onset of an attack 1 to 2 days before anterior chamber cell and flare are evident on slit-lamp biomicroscopy. Use of laser photometry may help to determine when initial breakdown of the blood-aqueous barrier occurs in relation to the development of symptoms and clinical signs of inflammation. Vision may transiently decrease during an acute episode as a result of anterior chamber inflammation or less often because of associated cystoid macular edema. A fibrin clot may form in the anterior chamber (Fig. 19-1, *B*). Posterior synechiae commonly develop unless attacks are treated

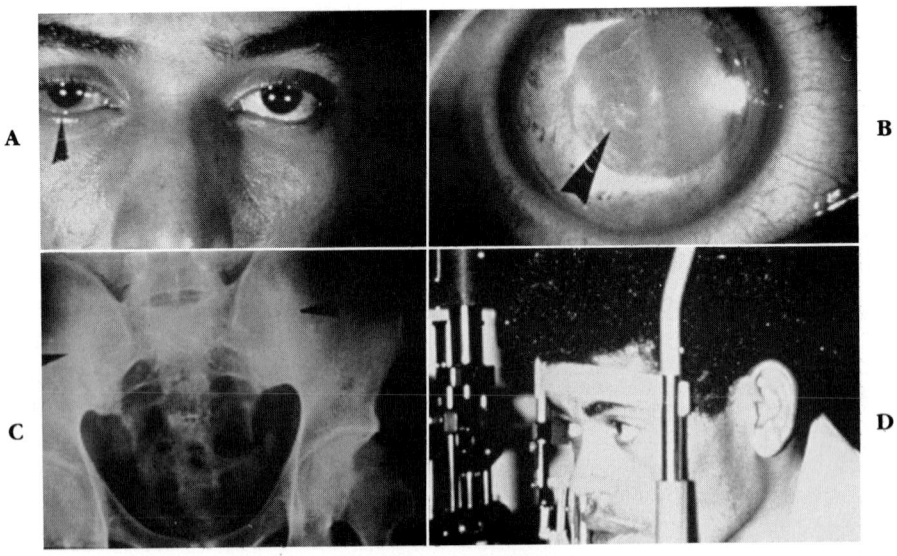


**Fig. 19-1. A,** Unilateral redness caused by iritis associated with ankylosing spondylitis. **B,** Fibrin clot in anterior chamber in iritis associated with ankylosing spondylitis. **C,** X-ray film of sacroiliac joints demonstrating increased radiodensity caused by ankylosing spondylitis. **D,** Flexed neck caused by ankylosis of cervical spine in ankylosing spondylitis. (Courtesy Fernando Oréfice, M.D., and Rubens Belfort, Jr., M.D.) (See Color Plate 35.)

promptly with corticosteroids and cycloplegics (Fig. 19-2).

Ankylosing spondylitis has been reported to affect men 2.5 to 3 times more frequently than women. Women may have a milder disease that may present with more peripheral joint manifestations. It is a common disorder that affects 0.1% of white adults.[20] Because HLA-B27 antigen is dominantly inherited and expressed, 50% of offspring will carry the gene, but the disease will be manifest in only 10% of the offspring. Approximately 96% with ankylosing spondylitis have the HLA-B27 antigen compared with 6% to 14% of a control white population without ankylosing spondylitis. HLA-B27 is found in 0 to 4% of African-Americans. Thus, the relative risk for ankylosing spondylitis in patients with the HLA-B27 antigen is as high as 100. Nevertheless, only 1.3% of all HLA-B27 positive patients with have the disease.

Sarcroilitis may be asymptomatic early in the course of disease, but it can be associated with severe lower back pain and debilitating stiffness and decreased range of motion. Radiographic films of the sacroiliac joints show blurring of the joint followed by sclerotic changes and eventually obliteration as the disease progresses (Fig. 19-1, *C*). A common mistake in the initial evaluation of patients with possible ankylosing spondylitis is to order lumbar-sacral spine films instead of radiographs of the sacroiliac joints. In severe disease, however, patients develop a fusion of the spine that begins in the lumbar region but can involve all parts of the spine. This fusion leads to back pain, stiffness, and in severe cases, may cause pulmonary restriction and a stiff flexed neck making positioning for slit-lamp biomicroscopy difficult (Fig. 19-1, *D*). Interesting, the associated uveitis does not appear to correlate with severity of the underlying spondylitis. Aortic insufficiency, cardiomegaly, and conduction defects are also associated with this disease.

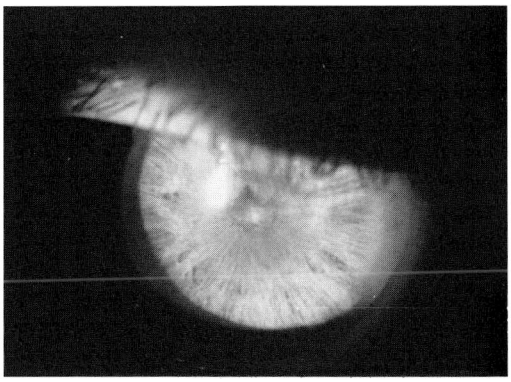

**Fig. 19-2.** Occluded pupil in patient with ankylosing spondylitis and recurrent iritis.

**Etiology.** The reason for the association between HLA-B27 and ankylosing spondylitis remains unknown. Some data suggest that environmental triggers such as infection with Gram-negative bacteria are important for the development of the disease. This information has lead to several theories. One hypothesis suggests that HLA-B27 is a receptor for the infectious agent. A second hypothesis suggests that HLA-B27 may cross-react with foreign antigens and induce tolerance. Others have suggested that HLA-B27 is a marker for an immune response gene that determines susceptibility to an environmental stimulus.

**Treatment.** It is important to make the diagnosis of ankylosing spondylitis in patients with uveitis because if the disease is recognized and treated early, spinal deformity can be prevented. Treatment usually involves physical therapy and antiinflammatory drugs including nonsteroidal antiinflammatory drugs (NSAIDS). NSAIDS may have some role in treating the uveitis associated with this disorder; however, data from large controlled trials are lacking.

### Reiter's syndrome

Reiter's syndrome is a systemic disorder characterized by arthritis, conjunctivitis, and urethritis. It was first described in 1818 but is named after Reiter who described the entity in 1916.[21] Reiter's syndrome is the most common cause of inflammatory oligoarthropathy in young males, and similar to ankylosing spondylitis it is related to both HLA-B27 and to a specific infection that may trigger the disease. The disease develops in at least 1% of patients with nonspecific urethritis and occurs in about 2% of patients after *Shigella* dysentery.

Many patients do not manifest the classic triad of arthritis, conjunctivitis, and urethritis. In addition, many of the findings of Reiter's syndrome are easily missed. For example, urethritis may be mild and missed. Other systemic associations include a scaling skin eruption called keratoderma blennorrhagicum, balanitis, and an aphthous stomatitis. Rheumatologic features of the disease include arthral-

**Box 19-1**
**Reiter's syndrome**

**MAJOR CRITERIA**

Polyarthritis
Conjunctivitis, iridocyclitis
Urethritis
Keratoderma blennorrhagica, balanitis circinata

Reiter's syndrome is:
Definite if ≥3 major criteria or 2 major and ≥3 minor
Probable if 2 major and 2 minor
Possible if 2 major and 1 minor

**MINOR CRITERIA**

Fasciitis, tendonitis, sacroiliitis, spondylitis
Keratitis
Cystitis, prostatitis
Oral mucosal lesions, psoriasis-like rash, nail changes
Diarrhea, leukocytosis, increased serum globulins, inflammation in the synovial fluid

Modified from Lee DA, Barker SM, Su WPD et al: The clinical diagnosis of Reiter's syndrome, *Ophthalmology* 93:350-356, 1986.

gias, plantar fasciitis, and tenosynovitis. About 20% of patients with Reiter's syndrome develop sacroiliitis and ascending spinal disease similar to ankylosing spondylitis. Hyperkeratotic skin lesions occur and may be indistinguishable from psoriasis. A number of classification systems have been proposed for Reiter's syndrome (Box 19-1),[22] but none are used uniformly in clinical practice.

In one review, arthritis was the presenting symptom in 25% of patients and genitourinary symptoms in 19%.[22] As the syndrome progresses, 94% of patients developed arthritis at some point, mostly in the joints of the hands, wrists, feet, and knees. Sacroiliitis occurred in 19% of cases, and almost any joint can be involved. Urethritis occurred in 75% of cases with cystitis, orchitis, vaginitis, and epididymitis occurring in occasional patients. Oral ulcers occurred in 19% of patients, external genital lesions in 39%. Skin lesions are common in Reiter's syndrome; they are seen in about 20% of patients but occur rarely in patients with ankylosing spondylitis.

Conjunctivitis is the most common ocular finding in patients with Reiter's syndrome and occur in 30% to 60% of patients. Some patients develop a mucoid discharge, but the conjunctivitis is usually not chronic. Iritis and keratitis are less common. Iritis occurs in 3% to 12% of patients and is nongranulomatous and mild. The keratitis is characterized by multifocal punctate subepithelial and anterior stroma infiltrates. A small pannus may also develop.

As stated previously, Reiter's syndrome may occur after gram-negative dysentery or after nongonococcal urethritis as a result of *Chlamydia trachomatis* and *Ureaplasma urealyticum*.[23] Nevertheless, treatment of the dysentery does not appear to alter the development or course of the syndrome. Most patients have signs of this syndrome 2 to 4 weeks after the onset of dysentery; however, the full syndrome may take years to develop.[22]

The diagnosis of Reiter's syndrome is based on clinical findings in association with HLA-B27 haplotype. Rheumatoid factor and autoantibodies are usually absent. The ocular disease associated with Reiter's syndrome is usually mild and can be treated with topical corticosteroids and mydriatic agents. However, the joint involvement may lead to significant long-term dysfunction and require treatment with NSAIDS. Immunosuppressive therapy with agents such as azathioprine and methotrexate may be required for systemic sequellae.

### Juvenile rheumatoid arthritis

Until recently, the term *juvenile rheumatoid arthritis* (JRA) was inappropriately used to describe all forms of childhood arthritis. As in adults, arthritis in children may be associated with infections such as Lyme disease, psoriasis, inflammatory bowel disease, or other systemic diseases. The diagnosis of JRA is based on the presence of arthritis in a child under the age of 16 and is usually found by a negative rheumatoid factor test result; there is no other known cause for the joint disease.[24] The joint inflammation may be polyarticular or pauciarticular, and the majority of patients are rheumatoid factor negative. A systemic form of JRA is characterized by a symmetric polyarthritis with an associated fever, rash, hepatosplenomegaly, and leukocytosis.

**Diagnosis.** Determination of the subclassification of JRA is important to determine the risk for developing uveitis. Children with uveitis are often asymptomatic and rarely complain of ocular symptoms, especially if the disease is uniocular. Uveitis is rare in children with systemic JRA.[25,26] Patients with polyarticular arthritis only occasionally develop uveitis. In contrast, patients with the pauciarticular form of JRA are at much higher risk for the development of ocular inflammation. Girls with pauciarticular arthritis and a positive result of an ANA test are at highest risk for developing chronic iridocyclitis.[24] A higher risk of uveitis is also associated with arthritis sparing the wrists but involving a lower extremity joint. Fourteen percent of girls in this high risk group will develop chronic anterior uveitis.

A group of boys with pauciarticular arthritis are also at increased risk to develop anterior uveitis.[27] Seventy-five percent of boys with pauciarticular arthritis are HLA-B27 positive, and the ocular inflammation they develop is similar in appearance to that of ankylosing spondylitis. The uveitis is characterized by an acute, episodic, nongranulomatous anterior uveitis, and some of these boys go on to develop ankylosing spondylitis later in life.[27]

Unlike males who develop uveitis, girls with JRA tend to develop chronic indolent disease, which can cause permanent ocular damage before it is recognized. In fact, the inflammation is clinically silent in over 50% of patients. Therefore girls with pauciarticular arthritis with test results that are ANA positive and rheumatoid factor negative should be screened every 3 to 4 months for the development of chronic smoldering uveitis. Parents should be told that a red eye should not be dismissed as conjunctivitis. Frequently, the first sign of uveitis in these girls is an irregular pupil as a result of posterior synechiae.

The chronic uveitis in JRA is characterized by anterior chamber cells and flare. Usually, patients only have 1 to 2+ cells, and once the uveitis has developed, chronic flare is the rule. Anterior chamber cells and not flare should be used to determine the severity of disease and the need for therapy. The number of cells will fluctuate with the severity of inflammation and diminish with corticosteroid therapy. Similar to the uveitis associated with other arthropathies, the severity of the uveitis is unrelated to the severity of the underlying joint disease. Although the joint disease often diminishes with age, ocular disease frequently persists into adulthood. Chronic inflammation may lead to band keratopathy, posterior synechiae, cataract, hypotony, and glaucoma. Glaucoma has been reported in up to 20% of eyes and may be caused by pupillary block or from chronic inflammatory disease with presumed damage to the trabecular meshwork.[28] The band keratopathy occurs in over half of cases and can cause significant visual disturbance (Fig. 19-3).[27] Cataract occurs in at least 60% of eyes, and in young patients may lead to amblyopia. Chronic inflammation in the presence of posterior synechiae and a small pupil can lead to the development of a fibrin membrane over the pupil. Finally, although the ocular inflammatory disease associated with JRA primarily involves the anterior segment, vitritis, macular edema, and macular folds may occur. Therefore visual loss may be caused by multiple factors in patients with JRA, and a thorough evaluation is necessary to develop an appropriate therapeutic approach.

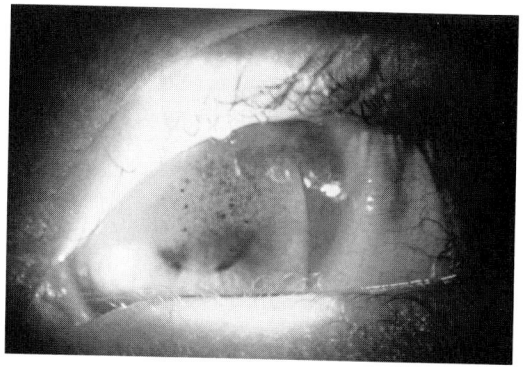

**Fig. 19-3.** Band keratopathy in patient with long-standing pauciarticular juvenile rheumatoid arthritis and chronic iritis.

The joint disease in patients who develop acute uveitis has an average age of onset of 7.5 to 9 years.[24,27] In contrast, patients with chronic uveitis develop joint symptoms earlier in life, with an average age of onset of 4 to 6.3 years. In one study, half the patients had chronic uveitis by age 6.[28] Joint inflammation usually precedes ocular disease by several years or more, but iritis can precede the joint symptoms by months to years.[27]

**Pathology.** Pathologic studies have been performed only on a few eyes with JRA.[29,30] Histologic findings show that the inflammation predominantly involves the iris and ciliary body. Plasma cells and lymphocytes are the most common inflammatory cells, and scattered giant cells have been noted. A similar histologic picture is seen in the involved joints of these patients. In view of the association between antinuclear antibodies and other autoantibodies with JRA, some have hypothesized that infiltrating plasma cells are responsible for local synthesis of autoantibodies against ocular antigens.[30] However, these proposed autoantibodies or ocular antigens have not been identified.

**Differential diagnosis.** Ocular sarcoidosis in children is the disease that most closely mimics JRA. Children with sarcoidosis develop arthritis and skin lesions and often lack radiographic evidence of pulmonary disease. JRA can be distinguished from sarcoidosis by the presence of a positive ANA test result, the characteristic distribution of involved joints, the nongranulomatous inflammation limited primarily to the anterior segment of the eye, and the absence of systemic symptoms and signs. Nevertheless, early in the course of JRA, children may have no history of joint disease and present only with chronic uveitis and band keratopathy. Other diseases to consider include Lyme disease, psoriatic arthritis, juvenile Reiter's syndrome, ankylosing spondylitis, inflammatory bowel disease–associated anterior uveitis, Kawasaki disease, trauma, and keratouveitis caused by herpes simplex or herpes zoster infection.

**Treatment.** Patients with chronic anterior uveitis associated with JRA need to be seen regularly, no less than every 3 months. Topical corticosteroids remain the mainstay of therapy.[31,32] Corticosteroid therapy should be used to decrease the number of anterior chamber cells, but chronic flare in the absence of cells should not be treated. Glaucoma and cataract are frequent side effects of topical steroids in children with JRA. Especially in young patients, cataracts may lead to the development of amblyopia and require prompt surgical removal.

Chylack[3] studied 210 patients with JRA and found that the uveitis responded to short courses of topical corticosteroids in 39% of cases. However, 61% of cases did not respond to corticosteroids or require prolonged treatment. Repeated periocular injections of depot preparations of corticosteroids are needed to manage some cases of chronic active inflammation that cannot be controlled with topical corticosteroids alone. For most children, this requires general anesthesia for each injection. Short courses of oral corticosteroids can be tried, but we do not favor the long-term use of oral corticosteroids in children because of the overwhelming side effects on growth and bone formation. Alternate-day therapy may decrease the side effects and may be tried for unusually severe ocular disease requiring prolonged therapy.

NSAIDS may allow a reduction in the dose of corticosteroids required to treat chronic uveitis.[33] Tolmetin or naproxen are the NSAIDS most commonly used in children. A number of other immunosuppressive agents including azathioprine, chlorambucil, cyclophosphamide, and methotrexate have been used to treat severe uveitis associated with JRA. We are hesitant to use many of the cytotoxic agents in children for fear of inducing a secondary malignancy. A double-masked trial of methotrexate versus placebo in the treatment of resistant JRA showed that joint disease improved with methotrexate therapy; however, the study did not address the response of the uveitis.[34] We have found cyclosporine useful for the treatment of many forms of childhood uveitis but have rarely treated children with JRA with this agent.

Surgery is often needed in the management of JRA-associated uveitis. Cataracts are common in children with JRA and require surgical removal. Cataract surgery should only be performed in eyes that have been "quiet" for at least 3 months. Cataract extraction may be performed with either an extracapsular approach or a pars plana lensectomy.[35,36] The need for a secondary surgical procedure appears to be decreased in patients undergoing a pars plana lensectomy with vitrectomy.[28] Many uveitis specialists also recommend the removal of the posterior capsule at the time of surgery because a secondary laser posterior capsulotomy may be difficult to perform in children.

Foster and Barrett[37] recently reported their surgical experience in patients with JRA. Cataracts were common in their patients and developed in 13 (18%) of 72 patients during follow-up. Cataract extraction was performed with a phacoemulsification extracapsular cataract extraction followed by a pars plana vitrectomy. The authors emphasized the need for aggressive antiinflammatory therapy both before and after surgery. The average postoperative visual acuity in this study was 20/40.

Medical management of glaucoma in patients with JRA is problematic. Topical β blockers and sympathomimetic agents control intraocular pressure in some patients, but many require carbonic anhydrase inhibitors. Surgical therapy is required for a number of patients that fail medical management. Laser iridectomy is indicated for glaucoma caused by pupillary block with iris bombe. In patients with secondary glaucoma caused by chronic intraocular inflammation, the success of traditional surgery with trabeculectomy is poor.[38] Filtering devices such as Molteno implants may improve the prognosis. Cyclocryotherapy should only be used when other surgical procedures have failed to control the pressure.

Finally, band keratopathy is seen in 77% of patients with severe JRA-associated iridocyclitis.[26] This band keratopathy can be treated with chemical chelation with topical application of 0.37M ethylenediamine tetraacetic acid solution after debridement of the epithelium with 70% isopropyl alcohol and scraping. The excimer laser may have some role in the management of this complication in the future.

### Psoriatic arthropathy

Psoriasis is a skin disease caused by hyperproliferation of the epidermis with resultant scaling. Uveitis occurs predominantly in patients who develop arthropathy. About 20% of patients with psoriasis develop psoriatic arthropathy, and about 20% of these patients develop uveitis, sacroiliitis, and ascending spine disease.[39] The arthropathy usually involves the distal joints of the hands and feet as well as the sacroiliac joints. The uveitis predominantly involves the anterior segment of the eye and is similar to HLA-B27–associated disease. Because psoriasis is a common disorder, not all anterior uveitis that occur in patients with psoriasis will be causally related, especially if the patient does not have arthritis. The psoriasis and arthropathy in these patients are treated separately. The uveitis tends to respond well to standard therapy with topical corticosteroids and a drop to induce cycloplegia and mydriasis.

### Inflammatory bowel disease

Patients with both ulcerative colitis and Crohn's disease can develop uveitis.[40,41] About 5% of patients with ulcerative colitis will develop ocular disease. Conjunctivitis, episcleritis, and anterior uveitis are most commonly described; however, posterior uveitis may also occur. Similar ocular inflammatory disease has been associated with Crohn's disease. The ophthalmologist should ask patients with anterior uveitis whether they have recurrent diarrhea, bloody diarrhea, or abdominal cramping. Although the uveitis often responds to topical corticosteroids, early diagnosis of inflammatory bowel disease will lead to prompt treatment for the gastrointestinal complications that frequently occur.

### Whipple's disease

Whipple's disease is a systemic disorder characterized by malabsorption causing chronic diarrhea. Anterior uveitis and vitritis have been rarely reported in patients with Whipple's disease.[42] However, because antibiotic therapy can effectively treat this disease, it is important to diagnose Whipple's disease in uveitis patients with gastrointestinal symptoms.

## DISEASE ASSOCIATIONS

### Fuchs' heterochromic iridocyclitis

The association of iris heterochromia and cataract was initially described by Lawrence in 1843.[43] In 1906 Fuchs described seven patients with heterochromic iridocyclitis[44] and later described 38 patients with the disease and reported on the pathologic features of six eyes. The classic hallmark of Fuchs' heterochromic iridocyclitis is, as the name suggests, iris heterochromia. However, this classic finding may be difficult to perceive. It is easiest to see in blue-eyed patients, in whom the affected eye appears more intensely blue.[45] In addition, 7% to 15% of patients have bilateral involvement, and there is no obvious heterochromia in these patients. A more consistent finding appears to

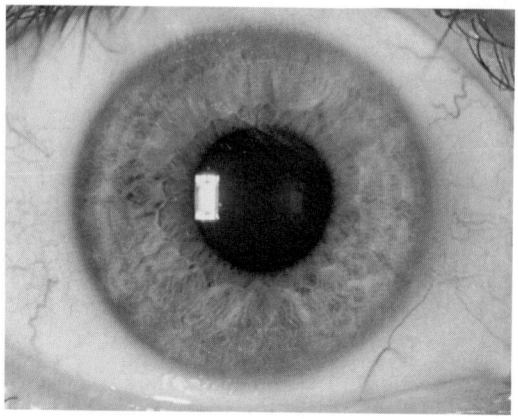

**Fig. 19-4.** Photograph of iris in patient with Fuchs' heterochromic iridocyclitis demonstrating iris stromal abnormalities.

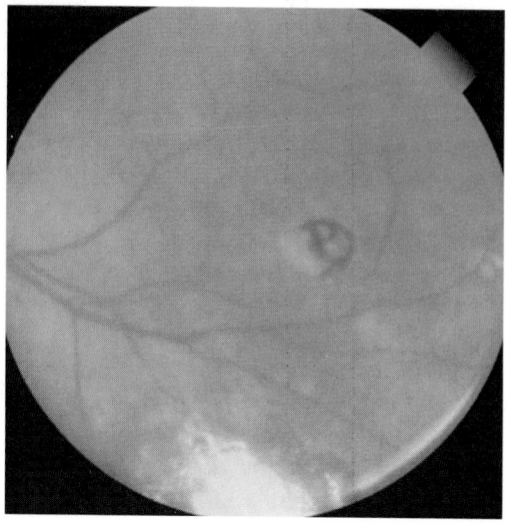

**Fig. 19-5.** Chorioretinal scar consistent with toxoplasmosis observed in patient shown in Fig. 19-4. (Courtesy Rubens Belfort, Jr., M.D.)

be blurring of the iris stroma and loss of detail and density of the iris surface that can only be seen on careful slit-lamp biomicroscopy (Fig. 19-4).[45,46] Fuchs observed that most patients with this disorder develop cataracts.

The typical patient is young and presents with iris heterochromia and a mild disturbance of vision. Pain and redness are rare. Slit-lamp examination shows small stellate keratic precipitates (KP) with fine filaments that are uniformly scattered over the endothelium, unlike most other cases of anterior uveitis in which the precipitates occur predominantly on the lower half of the cornea. Anterior chamber inflammation is mild, and low-grade vitritis may be seen. The posterior segment of the eye is usually unaffected, although cystoid macular edema has been reported in a few cases. Abnormal vessels bridging the anterior chamber angle are frequently described, but iris neovascularization and neovascular glaucoma are rare.[47] It is well documented that hyphema is likely to occur after intraocular surgery. Amsler[48] first noted the occurrence of hyphema after paracentesis. Anterior chamber paracentesis was initially proposed as a diagnostic test for Fuchs' heterochromic iridocyclitis, but it appears unwarranted for this purpose.[47]

Many patients with Fuchs' heterochromic iridocyclitis are unaware of their disease until their vision decreases because of cataract or progressive glaucoma. Rarely, vitreous inflammation is severe enough to cause floaters. The presence of fine evenly distributed KP in a white eye with mild anterior chamber cells and flare, cataract, and increased intraocular pressure should suggest the diagnosis. Patients often note that one iris has been lighter in color for many years. Brown eyes become less brown and blue eyes appear more blue with this disorder, because the heterochromia is due to a loss of anterior iris pigment. Gray eyes may appear green.

The differential diagnosis of Fuchs' heterochromic iridocyclitis includes disorders that produce iris heterochromia. Malignant melanoma of the iris, Horner's syndrome, chronic anterior uveitis with iris atrophy caused by infections such as herpes zoster should all be considered. In addition, Posner-Schlossman syndrome and neovascular glaucoma may cause ocular disease that looks like Fuchs' heterochromic iridocyclitis.

Fuchs described peripheral chorioretinal scars in some patients with this disease. Several authors have now associated Fuchs' heterochromic iridocyclitis with toxoplasmosis (Fig. 19-5). Ocular toxoplasmosis may cause fine KP and anterior uveitis and mimic Fuchs' heterochromic iridocyclitis. This would explain why many patients with Fuchs' lack findings of toxoplasmosis. Others suggest that infection with toxoplasmosis may be causally related to the development of the disorder. Chorioretinal scars consistent with ocular histoplasmosis have also been noted, but a causal relationship between infectious agents and Fuchs' heterochromic iridocyclitis is unproven. Others have proposed that a lack of normal sympathetic innervation and neurogenic factors cause the findings associated with the disease, but again these associations are unproven.[47]

The finding of infiltrating plasma cells and lymphocytes on pathologic examination of ocular specimens from patients with Fuchs' iridocyclitis suggests an inflammatory cause for the disease.[49] Electron microscopy of iris biopsy specimens showed both a decrease in the number of stromal melanocytes and a decrease in melanosome size.[50] Plasma cells, mast cells, and lymphocytes were present in the tissue, but no infectious organisms were seen. Although Fuchs' heterochromic iridocyclitis may be a single pathologic entity with a single cause, much of the evidence suggests that many cases of Fuchs' heterochromic iridocyclitis represent a common ocular response that can develop from a variety of etiologic insults.

Fuchs' heterochromic iridocyclitis is generally chronic. Although topical corticosteroids can decrease the clinical signs of inflammation, long-term topical therapy is often unnecessary and may serve only to hasten cataract formation and induce glaucoma in steroid responders. Cataracts can be safely removed in patients with Fuchs' heterochromic iridocyclitis; however, the glaucoma associated with the disease may not be easily controlled and can result in significant and permanent visual loss. Uveitis in these patients must be controlled. Although medications can control the glaucoma, surgery is often required but is fraught with the complications and difficulties associated with glaucoma surgery in other patients with uveitis.[46,47]

### Kawasaki disease

Kawasaki disease, also called mucocutaneous lymph node syndrome, is a disease of children and young adults, characterized by an erythematous and desquamative exanthem (Fig. 19-6, *A*), oral mucosal erythema (Fig. 19-6, *B*), conjunctivitis, fever, and an asymmetric cervical adenopathy.[51] Anterior uveitis has also been noted in many patients with this disorder. Although the cause is unknown, patients with active Kawasaki disease have an antibody to γ interferon-activated endothelial cells from the umbilical vein that express major histocompatibility complex class II antigens.[52] In one study, 66% of patients had evidence of anterior uveitis that occurred most commonly during the first week of illness.[53] The uveitis does not appear to be severe or chronic and usually resolves without therapy. Optic disc edema and dilated retinal veins may also be seen (Fig. 19-6, *C* and *D*).

### Anterior uveitis associated with renal disease

Anterior uveitis has been associated with acute interstitial nephritis.[54] Patients usually present with an acute uveitis and later develop manifestations of acute interstitial nephritis with cellular casts in the urine. Renal biopsy results show infiltration with eosinophils and mononuclear cells. The nephritis usually responds to corticosteroid therapy. Anterior uveitis has also been reported in patients with IgA nephropathy.[55] This disease often occurs in children and is associated with an upper respiratory tract infection. The uveitis appears to occur with the pulmonary disease and responds to standard therapy with topical corticosteroids and mydriatic and cycloplegic drops.

### Glaucomatous cyclitic crisis

Glaucomatous cyclitic crisis, also known as Posner-Schlossman syndrome, is an inflammatory glaucoma manifested by fine KP, mydriasis, and elevated intraocular pressure.[56] Conglomerates of inflammatory cells are occasionally noted in the anterior chamber angle, and an accompanying decrease in aqueous outflow has been documented. Episodes are treated with topical corticosteroids, β-blockers, and carbonic anhydrase inhibitors.

### Schwartz syndrome

Rhegmatogenous retinal detachment is frequently associated with a mild reduction in the intraocular pressure. In some cases, intraocular pressure is elevated and associated with anterior uveitis. This syndrome of increased intraocular pressure, an open anterior chamber angle, and anterior segment inflammation is termed Schwartz syndrome.[57] It remains unclear whether the increased intraocular pressure is secondary to the anterior uveitis, concomitant damage to the trabecular meshwork, or blockage of the trabecular meshwork from retinal pigment epithelium or components of the photoreceptors.[58] It should also be noted that anterior uveitis is a frequent finding in blunt ocular trauma and usually resolves with topical corticosteroids.

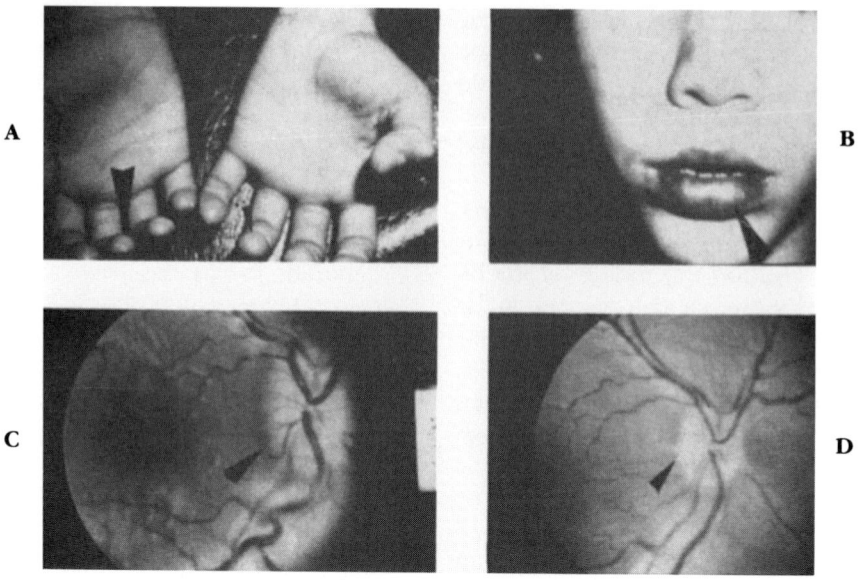


**Fig. 19-6. A,** Distal cutaneous erythematous lesions seen in patient with Kawasaki disease. **B,** Oral mucocutaneous lesions in patient with disease. **C,** Papilledema and dilated retinal veins in patient with Kawasaki disease that **(D)** resolves after acute phase of disease. (Courtesy Fernando Oréfice, M.D., and Rubens Belfort, Jr., M.D.)

### Anterior segment ischemia

Anterior segment ischemia caused by carotid artery insufficiency may simulate an anterior uveitis in older patients with the presence of cells and flare. The amount of flare is often out of proportion to the number of cells in the anterior chamber when compared with other types of anterior uveitis. The pupil is poorly reactive, and patients often complain of dull, deep, and chronic pain. Anterior segment ischemia is often associated with other signs of ischemia such as venous stasis and neovascularization.[59] Therapy should be directed toward improving the ischemia rather than treating the secondary ocular findings.

### Lens-induced anterior uveitis

Anterior uveitis occurs in association with several forms of lens-induced glaucoma. Phacolytic glaucoma occurs when a hypermature cataract leaks liquefied cortical material into the anterior chamber. Macrophages are found in the aqueous humor, although KP is rare.[60] Treatment involves suppressing the inflammation with topical corticosteroids and removing the cataract. Phacoantigenic glaucoma occurs after rupture of the lens capsule and is characterized by conjunctival chemosis and anterior segment inflammation that develops within days to weeks after the capsular disruption. A phacotoxic glaucoma may also occur after recent cataract extraction or traumatic rupture of the lens capsule.[61] In these cases, inflammation is treated with topical, periocular, or systemic corticosteroids, in addition to antiglaucoma medications. These cases must be distinguished from endophthalmitis especially in the context of recent trauma or ocular surgery.

### Anterior uveitis associated with AIDS

Anterior uveitis is found in a number of patients with AIDS.[62] The anterior uveitis is often associated with other infectious diseases such as syphilis, cytomegalovirus retinitis, toxoplasmosis, herpes simplex, or herpes zoster. A mild anterior uveitis may be associated with HIV infection in the absence of coinfection. In addition, anterior uveitis may result as an adverse reaction to one of the many medications that patients with AIDS receive. As stated earlier, anterior uveitis, occasionally with hypopyon, has been associated with rifabutin use in patients with AIDS.[5-7,63]

### Other disease associations

In addition to the disorders described here, anterior uveitis can occur in many forms of uveitis. Infectious causes of uveitis such as syphilis, herpes simplex virus keratitis, herpes zoster infection, and toxoplasmosis are frequently accompanied by an anterior uveitis. Noninfectious causes of uveitis such as Behçet's disease, sarcoidosis, and multiple sclerosis are also associated with anterior segment inflammation. Anterior uveitis may also be caused by postoperative infection. Acute bacterial endophthalmitis may present with a hypopyon. *Propionibacterium acnes* infection has been associated with an indolent smoldering anterior uveitis after cataract surgery. Anterior uveitis may also be a sign of corneal allograft rejection, especially when seen in conjunction with corneal inflammation such as a Koudadoust line. Anterior uveitis can occur after immunization or vaccination and may develop as a toxic effect of certain medications.[5,63,64] Finally, a number of malignancies such as leukemia, retinoblastoma, and intraocular lymphoma may masquerade as an idiopathic anterior uveitis.[65,66] These entities are discussed in detail in Chapter 29.

## REFERENCES


1. Wakefield D, Dunlop I, McClusky PJ et al: Uveitis: aetiology and disease associations in an Australian population, *Aust NZ J Ophthalmol* 14:181-187, 1986.
2. Vedot E, Barth E, Billet P: Epidemiology of uveitis: preliminary results of a prospective study in Savoy, In Sarri KM, editor: Uveitis update, Amsterdam, 1984, Elsevier, pp 13-16.
3. Rothova A, Veenedaal WG, Linssen A et al: Clinical features of acute anterior uveitis, *Am J Ophthalmol* 103:137-145, 1987.
4. Guex-Crosier Y, Pittet N, Herbort CP: Evaluation of laser flare-cell photometry in the appraisal and management of intraocular inflammation in uveitis, *Ophthalmology* 101(4):728-735, 1994.
5. Frank MO, Graham MB, Wispelway B: Rifabutin and uveitis, *N Engl J Med* 330:868, 1994, [letter].
6. Jacobs DS, Piliero PJ, Kuperwaser MG et al: Acute uveitis associated with rifabutin use in patients with human immunodeficiency virus infection, *Am J Ophthalmol* 118:716-722, 1994.
7. Saran BR, Maguire AM, Nichols C et al: Hypopyon uveitis in patients with acquired immunodeficiency syndrome treated for systemic *Mycobacterium avium* complex infection with rifabutin, *Am J Ophthalmol* 112:1159-1165, 1994.
8. Fong DS, Raizman MB: Spontaneous hyphema associated with anterior uveitis, *Br J Ophthalmol* 77(10):635-638, 1993.
9. Whitcup SM, Wakefield D, Li Q et al: Endothelial leukocyte adhesion molecule-1 in endotoxin-induced uveitis, *Invest Ophthalmol Vis Sci* 33(9):2626-2630, 1992.
10. Whitcup SM, DeBarge LR, Rosen H et al: Monoclonal antibody against CD11b/CD18 inhibits endotoxin-induced uveitis, *Invest Ophthalmol Vis Sci* 34(3):673-681, 1993.
11. Elner VM, Elner SG, Pavilack MA et al: Intercellular adhesion molecule-1 in human corneal endothelium: mudulation and function, *Am J Pathol* 138:525-536, 1991.
12. Wakefield D, Montanaro A, McCluskey P: Acute anterior uveitis and HLA-B27, *Surv Ophthalmol* 36(3):223-232, 1991.
13. Wakefield D, Abi-Hanna D: HLA antigens and their significance in the pathogenesis of anterior uveitis: a mini review, *Curr Eye Res* 5:465-473, 1986.
14. Mondino BJ, Rao H: Hemolytic complement activity in aqueous humor, *Arch Ophthalmol* 101:465-468, 1983.
15. Mondino BJ, Sumner H: Anaphylatoxin levels in human aqueous humor, *Invest Ophthalmol Vis Sci* 27:1288-1292, 1986.
16. Sen DK, Sarin GS, Mathur MD: Serum fibrin degradation products in acute idiopathic anterior uveitis, *Acta Ophthalmol* 64:632-636, 1986.
17. Wakefield D, McCluskey P, Palladinetti P: Distribution of lymphocytes and cell adhesion molecules in iris biopsy specimens from patients with uveitis, *Arch Ophthalmol* 110(1):121-125, 1992.
18. Brewerton DA, Caffrey M, Hart FD et al: Ankylosing spondylitis and HLA-B27, *Lancet* 1:904-907, 1973.
19. Ebringer R, White L, McCoy R et al: Seasonal variation in acute anterior uveitis: differences between HLA-B27 positive and HLA-B27 negative disease. *Br J Ophthalmol* 69:202-204, 1985.
20. Masi AT: Epidemiology of B27 associated disease, *Ann Rheum Dis* 38:131-134, 1979.
21. Reiter H: Uber eine bisher unerkannte Spirochäteninfektion, *Dtsch Med Wochenschr* 42:1535-1536, 1916.
22. Lee DA, Barker SM, Su WPD et al: The clinical diagnosis of Reiter's syndrome, *Ophthalmology* 93:350-356, 1986.
23. Keat A: Reiter's syndrome and reactive arthritis in perspective, *N Engl J Med* 39:1606-1615, 1983.
24. Cassidy JT, Levinson JE, Bass JC et al: A study of classification criteria for a diagnosis of juvenile rheumatoid arthritis, *Arthritis Rheum* 29:274-281, 1986.
25. Rosenberg AM: Uveitis associated with juvenile rheumatoid arthritis, *Semin Arthritis Rheum* 16:158-173, 1987.
26. Wolf MD, Lichter PR, Ragsdale CG: Prognostic factors in the uveitis of juvenile rheumatoid arthritis, *Ophthalmology* 94:1242-1247, 1987.
27. Smiley WK: The eye in juvenile rheumatoid arthritis, *Trans Ophthalmol Soc UK* 94:817-829, 1974.
28. Key SW III, Kimura SJ: Iridocyclitis associated with juvenile rheumatoid arthritis, *Am J Ophthalmol* 80:425-429, 1975.
29. Merriam JC, Chylack LT, Albert DM: Early onset pauciarticular juvenile rheumatoid arthritis: a histopathologic study, *Arch Ophthalmol* 101:1085-1092, 1983.
30. Sabates R, Smith T, Apple D: Ocular histopathology in juvenile rheumatoid arthritis, *Ann Ophthalmol* 1979: 733-737, 1979.
31. Kanski JJ: Anterior uveitis in juvenile rheumatoid arthritis, *Arch Ophthalmol* 95:1794-1797, 1977.
32. Chylack LT: The ocular manifestations of juvenile rheumatoid arthritis, *Arthritis Rheum* 20:217-223, 1977.
33. Olson NY, Lindsley CB, Godfrey WA: Nonsteroidal antiinflammatory drug therapy in chronic childhood iridocyclitis, *Am J Dis Child* 142:1289-1292, 1988.
34. Giannini EH, Brower EJ, Kuzmind N et al: Methotrexate in resistant juvenile rheumatoid arthritis. Results of the

U.S.A.-U.S.S.R. double-blind, placebo-controlled trial, *N Engl J Med* 326:1043-1049, 1992.
35. Diamond JG, Kaplan HG: Lensectomy and vitrectomy for complicated cataract secondary to uveitis, *Arch Ophthalmol* 96:1798-1804, 1978.
36. Praeger DL, Schneider HA, Sakowski AD et al: Kelman procedure in the treatment of complicated cataract of the uveitis of Still's disease, *Trans Ophthalmol Soc UK* 96:168-171, 1976.
37. Foster CS, Barrett F: Cataract development and cataract surgery in patients with juvenile rheumatoid arthritis-associated iridocyclitis, *Ophthalmology* 100:809-817, 1993.
38. O'Brien JM, Albert DM: Therapeutic approaches for ophthalmic problems in juvenile rheumatoid arthritis, *Rheum Dis Clin North Am* 15:413-437, 1989.
39. Calin A: The spondyloarthropathies. In Wyngaarden JB, Smith LH Jr, Bennett JC, editors: *Cecil textbook of medicine,* ed 19, Philadelphia, 1992, WB Saunders, pp 1515-1521.
40. Ellis PP, Gentry JH: Ocular complications of ulcerative colitis, *Am J Ophthalmol* 58:779-784, 1964.
41. Duker JS, Brown GC, Brooks L: Retinovasculitis in Crohn's disease, *Am J Ophthalmol* 103:654-668, 1987.
42. Selsky EJ, Knox DL, Maumanee AE et al: Ocular involvement in Whipple's disease, *Retina* 4:103-106, 1984.
43. Lawrence W: Changes in colour in the iris. In Hays I, editor: *A treatise on diseases of the eye,* Philadelphia, 1843, Lea & Blanchard, pp 411-416.
44. Fuchs E: Über Komplicaationen der Heterochromie, *Z Augenheilkd* 15:191-212, 1906.
45. Kimura SJ, Hogan MJ, Thygeson P: Fuchs' syndrome of heterochromic cyclitis, *Arch Ophthalmol* 54:179-186, 1955.
46. Liesegang TJ: Clinical features and prognosis in Fuchs' uveitis syndrome, *Arch Ophthalmol* 100:1622-1626, 1982.
47. Jones NP: Fuchs' heterochromic uveitis: an update, *Surv Ophthalmol* 37:253-272, 1993.
48. Amsler M: New clinical aspects of the vegetative eye, *Trans Ophthalmol Soc UK* 68:45-74, 1948.
49. Goldberg MF, Erozan YS, Duke JR et al: Cytopathologic and histopathologic aspects of Fuchs' heterochromic iridocyclitis, *Arch Ophthalmol* 74:604-609, 1965.
50. McCartney AC, Bull TB, Spalton DJ: Fuchs' heterochromic cyclitis: an electron microscopy study, *Trans Ophthalmol Soc UK* 105:324-329, 1986.
51. Bligard CA: Kawasaki disease and its diagnosis, *Pediatr Dermatol* 4:75-84, 1987.
52. Leung DY, Collins T, Lapierre LA et al: Immunoglobulin M antibodies present in the acute phase of Kawasaki syndrome lyse cultured vascular endothelial cells stimulated by gamma interferon, *J Clin Invest* 77:1428-1435, 1986.
53. Burns JC, Joffe L, Sargent RA et al: Anterior uveitis associated with Kawasaki syndrome, *Pediatr Infect Dis* 4:258-261, 1985.
54. Gafter U, Ben-Basat M, Zevin D et al: Anterior uveitis, a presenting symptom in acute interstitial nephritis, *Nephron* 42:249-251, 1986.
55. Moller-Jensen J, Marthinsen L, Linne T: Anterior uveitis in IgA nephropathy, *Am J Ophthalmol* 108:604-605, 1989.
56. Posner A, Schlossman A: Syndrome of unilateral recurrent attacks of glaucoma with cyclitic symptoms, *Arch Ophthalmol* 39:517-528, 1948.
57. Schwartz A: Chronic open-angle glaucoma secondary to rhegmatoenous retinal detachment, *Am J Ophthalmol* 75:205-211, 1973.
58. Matsuo N, Takabatake M, Ueno H et al: Photoreceptor outer segments in the aqueous humor in rhegmatogenous retinal detachment, *Am J Ophthalmol* 101:673-679, 1986.
59. Jacobs NA, Ridgway AE: Syndrome of ischaemic ocular inflammation: six cases and a review, *Br J Ophthalmol* 69:682-687, 1985.
60. Epstein DL, Jedziniak JA, Grant WM: Identification of heavy molecular weight protein in aqueous humor in human phacolytic glaucoma, *Invest Ophthalmol* 17: 398-402, 1978.
61. Irvine SR, Irvine AR Jr: Lens-induced uveitis and glaucoma. II. The "phacotoxic" reaction, *Am J Ophthalmol* 35:370-375, 1952.
62. Shuler JD, Engstrom RE, Holland GN: External ocular disease and anterior segment disorders associated with AIDS, *Int Ophthalmol Clin* 29:98-104, 1989.
63. Fuller JD, Stanfield LE, Craven DE: Rifabutin prophylaxis and uveitis, *N Engl J Med* 330:1315-6, 1994, [letter, comment].
64. Yeomans SM, Knox DL, Green WR et al: Ocular inflammatory pseudotumor associated with propranolol therapy, *Ophthalmology* 90:1422-1425, 1983.
65. Woog JJ, Chess J, Albert DM et al: Metastatic carcinoma of the iris simulating iridocyclitis, *Br J Ophthalmol* 68:167-173, 1984.
66. Hertler AA, Rosenwasser GO, Gluck WL: Isolated anterior chamber relapse in acute monoblastic leukemia, *Am J Hematol* 23:401-403, 1986.

# CHAPTER 20

# Intermediate Uveitis

Intermediate uveitis is a diagnosis based on the anatomic location of ocular inflammation; it is not a distinct clinicopathologic condition. The diagnosis of intermediate uveitis is made when ocular inflammation primarily involves the vitreous and peripheral retina. Intermediate uveitis was first described as *chronic cyclitis* by Fuchs in 1908.[1] The clinical description of intermediate uveitis was further elucidated by Schepens[2] in 1950 when he described patients with a *peripheral uveitis* characterized by inflammation centered around the vasculature and exudative changes in the retinal periphery. In 1960, Brockhurst and colleagues[3] described additional patients with peripheral vascular abnormalities and an exudate along the ora serrata and pars plana, and Welch and colleagues[4] used the term *pars planitis* to describe an inflammation characterized by the white accumulation on the pars plana. Other terms used in the literature to describe patients with intermediate uveitis include *vitritis, peripheral exudative retinitis, cyclochorioretinitis, chronic posterior cyclitis,* and *peripheral uveoretinitis.* Unfortunately, there is still confusion and controversy, even among uveitis specialists, on how to classify patients with this anatomic distribution of intraocular inflammation.

We use the term *intermediate uveitis,* as suggested by the International Uveitis Study Group, to classify patients with intraocular inflammation predominantly involving the vitreous and peripheral retina. This diagnosis is used by some specialists only if a more specific diagnosis cannot be made. Specific diseases such as sarcoidosis and multiple sclerosis are known to cause an intermediate uveitis, and we will often classify patients as having an intermediate uveitis associated with sarcoidosis or associated with multiple sclerosis, when an underlying disease can be identified. We also use the term *pars planitis* to describe a subset of patients with intermediate uveitis when a white opacity (commonly called a *snowbank*) occurs over the pars plana and ora serrata. Although pars planitis probably does not represent a distinct clinical entity from intermediate uveitis, patients with pars planitis often have worse vitritis, more severe macular edema, and a worse prognosis than patients with intermediate uveitis who do not have a pars plana exudate.[5]

## EPIDEMIOLOGY

Intermediate uveitis accounts for approximately 4% to 8% of uveitis cases in a referral practice.[6–8] Approximately 15% of the uveitis cases referred to us at the National Institutes of Health (NIH) are diagnosed with intermediate uveitis. Although the incidence of uveitis in children is low, intermediate uveitis may account for up to 25% of cases.[9] Cases of intermediate uveitis have been reported in young children and the elderly; however, the disease tends to mostly affect younger patients, typically in their teens to their forties.[7] There does not appear to be a sex or race predilection for the disease. There have been occasional reports of intermediate uveitis occurring in families, suggesting that either hereditary or environmental factors may predispose one to develop the disease. HLA associations have been identified in patients with multiple sclerosis and intermediate uveitis, but no other common HLA haplotypes have been found in patients with intermediate uveitis.[10] Intermediate uveitis has been described in families. In 1963, Kimura and Hogan[11] first reported multiple family members with intermediate uveitis. There are only about a dozen cases of familial intermediate uveitis of which we are aware, and a number of these have been reported.[9,12-14] In one case of familial pars planitis, the two affected brothers were not twins but had identical HLA.[12] Although the disease is typically diagnosed in young adults, 20% of children with uveitis will have pars planitis.[15]

## CLINICAL MANIFESTATIONS

In our experience, most patients present with blurred vision and/or floaters. Pain and photophobia are rare. Early in the course of the disease, visual acuity is often reduced to the 20/40 range as a result of a moderate vitritis and cystoid macular edema. However, if inflammation is not well controlled, severe visual loss can ensue associated with chronic cystoid macular edema, glaucoma, inflammatory changes in the retina, and retinal detachment. We have seen sudden loss of vision in several patients after vitreous hemorrhage. Seventy to eighty percent of patients have bilateral involvement at the time of presentation, and approximately one third of patients who start with unilateral disease will later develop bilateral involvement.[5,7]

Many adults have minimal anterior segment inflammation[16]; the exception is intermediate uveitis associated with multiple sclerosis when patients typically develop a granulomatous anterior uveitis with formation of mutton-fat keratic precipitates. Anterior segment inflammation is more common in children with uveitis when there may be a moderate degree of anterior chamber cells with posterior synechiae. Brockhurst and colleagues[3] noted peripheral anterior synechiae in 24% of patients and posterior synechiae in 18%. Band keratopathy may be seen in children. Occasionally patients may present with significant anterior segment inflammation with pain and photophobia and only later develop signs typical of an intermediate uveitis.

Autoimmune endotheliopathy is a rare finding associated with pars planitis. Khodadoust and colleagues[17] reported 4 of 10 patients with pars planitis who demonstrated areas of peripheral corneal edema with keratic precipitates arranged linearly on the border between edematous and normal cornea. This morphologic finding was reminiscent of a corneal graft endothelial rejection line. Although other investigators have not observed this finding as frequently as Khodadoust, the possible association of an autoimmune phenomenon is intriguing.

Glaucoma has been described as a cause of severe visual loss in patients with intermediate uveitis. In a study of 182 eyes with intermediate uveitis, glaucoma was diagnosed in 15 (8%).[18] However, 11 of the 15 glaucoma cases were thought to be related to corticosteroid use, and only 4 of the 182 eyes (2%) had disease-induced glaucoma. Cataract is a more common finding in these patients; it develops as a result of the ocular inflammatory disease and corticosteroid therapy. Similar to other cataracts in uveitis patients, posterior subcapsular cataract is the most common lenticular opacity found in patients with intermediate uveitis.

The most characteristic findings in this disease are in the vitreous and peripheral retina. Vitreous cells are always present in active intermediate uveitis. Some patients may only have 1+ cells, but the absence of cellular activity in the vitreous precludes a diagnosis of an active intermediate uveitis. White and yellow colored aggregates of inflammatory cells called vitreous snowballs tend to accumulate in the inferior vitreous. Occasionally, the vitritis is dense enough to obscure the retina entirely. This dense vitritis must be differentiated from vitreous hemorrhage that may also occur as a result of neovascularization usually in the vitreous base or peripheral retina.

Brockhurst and colleagues[3] described the early stages of peripheral uveitis as the accumulation of yellow gray exudates at the ora serrata. Although this clinical finding is not required for a diagnosis of intermediate uveitis, it is the major clinical feature in the subset of intermediate uveitis that we call pars planitis. Not all patients with intermediate uveitis have a snowbank and as some patients may have it in one eye only, the inferior white snowbank is an important finding but not an absolute requirement. As the disease progresses, Brockhurst and colleagues note that these exudates coalesce to form the material that is commonly referred to as a snowbank. This is usually located inferiorly only, but in rare patients it can extend for 360 degrees. The snowbank may be discontinuous. It may form a fine band along the ora serrata or be broad and extend onto both the peripheral retina and the pars plana. The snowbank can be dense and extend several millimeters into the vitreous and is usually best seen with scleral depression (see Fig. 4-12). However, a high dense snowbank on the pars plana can often be better seen with the indirect ophthalmoscope without using the 20 D lens while the patient looks down. Although this material has been termed an exudate, it is probably a fibroglial mass and not a true protein exudate as will be discussed later. When a snowbank is observed, the area should be carefully examined for the presence of neovascularization because these areas are a source of potential vitreous hemorrhage.

The peripheral retinal vascular abnormalities may be obscured by the dense vitreal inflammation in some patients. When the vitreous is fairly clear, sheathing or obliteration of the small peripheral venules can be seen. Periarteritis of the small arteries is found less commonly. The perivasculitis is often associated with whitish infiltrates of the peripheral retina. In rare cases, the peripheral neovascularization can evolve into a vascular cyclitic membrane (Fig. 20-1).

Many patients have a mild course of intermediate uveitis or pars planitis and do not have a loss of visual acuity. However, when visual acuity does decrease early in the disease process, cystoid macular edema is the most common cause. Fluorescein angiography or clinical examination reveals cystoid macular edema. In addition, there is often diffuse retinal vascular leakage and optic disc edema when the disease is active. Interestingly, optic disc edema occurs in 50% of children with this entity.[19]

Vitreous hemorrhage from peripheral neovascularization may occur in a small percentage of patients.[3] In many cases the hemorrhage will clear, but in some patients a nonclearing hemorrhage will require surgical intervention. We have observed one patient in whom the neovascularization extended well into the posterior pole leading to recurrent vitreous hemorrhages (Fig. 20-2). Rhegmatogenous retinal detachment can occur from vitreoretinal traction; it occurs in 3.7% to 22% of patients depending on the published series.[3,7] In our experience, rhegmatogenous retinal detachment is an uncommon complication of intermediate uveitis that occurs in less than 3% of patients. Retinal detachments when they occur tend to develop later in the disease process, as persistent vitreal inflammation leads to vitreal contraction and retinal traction. In addition to rhegmatogenous retinal detachments, nonrhegmatogenous retinal detachments associated with choroidal detachments have been described by Brockhurst and colleagues.[3]

Although macular edema is the most common cause of visual loss in intermediate uveitis and is present in most of the patients who are referred to us, other series have reported an

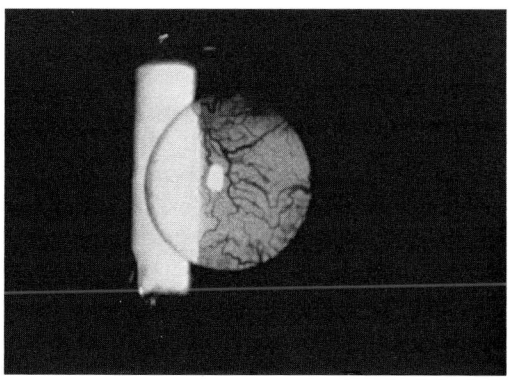

**Fig. 20-1.** Retroillumination photograph demonstrates vascular cyclitic membrane in patient with pars planitis. (Courtesy Rubens Belfort, Jr., M.D.)

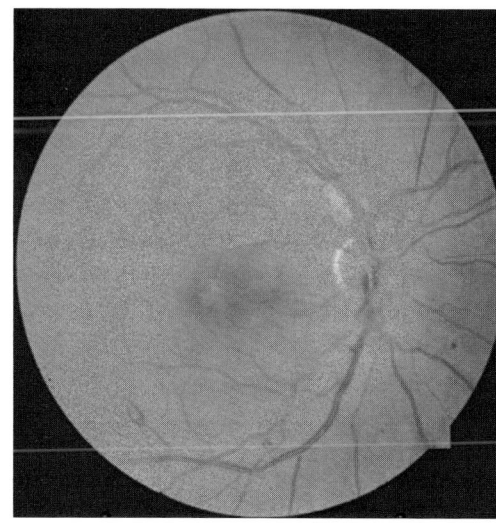

**Fig. 20-2.** Retinal photograph demonstrates small areas of neovascularization in posterior pole in patient with pars planitis and recurrent vitreous hemorrhages.

incidence of macular edema ranging from 28% to 50%.[5,7,20] Long-standing macular edema can lead to the development of retinal pigment epithelial stippling in the macula and may be a subtle sign of previous edema in chronic cases of intermediate uveitis. Unfortunately, this postcystoid macular degeneration can be a cause of severe visual loss in these patients.

Disc edema, optic atrophy, and optic disc neovascularization have been reported in patients with intermediate uveitis. Neovascularization of the disc is associated with severe retinal ischemia but responds to panretinal laser photocoagulation.[21] Phthisis bulbi may be the final outcome of an eye with chronic poorly controlled intermediate uveitis. Oftentimes these eyes have had total retinal detachments, proliferative vitreoretinopathy, or a cyclitic membrane leading to ciliary body traction and hypotony.[22]

## PROGNOSIS

Brockhurst and colleagues[3] originally described five possible types of intermediate uveitis; 28% of their patients had a benign course during which the inflammation subsided with good visual outcome. In fact, Schlaegel[5] has stated that 80% of patients with intermediate uveitis of the pars planitis subtype need no therapy, and we have seen a number of patients with intermediate uveitis with or without pars plana exudates who have low-grade inflammation but never develop macular edema or decreased visual acuity. However, patients in Brockhurst's second group developed choroidal and serous retinal detachments. Patients in the third group developed vascularized high snowbanks that eventually formed cyclitic membranes that led to retinal detachments or glaucoma. Patients in the fourth group had significant vascular obliteration that led to visual field loss and optic atrophy. The fifth group, accounting for 46% of his patients, developed chronic smoldering inflammation.

In a later article, Brockhurst and Schepens[23] condensed the classification into four groups: benign (31%), mild chronic (49%), severe chronic (15%), and relentlessly progressive (10%). In an article published 10 years later, Smith and colleagues[7] found that 19% of intermediate uveitis patients had mild disease, 42% had moderate inflammation, and 39% had severe inflammation. Clearly, the exact percentage of patients in any given category is dependent on the patient populations of the institutions in which the studies are performed. Tertiary referral centers will have more severe disease than primary care institutions. For example, Brockhurst and Schepens reported retinal detachments in 50% of their patients; however, patients with intermediate uveitis and retinal detachments were probably preferentially referred to their retina practice. We have found retinal detachment to occur rarely in patients with intermediate uveitis, but this may reflect the positive effect of therapy with corticosteroids.

Accurate data on the overall prognosis of patients with intermediate uveitis are not available despite the large number of case series published in the literature. At the time of presentation, half the patients have a visual acuity of 20/30 or better.[5] Nevertheless, the disease can produce long-term visual disability in over one third of patients.[7] Schlaegel and Weber[24] found that two thirds of eyes in patients treated with corticosteroids maintained visual acuity of 20/40 or better. The presence of pars plana exudation or snowbanks may be of some prognostic value. Henderly and colleagues[5] observed that eyes with pars plana exudates had more vitritis and macular edema, although the difference was not statistically significant. In addition, severity of disease appears to be more related to visual outcome than length of disease.[7,25]

Although inflammatory disease does remit in some patients, Smith and colleagues[7] found only a 5% remission rate in patients who were followed from 4 to 26 years. Similarly, Hogan and colleagues[1] reported only one remission of 56 cases followed from 1 to 9 years. Patients with intermediate uveitis are often told that their disease will "burn out" after a number of years, and although many patients may maintain useful vision, the disease is usually characterized by either a chronically active course or a course of exacerbations interceded by apparent remissions. In fact, Aaberg[19] has stated that ophthalmologists rarely observe a permanent spontaneous resolution of the disease.

## DIFFERENTIAL DIAGNOSIS

Although intermediate uveitis may exist as an isolated idiopathic disorder, a number of underlying diseases are associated with the disease. Evidence of systemic disorders was found in 83 patients with intermediate uveitis.[26] Of these 26 patients, 10 had presumed sarcoidosis, 6 had multiple sclerosis, 2 had optic neuritis, 2 had inflammatory bowel disease, 4 had thyroid abnormalities, and 2 had histories consistent with Epstein-Barr virus infection. Recently, infectious diseases have been associated with intermediate uveitis. Intermediate uveitis has recently been reported in patients with Lyme disease[27,28] and HTLV-1 infection.[29] A list of the diagnoses associated with intermediate uveitis can be found in Box 20-1. Many of these disorders are discussed in detail elsewhere in the book. Sarcoidosis is discussed in Chapter 21, multiple sclerosis in Chapter 29, Lyme disease in Chapter 10, toxocariasis in Chapter 16, intraocular lymphoma in Chapter 29, and iridocyclitis and Irvine Gass syndrome in Chapter 19.

**Box 20-1**
**Differential diagnosis of intermediate uveitis**

Sarcoidosis
Multiple sclerosis
Inflammatory bowel disease
Lyme disease
Toxocariasis
Intraocular lymphoma
Whipple's disease
Iridocyclitis
Multifocal choroiditis
Irvine Gass syndrome
Amyloidosis
HTLV-1

Our diagnostic evaluation of patients with intermediate uveitis includes a thorough evaluation for sarcoidosis including a chest x-ray, serum angiotensin converting enzyme level, serum calcium level, pulmonary function testing, and a gallium scan. Patients with a history of chronic or bloody diarrhea are referred to a gastroenterologist for evaluation for inflammatory bowel disease. A neurologic history and examination are performed and a magnetic resonance imaging (MRI) scan is performed in patients suspected of having multiple sclerosis. Patients with a history of a rash and who live in an endemic area for Lyme disease, especially with a history of chronic arthritis, receive a Lyme serologic test. If the inflammation is unilateral, a toxocara serology is performed especially in younger patients. Intraocular lymphoma is suspected in older patients who undergo an MRI of the brain, lumbar puncture for cytologic evaluation of the cerebral spinal fluid, and a diagnostic vitrectomy. Other tests are ordered on the basis of a clinical suspicion of a specific disorder.

We usually will obtain a fluorescein angiogram on these patients for two reasons: (1) to assess the presence and extent of cystoid macular edema and (2) to examine the retinal vasculature for signs of perivasculitis including staining of the vessel wall and vascular leakage of dye (Fig. 20-3, *A* and 20-3, *B*). Ultrasonography can demonstrate cyclitic membranes or the

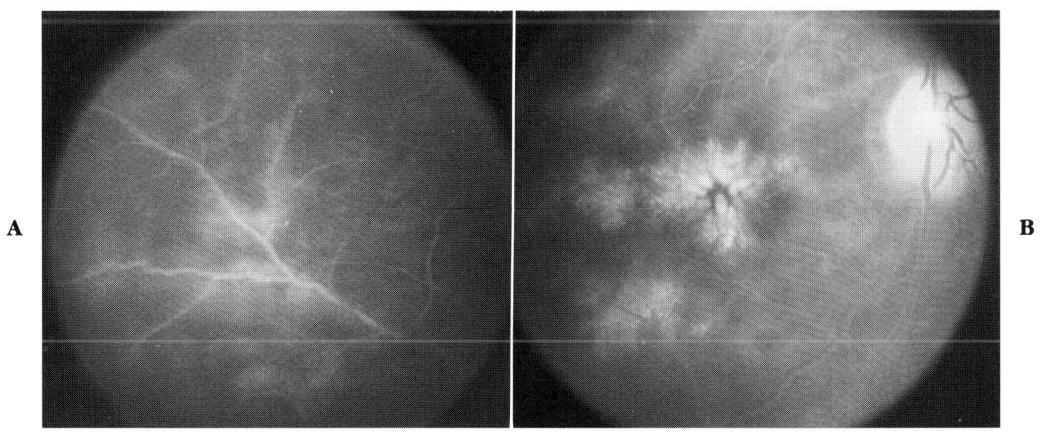


**Fig. 20-3. A,** Late phase of fluorescein angiogram from patient with intermediate uveitis shows substantial leakage of dye from peripheral retinal vessels. **B,** Late phase of fluorescein angiogram from patient with pars planitis shows vascular leakage and prominent cystoid macular edema.

extent of vitreous debris when the view of the posterior pole is obscured by cataract.

## ETIOLOGY

The cause of intermediate uveitis and pars planitis has not been elucidated. Evidence suggests that patients with intermediate uveitis probably do not all have the same disease. Although intermediate uveitis is a fairly common condition in uveitis clinics, the limited amount of pathologic material that has been studied has prevented a thorough clinicopathologic classification of the disease process.

The exudate deposited in eyes with intermediate uveitis of the pars planitis subtype typically localizes to a broad area of the inferior pars plana (see Fig. 4-12). The inferior location of the exudate is attributed to gravity. A diffuse phlebitis leads to breakdown of the blood-ocular barrier and release of inflammatory cells, cytokines, and other inflammatory mediators that settle inferiorly.[30] Gross pathologic examination of the peripheral "snowbank" in pars planitis shows exudate deposited on the peripheral retina and pars plana (Fig. 20-4). Histologic examination of this snowbank reveals a collapsed vitreous, blood vessels, fibroglial cells including fibrous astrocytes, and scattered inflammatory cells, predominantly lymphocytes (Fig. 20-5).[22] Peripheral veins show lymphocytic cuffing and infiltration. The vascular component of the snowbank is continuous with the retina in some cases; this suggests that the neovascularization associated with pars planitis may be the result of retinal vessels extending through breaks in the inner limiting membrane of the vitreous base.[22] Only mild inflammation is noted in the choroid and ciliary body suggesting that the inflammatory process in intermediate uveitis primarily involves the vitreous base and peripheral retina and not the uvea.

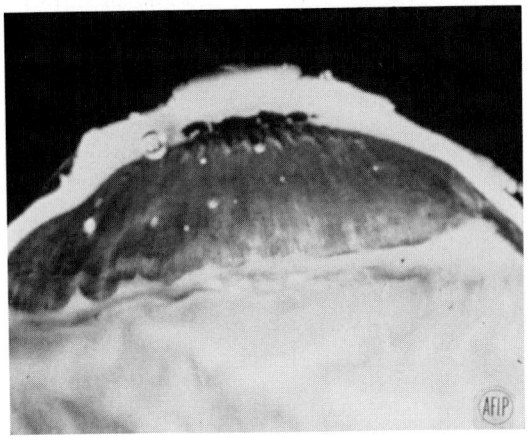


**Fig. 20-4.** Gross pathology of peripheral snowbank in pars planitis. (Courtesy Lorenz Zimmerman, M.D.)

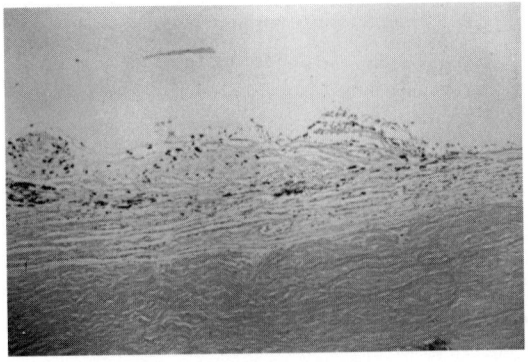

**Fig. 20-5.** Histopathologic section of snowbank in patient with pars planitis shows fibroglial cells, including fibrous astrocytes on surface of peripheral retina and in pars plana. Infiltrating inflammatory cells, predominantly lymphocytes, also can be seen. (Hematoxylin and eosin stain; original magnification ×50.)

The vitreous snowballs in patients with intermediate uveitis are composed of epithelioid cells and multinucleated giant cells. Green and colleagues[31] noted that these cells are absent from the uvea suggesting that the vitreous may be the primary site of inflammation. We have had the chance to study an eye from a case of familial pars planitis. Histologic examination revealed glial tissue in the snowbank and extensive peripheral vascular disease with perivascular infiltration of lymphocytes and expression of MHC class II antigen on the vascular endothelium.[12] There was no substantial choroidal inflammation, again suggesting that pars planitis is a peripheral retinitis or vitritis and not a choroiditis. Studies of eyes with intermediate uveitis without pars plana exudate are sparse; this makes clinicopathologic correlation between the two disease types difficult.

The association of intermediate uveitis with autoimmune diseases such as multiple sclerosis suggest that at least some cases of the disorder are autoimmune in nature. Intermediate uveitis is thought to be a primary peripheral retinal perivasculitis. Once begun, the process of vascular occlusion and inflammation may lead to vitritis and snowbank formation in some cases. Although others, like Khodadoust and colleagues[17] have hypothesized that intermediate uveitis is primarily a vitreal inflammation, they note that the inflammation appears to start adjacent to involved vascular tissue. Interestingly, injection of hyaluronic acid into the vitreous of monkeys induces a clinical picture similar to pars planitis.[32] Furthermore, Gartner[33] demonstrated that the vitreous contains cellular remnants that may be the antigenic stimulus in pars planitis. More recently, Kaplan and colleagues[34] have noted a protein from the serum of patients with active intermediate uveitis that may be a marker for the disease.

However, none of these theories fully explain the familial association with intermediate uveitis, the association of this disorder with certain systemic diseases such as sarcoidosis, inflammatory bowel disease, and multiple sclerosis, or the cause of cystoid macular edema. It is our feeling that the periphlebitis and breakdown of the blood-ocular barrier is the initiating event in many cases. Increased levels of immune markers such as soluble interleukin-2 receptors and ICAM-1 have been found in the serum of patients with intermediate uveitis.[35,36] However, the specific cause of this vascular disease is multifactorial and probably differs from case to case.

## TREATMENT

Because intermediate uveitis is a disorder associated with a number of underlying diseases, the first step in the treatment is to exclude the possibility of an underlying infectious disease or malignancy. Both Lyme disease and intraocular lymphoma are in the differential diagnosis of intermediate uveitis and should be ruled out before treatment with immunosuppressive therapy is begun. The second step is to decide whether therapy is needed. In general, similar to an approach detailed by Kaplan,[37] we have not treated eyes with visual acuity better than 20/40. There are exceptions to this rule. Eyes with extensive neovascularization of the peripheral snowbank or eyes with substantial vasculitis are often treated despite good vision. Nevertheless, we have a number of cases of intermediate uveitis with mild vitritis, periphlebitis, and cystoid macular edema that maintain good vision for years without therapy and the resultant side effects. Whether these patients in the long run are better served by more aggressive antiinflammatory therapy early on is unknown.

Corticosteroids are the mainstay of therapy as they are for most forms of uveitis. Although topical corticosteroids are effective for the treatment of anterior uveitis, we have found them ineffective for the treatment of intermediate uveitis in the phakic patient. In aphakic patients, large doses of topical corticosteroids may yield enough concentration of the drug in the vitreous to treat mild disease. Most patients, however, will require either systemic therapy or periocular injections. Periocular corticosteroids are very effective in treating many cases of intermediate uveitis especially for uniocular disease. We prefer to use injections of 40 mg of triamcinolone given retroseptally through the lower lid or into the subtenons space superotemporally. We emphasize that two or three injections given over a 6- to 8-week period should be tried before the technique is deemed ineffective. We have also given bilateral periocular corticosteroid injections to children and some adults with intermediate uveitis under general anesthesia and have found this approach quite helpful.

Systemic corticosteroids are used for most cases of bilateral intermediate uveitis or unilocular disease resistant to periocular corticosteroids. We start patients on one half to 1 mg/Kg/day of prednisone and then taper the prednisone on the basis of the clinical response. Patients should have a purified protein derivative test before immunosuppressive therapy is started to determine if antituberculous medications are needed. In addition, patients should be placed on antiulcer medications such as an H-2 blocker. We typically prescribe ranitidine 150 mg taken orally twice a day.

For patients who are resistant to corticosteroid therapy or who require chronic corticosteroid treatment for their disease, we will add an immunosuppressive agent. At the NIH, we tend to use cyclosporine as our first line steroid-sparing agent; it has demonstrated good therapeutic efficacy in patients with intermediate uveitis. The major side effects of cyclosporine include renal toxicity and hypertension (see Chapter 8); however, by carefully watching patients for signs of toxicity and adjusting the dose of cyclosporine when needed, we have been able to maintain patients on cyclosporine for up to 10 years. Other immunosuppressive agents that have been used for treating intermediate uveitis include azathioprine and methotrexate. We tend to avoid the use of cyclophosphamide for the treatment of this disorder because of the significant adverse effects such as bladder cancer that are associated with its use.

Two surgical therapies have been used for the treatment of intermediate uveitis: cryotherapy and vitrectomy. Cryotherapy applied to the pars plana exudate is thought to be effective in the treatment of pars planitis. The rationale for cryotherapy is that it destroys the vascular component of the peripheral retinitis or vitritis and eliminates the entrance site for inflammatory mediators into the eye.[19] Cryotherapy is often combined with periocular corticosteroid injections. The effect of cryotherapy is evident within several weeks and lasts for 3 to 6 months. A second treatment may be given if the first treatment was effective.

Well-controlled masked clinical trials of cryotherapy are lacking in the literature. Devenyi and colleagues[38] reported the use of cryotherapy in 27 eyes with steroid-resistant intermediate uveitis and neovascularization of the vitreous base. Patients were followed up from 2 to 12 years, and vitritis was eliminated in 78% of patients. In addition, cryotherapy eliminated the need for corticosteroid therapy in 90% of eyes. Complications included transient increased vitreal inflammation, decreased accommodation, cataract, and hyphema. Some specialists have stopped using cryotherapy for the treatment of intermediate uveitis because of a reported increased incidence of posttreatment retinal detachment. Currently, we limit the use of cryotherapy to patients with intermediate uveitis, neovascularization of the vitreous base, and a history of vitreous hemorrhage.

Decreased inflammatory disease has been reported after pars plana vitrectomy for chronic inflammation in patients with intermediate uveitis, possibly because the inflammatory mediators were removed from the eye.[39] Bacskulin and Eckardt[40] reported significant improvement in 12 of 19 eyes with chronic uveitis treated with vitrectomy. Cystoid macular edema was reduced in 7 of 8 eyes, and in two thirds of cases the intensity of the inflammation decreased so that the dose of corticosteroids could be reduced postoperatively. Miller and colleagues[41] reported significant visual improvement in patients undergoing vitrectomy for intermediate uveitis. However, six (50%) eyes required further surgery after the development of retinal detachment, recurrent vitreous hemorrhage, or cataract formation. We have been less convinced of the therapeutic efficacy of pars plana vitrectomy in patients with chronic uveitis and reserve vitrectomy for patients with persistent vitreous hemorrhage or dense vitreous debris that does not clear with medical therapy.

Cataracts are a frequent complication of intermediate uveitis; they result from both chronic inflammation and corticosteroid therapy. Extreme vigilance in controlling ocular inflammation preoperatively is a key to successful and safe cataract extraction in these patients.[42] Use of systemic corticosteroids is also required after surgery. Patients with intermediate uveitis often have an exacerbation of inflammatory activity starting about 3 days postoperatively. It is therefore necessary to see these patients almost on a daily basis in the early postoperative period so that increased inflammatory activity can be promptly recognized and appropriately treated.

Should patients with intermediate uveitis

who are undergoing cataract surgery have intraocular lens placement? Michelson and colleagues[43] reported on 15 eyes in 8 patients with intermediate uveitis who were undergoing cataract extraction with intraocular lens placement. Despite having quiescent disease for at least 6 months before surgery, 40% had a final visual acuity worse than 20/40. Complications included debris on the intraocular lens requiring multiple yttrium-aluminum-garnet laser procedures to clear off the anterior surface. It is our opinion that patients with intermediate uveitis characterized by chronic relapsing inflammatory disease, cystoid macular edema, and substantial posterior synechiae are better served by aphakic correction or contact lenses than an intraocular lens. We are currently investigating whether surface modified intraocular lenses coated with heparin can improve the prognosis for intraocular lens placement in these patients.

### Case 20-1

An 8-year-old boy presented with a 1-year history of progressive unilateral visual loss. Examination revealed a visual acuity of 20/100, 2+ vitreal cells and haze, and a pars plana exudate (snowbank) and a diagnosis of intermediate uveitis of the pars planitis subtype. He received cryopexy to the snowbank and a periocular injection of 40 mg of methylprednisolone acetate (Depo-Medrol). Over the next 2 weeks, his visual acuity improved from 20/100 to 20/30 with a concurrent reduction in inflammation. Visual acuity remained stable for the next 9 months, but intraocular inflammation began to recur. One year after the first cryopexy and periocular injection with corticosteroids, vision decreased to 20/80. The patient was treated with a second cryopexy and periocular injection of corticosteroids. Vision again improved to 20/30, but 1 year later the vision again fell to 20/80. A third cryopexy and periocular corticosteroid injection had no effect. However, two additional periocular injections lead to decreased ocular inflammation and improvement of vision to 20/30.

### Case 20-2

An 11-year-old girl developed bilateral intermediate uveitis with pars plana exudates that resulted in decreased vision in both eyes. She was treated with systemic prednisone, and visual acuity improved. The patient, however, developed intolerable weight gain, mood changes, and gastrointestinal distress, and the prednisone therapy was discontinued. The patient received three periocular injections of corticosteroids without improvement in vision. Cryotherapy to one eye similarly had no effect. Two years after the start of the disease, the patient was left with bilateral cystoid macular edema, moderate vitritis, and visual acuity of 20/50 OD and 20/80 OS.

The patient was started on cyclosporine at a dose of 4 mg/kg daily and bromocriptine at 10 mg/day. Over the next 2 months the vitreal inflammation and cystoid macular edema resolved, and the visual acuity improved to 20/20 in the right eye and 20/32 in the left eye. The patient tolerated these medications without problems, and she continued on this therapeutic regimen.

## REFERENCES


1. Hogan MJ, Kimura SJ, O'Connor GR et al: Peripheral retinitis and chronic cyclitis in children, *Trans Ophthalmol Soc UK* 85:39-52, 1965.
2. Schepens CL: L'inflammation de la region de l'ora serrata et ses sequelles, *Bull Soc Ophthalmol Fr* 73:113-124, 1950.
3. Brockhurst RJ, Schepens CL, Okamura ID: Uveitis II. Peripheral uveitis: clinical description, complications and differential diagnosis, *Am J Ophthalmol* 49:1257-1266, 1960.
4. Welch RB, Maumenee AE, Wahlen HE: Peripheral posterior segment inflammation, vitreous opacities, and edema of the posterior pole, *Arch Ophthalmol* 64:540-549, 1960.
5. Henderly DE, Haymond RS, Rao NS et al: The significance of the pars plana exudate in pars planitis, *Am J Ophthalmol* 103:669-671, 1987.
6. Schlaegel TF Jr: Differential diagnosis of uveitis, *Ophthalmol Digest* 35:34, 1973.
7. Smith RE, Godfrey WA, Kimura SJ: Chronic cyclitis. I. Course and visual prognosis, *Trans Am Acad Ophthalmol Otolaryngol* 77:760-768, 1973.
8. Van Metre TE: Role of the allergist in diagnosis and management of patients with uveitis, *JAMA* 195:167-172, 1966.
9. Giles CL: Uveitis in childhood. In Tasman W, Jaeger EA, editors: *Duane's clinical ophthalmology*, Philadelphia, 1981, JB Lippincott, pp 1-8.
10. Arocker-Mettinger E, Mayr WR, Huber SV et al: Do HLA antigens play a role in intermediate uveitis? *Vox Sang* 63(4):282-284, 1992.
11. Kimura SJ, Hogan MJ: Chronic cyclitis, *Arch Ophthalmol* 71:193-201, 1964.
12. Wetzig RP, Chan CC, Nussenblatt RB et al: Clinical and immunopathological studies of pars planitis in a family, *Br J Ophthalmol* 72:5-10, 1988.
13. Culbertson WW, Giles CL, West CW et al: Familial pars planitis, *Retina* 3:179-181, 1983.
14. Augsburger JJ, Annesley WH, Sergott RC et al: Familial pars planitis, *Ann Ophthalmol* 13:553-557, 1981.
15. Schlaegel TF: *Ocular toxoplasmosis and pars planitis*, New York, 1978, Grune & Stratton.
16. Capone A Jr, Aaberg TM: Intermediate uveitis. In Albert DM, Jacobiec FA, editors: *Principles and practice of ophthalmology*, Philadelphia, 1994, WB Saunders, pp 423-442.

17. Khodadoust AA, Karnama Y, Stoessel KM et al: Pars planitis, an autoimmune endotheliopathy, *Am J Ophthalmol* 102:633-639, 1986.
18. Smith RE, Godfrey WA, Kimura SJ: Complications of chronic cyclitis, *Am J Ophthalmol* 82:277-282, 1976.
19. Aaberg TM: The enigma of pars planitis, *Am J Ophthalmol* 103:828-830, 1987.
20. Hogan MJ, Kimura SJ, O'Connor GR: Peripheral retinitis and chronic cyclitis in children, *Trans Ophthalmol Soc UK* 85:39-52, 1965.
21. Felder KS, Brockhurst RJ: Neovascular fundus abnormalities in peripheral uveitis, *Arch Ophthalmol* 100: 750-754, 1982.
22. Pederson JE, Kenyon KR, Green WR et al: Pathology of pars planitis, *Am J Ophthalmol* 86:762-774, 1978.
23. Brockhurst RJ, Schepens CL: Uveitis IV. Peripheral uveitis: the complications of retinal detachment, *Arch Ophthalmol* 80:747-753, 1968.
24. Schlaegel TF, Weber JC: Corticosteroids for pars planitis, *Surv Ophthalmol* 22:120-130, 1977.
25. Chester GH, Blach RK, Cleary PE: Inflammation in the region of the vitreous base: pars planitis, *Trans Ophthalmol Soc UK* 96:151-157, 1976.
26. Boskovich SA, Lowder CY, Meisler DM et al: Systemic diseases associated with intermediate uveitis, *Cleve Clin J Med* 60(6):460-465, 1993.
27. Breeveld J, Rothova A, Kuiper H: Intermediate uveitis and Lyme borreliosis, *Br J Ophthalmol* 76(3):181-182, 1992.
28. Guex CY, Herbort CP: Lyme disease in Switzerland: ocular involvement, *Klin Monatsbl Augenheilkd* 200(5):545-546, 1992.
29. Mochizuki M, Watanabe T, Yamaguchi K et al: Uveitis associated with human T-cell lymphotropic virus type I, *Am J Ophthalmol* 114(2):123-129, 1992.
30. Deschenes J, Freeman W, Char DH et al: Lymphocyte subpopulations in uveitis, *Arch Ophthalmol* 104:233-236, 1986.
31. Green WR, Kincaid MC, Michels GG et al: Pars planitis, *Trans Ophthalmol Soc UK* 101:361-367, 1981.
32. Hultsch E: Peripheral uveitis in the owl monkey, *Mod Probl Ophthalmol* 18:247-251, 1977.
33. Gartner J: The vitreous base of the human eye and 'pars planitis': electron microscopic observations, *Mod Probl Ophthalmol* 10:250-255, 1972.
34. Bora NS, Gobleman CL, Cirrito TP et al: Correlation of serum and plasma P-36 with active pars planitis, *Invest Ophthalmol Vis Sci* 34(suppl):973, 1993.
35. Murray PI, Young DW: Soluble interleukin-2 receptors in retinal vasculitis, *Curr Eye Res* 11 Suppl:193-195, 1992.
36. Arocker-Mettinger E, Steurer-Georgiew L, Steurer M et al: Circulating ICAM-1 levels in serum of uveitis patients, *Curr Eye Res* 11 Suppl:161-166, 1992.
37. Kaplan HJ: Intermediate uveitis (pars planitis, chronic cyclitis)—a four step approach to treatment. In Saari KM, editor: *Uveitis update,* Amsterdam, 1984, Excerpta Medica, pp 169-172.
38. Devenyi RG, Mieler WF, Lambrou FH et al: Cryopexy of the vitreous base in the management of peripheral uveitis, *Am J Ophthalmol* 106:135-138, 1988.
39. Kaplan HJ: Surgical treatment of intermediate uveitis, *Dev Ophthalmol* 23(185):185-189, 1992.
40. Bacskulin A, Eckardt C: Results of pars plana vitrectomy in chronic uveitis in childhood, *Ophthalmologe* 90:434-439, 1993.
41. Miller WF, Will BR, Lewis H et al: Vitrectomy in the management of peripheral uveitis, *Ophthalmology* 95:859-864, 1988.
42. Foster CS: Vitrectomy in the management of uveitis, *Ophthalmology* 95:1011-1012, 1988.
43. Michelson JB, Friedlander MH, Nozik RA: Lens implant surgery in pars planitis, *Ophthalmology* 97:1023-1026, 1990.

# CHAPTER 21

# Sarcoidosis

Sarcoidosis is a multisystem granulomatous disease that can affect almost every organ in the body. The most common organs involved in sarcoidosis are the lung, thoracic lymph nodes, and skin. The adrenal glands, which produce corticosteroids, are the only organs not affected by this disease. Sarcoidosis was initially described as a dermatologic disease by Hutchinson in 1869, and Boeck used the term *sarkoid* to describe the skin biopsies that had a histologic appearance similar to sarcomas.[1] Uveitis was described in patients with sarcoidosis in the early 1900s, and in 1936 sarcoid uveitis associated with a facial nerve palsy and uveoparotid fever was termed *Heerfordt's syndrome.*[2] Although the cause of sarcoidosis remains unknown, it is important to make the diagnosis of sarcoidosis in patients with uveitis not only to allow appropriate therapy for the eye disease, but also to alert the physician to the possible systemic manifestations that may also require treatment.

## EPIDEMIOLOGY

Epidemiologic studies of sarcoidosis are prone to considerable error because of variability in the criteria for diagnosis. Nevertheless, there are substantial differences in the yearly incidence rate in differing parts of the world, from 0.2 per 100,000 in Japan and Spain to 64 per 100,000 in Sweden.[3,4] In the United States, the age-adjusted annual incidence in African-Americans is 82 per 100,000 and in whites is 8 per 100,000.[5] In addition, African-Americans with chronic sarcoidosis are more likely to develop ocular manifestations than whites.[6] Systemic sarcoidosis does not appear to have a sex predilection.[5]

## ETIOLOGY

Although the cause of sarcoidosis remains unknown, a number of recent studies have elucidated the immunologic basis for the disease pathogenesis. The macrophage is hypothesized to initiate the inflammatory response in sarcoidosis.[7–10] Possibly in response to presentation of an unknown antigen, macrophages are thought to release cytokines such as interleukin-1 that cause the infiltration of T-helper lymphocytes. These lymphocytes will also release cytokines and recruit other inflammatory cells to the site of inflammation. In response to these events, granulomas are formed and immunoglobulins produced in large quantities by stimulated B lymphocytes and released into the circulation. The immunohistochemical staining of one eye with sarcoidosis showed granulomas in the choroid and anterior uvea composed of macrophages and T-helper cells.[11]

Although the primary involvement of the lung in sarcoidosis suggests sensitization and a resultant immune response to an endogenous lung antigen or an inhaled infectious agent or other antigen, no study has successfully shown a consistent relationship to a causative agent. An alternative hypothesis suggests that sarcoidosis is an abnormal immune response directed against one of many different antigens in a patient with a hereditary or acquired abnormality of the immune system. There are a number of immune defects

**Table 21-1.** Uveitis associated with sarcoidosis

| | |
|---|---|
| **DIAGNOSTIC CRITERIA** | |
| Suspected sarcoidosis | Hilar adenopathy, erythema nodosum, increased serum ACE, positive lung or lacrimal or salivary gland gallium scan, increased serum globulin, increased serum or urinary calcium, lymphadenopathy, decreased lung diffusing capacity |
| Definite sarcoidosis | Histologic confirmation of noncaseating granulomas |
| Associated findings | Uveitis, arthritis, neurologic signs, anemia, decreased pulmonary function, lymphadenopathy |
| **OCULAR FINDINGS** | |
| Common | Acute nongranulomatous or chronic granulomatous iridocyclitis, vitritis, vitreal snowballs, macular edema, perivenous sheathing, small yellow choroidal and retinal pigment epithelial patches of inflammation, optic disc swelling, retinal neovascularization |
| Rare | Large choroidal granulomas, subretinal neovascularization, optic neuropathy |

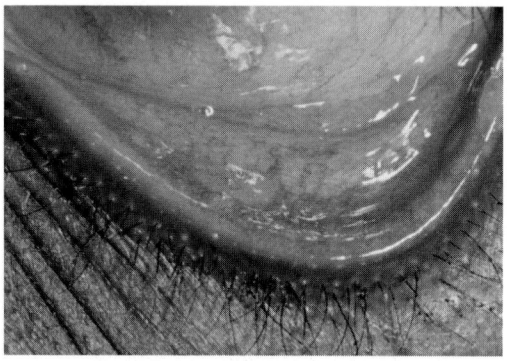

**Fig. 21-1.** Biopsy proven conjunctival granulomas in patient with sarcoidosis. (See Color Plate 36.)

in patients with sarcoidosis. Delayed-type hypersensitivity is depressed causing anergy on skin testing, and a generally depressed cellular immunity has been reported.

## CLINICAL MANIFESTATIONS

Most patients with sarcoidosis present with respiratory symptoms, although some have generalized symptoms such as fever, fatigue, or weight loss. Many patients with sarcoidosis are asymptomatic at the time of diagnosis and are only recognized after an abnormal chest x-ray or laboratory test result. Sarcoid uveitis is diagnosed when ocular inflammation is found in a patient with extraocular findings diagnostic of sarcoidosis. The definitive diagnosis of sarcoidosis requires the demonstration of a noncaseating, granulomatous, noninfectious inflammatory process on biopsy; however, a number of laboratory and other diagnostic tests can strongly support the diagnosis.

Ophthalmic involvement occurred in 50% of patients with sarcoidosis in one report,[12] but most series report eye findings in about 25% of patients.[6,13,14] The common ocular findings in patients with sarcoidosis are listed in Table 21-1. Twenty-six percent of patients with chronic systemic sarcoidosis have ophthalmic involvement at some point during the course of their disease.[6] Ocular disease is usually bilateral but may be unilateral or markedly asymmetric. It is important to examine both the conjunctiva and lacrimal gland in patients with possible sarcoidosis. The palpebral conjunctiva should be carefully scrutinized for sarcoid granulomas (Fig. 21-1), which are seen in 7% to 17% of patients with ophthalmic involvement.[6,13,14] The lacrimal gland, which is clinically involved in 7% to 26% of patients with ocular sarcoidosis,[6,13,14] should also be examined for possible enlargement as a result of the disease. Although a positive conjunctival biopsy for sarcoidosis does not correlate with the presence of anterior uveitis in sarcoidosis,[15] the demonstration of a noncaseating granuloma in the conjunctiva can be diagnostic.

### Anterior uveitis

Anterior uveitis is the most common ocular manifestation and occurs in almost two thirds of patients with ocular sarcoidosis. From 53% to 60% of patients with ocular sarcoidosis will have a chronic granulomatous uveitis.[6,13,14] Most of these patients will have mutton-fat keratic precipitates (KP) that may be extremely large and dense as shown in Fig. 21-2. Iris nodules, although characteristic for granulomatous inflammation, occur in only 11% of all patients with ocular sarcoidosis (Fig. 21-3).[13] Occasionally, an iris nodule can enlarge to the point that it resembles a tumor. Although the

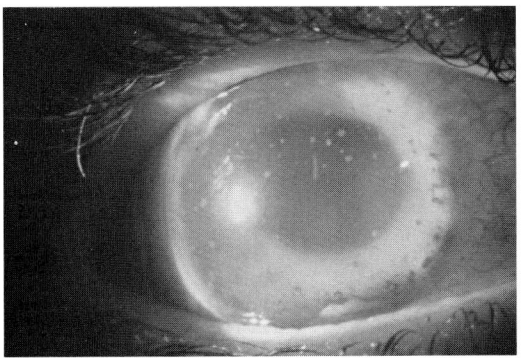

**Fig. 21-2.** Large granulomatous mutton-fat keratic precipitates in patient with chronic uveitis and sarcoidosis. (See Color Plate 37.)

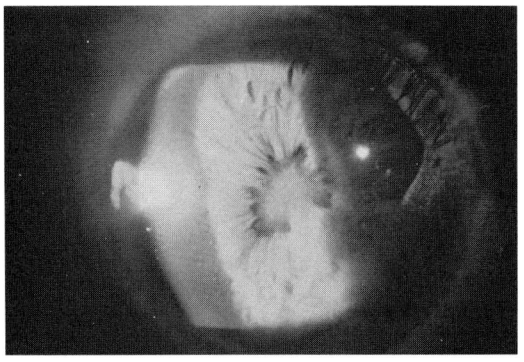

**Fig. 21-3.** Chronic anterior uveitis in patient with sarcoidosis leading to posterior synechiae formation. Iris granuloma is also seen at 4 o'clock position.

presence of other signs of inflammation and the yellow color of the lesion may be reassuring, only a decrease in the size of the lesion after corticosteroid therapy can prove that the nodule is inflammatory and not malignant.

This chronic form of anterior inflammation generally occurs in patients with sarcoidosis in the fourth through sixth decade[14] and results in secondary damage to the eye including cataract and glaucoma. The incidence of both of these complications is difficult to estimate from the literature as there is an increasing incidence of both cataracts and glaucoma with an increasing duration of the chronic inflammation. The prevalence of cataracts in chronic sarcoid uveitis is 8% to 17%, and the prevalence of glaucoma varies from 11% to 23%.[6,13,14] Both pupillary block and trabecular meshwork damage can cause glaucoma in these patients and may exist simultaneously. In contrast, chronic inflammation will occasionally lead to hypotony and phthisis.[11,16]

Acute iridocyclitis of limited duration associated with small fine KP occurs in 15% to 45% of patients with ocular sarcoidosis.[6,13,14] Even among patients with chronic systemic sarcoidosis, those patients with anterior iridocyclitis frequently have one attack early in the course of their disease and no further recurrences. Some patients will develop a pattern of acute recurrent uveitis without granulomatous signs. Therefore, although granulomatous uveitis is the more common presentation of ocular sarcoidosis, even a patient with recurrent anterior iritis may have sarcoidosis as an underlying cause. We have followed up on several patients with recurrent anterior uveitis who developed mild vitritis years later along with systemic manifestations of sarcoidosis. As will be discussed later, there is little proof at this time that the lesions of acute iritis in patients with sarcoidosis are due to the same pathologic process that is responsible for the noncaseating granulomas of the thorax.

### Posterior segment findings

Inflammation of the vitreous, retina, and choroid is less common but more visually disabling than inflammation in the anterior segment and occurs in 6% to 33% of patients with sarcoidosis.[6,13,14] Many of these patients will also have anterior inflammation. The presence of clumps of cells and proteinaceous debris called snowballs in the vitreous should suggest the diagnosis of sarcoidosis. Often these snowballs are located inferiorly and lie on the retinal surface anterior to the equator. The classic "candle wax dripping" (en taches de bougie) along the retinal veins is not frequently seen (Fig. 21-4), but many patients with posterior inflammation will have perivenous sheathing.[13,17] In contrast, periarterial sheathing is rarely observed. Small areas of peripheral venous occlusion have been reported, but large vein occlusions are uncommon. Deep yellow choroidal lesions consistent with Dalen-Fuchs nodules and mottling of the pigment epithelium occur in 36% of these patients (Fig. 21-5) and are more common than true elevated choroidal granuloma.[17] These smaller lesions are probably small choroidal granulomas that evolve and lead to secondary pigment epithelial alterations. They are similar in appearance and histology to the Dalen-Fuchs nodules of sympathetic ophthalmia, although the lesions may be somewhat larger in sarcoidosis than in sympa-

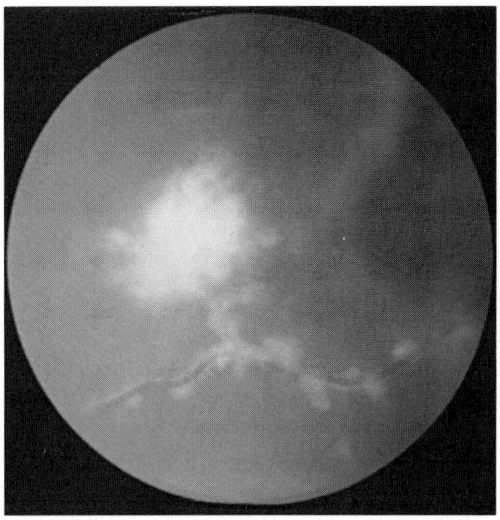

**Fig. 21-4.** Peripheral perivenous sheathing (candle wax drippings) and peripheral retinal exudate in sarcoidosis.

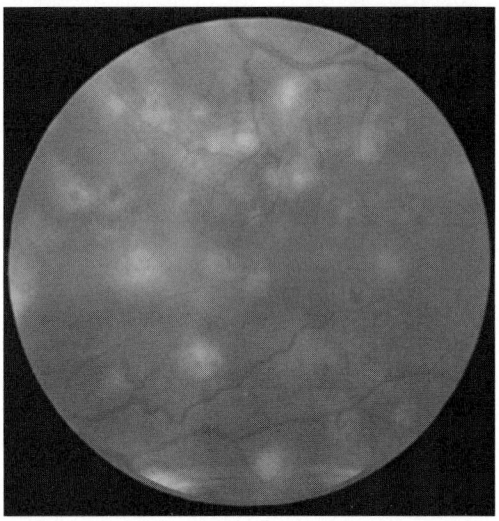

**Fig. 21-5.** Multiple chorioretinal lesions in fundus of patient with sarcoidosis.

thetic ophthalmia. Large granulomas of the choroid can also occur and may resemble choroidal tumors.[18,19] These appear as yellow white or yellow grey discrete elevated masses. Large granulomas can have overlying serous retinal detachments and will cause decreased acuity if they involve the fovea (Fig. 21-6). These lesions will block fluorescence in the early stages of a fluorescein angiogram and will stain in the late phase. If these lesions occur under the macula, one needs to be concerned about the development of a submacular neovascular net extending from the granuloma.

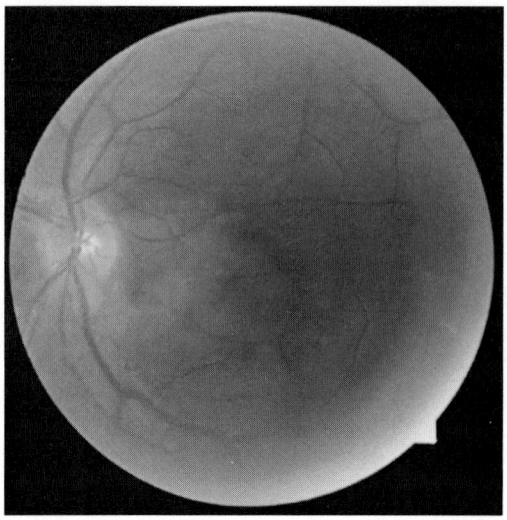

**Fig. 21-6.** Photograph of choroidal granuloma with associated serous retinal detachment in patient with sarcoidosis.

Chronic cystoid macular edema is usually the cause of decreased acuity in patients with posterior uveitis and sarcoidosis. However, the vitreous opacities can occasionally be sufficiently dense in this disease to contribute to a decrease in visual acuity. Nevertheless, we have been surprised that visual acuity is only minimally affected in most uveitis patients with even dense vitreous opacity as long as the macula and optic nerve are uninvolved. Neovascularization of the optic disc occurs in approximately 15% of patients with posterior uveitis related to sarcoidosis.[17] In our experience, prompt steroid therapy will frequently lead to a involution of these vessels, which implies that the ischemic stimulus that promoted the neovascularization is reversible and related to the inflammation. If there is significant peripheral vascular ischemia or neovascularization, therapy with antiinflammatory drugs may not be adequate, and photocoagulation may be indicated.

In contrast to retinal neovascularization, subretinal neovascularization in sarcoidosis is much less common and does not respond to medical therapy.[16,20,21] Case reports usually describe a peripapillary or macular subretinal neovascular membrane (Fig. 21-7). It is likely that choroidal inflammation with secondary retinal pigment epithelial damage leads to breaks in Bruch's membrane that permit the development of the neovascular net. The natural course of these vascular abnormalities is not

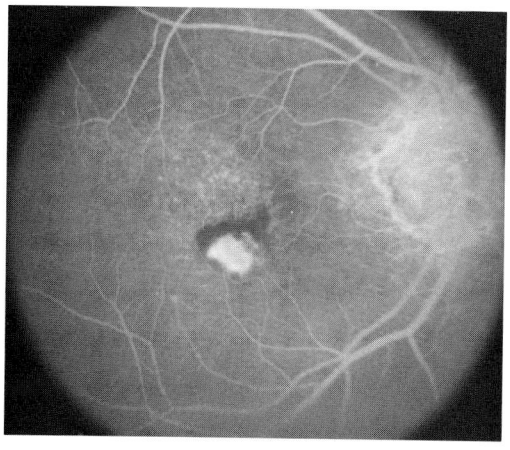

**Fig. 21-7.** Fluorescein angiogram of subretinal neovascular membrane in patient with sarcoidosis.

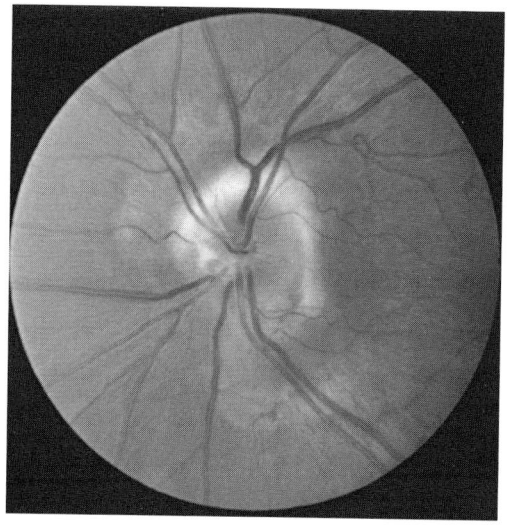

**Fig. 21-8.** Optic disc hyperemia and peripapillary fibrous ring in patient with sarcoidosis and history of optic disc swelling.

well defined, but they probably have a prognosis that is similar to subretinal membranes as a result of other causes.

Optic disc swelling occurs in 39% of patients with posterior uveitis, but it is usually mild and not associated with visual dysfunction.[17] The optic disc may also be hyperemic. Papilledema from sarcoid granulomas that invade the optic nerve can occur, but it is probably not the common cause of disc swelling as the optic disc swelling follows a course that parallels the severity of the posterior uveitis.[17] After the disc edema resolves, a peripapillary fibrous ring may remain (Fig. 21-8). Retrobulbar neuritis without any intraocular signs of inflammation has also been reported and is presumably related to direct involvement of the optic nerve by granulomatous inflammation.[22]

## Systemic involvement

Sarcoidosis is a systemic disease, and the other organ systems involved in this disease are listed in Table 21-2. Skin lesions are common in sarcoidosis, and a biopsy of granulomatous lesions can be diagnostic. Both erythema nodosum and granulomatous sarcoid nodules of the skin have been described. Erythema nodosum is a nodular subcutaneous inflammation that presents on the lower extremities and occasionally on the upper extremities or face. The nodules are elevated, red, and tender. It is a hypersensitivity reaction and occurs in drug allergies and in diseases such as streptococcal infection, colitis, and Behçet's disease as well as in sarcoidosis. The lesions of erythema nodosum are not granulomatous, and the condition is generally self-limited. It usually occurs in women with sarcoidosis in the second and third decade and is frequently associated with an acute presentation of sarcoidosis that also includes fever, arthralgia, hilar adenopathy, and iritis.[5] The granulomatous nodules of sarcoidosis in the skin appear as movable nontender subcutaneous nodules usually on the lower extremities. Biopsy of these lesions often reveals noncaseating granulomas diagnostic of sarcoidosis.

**Table 21-2.** Systemic involvement of sarcoidosis

| Locus | Incidence (%) |
|---|---|
| Hilar adenopathy | 74 |
| Lung parenchyma | 46 |
| Lymphadenopathy | 28 |
| Skin lesions (excluding erythema nodosum) | 18 |
| Erythema nodosum | 15 |
| Splenomegaly | 10 |
| Bone | 4 |
| Parotid | 6 |
| Central nervous system | 5 |

Modified from Siltzbach LE, James DG, Neville E et al: Course and prognosis of sarcoidosis around the world, *Am J Med* 57:847-852, 1974.

The arthritis of sarcoidosis can be either acute or chronic in nature. Twenty-one percent of North American whites with sarcoidosis have joint symptoms,[23] and the percentage in

African-Americans may be somewhat higher. Arthritis is most common during acute sarcoidosis, and the arthritis in these patients rarely becomes chronic. Although granulomas in the joint synovium may be seen, mild nongranulomatous synovitis is more common. Arthritis occurs less frequently in patients with chronic sarcoidosis, but these patients are more likely to have synovial granulomas.

A wide range of neurologic symptoms including cranial nerve palsies, neuropathy, myopathy, and aseptic meningitis can result from the meningoencephalitis of sarcoidosis. A lumbar puncture and central nervous system imaging studies are important to define the nature of the neurologic involvement that occurs in approximately 5% of patients with sarcoidosis.[5] Sarcoidosis that involves the base of the brain and chiasm may be clinically difficult to prove without a biopsy. The facial nerve is the cranial nerve most commonly involved in patients with sarcoidosis. Because Lyme disease is also a cause of facial nerve paresis, arthralgias, rash, and uveitis, it should be considered in the differential diagnosis of patients with these findings.

Although hilar adenopathy is a more frequent finding in sarcoidosis, splenomegaly and lymphadenopthy occur in 10% and 28% of patients with sarcoidosis, respectively.[5] These findings are detectable by physical examination and should be looked for in patients with possible sarcoidosis. Enlarged lymphoid organs are unusual in most types of endogenous uveitis and point to a clinical diagnosis of sarcoidosis.

Sarcoidosis is also a common cause of uveitis in children under the age of 5 years. The disease in these children is characterized by a granulomatous anterior uveitis, polyarticular arthritis, rash, and lymphadenopathy.[24] Posterior uveitis and orbital disease can also occur. Pulmonary disease occurs in only one third of younger patients, but these children often have skin and joint disease.[25] Finding an anterior uveitis and arthritis in a young child with a normal chest x-ray often leads to the misdiagnosis of juvenile arthritis. However, similar to patients with juvenile rheumatoid arthritis, the anterior uveitis may lead to permanent loss of vision, especially in young children susceptible to the development of amblyopia. In these children especially, aggressive therapy is often warranted. In older children the presentation and course of sarcoidosis more closely parallel that of adults.

One genetic disease that occurs in children that can mimic sarcoidosis is Blau syndrome, a disorder characterized by familial granulomatosis, arthritis, uveitis, and rash.[26] Although some of these patients may have elevated serum angiotensin-converting enzyme (ACE) levels, the disorder is otherwise clinically distinct. Patients with Blau syndrome may have camptodactyly and do not have pulmonary disease, hypercalcemia, or positive reactions to Kveim skin testing.

Although many patients with sarcoid uveitis maintain good visual acuity, permanent visual loss can occur despite appropriate therapy. In our patients with biopsy-proven ocular sarcoidosis, 14 (67%) of 21 had a visual acuity of 20/40 or worse in at least one eye. Visual acuity worse than 20/200 was most often caused by secondary glaucoma, and aggressive treatment of this complication is therefore warranted.

## PATHOLOGY

The definitive diagnosis of sarcoidosis requires the finding of noncaseating epithelioid cell granulomas on biopsy. The typical sarcoid granuloma consists of whorls of epithelioid cells surrounding multinucleated giant cells (Fig. 21-9). Mononuclear cells, fibroblasts, and lymphocytes may be found at the periphery of these nodules, and surrounding areas of fibrosis are common. True caseation, however, is absent. Although suggestive of sarcoidosis, these pathologic findings are nonspecific, and the presence of infectious agents or foreign bodies should be excluded. This may be accomplished with the use of cultures, special stains, and microscopic examination for foreign bodies under polarized light. Several types of inclusion bodies have been noted in biopsies of sarcoid granulomas. Asteroid bodies composed of vimentin intermediate filaments, Schaumann's bodies composed of aggregates of basophilic material and crystalline inclusions containing calcium carbonate crystals have all been described. Most histologic specimens from enucleated eyes have shown granulomas of the retina, choroid, or the region of the retinal pigment epithelium.[11,27] Histologic examination of the vitreous, perivascular and retinal infiltrates revealed epithelioid cells.[27] The deeper lesions at the level of the retinal pigment epithelium are granulomas like the

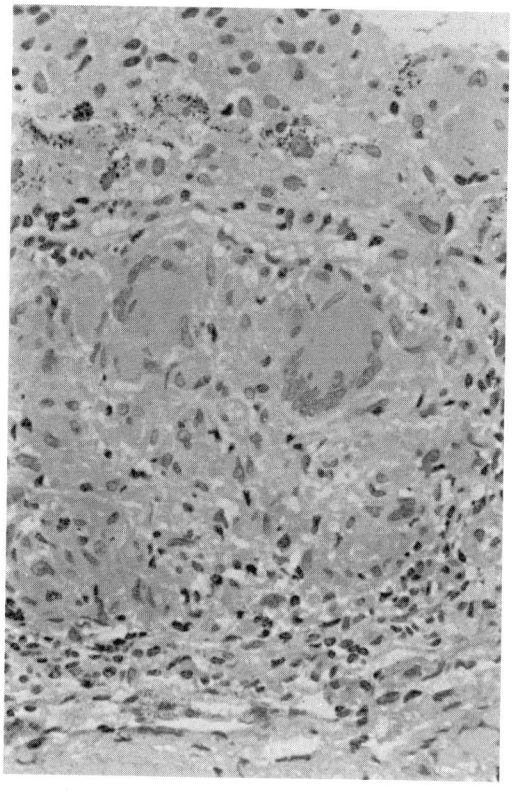

**Fig. 21-9.** Chorioretinal biopsy from patient with sarcoidosis shows inflammatory cell infiltration into retina with noncaseating granuloma. (Hematoxylin and eosin stain; original magnification ×400.) (Courtesy Chi-Chao Chan, M.D.)

Dalen-Fuchs' nodules of sympathetic ophthalmia. Choroidal involvement is infrequent, and Gass[27] has written that many lesions that have been called focal choroiditis in sarcoidosis may be granulomas below the pigment epithelium and not discretely involving the choroid. However, large choroidal granulomas do occur (Fig. 21-6).

The pathologic findings of the acute iritis of sarcoidosis can resemble erythema nodosum rather than the pulmonary granulomas that are prominent and diagnostic of sarcoidosis. Some suggest that iritis may be a hypersensitivity reaction of the eye that occurs in a number of diseases of diverse cause in a manner similar to the occurence of erythema nodosum in association with a variety of unrelated diseases. It is clear that the granulomatous reaction that is characteristic of sarcoidosis is not necessarily the cause of some of the clinical pathologic conditions but a secondary response to an underlying immune sensitization.

## DIAGNOSIS

Although the definitive diagnosis of sarcoidosis requires biopsy confirmation, the diagnosis of sarcoidosis can sometimes be made in patients with a characteristic clinical presentation. Asymptomatic patients between the ages of 20 and 40 years with bilateral symmetric hilar and paratracheal lymphadenopathy are likely to have sarcoidosis. This likelihood is increased in patients who also have arthralgias, erythema nodosum, or an associated uveitis. However, in most cases, a biopsy is needed to make the diagnosis.

Our diagnostic approach is to closely examine the skin, conjunctiva, and lacrimal glands for nodular lesions to biopsy. Biopsy of nodular skin lesions can show granulomas diagnostic for sarcoidosis; however, biopsy of lesions of erythema nodosum shows a nonspecific vasculitis and is not useful. The incidence of a positive conjunctival biopsy in patients with biopsy-proven sarcoidosis is 27% to 55% in patients without a discrete conjunctival lesion, but falls to 12% in patients in whom sarcoidosis is suspected.[15] Granulomas were found on biopsy of the lacrimal gland in 22% of patients with presumed ocular sarcoidosis.[28] The diagnostic yield of lacrimal gland biopsy is improved if there is increased uptake on a gallium scan or if the gland is clinically enlarged.

Ninety percent of sarcoidosis patients will have an abnormal chest x-ray, and transbronchial biopsy is often a sensitive and specific diagnostic test. Approximately 60% of patients with sarcoidosis show granulomas on transbronchial lung biopsy, even patients with a normal chest radiograph (stage 0 disease).[3] When there is a parencymal abnormality on the chest film, almost 90% of patients will have granulomas on transbronchial lung biopsy. However, some patients do require multiple biopsies to make the correct diagnosis.

Laboratory testing may be useful in the diagnosis of sarcoidosis. Transbronchial lung biopsy cannot be performed on all patients with a uveitis compatible with ocular sarcoidosis, and diagnostic tests can help determine which patients should undergo more invasive diagnostic procedures. ACE is predominantly produced in pulmonary macrophages and vascular endothelium, and serum ACE levels are elevated in 60% to 90% of patients with sarcoidosis with active disease.[29] Unfortunately serum ACE levels may be normal in patients with quiescent or isolated disease. In addition, ACE is produced by epitheliod cells present in granulomas associated with a number of diseases including tuberculosis, leprosy, silicosis, primary biliary cirrhosis, asbestosis, and histoplasmosis. ACE levels may be elevated in the aqueous humor of patients with ocular sarcoidosis,[30] or in the cerebral spinal fluid of patients with neurosarcoidosis. ACE levels may be high in normal children and are less useful as a diagnostic test for sarcoidosis in children.

Serum lysozyme levels may also be elevated in patients with sarcoidosis but are less specific than ACE and are rarely obtained. Hypercalcemia and hypercalciuria occur in some patients as a result of increased calcium absorption after increased production of 1,25-dihydroxycholecalciferol; they can be detected on routine laboratory tests. Lymphopenia and elevated liver enzymes, particularly the alkaline phosphatase, may also occur.

The Kveim skin test used to be an accepted method to diagnose sarcoidosis. Kveim antigen is prepared from the spleens of patients with proven sarcoidosis and is then injected intradermally into a patient with suspected sarcoidosis.[23] The presence of granulomatous inflammation in a skin biopsy performed 6 weeks after the injection was considered diagnostic of sarcoidosis. Although the Kveim test is positive in about 80% of patients with sarcoidosis, negative tests can occur in patients with more limited disease.[31] In addition, the fear of transmitting infectious agents has led to the decreased use of the test. Anergy on skin testing is also seen in about half of sarcoidosis patients and may help support the diagnosis.

The gallium scan, which detects concentrated radioactive gallium in areas of inflammation, can be useful for showing involvement of organs such as the lungs, lacrimal glands, and parotid glands (Fig. 21-10).[16,32] Bronchoalveolar lavage may show a lymphocytosis in patients with sarcoidosis. However, because bronchoalveolar lavage findings are not diagnostic of sarcoidosis, it is not commonly performed in the evaluation of sarcoidosis patients. Pulmonary function tests can be useful in evaluating patients with suspected sarcoidosis. Limited diffusing capacity, noted as a diminished carbon monoxide diffusion in the lung, can occur before radiographic abnormalities are seen on a chest x-ray. Diminished lung volumes are later seen with the development of restrictive lung disease. We retrospectively reviewed the records of 46 patients with biopsy-proven sarcoidosis at the NIH; 21 had uveitis. Only 61% of the patients with sarcoid uveitis had an abnormal chest x-ray, and only 36% had an elevated serum ACE level. The most sensitive diagnostic test in our patients was the pulmonary diffusing capacity, which was diminished in 78% of the patients we tested. Interestingly, there was no statistical difference in test results between sarcoidosis patients with or without uveitis. Our current diagnostic approach is to obtain pulmonary consultation for transbronchial biopsy in patients with suspected ocular sarcoidosis who have a decreased diffusing capacity especially if other diagnostic tests support the diagnosis.

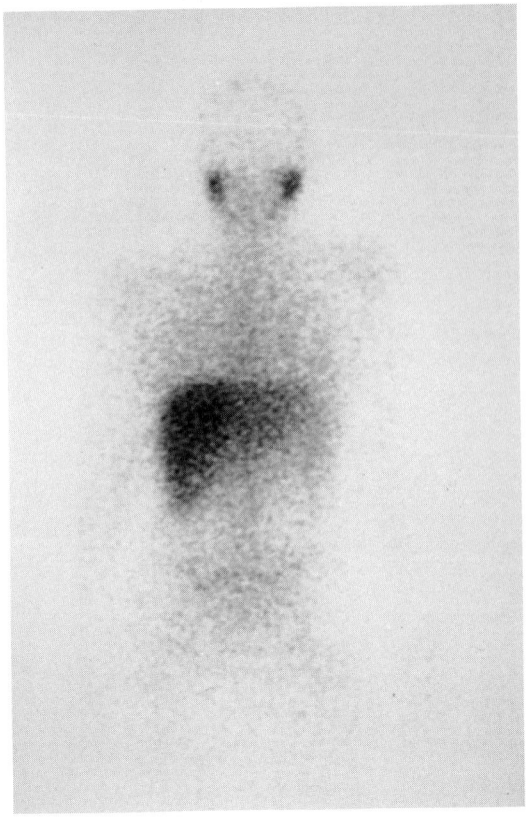

**Fig. 21-10.** Gallium scan of upper torso and head of patient with active systemic sarcoidosis demonstrates uptake in parotid gland.

## TREATMENT

Asymptomatic patients with hilar adenopathy do not require therapy and can be followed. The two main indications for therapy in patients with sarcoidosis are symptomatic pulmonary disease and uveitis. The mainstay of therapy for both systemic and ocular sarcoidosis are corticosteroids.[5,16] Internists must rely on a number of indicators of disease activity to guide their therapy. Doses of corticosteroids are adjusted depending on clinical symptoms and signs as well as pulmonary function tests, chest radiographs, serum ACE levels, and occasionally on results of broncheoalveoloar lavage. The ophthalmologist is fortunate in being able to judge the severity of disease by clinical examination, and as described in Chapter 8 therapy must be tailored to the severity of the ocular disease. Acute anterior inflammation is best managed by topical corticosteroids, but frequently periocular injections of corticosteroids are needed to control severe anterior uveitis complicated by iris nodules and glaucoma. The treatment of chronic anterior or posterior uveitis is more difficult. Systemic therapy is often required for bilateral chronic uveitis, and patients with chronic ocular inflammatory disease frequently require higher daily doses of oral corticosteroid than patients with chronic sarcoid pulmonary disease. However, sarcoidosis is very responsive to corticosteroids, and the use of high initial doses with slow tapering is effective in managing most patients. Two or three high doses of intravenous pulse corticosteroids (1 g of methylprednisolone) on sequential days may induce a more rapid remission. In cases of chronic sarcoidosis that require prolonged corticosteroid therapy, side effects often require the addition of a steroid-sparing drug. Cyclosporin A and other immunosuppressive agents such as chlorambucil and methotrexate have had therapeutic effects in patients with sarcoidosis. We have observed improvement of both the ocular and systemic manifestations of sarcoidosis after cyclosporine therapy,[16] but there is still no optimal safe long-term approach for the use of this drug. Supplementation with periocular steroids and pulse systemic steroids can assist in keeping the dose of cyclosporine low. Sarcoidosis involving the central nervous system may be resistant to treatment, and radiotherapy has been tried for unresponsive disease. Gelwan and colleagues[33] have reported the use of radiotherapy for cases of sarcoidosis involving the anterior visual pathway.

Sarcoidosis produces a high incidence of glaucoma and cataract, and surgical intervention is frequently required. Because of the changes in the anterior segment and the substantial vitreous opacities that often occur in sarcoidosis, some uveitis specialists prefer to use a pars plana lensectomy to remove the cataract. However, there are no data on the relative benefits of this procedure compared with extracapsular cataract extraction in patients with sarcoidosis. Patients with sarcoidosis frequently have severe exacerbations of their ocular inflammation in the immediate postoperative period, and the optic disc may not be seen for the first few days. This occurs with both pars plana lensectomy and extracapsular cataract extraction. This inflammatory response peaks about 48 hours after surgery and lasts for 5 or 6 days after the surgery, and patients with sarcoidosis should therefore be treated with high doses of systemic corticosteroids for the first week after surgery. The patient's immediate postoperative vision may be greatly decreased because of the vitreous haze, but it will improve as the vitritis resolves. The retinal and optic disc neovascularization that occurs in sarcoidosis frequently responds to oral corticosteroid therapy.[17] However, the subretinal neovascularization requires laser photocoagulation if it is in a treatable location.[16]

Fortunately, many patients with sarcoidosis show complete remission of their disease within several years. In cases when sarcoidosis regresses spontaneously, it rarely recurs. In all patients with ocular manifestations of sarcoidosis, the goal is to control the inflammatory disease and thereby prevent permanent visually impairing changes such as photoreceptor damage caused by chronic cystoid macular edema. The ideal therapy for all forms of sarcoidosis awaits discovery, but advances in the therapy of ocular sarcoidosis should follow both an improved understanding of the cause of systemic sarcoidosis and an insight into the relationship between the ocular manifestations and the systemic inflammatory disease.

**Case 21-1**

A 25-year-old white woman with sarcoidosis developed floaters and blurred vision in one eye. Examination revealed granulomatous KP, vitreous cells, fluff balls, and a choroidal granuloma in the posterior pole temporal to the macula. Vision was 20/200 primarily because of macular edema. The patient received a periocular depot steroid injection that resulted in a partial decrease in the inflammation but no visual improvement. Four additional injections given 3 weeks apart resulted in total clearing of the inflammation and an improvement in visual acuity to 20/25. The patient remained quiet for 6 months. The inflammation began to increase, and the vision dropped to 20/50. One periocular depot steroid injection resulted in resolution of the inflammation and a return of vision to 20/25. The patient has required one or two injections of periocular steroid every 6 months to maintain good vision in the affected eye. The other eye has remained normal.

## REFERENCES


1. Hunter DG, Foster CS: Systemic manifestations of sarcoidosis. In Albert DA, Jakobiec FA, editors: *Principles and practice of ophthalmology,* Philadelphia, 1994, WB Saunders, pp 3132-3142.
2. Bruins Slot WJ: Ziekte van Besnier-Boeck en Febris uveoparotidea (Heerfordt), *Ned Tijdshr Geneeskd* 80:2859-2870, 1936.
3. Fanburg BL: Sarcoidosis. In Wyngaarden JB, Smith LH Jr, Bennett JC, editors: *Cecil textbook of medicine,* ed 19, Philadelphia, 1992, WB Saunders, pp 430-435.
4. Bresnitz EA, Strom BL: Epidemiology of sarcoidosis, *Epidemiol Rev* 5:124-156, 1983.
5. Siltzbach LE, James DG, Neville et al: Course and prognosis of sarcoidosis around the world, *Am J Med* 57:847-852, 1974.
6. Jabs DA, Johns CJ: Ocular involvement in chronic sarcoidosis, *Am J Ophthalmol* 102:297-301, 1986.
7. Thomas PD, Hunninghake GW: Current concepts of the pathogenesis of sarcoidosis, *Am Rev Respir Dis* 135:747, 1987.
8. Crystal RG, Roberts WC, Hunninghake GW et al: Pulmonary sarcoidosis: a disease characterized and perpetuated by activated lung T-lymphocytes, *Ann Intern Med* 94:73-94, 1981.
9. Hunninghake GW, Crystal RG: Pulmonary sarcoidosis: a disorder mediated by excess helper T-lymphocyte activity at sites of disease activity, *N Engl J Med* 305:429-434, 1981.
10. Sememzato G, Pezzutto A, Pizzolo G: Immunohistological study in sarcoidosis: evaluation at different sites of disease activity, *Clin Immunol Immunopathol* 30:29-40, 1984.
11. Chan CC, Wetzig RP, Palestine AG et al: Immunohistopathology of ocular sarcoidosis: report of a case and discussion of immunopathogenesis, *Arch Ophthalmol* 105:1398-1402, 1987.
12. Crick RP, Hoyle C, Smellie H: The eyes in sarcoidosis, *Br J Ophthalmol* 45:461-481, 1961.
13. Obenauf CD, Shaw HE, Sydnor CF et al: Sarcoidosis and its ophthalmic manifestations, *Am J Ophthalmol* 86: 648-655, 1978.
14. James DG, Neville E, Langley DA: Ocular sarcoidosis, *Trans Ophthal Soc UK* 96:133-139, 1976.
15. Nichols CW, Eagle RC, Yanoff M et al: Conjunctival biopsy as an aid in the evaluation of the patient with suspected sarcoidosis, *Ophthalmology* 87:287-291, 1980.
16. Palestine AG, Nussenblatt RB, Chan CC: Treatment of intraocular complications of sarcoidosis, *Ann NY Acad of Med* 465:564-573, 1986.
17. Spalton DJ, Sanders MD: Fundus changes in histologically confirmed sarcoidosis, *Br J Ophthalmol* 65:348-358, 1981.
18. Marcus DF, Bovino JA, Burton TC: Sarcoid granuloma of the choroid, *Ophthalmology* 89:1326-1330, 1982.
19. Campo RV, Aaberg TM: Choroidal granuloma in sarcoidosis, *Am J Ophthalmol* 97:419-427, 1984.
20. Frank KW, Weiss H: Unusual clinical and histopathologic findings in ocular sarcoidosis, *Br J Ophthalmol* 67:8-16, 1983.
21. Gragoudas ES, Regan CDJ: Peripapillary subretinal neovascularization in presumed sarcoidosis, *Arch Ophthalmol* 99:1194-1197, 1981.
22. Rush JA: Retrobulbar optic neuropathy in sarcoidosis, *Ann Ophthalmol* 12:390-394, 1980.
23. Mitchell DN, Scadding JG, Heard BE et al: Sarcoidosis: histopathological definition and clinical diagnosis, *J Clin Path* 30:395-408, 1977.
24. Hoover DL, Khan JA, Giangiacomo J: Pediatric ocular sarcoidosis, *Surv Ophthalmol* 30:215, 1986.
25. Perruquet JL, Harrington TM, Davis DE et al: Sarcoid arthritis in a North American Caucasian population, *J Rheumatol* 11:521-525, 1984.
26. Raphael SA, Blau EB, Zhang WH et al: Analysis of a large kindred with Blau syndrome for HLA, autoimmunity, and sarcoidosis, *Am J Dis Child* 147:842-848, 1993.
27. Gass JDM, Olson CL: Sarcoidosis with optic nerve and retinal involvement, *Arch Ophthalmol* 94:945-950, 1976.
28. Cohen KL, Peiffer RL, Powell DA: Sarcoidosis and ocular disease in a young child, *Arch Ophthalmol* 99:422-424, 1981.
29. Lieberman J: Enzymes in sarcoidosis: angiotensin converting enzyme (ACE), *Clin Lab Med* 9:745, 1989.
30. Weinreb RN, Sandman R, Ryder MI et al: Angiotensin converting enzyme activity in human aqueous humor, *Arch Ophthalmol* 34:103, 1985.
31. Munro CS, Mitchell DN: The Kveim response: still useful, still a puzzle, *Thorax* 42:321, 1987.
32. Weinreb RN: Diagnosing sarcoidosis by transconjunctival biopsy of the lacrimal gland, *Am J Ophthalmol* 97:573-576, 1984.
33. Gelwan MJ, Kellen RI, Burde RM et al: Sarcoidosis of the anterior visual pathway: successes and failures, *J Neurol Neurosurg* 51:1473, 1988.

# CHAPTER 22

# Sympathetic Ophthalmia

Sympathetic ophthalmia probably is the intraocular inflammatory condition best known to practitioners outside of ophthalmology. It has stimulated enormous interest within our field as well since its clinical description by MacKenzie[1] early in the nineteenth century. The number of patients afflicted with this problem per year is relatively small, but the dread of losing not only the involved eye but the contralateral, untouched eye as well in a potentially sight-threatening process is indeed great, and justifiably so. Further, the potential mechanisms to explain such a process are many, which has provided the more intellectually (and imaginatively) inclined with ample material for thought. Newer observations have certainly helped place this disorder in perspective.

## CLINICAL APPEARANCE

Sympathetic ophthalmia is a bilateral granulomatous uveitis that occurs after either intentional or unintentional penetrating trauma to one eye. Therefore trauma to one eye (the exciting eye) will result not only in an inflammatory response in that eye but in the contralateral one (the sympathizing eye) as well. The disease can begin as early as several days after the penetrating insult to decades later, with the clinical diagnosis becoming apparent in 80% of cases some 3 months after injury to the exciting eye.[2] Sympathetic ophthalmia occurs more often after nonsurgical trauma, with Liddy and Stuart[3] reporting the disorder occurring in 0.2% of nonsurgical wounds whereas Holland[4] found the disorder in 0.5% of eyes with trauma. Marak[2] has estimated the incidence of this disease to be less than 10 cases/100,000 surgical penetrating wounds. In a review by Gass,[5] in which 26 eye pathology laboratories were surveyed for a 5-year period from 1975-1980 sympathetic ophthalmia was diagnosed in 53 eyes (two of 1000 eyes examined); 55% were posttraumatic. In the same report a survey of 34 retinal surgeons who had performed 14,915 vitrectomies disclosed that sympathetic ophthalmia occurred in nine eyes (incidence of 0.06%), with one case having vitrectomy as the only operative procedure performed (incidence of 0.01%).

Very few, if any, cases of sympathetic ophthalmia were seen as a result of ocular trauma suffered during the Vietnam conflict. This is in contrast to the older literature of this century suggesting an incidence of about 2%,[6] and it was believed that 16% of ocular injuries during the American Civil War resulted in sympathetic ophthalmia. It is thought to be more common in males—almost certainly because of the higher incidence of ocular trauma. As well it is thought more common in lighter-skinned ethnic groups, but this may be because of better reporting and recognition of the disease.

We have followed up 29 patients with sympathetic ophthalmia during the past few years. Most of these patients—13 males and 16 females—are white, with an age range from 6 to

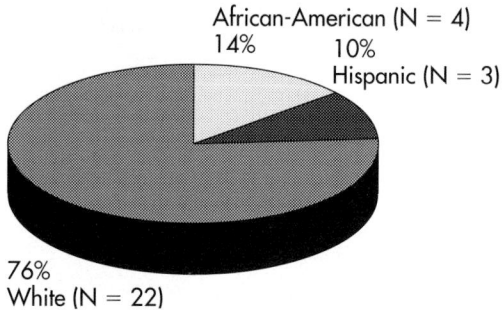


**Fig. 22-1.** Racial distribution of patients with sympathetic ophthalmia seen at National Eye Institute.

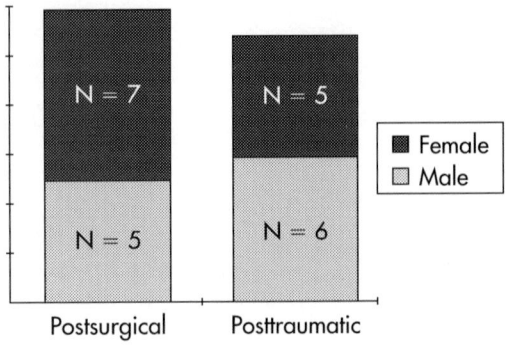


**Fig. 22-2.** Distribution of patients at National Eye Institute in whom sympathetic ophthalmia developed after surgery and after trauma.

70 years (average age 41 years) (Fig. 22-1). In 12 of the patients, the disease developed after multiple surgeries, and the disease tended to develop after this type of trauma more frequently in females than in males (Fig. 22-2). Hakin and associates[7] have reported their experience with 18 patients; 15 of the cases followed trauma, 11 of which occurred after a known penetrating wound, with the other 4 having undergone a posterior scleral rupture. Three cases occurred after retinal detachment, with patients on the average having three surgical interventions. Surgical trauma, particularly vitrectomy, is well recognized as an antecedent event to sympathetic ophthalmia.[5,8-10]

### Classic presentation

In the classic case the inflammatory response seen in the anterior chamber is granulomatous, with mutton-fat keratic precipitates on the corneal endothelium and findings of an acute anterior uveitis. However, the anterior chamber inflammatory response can be relatively mild, with the inflammation taking on a nongranulomatous appearance as well. There is generally a moderate to severe vitritis accompanied by changes in the posterior segment. Of particular note are multiple white-yellow lesions in the periphery, which sometimes become confluent (Fig. 22-3). These represent the clinical appearance of a Dalen-Fuchs nodule, a histologic finding. Swelling of the disc (papillitis) can be prominent, and circumpapillary choroidal lesions can also occur. Retinal involvement is not an uncommon finding in sympathetic ophthalmia, although this involvement, classically thought of as a choroidal disease, has been amply corroborated by histologic findings (see following discussion). Although rare, subretinal neovascularization has been reported to occur in sympathetic ophthalmia,[11] as it has been in the Vogt-Koyanagi-Harada syndrome (VKH) (see Chapter 23) (see Fig. 22-3).

A small number of patients with sympathetic ophthalmia report or demonstrate extraocular findings not dissimilar from those seen in VKH (see Chapter 23), such as cells in the cerebrospinal fluid, hearing disturbances, and hair and skin changes. These extraocular findings are rare in sympathetic ophthalmia when compared with VKH, in which they are fairly common symptoms that are important indicators in making the diagnosis. They are also important in the conceptualization of autoimmune disease, because sympathetic ophthalmia is the only disease in which we know when a specific event leading to autosensitization has occurred. The development of extraocular signs must be secondary to ocular immunization.

It should be noted that the clinical appearance of sympathetic ophthalmia comprises a spectrum that ranges from the very mild to the severe. Lewis and coworkers[12] reported a case of sympathetic ophthalmia after trauma and vitrectomy that was confined to the posterior segment in such a way that it resembled focal lesions of acute posterior multifocal placoid pigment epitheliopathy (APMPPE) (see Chapter 28). A mild anterior uveitis has also been reported, but this has not been our experience. Carrying the concept to the extreme, some have proposed the notion of an unilateral sympathetic ophthalmia. It is quite possible that the sympathizing response may be so mild as to disappear with minimal or no sequelae, and the

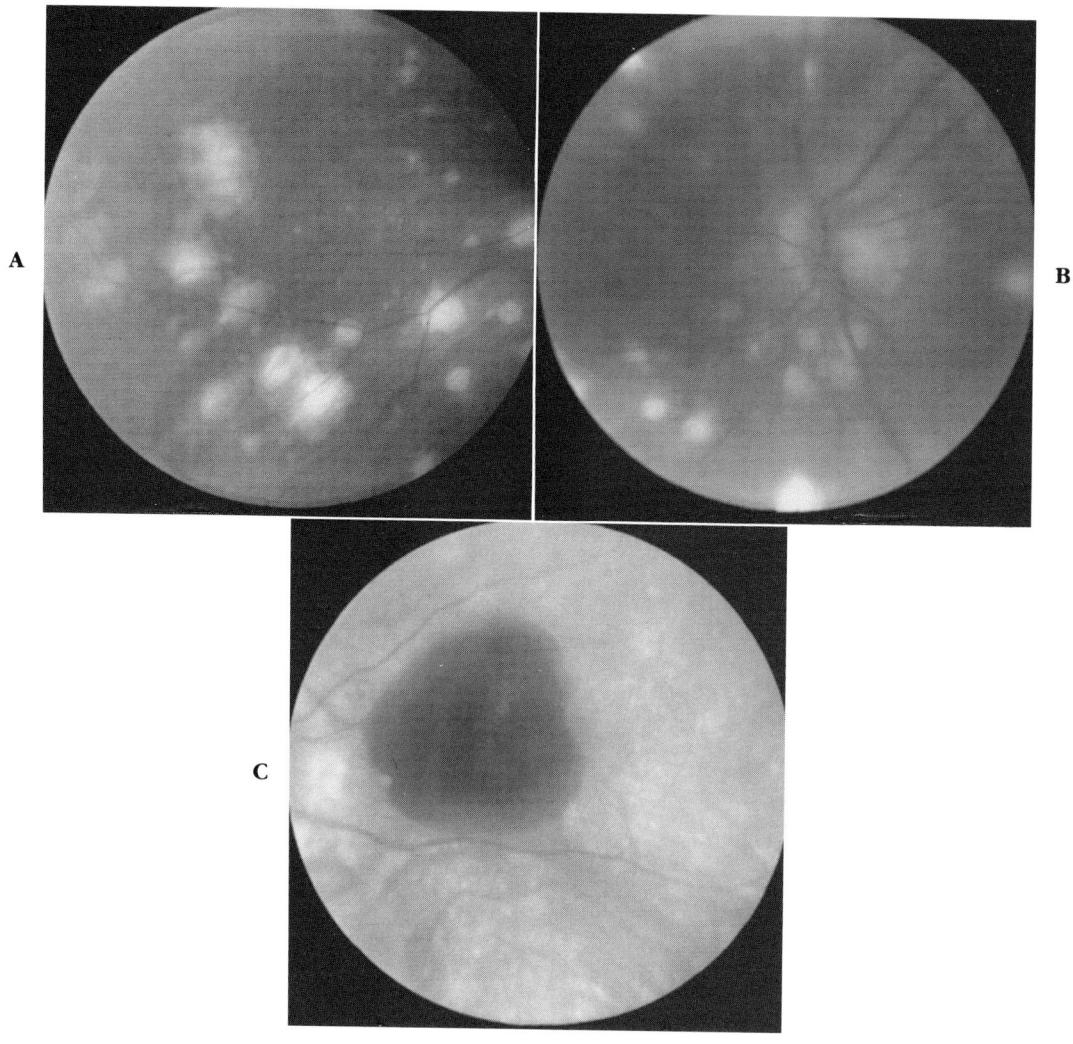


**Fig. 22-3. A,** Multiple cream-colored lesions that correspond to histologic diagnosis of Dalen-Fuchs nodules. They characteristically tend to be strewn throughout periphery and can extend to disc and at times into posterior pole **(B)**. Initially, they appear to have "substance" to them, raising overlying retina. With time they appear atrophic. Although considerably less common in sympathetic ophthalmia than in VKH (see Chapter 23), subretinal neovascularization with resultant hemorrhage **(C)** can occur, in this case nasal to disc in a one-eyed patient and not affecting vision.

spectrum of the histologic response seen would support this concept. However, if no inflammatory disease is noted, or if none is seen on a histologic specimen, it therefore seems inappropriate to use the term *sympathetic ophthalmia* to describe the disease under observation. Marak[2] describes a phenomenon he has called sympathetic irritation, which occurs in the fellow eye after injury to or disease in one eye. About one third of these patients may have cells and flare in the anterior chamber, with 67% of the patients complaining of photophobia and a smaller number having perilimbal or conjunctival injection, or both. The distinction between this entity and "mild" sympathetic ophthalmia to us seems quite unclear.

## Sequelae

The sequelae of the inflammation noted in sympathetic ophthalmia are quite variable, depending on the severity of the ocular inflammation and whether therapy has been instituted (see later discussion of therapy). Secondary glaucoma and cataract can result from the inflammatory process, as well as retinal and optic atrophy in association with retinal detachment and/or subretinal alterations such as fibrosis and underlying choroidal atrophy.

Several ocular entities have been associated with sympathetic ophthalmia. Phacoanaphylaxis has been observed,[13] and Blodi[14] noted its occurrence in 23% of eyes with sympathetic ophthalmia. He believed that the presence of the two entities in the same eye reflected the fact that these patients have a predisposition for autoimmune phenomena. In Lubin and coworkers' excellent review of 105 cases,[15] they found an incidence of 46%. It should be noted that both entities can be found in the sympathizing (noninjured) eye as well,[16] and the phacoanaphylaxis can be a confounding element in attempting to make the diagnosis of sympathetic ophthalmia (see later discussion).

Malignant melanoma has also been associated with sympathetic ophthalmia.[17,18] In 400 cases of sympathetic ophthalmia evaluated by Easom[19] at the Armed Forces Institute of Pathology, 7 were found to involve a malignant melanoma. Fries and colleagues[20] reported sympathetic ophthalmia after helium ion irradiation of a choroidal melanoma, whereas Margo and Pautler[21] reported the development of a granulomatous bilateral uveitis after therapy with proton-beam irradiation. In the latter case the authors stress the fact that the sutures securing the four tantalum rings to the sclera did not penetrate the uvea.

Sympathetic ophthalmia has been reported to occur after cyclocryotherapy.[22] Edward and colleagues[23] reported a case after noncontact neodymium:YAG cyclotherapy; and Lam and coworkers[24] reported three others. Tessler and group discussed this problem recently.[25] Harrison[26] discussed the development of sympathetic ophthalmia in a patient who underwent cyclocryotherapy for neovascular glaucoma. No penetration of the sclera was noted.

Cataract surgery has been rarely mentioned as an inciting cause of this entity.[27] In one report[28] the disease occurred 3 months after an intracapsular cataract extraction and anterior chamber lens placement that had the immediate postoperative problem of flat chamber, pupillary block, and wound dehiscence, with one of the haptics protruding into the subconjunctival space. Vitrectomy and removal of the lens resulted in control of the disease and improvement of vision.

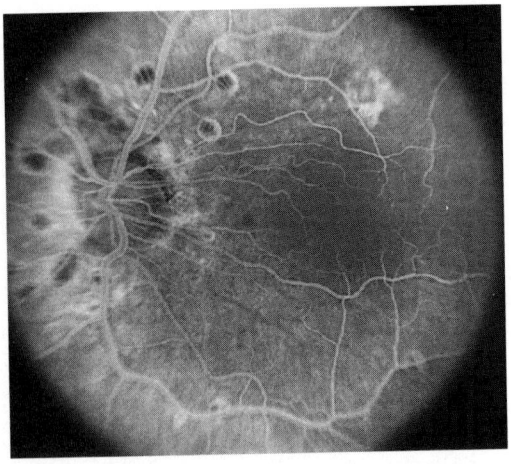

**Fig. 22-4.** Fluorescein angiogram showing initial blockage of Dalen-Fuchs nodules, with ultimate hyperfluorescence of lesion.

## TESTS AND IMMUNOLOGIC CHARACTERISTICS

Clinical testing of patients will help to put into perspective the amount and severity of sympathetic ophthalmia but will not help make the diagnosis. Fluoroscein angiography is useful in evaluating the degree of posterior segment disease. Spitznas[29] noted that the fluorescein angiogram obtained during the acute stage of sympathetic ophthalmia reflects an exudative process, with multiple subretinal enlarging hyperfluorescent spots and pooling of dye (Fig. 22-4). Although Spitznas thought that the retinal vasculature was not involved, we have seen evidence of late staining of the retinal vessels. During the cicatricial phase there is a coarsening of the pigment pattern in the fundus. The areas that are believed to correspond to Dalen-Fuchs nodules will, in the later stages of the disease, become atrophic and appear on the angiogram as window defects.

As might be expected, findings on both the electroretinogram and electrooculogram can be affected by the disease. Dreyer and associates[30] observed changes in the photopic cone b-wave amplitudes and scotopic rod b-wave amplitudes during acute disease, with improvement in these functions after successful therapy.

The histologic features of sympathetic ophthalmia, which are rather distinctive, were first described by Fuchs in 1905.[31] In the full-blown picture the choroid is markedly thickened by a sea of lymphocytes, with a granulomatous non-

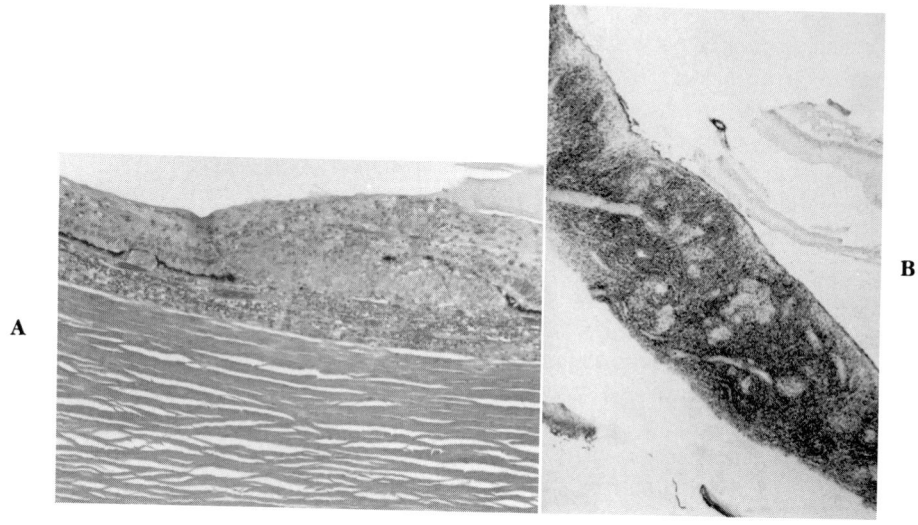


**Fig. 22-5. A,** Markedly thickened choroid with nonnecrotizing granulomatous inflammation surrounded by lymphocytes, which is typical of sympathetic ophthalmia. **B,** Immunohistochemical techniques reveal dark areas of cells that bear OKT3 marking, indicating that they are mature T cells. Central areas that have no black staining represent areas of granulomatous reaction. Retina can be seen above choroid.

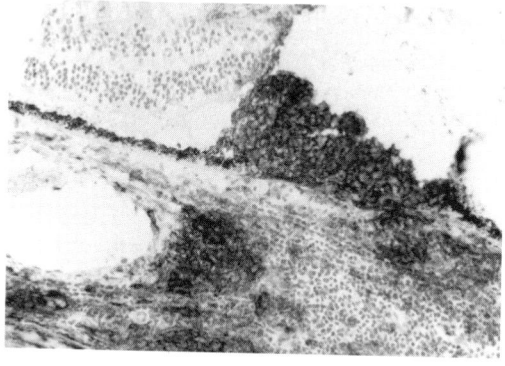

**Fig. 22-6.** Immunohistochemical staining of Dalen-Fuchs nodule with monoclonal antibody OKM1, which is specific for macrophages. Note that most cells in this particular nodule are of that lineage, with smaller area of macrophages in choroid.

necrotizing reaction the predominant feature (Fig. 22-5). In general, the choriocapillaris tends to be spared, although this is not always the case. The infiltrate in the choroid can also have large numbers of eosinophils. Although plasma cell infiltration into the choroid was thought not to be a part of the disease, these cells were noted in 85.7% of the cases Lubin and coworkers[15] reviewed. Marak and colleagues[32] reported the presence of more choroidal granulomas and eosinophils in African-American than in white patients, but no differences have been noted between Chinese patients and those from the United States.[33] As already noted, retinal changes are not rare. Croxatto and coworkers[34] described retinal detachment and retinal perivasculitis in 50% of the 100 eyes with sympathetic ophthalmia they examined, whereas 18% had mild inflammatory infiltrates into the retina.

### Dalen-Fuchs nodules

A typical but by no means pathognomonic finding in sympathetic ophthalmia is that of Dalen-Fuchs nodules (Fig. 22-6), which occur in about one third of eyes with sympathetic ophthalmia.[15] On fluorescein angiography, the lesion may block early (i.e., become hypofluorescent) and then stain late (i.e., hyperfluorescence).[35] As the lesions mature, with ultimate disruption of the retinal pigment epithelium (RPE) and probably a decrease in the inflammatory process, these lesions may simply show as window defects. These lesions were thought by Fuchs[31] to represent RPE cells that had migrated and transformed. Although early Dalen-Fuchs nodules may represent such a phenomenon,[36] Jakobiec and coworkers[37] and Chan and colleagues[38,39] have used monoclonal antibodies and structural analysis to demonstrate that Dalen-Fuchs nodules were made up of a mixture of $Ia^+$, $OKM1^+$ cells (presumably histiocytes) and depigmented RPE cells, which were $Ia^-$ and $OKM1^-$. These authors' conclusions, which were similar for the epithelioid cells seen in the choroid itself, were corroborated by Rao and coworkers.[40] The subsets of infiltrating lymphocytes into the choroid have been identified with use of immunohistochemical techniques. Jakobiec and colleagues[37] noted that the predominant T cell was of the $CD8^+$ (OKT8) subset (suppressor/cytotoxic cell) in the choroid of an eye removed 1½ years after the initial surgical trauma. Chan and coworkers[38] evaluated an eye enucleated for the disease only several months after the initial nonsurgical trauma and found that the predominant T cell was the CD4 (Leu-3a) subset, the helper/inducer subset. The sympathizing eye of the same case ultimately came to be studied,[38] and in this eye the predominant T-cell subset had changed to the suppressor/cytotoxic ($CD8^+$) subset as had been seen in Jakobiec and coworkers' case. The interpretation of the observations is that the human eye's inflammatory response in this disease parallels that seen in the experimentally induced uveitis model in lower mammals (see Chapter 2). That is, there is a dynamic, changing cellular immune response that is initiated by the helper T cell. As the disease progresses, the body attempts to down-regulate the immune response, and this is done by an influx of large numbers of the suppressor subset of T cell.

The foregoing scenario, however, may not explain all cases. Several authors[34,39,41,42] have stressed that the classic findings just outlined represent one point in a spectrum of disease that clinically is recognized as sympathetic ophthalmia. A recent immunohistochemical study was completed in 29 cases of sympathetic ophthalmia.[43] In 20 eyes, T cells predominated in the choroidal infiltration, whereas in four cases—all male patients—it was B cells that were predominantly found. The presence of B cells was correlated to long-term disease (more than 9 months) and phthisical changes. It has classically been taught that the presence of B cells in the choroid of an eye with sympathetic ophthalmia is extremely rare. The authors of this study suggest that these findings may reflect a secondary pathologic process. They further speculate on these findings from a therapeutic point of view. It could be argued that in light of these observations, cytotoxic agents as opposed to more T-cell specific drugs (e.g., cyclosporine, FK506) may be a more logical choice for those patients who do not respond to steroid therapy.

There is no established and accepted laboratory test for sympathetic ophthalmia. Sen and coworkers[44] measured the level of serum $\beta_2$-microglobulin levels in the blood of patients with sympathetic ophthalmia. They found levels to be high in these patients as compared with those with traumatic uveitis and with control subjects. The levels appeared to be higher at the initial stages of the disease and reflected the severity of the disease. These results need to be corroborated.

### Sympathetic ophthalmia and Vogt-Koyanagi-Harada syndrome

The question arises whether sympathetic ophthalmia can be distinguished histologically from VKH. It would appear that the two entities represent the spectrum of very similar inflammatory responses.[45] It is thought that "classic" sympathetic ophthalmia neither involves the choriocapillaris nor has chorioretinal scarring, both of which are common in VKH. Although these changes can be seen in sympathetic ophthalmia,[2] they probably occur in fewer patients. In addition, the lack of chorioretinal scarring and obliteration of the choriocapillaris in eyes with sympathetic ophthalmia (a phenomenon seen late) may reflect the fact that eyes with sympathetic ophthalmia are usually removed early in the course of the inflammatory disease. In contrast the eyes with VKH that have been studied were removed late in the course of the disease. Is the inflammatory response seen in sympathetic ophthalmia unique to this entity? Chan and coinvestigators[46] evaluated the cellular composition of granulomas of sympathetic ophthalmia and sarcoidosis. Most of the cells within the lesions were found to be identical and were mainly cells from bone-derived monocytes (Table 22-1). It has been suggested that Dalen-Fuchs nodules in sarcoidosis are larger.

A complicating factor is the presence of phacoanaphylaxis. Easom and Zimmerman[47] reported cases in which the clinical diagnosis in the exciting eye was thought to be sympathetic ophthalmia, but histologic confirmation could not be obtained; the so-called sympathizing eye showed evidence only of phacoanaphylaxis rather than the alterations typical of the suspected disorder. Although it is not always the

**Table 22-1.** Sympathetic ophthalmia versus sarcoidosis

| Disease | Uveitis | Dalen-Fuchs | Other |
|---|---|---|---|
| **HISTOPATHOLOGY** | | | |
| Sarcoidosis | Focal or diffuse granulomatous | Some larger | "Snowbanking" conjunctival nodules |
| Sympathetic ophthalmia | Diffuse | Many | Sparing of choriocapillaris; retina may not be involved |

| Disease | T cells | T Helper cells | T Suppressor cells | B cells | Macrophages |
|---|---|---|---|---|---|
| **IMMUNOPATHOLOGY** | | | | | |
| Sarcoidosis | Majority | Many | Some | A few | In granuloma and Dalen-Fuchs |
| Sympathetic ophthalmia | Majority | Early—more; late—less | Early—less; late—more | Some | In granuloma and Dalen-Fuchs |

case, de Veer[13] has emphasized that in phacoanaphylaxis, the first eye involved has already become quiet by the time the second eye is involved. This is in contradistinction to sympathetic ophthalmia, in which both eyes are inflamed at the same time. A history of penetrating trauma is imperative. If this is not available or if it is not clear whether ocular penetration occurred, then the diagnosis becomes even more difficult to make. VKH and sarcoidosis perhaps most resemble the disorder, but the diagnosis of such localized posterior segment disorders as APMPPE (see Chapter 28) must also be considered.

The concept that an autoimmune inflammatory response is at the basis of sympathetic ophthalmia is not new, having been proposed by Elschnig in 1910.[48] For years the notion was that uveal pigment was the antigenic stimulus for this disease. A report by Woods[49] in 1921 outlined the interesting observation that patients who had sustained ocular trauma without resultant sympathetic ophthalmia had circulating antibodies to uveal pigment but that in all cases of sympathetic ophthalmia, circulating antibodies were absent. Furthermore, one of these latter cases demonstrated a cellular immune response to uveal pigment as measured with an intradermal skin test. These observations are striking, considering our knowledge of the predominant T-cell response in the eye. In vitro cell-culturing techniques have been used to evaluate cell-mediated anamnestic responses of lymphocytes from patients with sympathetic ophthalmia, and these patients demonstrated a positive response to uveal or uveoretinal preparations.[50,51]

Of interest was Marak and coworkers' observations[52] that blastogenic activity of lymphocytes from a small group of patients with sympathetic ophthalmia could be elicited only with RPE and retinal antigens but not with antigens from the choroid. De Smet and colleagues[53] tested two patient populations, one from the National Eye Institute's clinic and the other from an uveitis clinic in Japan. Patients with sympathetic ophthalmia were tested for their cellular immune response to both the S-antigen and the interphotoreceptor retinoid-binding protein (IRBP). Patients' lymphocytes were found to respond to several autoantigens and to several fragments. Chan and colleagues,[54] using the ELISA system, found no circulating antiretinal S-antigen antibodies. However, when serum from patients with sympathetic ophthalmia was placed over normal human retinal tissue, a few showed antiretinal antibodies directed against the outer segments of the photoreceptors and against Müller cells. However, the titer of the antiretinal antibodies and the number of patients with these circulating antibodies were considerably higher in the VKH group than in the sympathetic group. An association between HLA-A11 and sympathetic ophthalmia has been suggested.[55] However, the study reports the results in a population that is multiethnic and multiracial, making the validity of the results most difficult to evaluate. Davis and colleagues[56] found a strong association between HLA-DR4, DRw53, and Bw54 with both VKH and sympathetic ophthalmia, but in the latter disease the small number of patients precluded statistical analysis.

No exact experimental model for sympathetic ophthalmia yet exists. The induction of uveitis with the ocular antigens IRBP and S-antigen will produce a disease in monkeys and mice that has many characteristics of sympathetic ophthalmia, including Dalen-Fuchs nodules (see Fig. 22-6 and Chapter 2). However, although there may some choroidal involvement, the disease induced in these animals is essentially retinal in nature. Another important factor in the development of the human disorder is that penetrating trauma may permit the development of intraocular lymphatics and the presentation of ocular antigens to the systemic immune system in a way different from the usual.[57]

Is it then possible to develop a working hypothesis to explain the development of sympathetic ophthalmia? The dominant T-cell response certainly seems clear. But what of the precipitating factors leading to the disease? An autoimmune role still seems quite attractive, based on the type of disease in the monkey that is induced with retinal antigens. It is possible to hypothesize that the perforating injury permits several events to take place (Fig. 22-7). The first is that drainage of antigen from the eye can occur via the lymphatics, an event that does not occur under normal conditions. The second is that small amounts of adjuvant, such as bacterial cell wall or other immunostimulators, might now enter

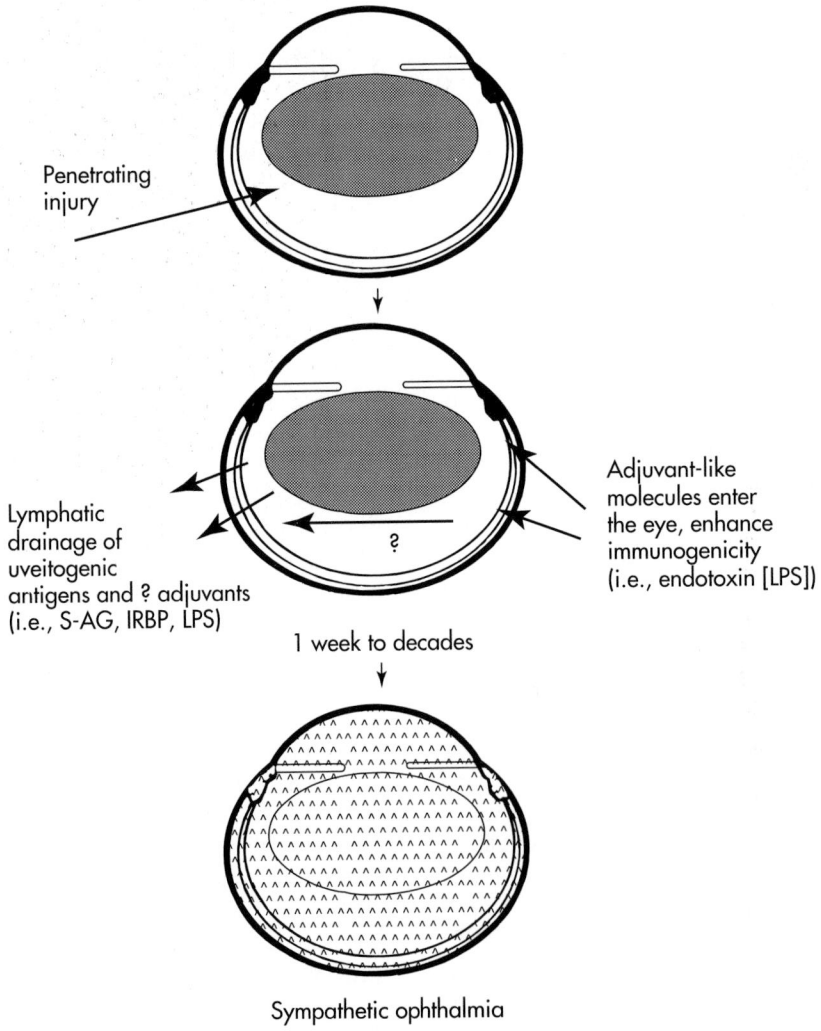


**Fig. 22-7.** Hypothesis explaining development of sympathetic ophthalmia.

the eye. These products may come from already killed bacteria on the skin (such as *Propioni bacterium acnes*), and therefore active proliferation of the organism is not significant to the hypothesis. Rather, these products may profoundly "upgrade" the local immune response, causing it to bypass certain inherent suppressor mechanisms in genetically prone persons. This leads then to the inflammatory kinetic process that ultimately we recognize as sympathetic ophthalmia.

## THERAPY

Enucleation of an injured eye before the sympathizing eye becomes involved is the only known way to prevent sympathetic ophthalmia. Enucleation has classically been taught not to have any effect on the course of the sympathizing eye once the disease has begun. Indeed, experience from the presteroid era suggested that enucleation did not help in improving the patient's ultimate visual outcome.[58] However, Lubin and coworkers' review[15] would suggest that enucleation within 2 weeks of the initiation of the inflammatory response may beneficially affect the visual outcome of the remaining eye. Reynard and associates,[59] in their retrospective clinicopathologic study, also noted that enucleation within 2 weeks of the beginning of symptoms resulted in a fairly benign course. We would, however, hesitate to suggest early enucleation of any eye with any prognosis for useful vision. It may be that the exciting eye's visual acuity could be superior to that obtained in the sympathizing eye. Brackup and coworkers[60] evaluated 50 eyes not removed within 2 weeks of injury and that had suffered global rupture, with visual acuities of no better than hand motion. Seventeen of the eyes were removed, nine of them being painful. The other 33 eyes were not removed and remained comfortable for a mean follow-up of 66 months. Of interest was that there were no cases of sympathetic ophthalmia.

The decision as to when to treat a patient with sympathetic ophthalmia with immunosuppressive therapy usually is not problematic. The patient is first seen with a marked, bilateral inflammation and decrease in vision. On rare occasions, although an inflammatory response can be observed, the patient's vision remains good, and the practitioner may need to follow other parameters, such as changing visual fields, to decide whether a therapeutic intervention is indicated.

### Corticosteroids

If the decision has been made to intervene with antiinflammatory therapy, the initial approach, in most cases, should be systemic corticosteroids. They should be given at a dosage of at least 1 to 1.5 mg/kg of prednisone or equivalent on a daily basis. Some would recommend giving even higher dosages, from 100 to 200 mg/day of prednisone.[2] The practitioner must set both clinical guidelines and a time frame in which to see the patient. What one considers a reasonable improvement is quite dependent on the seriousness of the inflammatory response. Usually 3 months is a reasonable time frame in which to evaluate whether a therapeutic approach has worked. This approach should be effective with most patients. A slow taper should then be initiated. Control of inflammatory disease can be achieved in some patients at 15 to 20 mg/day of prednisone or an alternate-day dosing schedule if given for an extended period of time, such as a year. If this dosage is effective, it would seem reasonable to continue this approach, because any therapeutic intervention will have secondary effects and the potential side effects seen at this level of prednisone are probably less than those seen with other modalities. In Makley and Azar's long-term follow-up[61] (average of 10.6 years) of patients with sympathetic ophthalmia treated with steroids, 65% of eyes were 20/60 or better. Relapses were common, and secondary glaucoma, cataract, retinal detachment, and choroidal scarring were noted as sequelae. Reynard and colleagues[59] found as well that corticosteroid therapy was associated with a good visual outcome.

In some patients, however, the disease will not remain quiescent with this dosage reduction plan. Spitznas[29] found that transitory hyperopia was an indicator of disease activity, whereas Schlaegel[62] suggested that the degree of papillitis is also an excellent indicator of activity. In addition, there are children, older patients, and those with brittle diabetes for whom long-term steroid therapy may not be a viable approach. To deal with this eventuality, the International Uveitis Study Group many years ago suggested that cytotoxic agents may be appro-

**Table 22-2.** Summary of cyclosporine-treated patients with sympathetic ophthalmia

| Patient no. | Age/sex/race | Pretreatment VA | Posttreatment VA | Postsurgery or trauma | Length of CsA therapy |
|---|---|---|---|---|---|
| 1 | 43/F/AA | 20/200, – | 20/25, – | Surgery | 4 yr |
| 2 | 32/M/AA | LP, 20/200 | LP, 20/30 | Trauma | 3 yr |
| 3 | 62/M/W | 20/200, – | 20/25, – | Trauma | 3 yr |
| 4 | 41/F/W | 20/60, – | 20/60, – | Surgery | 1 yr |
| 5 | 6/M/AA | –, HM | –, NLP | Trauma | 6 mo |

*AA,* African-American; *CsA,* cyclosporine; *F,* female; *HM,* hand movement; *LP,* light perception; *M,* male; *NLP,* no light perception; *VA,* visual acuity; *W,* white.

priate in cases of steroid-resistant sympathetic ophthalmia (see Chapter 8). However, the greater recognition of the long-term hazards associated with this therapeutic approach has made this modality less popular. Of particular concern are the hazards of late neoplasm or chromosomal abnormalities. Tessler and Jennings[63] have suggested another approach with chlorambucil (an alkylating agent) – that of a high-dose short-term approach. Five patients with sympathetic ophthalmia each had a sustained remission after an average therapy duration of 11 weeks and a total average dose of 0.9 g. In the relatively short follow-up period (mean 4.5 years), no malignant processes occurred.

### Cyclosporine

We have used cyclosporine as a second-line drug in the treatment of sympathetic ophthalmia, that is, after corticosteroids but before cytotoxic agents. Typically its use would be in patients whose disease responds to steroid therapy, but in whom the maintenance dosage needed to remain in remission is quite high, or in patients who are steroid responders. To date, some five patients with sympathetic ophthalmia have met the criteria outlined and have been placed on cyclosporine therapy. The results of the visual acuity response can be seen in Table 22-2 (see Case 22-1). In the main we have noted that the inflammatory response appears to respond well to cyclosporine (see guidelines for therapy in Chapter 8). On the basis of recent immunohistochemical studies already mentioned[43] that show the presence of B cells in patients with long-term disease, one could argue for the initial use of cytotoxic agents. However, our continued preference for cyclosporine is based on the following: most of the specimens examined show the predominance of T cells; patients have responded well to a steroid/cyclosporine regimen; and the potential for long-term side effects is arguably less with cyclosporine than with cytotoxic agents.

An overall review of our 32 patients showed that 16 had a final visual acuity of 20/40 or better in at least one eye. A good visual outcome was associated with early aggressive immunotherapy. A poor visual outcome was associated with glaucoma, macular scarring, and persistent inflammation.[64]

In Hakin and colleagues' series of 18 patients with sympathetic ophthalmia,[7] azathioprine or cyclosporine, or both, were used in addition to steroids. Ten of the 18 patients saw 6/9 or better with their sympathizing eye. A poor visual outcome was due to cystoid macular edema, as well as lens opacities, and six patients needed antiglaucomatous therapy during the course of their therapy.

#### Case 22-1

A 62-year-old man suffered a hunting injury that caused bilateral inflammatory response several months after the trauma. Enucleation of the exciting eye demonstrated histologic alterations typical of sympathetic ophthalmia. His inflammatory disease responded to high-dose prednisone (80 mg/day), but he could not continue with this regimen because of side effects, and at lower dosages of prednisone the disease recurred. His vision was 20/200. He was begun on a regimen of cyclosporine as the sole therapeutic agent, and his vision improved to 20/40. There was a slow drop in his vision in his eye because of a cataract. The patient underwent cataract extraction (without intraocular lens [IOL]), and his vision stabilized at the 20/30 range. He has had no major recurrence of his disease while receiving cyclosporine therapy. He did, however, develop hypertension and renal toxicity due to the cyclosporine. This necessitated a progressive decrease in cyclosporine and the addition of low-dose prednisone. His vision remains stable, and he is undergoing very slow tapering of the cyclosporine.

**Comment 22-1** Starting this patient on a dose of cyclosporine that is needed when used as a sole therapeutic agent, although effective, will result in renal toxicity, particularly in the older-aged patient, whose renal reserve is less. Careful monitoring of renal function and combining low-dose cyclosporine with prednisone are mandatory.

### Case 22-2

A 36-year-old myopic white woman noted spots in front of her right eye followed by a sudden decrease in vision in that eye. She was diagnosed as having a total retinal detachment and underwent surgical repair of the detachment. The postoperative course was difficult and included a vitreal hemorrhage. She underwent repeat surgery, which included an attempt to reattach the retina, coupled with a vitrectomy. The retina could not be reattached, and although immediately after surgery the media was clear, a repeat vitreal hemorrhage was noted some weeks later.

Approximately 13 months after the initial problem in the right eye, it was noted that a small peripheral tear was present in the left eye. This was treated with laser. Several weeks after this intervention, she noted that the right eye was painful and the left eye had a large number of floaters. The left eye had multiple yellow lesions extending from the area of laser therapy, associated with a vitreal inflammatory response. The vision was 20/20. The clinical impression was that of sympathetic ophthalmia. Enucleation of the blind, painful right eye was carried out, and histologic evaluation of this eye confirmed the clinical impression. Because of the good vision in the left eye, it was elected to follow up the patient's condition. Baseline visual fields and electroretinogram were obtained. Although her vision remained 20/20, the visual field was noted to become increasingly more constricted and the electroretinogram (ERG) showed a change from baseline as well. The patient also noted subjective changes in her vision. In spite of the good visual acuity, it was elected to treat these alterations with steroids. The subjective alterations disappeared, but no improvement in the visual-field changes were seen, although there was no further progression.

## REFERENCES


1. MacKenzie W: *A practical treatise on disease of the eye,* London, 1830, Longmans.
2. Marak GE Jr: Recent advances in sympathetic ophthalmia, *Surv Ophthalmol* 24:141-156, 1979.
3. Liddy N, Stuart J: Sympathetic ophthalmia in Canada, *Can J Ophthalmol* 7:157-159, 1972.
4. Holland G: About the indication and time for surgical removal of an injured eye, *Klin Monatsbl Augenheilkd* 145:732-740, 1964.
5. Gass JDM: Sympathetic ophthalmia following vitrectomy, *Am J Ophthalmol* 93:552-558, 1982.
6. Duke-Elder WS, Perkins EA: Diseases of the uveal tract. In Duke-Elder WS, editor: *System of ophthalmology,* vol 9, St Louis, 1966, Mosby.
7. Hakin KN, Pearson RV, Lightman SL: Sympathetic ophthalmia: visual results with modern immunosuppressive therapy, *Eye* 6:453-455, 1992.
8. Smith RS, Webb R, van Heusen WAJ: Sympathetic ophthalmia as a complication of pars plana vitrectomy, *Perspect Ophthalmol* 2:117-120, 1978.
9. Green WR, Maumenee AE, Sanders TE: Sympathetic uveitis following evisceration, *Trans Am Acad Ophthalmol Otolaryngol* 76:625-644, 1972.
10. Awan KJ: Sympathetic uveitis in intraocular implant surgery, *J Ocular Ther Surg* 3:134-135, 1984.
11. Carney MD, Tessler HH, Peyman GA et al: Sympathetic ophthalmia and subretinal neovascularization, *Ann Ophthalmol* 22:184-186, 1990.
12. Lewis ML, Gass JDM, Spencer WH: Sympathetic uveitis after trauma and vitrectomy, *Arch Ophthalmol* 96:263-267, 1978.
13. de Veer JA: Bilateral endophthalmitis phacoanaphylactica, *Arch Ophthalmol* 49:607-632, 1953.
14. Blodi FC: Sympathetic uveitis as an allergic phenomenon, *Trans Am Acad Ophthalmol Otolaryngol* 63: 642-649, 1959.
15. Lubin JR, Albert DM, Weinstein M: Sixty-five years of sympathetic ophthalmia: a clinicopathologic review of 105 cases (1913-1978), *Ophthalmology* 87:109-121, 1980.
16. Allen JC: Sympathetic uveitis and phacoanaphylaxis, *Am J Ophthalmol* 63:280-283, 1967.
17. Romaine H: Malignant melanoma of the choroid with sympathetic ophthalmia, *Arch Ophthalmol* 42:102-103, 1949.
18. Melanowski WH: Contribution to the pathogenesis of sympathetic ophthalmia: a case of sympathetic ophthalmia due to intraocular melanosarcoma, *Klin Monatsbl Augenheilkd* 97:52-59, 1936.
19. Easom HA: Sympathetic ophthalmia associated with malignant melanoma, *Arch Ophthalmol* 70:786-790, 1963.
20. Fries PD, Char DH, Crawford JB et al: Sympathetic ophthalmia complicating helium ion irradiation of a choroidal melanoma, *Arch Ophthalmol* 105:1561-1564, 1987.
21. Margo CE, Pautler SE: Granulomatous uveitis after treatment of a choroidal melanoma with proton-beam irradiation, *Retina* 10:140-143, 1990.
22. Sabates R: Choroiditis compatible with the histopathological diagnosis of sympathetic ophthalmia following cyclocryotherapy of neovascular glaucoma, *Ophthalmic Surg* 19:176-182, 1988.
23. Edward DP, Brown SVL, Higginbotham E et al: Sympathetic ophthalmia following neodymium: YAG cyclotherapy, *Ophthalmic Surg* 20:544-546, 1989.
24. Lam S, Tessler HH, Lam BL et al: High incidence of sympathetic ophthalmia after contact and non-contact

neodymium: YAG cyclotherapy, *Ophthalmology* 99: 1818-1822, 1992.
25. Tessler HH, Lam S, Wilensky J et al: Sympathetic ophthalmia after non-contact neodymium: YAG cyclotherapy. In Dernouchamps JP, Verougstraete C, Caspers-Velu L et al, editors: *Recent advances in uveitis: Proceeding of the Third International Symposium on Uveitis,* Amsterdam, 1993, Kugler.
26. Harrison TJ: Sympathetic ophthalmia after cyclocryotherapy of neovascular glaucoma without ocular penetration, *Ophthalmic Surg* 24:44-46, 1993.
27. Glavici M: Sympathetic ophthalmia after a cataract operation, *Oftalmolgia* 36:397-401, 1992.
28. Lakhanpal V, Dogra MR, Jacobson MS: Sympathetic ophthalmia associated with anterior chamber intraocular lens implantation, *Ann Ophthalmol* 23:139-143, 1991.
29. Spitznas M: Fluorescein angiography of sympathetic ophthalmia, *Klin Monatsbl Augenheilkd* 169:195-200, 1976.
30. Dreyer WB Jr, Zegarra H, Zakov ZN, et al: Sympathetic ophthalmia, *Am J Ophthalmol* 92:816-823, 1981.
31. Fuchs E: Über sympathisierende Entzündung zuerst Bermerkunen über serose traumatische Iritis, *Albrecht von Graefes Arch Ophthalmol* 61:365-456, 1905.
32. Marak GE, Font RL, Zimmerman LE: Histologic variations related to race in sympathetic ophthalmia, *Am J Ophthalmol* 78:935-938, 1974.
33. Kuo PK, Lubin JR, Ni C et al: Sympathetic ophthalmia: a comparison of the histopathological features from a Chinese and American series, *Int Ophthalmol Clin* 22:125-139, 1982.
34. Croxatto JO, Rao NA, McLean IW et al: Atypical histopathologic features in sympathetic ophthalmia: a study of a hundred cases, *Int Ophthalmol* 3:129-135, 1981.
35. Allinson RW, Le TD, Kramer TR et al: Fluorescein angiographic appearance of Dalen-Fuchs nodules in sympathetic ophthalmia, *Ann Ophthalmol* 25:152-156, 1993.
36. Font RL, Fine BS, Messmer E et al: Light and electron microscopic study of Dalen-Fuchs nodules in sympathetic ophthalmia, *Ophthalmology* 90:66-75, 1983.
37. Jakobiec FA, Marboe CC, Knowles DM II et al: Human sympathetic ophthalmia: an analysis of the inflammatory infiltrate by hybridoma-monoclonal antibodies, immunochemistry, and correlative electron microscopy, *Ophthalmology* 90:76-95, 1983.
38. Chan CC, BenEzra D, Rodrigues MM et al: Immunohistochemistry and electron microscopy of choroidal infiltrates and Dalen-Fuchs nodules in sympathetic ophthalmia, *Ophthalmology* 92:580-590, 1985.
39. Chan CC, Nussenblatt RB, Fujikawa LS et al: Sympathetic ophthalmia: immunopathological findings, *Ophthalmology* 93:690-695, 1986.
40. Rao NA, Xu S, Font RL: Sympathetic ophthalmia: an immunohistochemical study of epithelioid and giant cells, *Ophthalmology* 92:1660-1662, 1985.
41. Rao NA, Marak GE: Sympathetic ophthalmia simulating Vogt-Koyanagi-Harada's disease: a clinico-pathologic study of four cases, *Jpn J Ophthalmol* 27:506-511, 1983.
42. Kaplan HJ, Waldrep JC, Chan WC et al: Human sympathetic ophthalmia: immunologic analysis of the vitreous and uvea, *Arch Ophthalmol* 104:240-244, 1986.
43. Shah DN, Piacentini MA, Burnier MN Jr et al: Inflammatory cellular kinetics in sympathetic ophthalmia: a study of 29 traumatized (exciting) eyes, *Ocular Immunol Inflamm* 1:255-262, 1993.
44. Sen DK, Sarin GS, Mathur MD: Serum beta-2 microglobulin level in sympathetic ophthalmitis, *Acta Ophthalmol (Copenh)* 68:200-204, 1990.
45. Goto H, Rao NA: Sympathetic ophthalmia and Vogt-Koyanagi-Harada syndrome, *Int Ophthalmol Clin* 30: 279-285, 1990.
46. Chan CC, BenEzra D, Hsu SM et al: Granulomas in sympathetic ophthalmia and sarcoidosis: immunohistochemical study, *Arch Ophthalmol* 103:198-202, 1985.
47. Easom HA, Zimmerman LE: Sympathetic ophthalmia and bilateral phacoanaphylaxis: a clinicopathologic correlation of the sympathogenic and sympathizing eyes, *Arch Ophthalmol* 72:9-15, 1964.
48. Elschnig A: Studies in sympathetic ophthalmia. II. The antigenic effect of eye pigments, *Albrecht von Graefes Arch Ophthalmol* 76:509-546, 1910.
49. Woods AC: Immune reactions following injuries to the uveal tract, *JAMA* 77:1317-1322, 1921.
50. Wong VG, Anderson R, O'Brien PJ: Sympathetic ophthalmia and lymphocyte transformation, *Am J Ophthalmol* 72:960-965, 1971.
51. Hammer H: Cellular hypersensitivity to uveal pigment confirmed by leucocyte migration tests in sympathetic ophthalmitis and the Vogt-Koyanagi-Harada syndrome, *Br J Ophthalmol* 58:773-776, 1974.
52. Marak GE Jr, Font RL, Johnson MC et al: Lymphocyte-stimulating activity of ocular tissues in sympathetic ophthalmia, *Invest Ophthalmol Vis Sci* 10:770-774, 1971.
53. de Smet MD, Yamamoto JH, Mochizuki M et al: Cellular immune responses of patients with uveitis to retinal antigens and their fragments, *Am J Ophthalmol* 110: 135-142, 1990.
54. Chan CC, Palestine AG, Nussenblatt RB et al: Anti-retinal autoantibodies in Vogt-Koyanagi-Harada syndrome, Behçet's disease, and sympathetic ophthalmia, *Ophthalmology* 92:1025-1028, 1985.
55. Reynard M, Shulman IA, Azen SP et al: Histocompatibility antigens in sympathetic ophthalmia, *Am J Ophthalmol* 95:216-221, 1983.
56. Davis JL, Mittal KK, Freidlin V et al: HLA associations and ancestry in Vogt-Koyanagi-Harada disease and sympathetic ophthalmia, *Ophthalmology* 97:1137-1142, 1990.
57. Rao NA, Robin J, Hartmann D et al: The role of the penetrating wound in the development of sympathetic ophthalmia: experimental observations, *Arch Ophthalmol* 101:102-104, 1983.
58. Winter FC: Sympathetic uveitis: a clinical and pathologic study of the visual result, *Am J Ophthalmol* 39:340-347, 1955.
59. Reynard M, Riffenburgh RS, Maes EF: Effect of corticosteroid treatment and enucleation on the visual prognosis of sympathetic ophthalmia, *Am J Ophthalmol* 96:290-294, 1983.

60. Brackup AB, Carter KD, Nerad JA et al: Long-term follow-up of severely injured eyes following globe rupture, *Ophthalmic Plast Reconstr Surg* 7:194-197, 1991.
61. Makley TA, Azar A: Sympathetic ophthalmia: a long term followup, *Arch Ophthalmol* 96:257-262, 1978.
62. Schlaegel TF Jr: Uveitis of suspected viral origin. In Duane T, editor: *Clinical Ophthalmology,* Hagerstown, Md, 1976, Harper & Row.
63. Tessler HH, Jennings T: High-dose short-term chlorambucil for intractable sympathetic ophthalmia and Behçet's disease, *Br J Ophthalmol* 74:353-357, 1990.
64. Chan CC, Roberge FG, Whitcup SM et al: Thirty two cases of sympathetic ophthalmia. A retrospective study at the National Eye Institute Bethesda, Md., from 1982-1992, *Arch Ophthalmol* 113:597-600, 1995.

# CHAPTER 23

# Vogt-Koyanagi-Harada Syndrome

The Vogt-Koyanagi-Harada syndrome (VKH) is a systemic disorder involving many organ systems, including the eyes, ears, skin, and meninges. It is a constellation of clinical signs and symptoms with no definitive confirmatory diagnostic tests yet available. Early reports describing this disorder can be found in the literature: Alfred Vogt[1] in 1906 presented one case, and Y. Koyanagi[2] in 1929 described in detail six cases of bilateral nontraumatic chronic iridocyclitis associated with poliosis, vitiligo, and dysacousia. Harada,[3] in 1926, described an essentially posterior uveitis with an exudative retinal detachment associated with a pleocytosis in the cerebrospinal fluid. As more of these cases were recognized, it became clear that many of the features seen in each of these entities overlapped. Babel[4] suggested that these symptoms were manifestations of the same underlying disorder and that only intensity and distribution varied from one patient to the next; it therefore seemed appropriate to call the entity the Vogt-Koyanagi-Harada syndrome, although it sometimes appears in the literature under other names, for example, uveomeningitis.

## CLINICAL ASPECTS

Although VKH has been reported throughout the world, it appears to be concentrated in certain racial and ethnic groups. It is a common type of endogenous uveitis in Japan, making up at least 8% of these cases.[5] The same holds true for certain parts of Latin America, particularly Brazil. It is, however, relatively uncommon in the United States and appears to be an exceedingly unusual diagnosis in persons of northern European extraction. Some years ago, when we reviewed our examinations of 78 patients with VKH (Fig. 23-1), we noted that most (77%) have been female. A similar observation has been made of patients in Latin America.[6] However, Ohno and coworkers,[7] in their series of 186 patients, reported that more males than females had the disease. In our series, 44% of the patients were African-Americans, 37% were white, 11% Hispanic, and 6% Oriental. Of interest is the fact that a very high percentage of the patients with VKH whom we have seen have American-Indian heritage, albeit sometimes distant. This observation is a most provocative one, because certainly this may be the unifying genetic bond between patients in the United States and those in the Orient. VKH is generally a disease of persons in the second to fourth decade of life, although the disease has been reported in children. Recently Lacerda[8] reported a case in a 7-year-old child.

### Systemic findings

VKH is a systemic disorder, and the extraocular findings are most important in securing the diagnosis. Perry and Font[9] have stressed that in those patients with the Harada form of the disease some extraocular findings, such as hair and skin alterations, are uncommon. However,

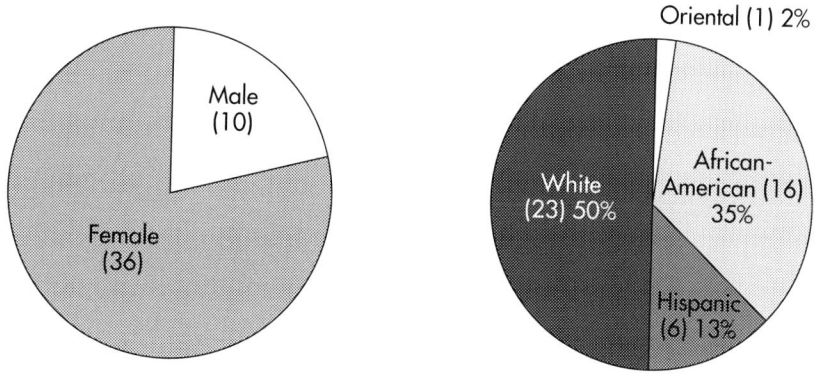


**Fig. 23-1.** Sex and ethnic distribution of 46 VKH patients seen at National Eye Institute.

in our mind, even patients with ocular lesions typical of this disorder cannot definitively be said to have VKH without these extraocular findings.

The disease may be preceded by a prodromal stage, in which the patient may complain of headache, orbital pain, stiff neck, and vertigo. There may be a fever as well. In Beniz and coworkers' group of mostly Hispanic patients,[10] headache was by far the most common neurologic complaint. Others[11,12] have reported presentation with a mild facial weakness, migrainelike headaches with a sensorimotor hemisyndrome, and cognitive brain dysfunction.

The patient complaining of central nervous system symptoms needs to be evaluated rapidly. A lumbar puncture will reveal a pleocytosis in 84% of cases,[7] with mostly lymphocytes and monocytes present. The cerebrospinal fluid glucose should show a normal relationship to the serum glucose level. The lumbar puncture should be performed early in the course of the disease inasmuch as the pleocytosis will ultimately disappear even though the inflammatory disease in the eye may continue.

The auditory difficulties associated with this disorder are central and will often occur concurrently with the ocular disease. The auditory disorder may be the presenting problem, however. The hearing loss usually involves the higher frequencies and may affect more than three quarters of the patients with the disorder. Dysacousia, which was observed in 74% of patients in one study,[7] may resolve after several months; however, we, as well as others, have noted that it may persist for years. Some patients will have tinnitus without an objective decrease in hearing. Detailed auditory testing, carried out by competent professionals, is important to rule out a noncentral reason for a decrease in hearing.

Skin lesions may be a prominent part of the disease complex as well. Some 72% of patients[7] report sensitivity to touch of both hair and skin during the active phase of their disease. Vitiligo and poliosis occur in a large number of patients (63% and 90%, respectively) during the convalescent stage, whereas alopecia was reported in 73% of one group of VKH patients studied[13] (Fig. 23-2). It should be noted that ethnic groups may manifest varying systemic symptoms, as suggested by Beniz and colleagues' study[10] in which the authors found dermatologic involvement only rarely in the mostly Hispanic group of VKH patients whose cases they followed. One area frequently overlooked during an examination for such changes is the axilla.

## Ocular findings

VKH is a bilateral ocular condition. Although only one eye may be inflamed initially, in 94% of cases the disease involves the second eye within 2 weeks. There is a tendency for the ocular disease to occur in spring and autumn.[7] The inflammatory disease is granulomatous in nature, with mutton-fat keratic precipitates on the corneal endothelium. Perilimbal vitiligo (Sugiura's sign) may be a striking feature, occurring in 85% of Oriental patients.[7] The inflammatory activity can be quite severe and involves both the anterior chamber and the anterior vitreous in about 56% of the cases. Nodules may be noted on the pupillary margin, as well as in the iris stroma (Fig. 23-3). An early finding in the disease is the shallowing of the anterior chamber and a moderate increase in

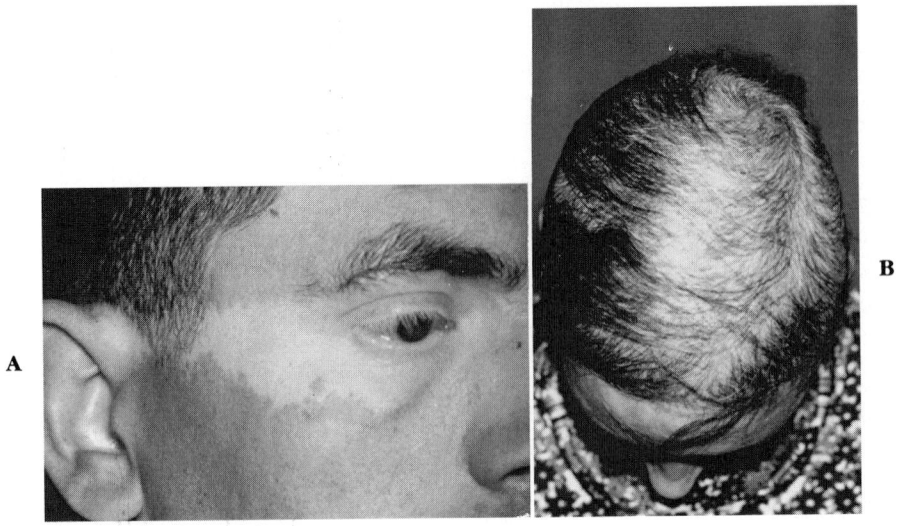


**Fig. 23-2. A,** Area of vitiligo and poliosis of cilia in patient with VKH. **B,** Alopecia in patient with VKH. Hair ultimately regrew. (**A,** Courtesy D. Cogan, M.D.)

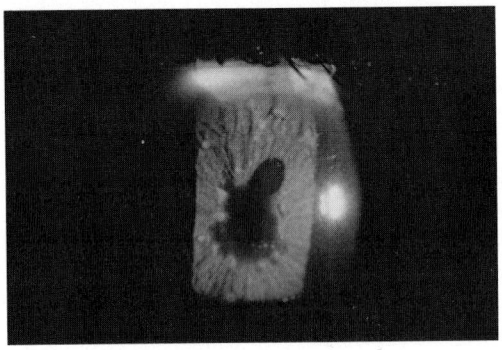

**Fig. 23-3.** Iris nodules and mutton-fat keratitic precipitates in patient with VKH.

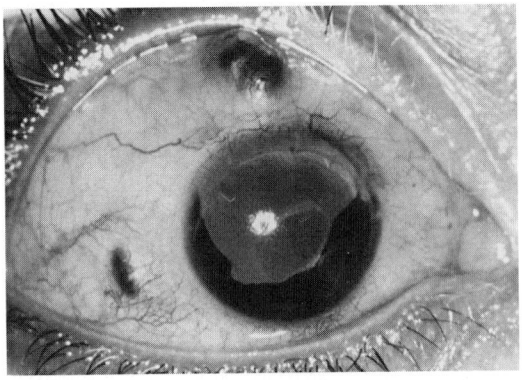

**Fig. 23-4.** Case of VKH with areas of focal scleritis and thinning of sclera anterior to insertion of recti muscles. There is a large sector iridectomy superiorly. (From Tabbara KF: Scleromalacia associated with Vogt-Koyanagi-Harada syndrome, *Am J Ophthalmol* 105: 694-695, 1988.)

intraocular pressure.[14] This appears to be related to a swelling of the ciliary processes, which has been noted to occur early in this disease.[15] This finding is apparent only with careful gonioscopic evaluation. Other patients, however, may have hypotony, probably a result of the edema of the ciliary body. A high incidence of neovascularization of the angle has been reported by one group of Japanese investigators,[16] but this has not been our personal experience. The severity of the inflammatory response is reflected by the fact that pupillary membranes often develop, and cataract formation occurs. The glaucoma associated with VKH can be difficult to control. In a series reported by Forster and coworkers,[17] 16 of 42 VKH patients required either surgical or medical therapy for their glaucoma, 9 having open-angle glaucoma and seven with angle closure due to pupillary block. A thickened iris is commonly noted in this disease. This is important for at least two reasons. The first is that laser iridotomies are very difficult to perform and often close quickly. The second is that the patient may experience angle closure with a plateau iris, which often adheres completely to the lens, making it impossible to bow forward as one would expect in a more typical case of iris bombé. A rare presentation in dark-skinned persons is scleral perforation, presumably at the site of emergence of the scleral nerves, which are involved as innocent bystanders in the immune response directed against the melanocytes surrounding them[18] (Fig. 23-4).

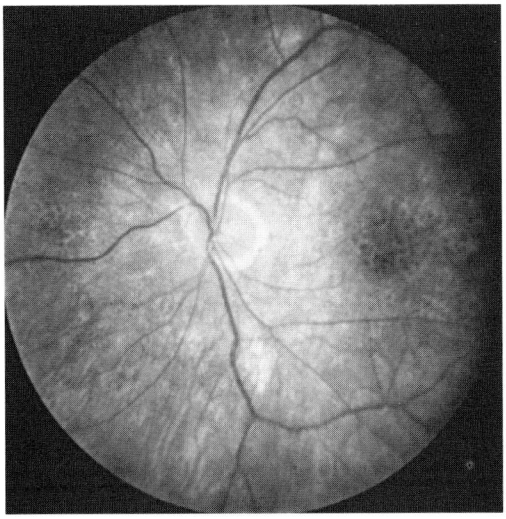

**Fig. 23-5.** Sunset glow fundus in Asian patient after inflammatory disease of posterior segment due to VKH. Note "blond" appearance of fundus. (Courtesy K. Masuda, M.D., and M. Mochizuki, M.D.)

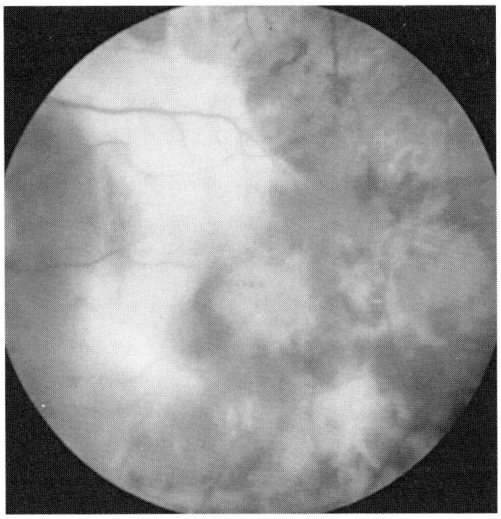

**Fig. 23-6.** Dramatic subretinal alterations with subretinal fibrosis can occur in severe posterior pole inflammatory attacks.

Severe and rather characteristic changes are noted to occur in the posterior portion of the eye as this disorder evolves. A swelling of the optic nerve head is seen early in 87% of the cases[7]; this is usually in concert with a severe vitreous inflammatory response. In addition, retinal edema may be one of the first signs of the disease and may be situated in the posterior pole. As the disease process continues, an exudative nonrhegmatogenous retinal detachment may occur, which is an important diagnostic finding. The inferior portion of the retina is most frequently involved. In the periphery of the retina, yellow-white, well-circumscribed lesions may appear, similar to those seen in sympathetic ophthalmia (see Chapter 22). It is thought that these are the clinical equivalent of Dalen-Fuchs nodules.

Several fundus alterations occur as the disease process continues. Neovascularization of the retina and optic nerve can be seen, with subsequent recurrent and clinically significant vitreous hemorrhages. Subretinal neovascularization of the macula can also occur. As well, extramacular disciform lesions have been reported,[19] presumably in areas of reactive proliferation of the retinal pigment epithelium (RPE) and perturbation of Bruch's membrane. Moorthy and coworkers[20] reported that subretinal neovascular membranes developed in 7 of 58 patients with VKH they were following up. They found that these seven affected patients showed more anterior and vitreous inflammation, as well as more pigmentary disturbances in the fundus. As to be expected, the visual outcomes for these patients were also significantly poorer than for those with less severe alterations.

The nonrhegmatogenous detachments frequently do not persist after the initial presentation, although the other signs of inflammation continue to be present—for example, "demarcation lines" representing the extent of previous detachments. Rhegmatogenous detachments may also occur in these eyes, and a constant surveillance for such changes is vital.

As the disease process begins to wane, characteristically a depigmentation of the posterior portion of the globe occurs. This "sunset glow" appearance to the fundus, which reflects the changes occurring at the level of the RPE or choroid, is seen commonly in Oriental patients. In the United States, the fundus of a white person with this disease has a more mottled appearance, as well as a profound loss of pigment, causing what is known as a "blond" fundus. At times profound subretinal changes, such as subretinal fibrosis, disciform scars, and RPE migration, can be quite striking (Figs. 23-5 to 23-7).

In the 78 VKH patients we reviewed, the disease manifests predominantly posterior pole changes. We have not noted patients with only anterior segment disorders. The wide

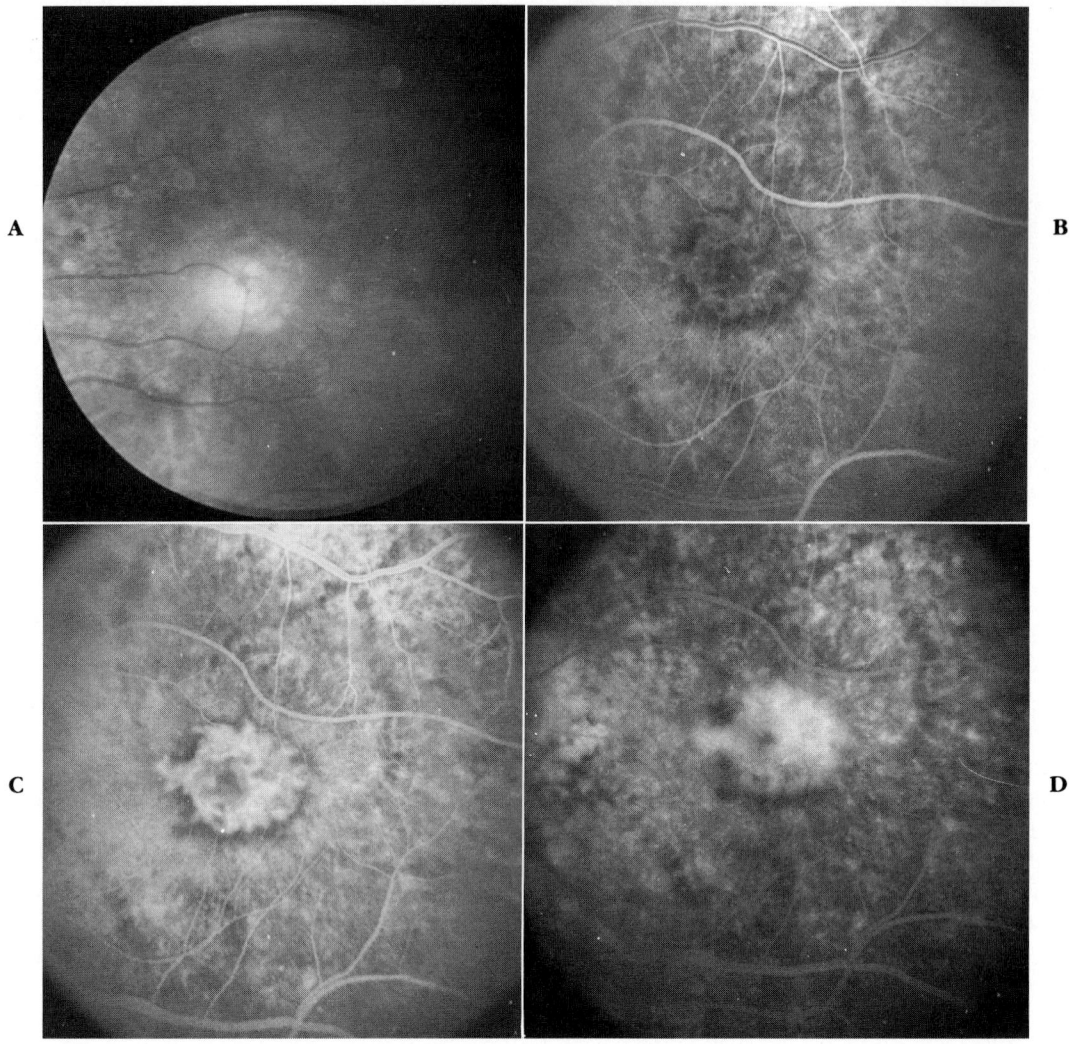


**Fig. 23-7. A,** to **D,** Hispanic female with poor vision in left eye after ongoing uveitis due to VKH. Fluorescein angiography findings demonstrated presence of subretinal neovascular net.

distribution of the visual acuities of 46 of these patients can be seen in Fig. 23-8. However, the acuities appear to be "bunched" at the extremes of the vision chart. A large number of the eyes demonstrate visual acuities that are 20/200 or worse, whereas a large portion of the eyes have a visual acuity of 20/40 or better. This reflects Ohno and coworkers' observations.[7] We have noted that our patients have had a far more persistent ocular inflammatory disease than is generally described in the literature. Rubsamen and Gass[21] found that in their series of 26 patients the disease recurred in 9 of 21 patients in the first 3 months, sometimes associated with a rapid taper of therapy. This may reflect referral patterns.

## Course of disease

The clinical course of VKH is quite variable. Some patients may have a limited period of severe ocular inflammatory activity, followed by a rapid depigmentation and no further episodes. Other patients, however, continue to have ongoing, chronic disease. It is this group that requires constant vigilance. Anterior segment alterations, such as cataract and secondary glaucoma, occur in about one third of the patients. With aggressive therapy, one can assume that the nonrhegmatogenous detachment will reattach. The reattachment usually results in reasonably good vision. However, a close evaluation of the retina will demonstrate changes, such as preretinal mem-

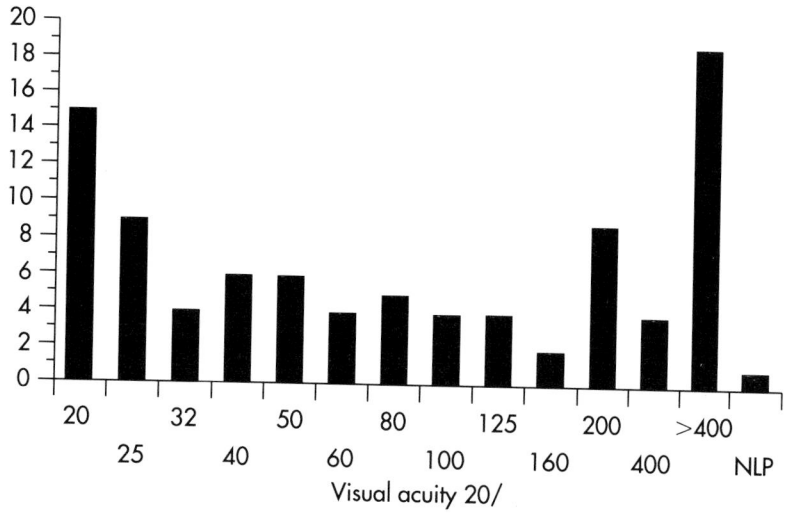


**Fig. 23-8.** Distribution of visual acuities in VKH patients seen at National Eye Institute.

branes, RPE stippling, and subtle folds in the retina precluding a return to previous levels of vision.

When patients manifest the classic acute findings of VKH, there is little difficulty in making the diagnosis. However, when the patient is examined at a later stage, the sequelae of the inflammatory disease cannot reliably help one in deciding what the original problem had been, particularly if the nonocular findings are absent. The problems faced in diagnosing this condition were considered by Kayazawa and Takahashi,[22] who described two patients, both of whom had multiple yellow-white placoid lesions and a decrease in vision. On the basis of fluorescein angiographic findings, one patient was believed to have acute posterior multifocal placoid pigment epitheliopathy (APMPPE). However, the fluorescein angiographic findings in the other patient showed multiple pin-point leaks, and later the fundus developed a "sunset glow" appearance. Rao and Marak[23] reported four patients with sympathetic ophthalmia, all with penetrating wounds, in whom there also developed two or more extraocular manifestations usually associated with VKH, that is, vitiligo, poliosis, dysacousia, and meningitis (see Chapter 22). Other disorders that can mimic VKH include sarcoidosis (see Chapter 21) (particularly if there is choroidal involvement and subretinal changes), and some of the white-dot syndromes (see Chapter 28).

The observer should set minimal ocular criteria for the diagnosis of this condition, because it is, in the main, a clinical decision. Our minimal criteria include a bilateral acute inflammatory response, with retinal edema, and typical pinpoint leakage at the level of the RPE early on, as noted on examination with fluorescein angiography (see next section). Disc edema (and leakage seen on the fluorescein angiogram) is an important confirmatory sign, and many patients will have a central nervous system pleocytosis early in the disease. The presence of other extraocular findings already enumerated are helpful but late in the disease may be missed. A history of Native-American heritage in patients is helpful information. We have no knowledge of the presence of Sugiura's sign in white patients with this disease.

## LABORATORY TESTS, ETIOLOGY, AND HISTOPATHOLOGY

Several tests can be performed to evaluate the alterations occurring in the eye as a result of the inflammatory disease. The use of fluorescein angiography is helpful in evaluating the extent of the disease in the posterior segment of the globe. Early in the disease, multiple pinpoint areas of leakage are noted at the level of the RPE. The later frames of the angiogram may show a large confluent area of leakage (Fig. 23-9), and late leakage of the disc usually occurs. Subretinal neovascularization can be evaluated best with use of fluorescein angiography (see Fig. 23-7). Manger and Ober[24] reported the presence of retinal arteriovenous anastamoses in a young female with VKH. By

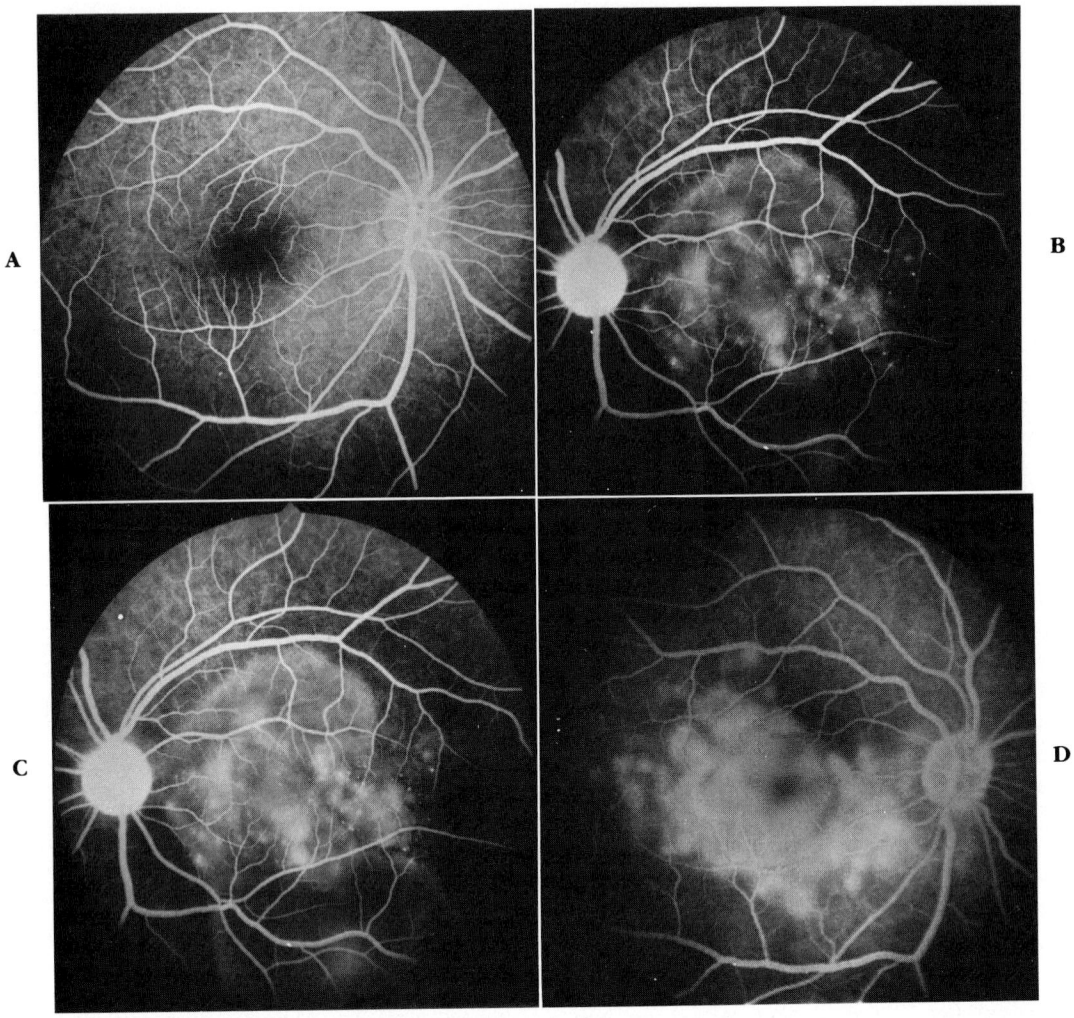


**Fig. 23-9.** Fluorescein angiograms of right eye (**A** and **D**) and left eye (**B** and **C**) of VKH patient, demonstrating pinpoint subretinal leakage, which later coalesces into large area of leakage.

using fluorescein angiography, they noted that these vessels were collaterals that developed in areas of damaged RPE.

The electroretinogram and electrooculogram findings show varying degrees of abnormalities, depending on the ocular disease. It is important to note that improvement in both tests may occur during certain time-points of the clinical course, with a worsening associated with a recurrence.[25] Although electrophysiologic testing and fluorescein angiography are helpful adjuncts, we have seen patients with dramatic alterations of the posterior pole who maintain very good vision in spite of poor test results.

Much attention has been placed on defining the immunoregulatory alteration that leads to VKH. Monoclonal antibodies directed to cell-surface markers of various components of the immune system and to markers of cellular activation that appear at times have been utilized to study this disorder. Okubo and coworkers[26] evaluated the various cellular immune components of 7 VKH patients with active uveitis as compared with those of 98 control subjects. They noted that the numbers of total T cells ($OKT3^+$), helper T cells ($OKT4^+$), and suppressor cells ($OKT11^+$) were lower in patients as compared with control subjects. Liu and Sun[27] reported that the CD4/CD8 ratio was increased in patients whose disease recurred, an observation seen previously by us when patients with uveitis were evaluated in the United States. However, in Okubo and coworkers' study[26] the number of cells bearing the antigen defined by the OKla antibody was elevated. Ia or DR expression can be taken as a sign of immune system activation. Ia expression can be enhanced by T-cell products released during the lymphokine cascade. In particular, interferon-γ is a powerful stimulus for la activation on cell-surface membranes and does not have antiviral activity. The presence of circulating interferon-γ was evaluated in VKH patients. Significantly increased interferon levels were detected in the blood of VKH patients 1 and 2 months after the initiation of ocular symptoms; further evaluation of the interferon present revealed it to be interferon-γ. Interferon-γ could not be detected in the cerebrospinal fluid in those patients whose blood samples showed positivity.[28] Similar observations have been made in diseases of putative autoimmune origin, such as systemic lupus erythematosus, rheumatoid arthritis, and Sjögren's syndrome.[29]

The evaluation of cell-surface markers of cerebrospinal fluid lymphocytes in VKH has been accomplished with use of antisera, as already described.[30] Results showed that 85% of the lymphocytes in the cerebrospinal fluid were $OKT11^+$, and 65% were $OKT4^+$, the antibody defining the helper T-cell subset, with this subset found in higher numbers in the peripheral blood of these patients when compared with that of control subjects.

### Antigen-specific immune responses

The notion that a specific antigen-driven immune response is occurring in this disorder remains an intriguing possibility. Initial hypotheses centered about the role of pigment as the antigen driving the immune response. Several reports observed positive in vitro immune phenomena when patients' lymphocytes were placed in an environment containing uveal extracts or pigment.[31] Most of these reports used a nonhuman, usually bovine, source for antigen, thereby raising the possibility that the positive test results were due to a sensitization against bovine antigens in meat-eating human beings. Yuasa and coworkers,[32] however, used human uveal preparations. They observed that 13 of 30 patients tested had positive macrophage migration inhibition test results, evidence that the immune system is capable of a memory response to the antigen(s). Maezawa and colleagues[33] evaluated the role of cytotoxic T cells in this disorder and how they may react against melanocyte-associated antigens. They noted that in the six VKH patients they studied, the cytotoxic T-cell component of the immune repertoire appeared to demonstrate specific killing against a P-36 melanoma cell line, which bears cross-reactive antigens with normal melanocytes. Further, they demonstrated that the monoclonal antibody, Leu-2a, specifically directed against the cytotoxic T-cell subset, blocked this reaction. They have recently observed that the cytotoxic activity depended on the presence of $DR^+$-adherent cells, and the activity could be augmented by the addition of interleukins into the in vitro system.[34]

The notion that pigment is the underlying agent seems difficult to accept. Rather, it may be that a membrane antigen is shared by the organs involved, namely the skin, meninges, inner ear, and the eye. All of these have elements derived from the neural crest.

The search for antigen-specific immune responses in the eye has also shown responses directed toward retinal elements rather than choroidal. Patients with this disorder have circulating lymphocytes that have been noted to have in vitro proliferative responses to the retinal S-antigen,[35] although this finding is by no means unique to this disorder. Chan and coworkers,[36] however, noted that sera from these patients had particularly unique properties. Using the avidin-biotin-peroxidase technique for the detection of retinal antibodies, they found particularly large titers of antiretinal antibodies in these patients' sera directed against the outer segments of photoreceptors and Müller cells. Considerably lower titers could be found in some patients with Behçet's disease and in a few with sympathetic ophthalmia. Whether this observation is reflective of a primary immune process or is a result of the severe posterior pole disease seen in these patients still remains to be evaluated. It will be interesting to see the cell-mediated responses of VKH patients to RPE-associated antigens, such as the melanin-associated protein (see Chapter 2 and following discussion). It is also of interest that nonspecific triggering mechanisms can lead to the full disease. We followed up a patient in whom typical VKH developed after the placement of a purified protein derivative (PPD) skin test (see Case 23-2). It is thought-provoking to speculate on the role of other exogenous triggering factors.

Because of the increased prevalence of this disorder in certain ethnic groups, it is logical to hypothesize an immunogenetic basis for this disease. Cases of siblings with this disorder have been reported,[37] as have monozygotic twins.[38] Ohno[28] evaluated the frequency of HLA antigens in Japanese patients with this disease as compared with control subjects. HLA-DR4 was present in 88% of patients but in only 32% of control subjects, with a calculated relative risk of 15.2. All (100%) the patients bore the supertypic DR antigen MT3 (HLA-B53) as compared with 53% of the control subjects, with a resultant relative risk of 74.5. Kunikane[39] reported an association with HLA-DQWa and Harada's disease in Japanese patients (relative risk 5.17), confirming Ohno's previous work with the same antigen. However, using two-dimensional electrophoresis and restriction fragment length polymorphism analysis, Kunikane noted that these antigen molecules differed in Japanese and white subjects tested. In typing 25 Han Chinese with VKH, Zhao and coworkers[40] found an association with HLA-DR4 (relative risk 16.0) and HLA-Dw53 (relative risk 34.2), similar to that seen in Japan. Zhang and coworkers[41] reported a strong association between VKH and HLA-DR4, with a calculated relative risk of 10.0, whereas a decreased frequency of HLA-DQw1 was seen in fewer patients. Numaga and colleagues,[42] using a polymerase chain reaction technique, demonstrated that the HLA-DR beta-1 in 19 of 20 patients had a specific amino acid sequence in positions 70 and 71. However, Yu and colleagues[43] found an association with HLA-B22, with a relative risk calculated at 8.69.

Davis and colleagues[44] evaluated the HLA associations of 23 American patients with VKH. A strong association was found with HLA-DR4 and HLA-DRw53. HLA-DQw3 was strongly associated with this disease, this antigen being in linkage disequilibrium with DR4. An interesting report by Rutzen and coworkers[45] described the development of VKH in monozygotic twins of Vietnamese ancestry. HLA typing disclosed HLA-DR4 positivity. In addition, the anecdotal association of VKH with Native-American ancestry was confirmed. In Martinez and colleagues' report[46] of North American VKH patients with Cherokee Indian ancestry, assay results in seven patients showed the HLA-DRw52 haplotype, five of whom were homozygous for this allele.

The concept that this disorder is of viral origin has been an attractive one for many, and numerous attempts have been made to substantiate this theory. However, studies aimed at isolating virus from either the eye[47] or the cerebrospinal fluid[48] have not met with success. Sunakawa and Okinami[49] determined anti–Epstein-Barr virus antibody levels in control subjects and in patients with panuveitis, including VKH patients, and found that the frequency of elevated titers was lower in the patient group than in the control group.

### Vogt-Koyanagi-Harada syndrome versus sympathetic ophthalmia

The histologic evaluation of VKH in several patients has appeared in the literature.[5] A major discussion point has been how this disorder differs from sympathetic ophthalmia (see Chapter 22). As in the latter condition, in VKH there is a marked thickening of the choroid, with macrophages and lymphocytes, as well as epithelioid cells that contain melanin. Unlike sympathetic ophthalmia, in VKH plasma cells are readily observed. Dalen-Fuchs nodules are present, and involvement of the choriocapillaris is more common—unlike the classic "sparing" of this portion of the choroid in sympathetic ophthalmia. Although much has been said about the histologic differences between sympathetic ophthalmia and VKH, it is clear that both represent a spectrum of disease and that, most of the time, standard histologic evaluation of the posterior globe cannot definitively differentiate one disease from the other.

Kahn and colleagues[50] used immunohistochemical techniques to study eyes enucleated from a patient with active VKH. They found that the uveal infiltrates were composed predominantly of T cells and HLA-DR$^+$ macrophages. Nondendritic CD1 (Leu-6)–positive cells were also seen. Emulsified chorioretinal tissue was processed for viral isolation and other tissue for isolation of *Treponema pallidum,* with no microorganisms identified. Sakamoto and colleagues[51] studied the eyes in two Japanese autopsy cases of this disease. They found that the choroidal infiltrate was made up mostly of T cells, with more helper/inducer (CD4$^+$) than suppressor/cytotoxic (CD8$^+$) cells. They also noted that major histocompatibility complex (MHC) class II molecules were expressed on both the choroidal melanocytes and the endothelium of the choriocapillaris.

Experimentally induced autoimmune uveoretinitis in monkeys bears a resemblance to

VKH.[52] After immunization with S-antigen, eyes showed both CD3- and CD19/CD22-positive lymphocytes. Class II MHC proteins and adhesion molecules were expressed on the surface of resident ocular cells. In addition to T cells, there is an influx of B cells and the development of subretinal fibrosis. Another fairly recent model of human disease, melanin-protein induced uveitis,[53] is a disease characterized by an anterior uveitis and bilateral uveal infiltrations with mainly $CD4^+$ lymphocytes as well as monocytes.[54] Of interest is that Cheung and coworkers[55] at the National Eye Institute (NEI) tested eight VKH patients for serum antimelanin antibodies, and all the patients had such antibodies.

## THERAPY

Medical management is the main therapeutic approach to VKH. The drug of choice remains corticosteroids. Usually given systemically for this bilateral condition, the dosage needed to effect a positive therapeutic result may be high. In severe cases, with bilateral retinal detachments and a dramatic drop in visual acuity, a beginning dosage at 100 to 120 mg or higher (e.g., 2 mg/kg) of prednisone can be used. It is clear that when such high dosages are used, the patient should preferably be hospitalized, with careful follow-up. Hayasaka and colleagues[56] reported using drip infusions of 200 mg of prednisolone per day. They have seen resolution of both intraocular and extraocular symptoms in most patients treated in this fashion. Their suggestion is that less steroid may be needed for the Harada type of the disease as compared with the Vogt-Koyanagi component of the disorder, although this has not been our own experience. In patients with particularly severe ocular disease, some practitioners use intravenous high-dose pulse steroid therapy (up to 1 g/day of methylprednisolone given for 3 days) followed by oral prednisone at levels of about 1 mg/kg/day.

The length of treatment and the rate of taper of therapy must be individualized to each case. Rubsamen and Gass[21] treated with steroid for 6 months on average and longer if the disease became chronic. In our experience with severe cases, corticosteroid therapy may continue for at least a year, with a slow, gradual taper occurring during this time. Recurrences are possible, and patients need to be monitored. The presence of new inflammatory cells in the vitreous or such extraocular complaints as headache should alert the treating physician's suspicion that the disorder may be recurring. However, the continued RPE perturbation or the increased prominence of the peripheral white spots may or may not represent true activity. Visual field testing can be helpful in such cases. Some patients regain and keep good vision only at doses of prednisone that are unacceptably high for long-term use. It is at this point, in our mind arbitrarily set at about 3 months, that we would consider other therapeutic alternatives. Although other immunosuppressive agents have been used, the number of patients thus treated is relatively small. Cytotoxic agents have not been used widely in the treatment of this disorder, but a positive therapeutic response to their administration has been reported.[57] We have noted that cyclosporine has been effective in the treatment of VKH patients with posterior pole involvement who were not able to continue systemic corticosteroid therapy because of side effects or the extremely high doses needed to maintain good vision (see Case 23-1).[58] Using this modality, we have been able to decrease dramatically the amount of steroid needed for treatment of the disease. Recently, Wakatsuki and coworkers[59] reported that combination cyclosporine and prednisone effectively treated a patient who required 200 mg or more of prednisone to control his disease, paralleling our experience. Others have also echoed its therapeutic efficacy but stressed the secondary effects and the possibility of disease relapse with drug withdrawal.[60] FK506[61] has been used in a small number of VKH patients with a positive therapeutic response but with the induction of a variety of adverse side effects.

Nonmedical methods of therapy have been employed in a small number of patients. Although usually not a primary therapeutic approach, drainage of the nonrhegmatogenous detachment might prove beneficial in some patients whose disease did not resolve with medical therapy.[62] It should be kept in mind that rhegmatogenous detachments can occur and need to be reattached as quickly as the inflammatory condition permits. Laser therapy for the neovascular lesions that arise as a result of the inflammatory disease is an important adjunct. Plasmapheresis has been used in a limited number of patients with initially good responses in some, but it is not clear whether this therapy will have a long-term beneficial response.

### Cataract extraction

Cataract extraction in VKH patients is a complicated issue. Moorthy and colleagues[63] found that cataracts developed over the course of therapy for 26 of 65 consecutive VKH patients. One can find reports in the literature suggesting that intraocular lens (IOL) placement after a planned extracapsular cataract extraction resulted in no exacerbation of the patient's disease and an improvement of visual acuity from the preoperative vision.[64] Although this clinical result certainly can happen, it behooves the treating physician to be highly critical in the evaluation of the VKH patient. Extensive synechiae may belie a tendency that will manifest after the surgery, with resultant lens capture by the iris, as well as the collection of myriad keratitic precipitates (KP) on the anterior and posterior surfaces of the lens, or the development of retrolental membranes necessitating repeated YAG procedures. Many patients who have undergone pars plana vitrectomies along with their cataract extraction adapt well to aphakic correction. This approach does (almost always) prevent the bound-down small pupil that makes it essentially impossible to visualize the posterior pole. With the bound-down pupil, changes in visual acuity become difficult to assess, and one must deal with the question of whether it is due to ongoing posterior segment inflammation, neovascular membrane, unrecognized glaucoma, or even a low-lying retinal detachment. Despite these concerns, certain well-chosen patients have shown benefit from IOL placement, but in our experience they comprise a small number of these patients. However, cataract extraction may result in a marked improvement in visual acuity and should be considered strongly in these patients.[63]

#### Case 23-1

A 39-year-old white woman with Native-American ancestry developed bilateral posterior uveitis with serous retinal detachments. Her vision fell to 20/400 OU. She began to have severe headaches. A lumbar puncture was performed, and 25/mm$^3$ mononuclear cells were noted. Soon after, a profound hearing loss developed in both ears, which was documented on audiogram. She was placed on a regimen of 120 mg/day of prednisone for 1 month, with no improvement in her condition. At this point the oral prednisone was tapered as quickly as was medically permissible, and the patient was placed on cyclosporine therapy. The response in both eyes was slow, but a constant decrease in inflammatory disease was followed by a gradual improvement in visual acuity OU. Her vision reached 20/40 OU. Some months after this vision was stabilized, an attempt was made to reduce and then stop the cyclosporine. Renewed intraocular inflammatory disease was observed. The patient's condition was stabilized on 10 mg prednisone coupled with 2 to 3 mg/kg day of cyclosporine, and this therapeutic schedule continues.

#### Case 23-2

A 17-year-old African-American woman with no Native-American ancestry was known to have to a positive PPD test reaction (but no radiologic evidence of tuberculosis), for which she was treated with isoniazid (INH) and paraaminosalicylic acid (PAS) for 1 year. The patient had no history of ocular disease. She underwent a repeat PPD test for a physical examination, and 5 days later her vision decreased to hand-motion vision in the right eye and counting-fingers vision left eye. She had bilateral serous retinal detachments with creamy deep spots throughout the fundus. She complained of intermittent tinnitus. As well, the site of the PPD test developed vitiligo, and a skin biopsy revealed a marked decrease in melanocytes in this region. A spinal tap was not performed. She was placed on a regimen of 120 mg of prednisone daily. Her visual acuity began to improve rapidly, and after 4 to 6 weeks her visual acuity returned to the 20/30 to 20/40 range. An audiologic evaluation failed to demonstrate a hearing loss. Results of the ocular examination showed that the retinal detachments resolved. However, striae in the macular region were seen in both eyes. She has maintained this good vision, with no recurrences, for 5 years after stopping all medication.

### REFERENCES

1. Vogt A: Frühzeitiges Ergrauen der Zilien und Bemerkungen üben den sogannten plözlichen Eintritt dieser Veränderung, *Klin Monatsbl Augenheilkd* 44: 228-242, 1906.
2. Koyanagi Y: Dysakusis, Alopecia un Poliosis bei schwerer Uveitis nicht traumatischen Ursprungs, *Klin Monatsbl Augenheilkd* 82:194-211, 1929.
3. Harada E: Clinical observations of nonsuppurative choroiditis, *Acta Soc Ophthalmol Jpn* 30:356, 1926.
4. Babel J: Syndrome de Vogt-Koyanagi, *Schweiz Med Wochenschr* 44:1136-1140, 1932.
5. Sugiura S: Vogt-Koyanagi-Harada disease, *Jpn J Ophthalmol* 22:9-35, 1978.

6. Belfort R Jr: Personal communication.
7. Ohno S, Minakawa R, Matsuda H: Clinical studies on Vogt-Koyanagi-Harada's disease, *Jpn J Ophthalmol* (in press).
8. Lacerda RR: Sindrome de Vogt-Koyanagi-Harada: descrição de um caso especial em criança de sete anos de idade, *Arq Bras Oftal* 57:46-48, 1994.
9. Perry HD, Font RL: Clinical and histopathologic observations in severe Vogt-Koyanagi-Harada syndrome, *Am J Ophthalmol* 83:242-254, 1977.
10. Beniz J, Forster DJ, Lean JS et al: Variations in clinical features of the Vogt-Koyanagi-Harada syndrome, *Retina* 11:275-280, 1991.
11. Ikeda M, Tsukagoshi H: Vogt-Koyanagi-Harada disease presenting meningoencephalitis: report of a case with magnetic resonance imaging, *Eur Neurol* 32:83-85, 1992.
12. Kätterer C, Kaeser HE, Steiger U: Rare form of uveitis with neurological symptoms: the Vogt-Koyanagi-Harada uveomeningoencephalitic syndrome, *Schweiz Med Wochenschr* 122:269-274, 1992.
13. Rosen E: Uveitis, with poliosis, vitiligo, alopecia and dysacousia, (Vogt-Koyanagi syndrome), *Arch Ophthalmol* 33:281-292, 1945.
14. Kimura R, Sakai M, Okabe H: Transient shallow anterior chamber as initial symptom in Harada's syndrome, *Arch Ophthalmol* 99:1604-1606, 1981.
15. Kimura R, Kasai M, Shoji K et al: Swollen ciliary processes as an initial symptom in Vogt-Koyanagi-Harada syndrome, *Am J Ophthalmol* 95:402-403, 1983.
16. Okinami S, Ogino N, Matsumura M et al: Neovascularization at the angle of anterior chamber in cases of uveitis—high incidence in Vogt-Koyanagi-Harada disease, *Nippon Ganka Gakkai Zasshi* 86:2186-2189, 1982.
17. Forster DJ, Rao NA, Hill RA et al: Incidence and management of glaucoma in Vogt-Koyanagi-Harada syndrome, *Ophthalmology* 100:613-618, 1993.
18. Tabbara KF: Scleromalacia associated with Vogt-Koyanagi-Harada syndrome, Am J Ophthalmol 105:694-695, 1988.
19. Ober RR, Smith RE, Ryan SJ: Subretinal neovascularization in the Vogt-Koyanagi-Harada syndrome, *Int Ophthalmol* 6:225-234, 1983.
20. Moorthy RS, Chong LP, Smith RE et al: Subretinal neovascular membranes in Vogt-Koyanagi-Harada syndrome, *Am J Ophthalmol* 116:164-170, 1993.
21. Rubsamen PE, Gass DM: Vogt-Koyanagi-Harada Syndrome: clinical course, therapy, and long-term visual outcome, *Arch Ophthalmol* 109:682-687, 1991.
22. Kayazawa F, Takahashi H: Acute posterior multifocal placoid pigment epitheliopathy and Harada's disease, *Ann Ophthalmol* 15:58-62, 1983.
23. Rao NA, Marak GE: Sympathetic ophthalmia simulating Vogt-Koyanagi-Harada's disease: a clinico-pathologic study of four cases, *Jpn J Ophthalmol* 27:506-511, 1983.
24. Manger CC III, Ober RR: Retinal arteriovenous anastomoses in the Vogt-Koyanagi-Harada syndrome, *Am J Ophthalmol* 89:186-191, 1980.
25. Nagaya T: Use of the electro-oculogram for diagnosing and following the development of Harada's disease, *Am J Ophthalmol* 74:99-109, 1972.
26. Okubo K, Kurimoto S, Okubo K et al: Surface markers of peripheral blood lymphocytes in Vogt-Koyanagi-Harada disease, *J Clin Lab Immunol* 17:49-52, 1985.
27. Liu T, Sun SM: Peripheral lymphocyte subsets in patients with Vogt-Koyanagi-Harada syndrome (VKH), *Chung Hua Yen Ko Tsa Chih* 29:138-140, 1993.
28. Ohno S: Immunological aspects of Behçet's and Vogt-Koyanagi-Harada's diseases, *Trans Ophthalmol Soc UK* 101:335-341, 1981.
29. Hooks JJ, Moutsopoulos HM, Geis SA et al: Immune interferon in the circulation of patients with autoimmune disease, *N Engl J Med* 301:5-8, 1979.
30. Okubo K, Kurimoto S, Okubo K et al: Surface markers studies of cerebrospinal fluid lymphocytes in Vogt-Koyanagi-Harada disease, *Nippon Ganka Gakkai Zasshi* 89:726-732, 1985.
31. Momoeda S: Lymphocyte transformation test in Vogt-Koyanagi-Harada syndrome, *Acta Soc Ophthalmol Jpn* 80:491-495, 1976.
32. Yuasa T, Murai Y, Hohki T et al: Lymphocyte transformation test and migration inhibition test of macrophages in Vogt-Koyanagi-Harada's syndrome, *Acta Soc Ophthalmol Jpn* 77:1652-1657, 1973.
33. Maezawa N, Yano A, Taniguchi M et al: The role of cytotoxic T lymphocytes in the pathogenesis of Vogt-Koyanagi-Harada disease, *Ophthalmologica* 185:179-186, 1982.
34. Maezawa N, Yano A: Requirement of la-positive nylon wool adherent cells for the activation of cytotoxic T lymphocytes specific for melanocyte-associated antigens in patients with Vogt-Koyanagi-Harada's disease, *Jpn J Ophthalmol* (in press).
35. Nussenblatt RB, Gery I, Ballintine EJ et al: Cellular immune responsiveness of uveitis patients to retinal S-antigen, *Am J Ophthalmol* 89:173-179, 1980.
36. Chan CC, Palestine AG, Nussenblatt RB et al: Anti-retinal auto-antibodies in Vogt-Koyanagi-Harada syndrome, Behçet's disease, and sympathetic ophthalmia, *Ophthalmology* 92:1025-1028, 1985.
37. Ashkenazi I, Gutman I, Melamed S et al: Vogt-Koyanagi-Harada syndrome in two siblings, *Metab Pediatr Syst Ophthalmol* 14:64-67, 1991.
38. Itho S, Kurimoto S, Kouno T: Vogt-Koyanagi-Harada disease in monozygotic twins, *Int Ophthalmol* 16:49-54, 1992.
39. Kunikane H: Analysis of HLA-DQWa antigen ethnic polymorphism among a Japanese and Caucasian population and an association with Harada's disease, *Hokkaido Igaku Zasshi* 61:672-681, 1986.
40. Zhao M, Youqin J, Abrahams IW: Association of HLA antigens with Vogt-Koyanagi-Harada syndrome in a Han Chinese population, *Arch Ophthalmol* 109:368-370, 1991.
41. Zhang XY, Wang XM, Hu TS: Profiling human leukocyte antigens in Vogt-Koyanagi-Harada syndrome, *Am J Ophthalmol* 113:567-572, 1992.
42. Numaga J, Matsuki K, Tokunaga K et al: Analysis of human leukocyte antigen HLA-DR beta amino acid sequence in Vogt-Koyanagi-Harada syndrome, *Invest Ophthalmol Vis Sci* 32:1958-1961, 1991.
43. Yu Q, Mao W, Xie C et al: HLA antigens and Vogt-Koyanagi-Harada's disease, *Yen Ko Hsueh Pao* 7:3-5, 1991.
44. Davis JL, Mittal KK, Freidlin V et al: HLA associations and ancestry in Vogt-Koyanagi-Harada disease and sympathetic ophthalmia, *Ophthalmology* 97:1137-1142, 1990.

45. Rutzen AR, Larrocea-Ortega G, Schwab IR et al: Simultaneous onset of Vogt-Koyanagi-Harada syndrome in monozygotic twins, *Am J Ophthalmol* 119: 239-240, 1995.
46. Martinez JA, Lopez PF, Sternberg P Jr et al: Vogt-Koyanagi-Harada syndrome in patients with Cherokee Indian Ancestry, *Am J Ophthalmol* 114:615-620, 1992.
47. Morris WR, Schlaegel TF Jr: Viruslike inclusion bodies in subretinal fluid in uveo-encephalitis, *Am J Ophthalmol* 58:940-945, 1964.
48. Moreira MB, Moreira CA: Virus search in cerebrospinal fluid in Vogt-Koyanagi syndrome: report of a case, *Arq Neuropsiquiatr* 42:408-410, 1984.
49. Sunakawa M, Okinami S: Epstein-Barr virus–related antibody pattern in uveitis, *Jpn J Ophthalmol* 29:423-428, 1985.
50. Kahn M, Pepose JS, Green WR: Immunocytologic findings in a case of Vogt-Koyanagi-Harada syndrome, *Ophthalmology* 100:1191-1198, 1993.
51. Sakamoto T, Murata T, Inomata H: Class II major histocompatibility complex on melanocytes of Vogt-Koyanagi-Harada disease, *Arch Ophthalmol* 109:1270-1274, 1991.
52. Fujino Y, Li Q, Chung H et al: Immunopathology of experimental autoimmune uveoretinitis in primates, *Autoimmunity* 13:303-309, 1992.
53. Broekhuyse RM, Kuhlman ED, Winkens HJ et al: Experimental autoimmune anterior uveitis (EAAU), a new form of experimental uveitis. I. Induction by a detergent-insoluble, intrinsic protein fraction of the retina pigment epithelium, *Exp Eye Res* 52:465-474, 1991.
54. Chan CC, Hikita N, Dastgheib K et al: Experimental melanin-protein induced uveitis in the Lewis rat: immunopathological processes, *Ophthalmology* (in press).
55. Cheung MK, Walton RC, Chan CC et al: Subretinal fibrosis in Vogt-Koyanagi-Harada syndrome, Invest Ophthalmol Vis Sci 36:5782, 1995.
56. Hayasaka S, Okabe H, Takahashi J: Systemic corticosteroid treatment in Vogt-Koyanagi-Harada disease, *Graefes Arch Clin Exp Ophthalmol* 218:9-13, 1982.
57. Limon S, Girard P, Bloch-Michel E et al: Les aspects actuels du syndrome du Vogt Koyanagi Harada: apropos de 9 cas, *J Fr Ophtalmol* 8:29-35, 1985.
58. Nussenblatt RB, Palestine AG, Chan CC: Cyclosporin A therapy in the treatment of intraocular inflammatory disease resistant to systemic corticosteroids and cytotoxic agents, *Am J Ophthalmol* 96:275-282, 1983.
59. Wakatsuki Y, Kogure M, Takahashi Y et al: The combination therapy of cyclosporin A and steroid in the severe case of Vogt-Koyanagi-Harada's disease, *Jpn J Ophthalmol* (in press).
60. Wakefield D, McCluskey P: Cyclosporine: a therapy in inflammatory eye disease, *J Ocular Pharmacol* 7:221-226, 1991.
61. Mochizuki M, Masuda K, Sakane T et al: A clinical trial of FK506 in refractory uveitis, *Am J Ophthalmol* 115:763-769, 1993.
62. Nozik R: Personal communication.
63. Moorthy RS, Rajeev B, Smith RE et al: Incidence and management of cataracts in Vogt-Koyanagi-Harada syndrome, *Am J Ophthalmol* 118:197-204, 1994.
64. Chung YM, Yeh TS: Intracular lens implantation following extracapsular cataract extraction in uveitis, *Ophthalmic Surg* 21:272-276, 1990.

# CHAPTER 24

# Birdshot Retinochoroidopathy

The spectrum of posterior uveitic entities is quite broad, with similar or identical entities known by various names in the literature. Attempts at better defining these entities is obviously a constant goal. Birdshot retinochoroidopathy fits the aforementioned spectrum. Laboratory tests, although not definitive, appear to help the clinician in making this diagnosis. This entity appears to have distinct characteristics; it occurs more frequently in whites of northern European extraction and has a strong genetic association.

## CLINICAL MANIFESTATIONS

Birdshot retinochoroidopathy was first described by Ryan and Maumenee[1] in 1980 and soon after by Gass in 1981,[2] who called it *vitiliginous chorioretinitis.* According to Gass—and this has been our experience as well—the onset is in healthy persons, more commonly women, with an onset somewhat later than other uveitic entities, from the third to the sixth decades. One recent report has described a patient with birdshot retinochoroidopathy as having psoriasis[3] and another with an autoimmune sensorineural hearing loss,[4] but these may be chance occurrences. This disorder affects about 5% of the patients with uveitis whom we see at the National Eye Institute. In our experience 62% of these patients are women, whose average age is 51 years. Patients report an increased number of floaters and often have difficulty with night vision or color distinctions. In the original description by Ryan and Maumenee, the key elements of the clinical presentation (see Box 24-1) are as follows:

- A nonpainful eye
- An anterior segment that is usually clear or with minimal inflammatory disease

**Box 24-1**
**Findings supporting diagnosis of birdshot retinochoroidopathy**

**PATIENT**

1. White
2. Female
3. Late 40s to 50s

**OCULAR EXAMINATION FINDINGS**

1. Quiet anterior chamber
2. Vitreal inflammation but no snowbanking
3. Retinal vascular leakage and cystoid macular edema
4. Deep circular cream-colored lesions, mostly in the posterior pole and surrounds
5. Bilateral
6. Low to moderate risk of subretinal neovascularization

**ADDITIONAL TESTS**

1. Abnormal electroretinogram (ERG) and electrooculogram (EOG) findings
2. Evidence of retinal autoimmunity
3. HLA-A29$^{+}$

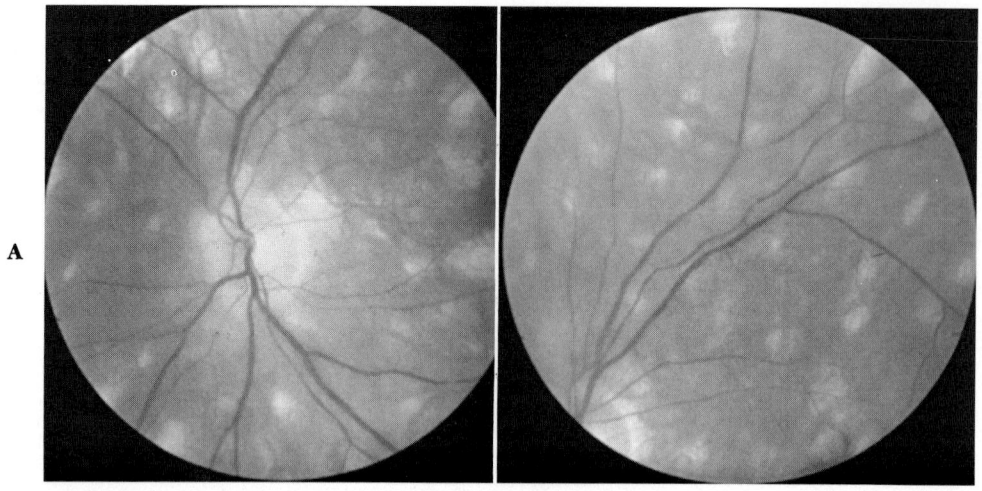


**Fig. 24-1.** Multiple cream-colored lesions, circular or oval, deep to retina, are seen in birdshot retinopathy. They tend to be clustered in posterior pole **(A)** out to midperiphery **(B).** (See Color Plate 38.)

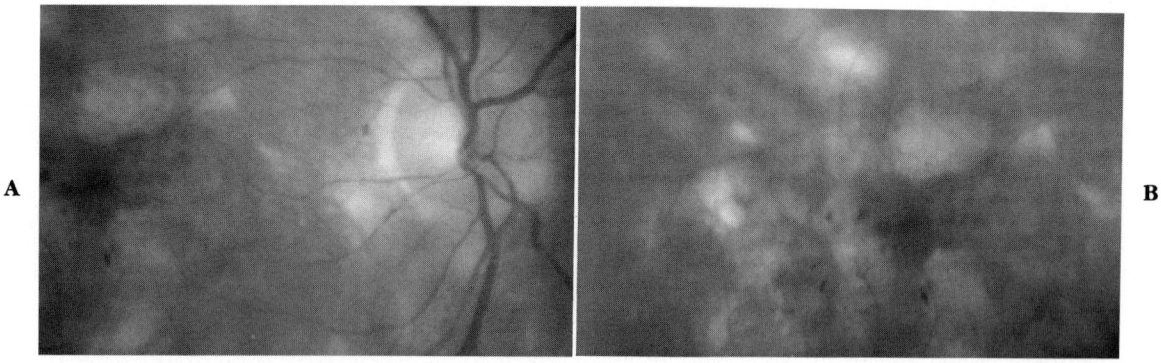


**Fig. 24-2. A** and **B,** High-magnification fundus photographs of lesions in long-standing disease. There is loss of retinal pigment epithelium in some areas, and choroidal vessels are apparent. (See Color Plate 39.)

- A significant vitritis, diffuse in nature, but with no snowbanking, distinguishing this entity from that of pars planitis
- Significant retinal vascular leakage, particularly in the posterior segment, leading in many cases to cystoid macula edema and, at times, to disc edema
- Distinctive, discrete, cream-colored or depigmented spots strewn throughout the fundus (Fig. 24-1)

Fuerst and colleagues[5] believed they could distinguish several patterns of birdshot-spot distribution in the nine patients they evaluated: those with macular sparing or macular predominance, those that were asymmetric with a concentration of spots particularly inferiorly, and those that were diffuse. In our experience the lesions tend to be present in the posterior pole and extend to the equator, but not in large part beyond that. The lesions themselves appear deep in the fundus, are circular or oval, and fairly large (at times 3/4 disc diameter in area). The lesions' edges are usually not sharply defined, and they frequently do not stand out as sharply demarcated lesions, particularly in a "blond" fundus. Often they are best observed with use of the indirect ophthalmoscope. The lesions themselves may have "substance" to them, which we have interpreted as being evidence of an active lesion, whereas with time they may flatten out, giving a more atrophic appearance (Fig. 24-2). The lesions can disappear. Usually the lesions in the posterior pole do not have a significant amount of pigment surrounding them and perhaps even less so in the periphery. The overlying retina may be quite normal, although in more advanced disease, an edematous or thinned retina can be

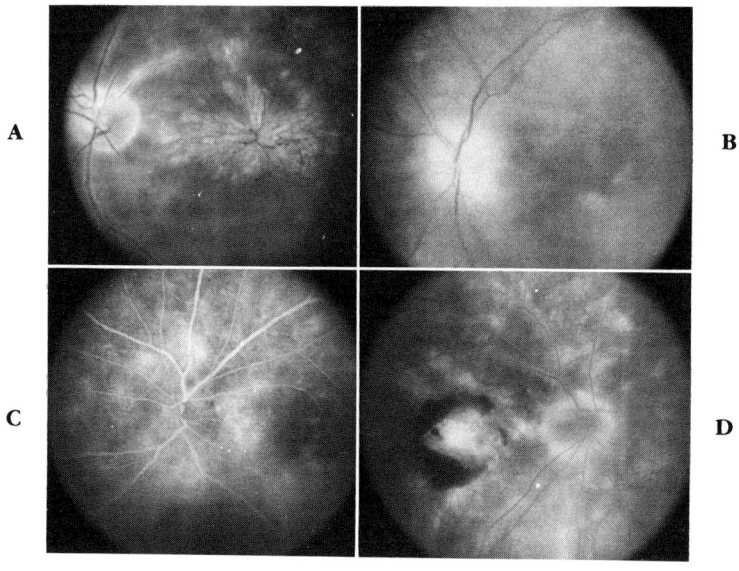


**Fig. 24-3.** Fluorescein angiogram changes in birdshot retinochoroidopathy. **A,** Macular edema and staining of retinal vessels. **B,** Late staining of disc. **C,** Areas of hyperfluorescence corresponding to birdshot lesions can sometimes be seen, but usually not. **D,** Subretinal neovascular net in macula of patient with birdshot retinochoroidopathy.

perceived. In the late stage of the disease, examination of the posterior segment reveals a strikingly blond fundus, suggestive in our minds of the involvement of the outer retina and the retinal pigment epithelium (RPE).

### Examination of macula

Examination of the macula is imperative inasmuch as cystoid edema is a significant sequela to this disease. Its presence is important in establishing the diagnosis and in deciding on a correct therapeutic approach. Patients with birdshot retinochoroidopathy have significant vitreal reaction, although visual acuity will often be quite good in spite of the opacities if cystoid edema is not present.

The use of fluorescein angiography is helpful in delineating the degree of retinal vascular leakage and the severity of the macular edema. This technique very dramatically underscores the rather marked retinal vascular component of this disease, as well as inflammatory disease affecting the optic nerve head. However, as Gass first noted—as have all the investigators reporting their findings concerning this disease—the cream-colored lesions are far more prominent ophthalmoscopically than with fluorescein angiography. Although mild hyperfluorescence may be noted in the later stage of the angiogram, early photographs in the angiogram may not demonstrate either hypofluorescence or hyperfluorescence (Fig. 24-3). Indocyanine green (ICG) is just beginning to be applied to study this disorder (Fig. 24-4). Lommatzsch and coworkers[6] studied choroidal blood flow using perfusion-pressure videoangiography in a patient with birdshot retinochoroidopathy. They found that in this patient fluorescein dye penetrated through the vessel walls of the large choroidal arterioles close to the short posterior ciliary arteries. These investigators thought that this leakage was the cause of the typical birdshot pattern seen in this disorder. It does not explain, however, why most patients initially may not have dramatic angiographic evidence of disease.

Problems with night vision and color discrimination are not uncommon complaints of these patients, sometimes despite excellent central visual acuity. These problems should not be taken lightly because alterations in retinal functions other than visual acuity can be demonstrated. In those reports investigating psychophysical and electrophysiologic testing of patients with this entity, all have noted disturbances in both the electroretinogram and the electrooculogram results. Fuerst and colleagues[5] reported that b-wave amplitudes were reduced with a disproportionate implicit-time

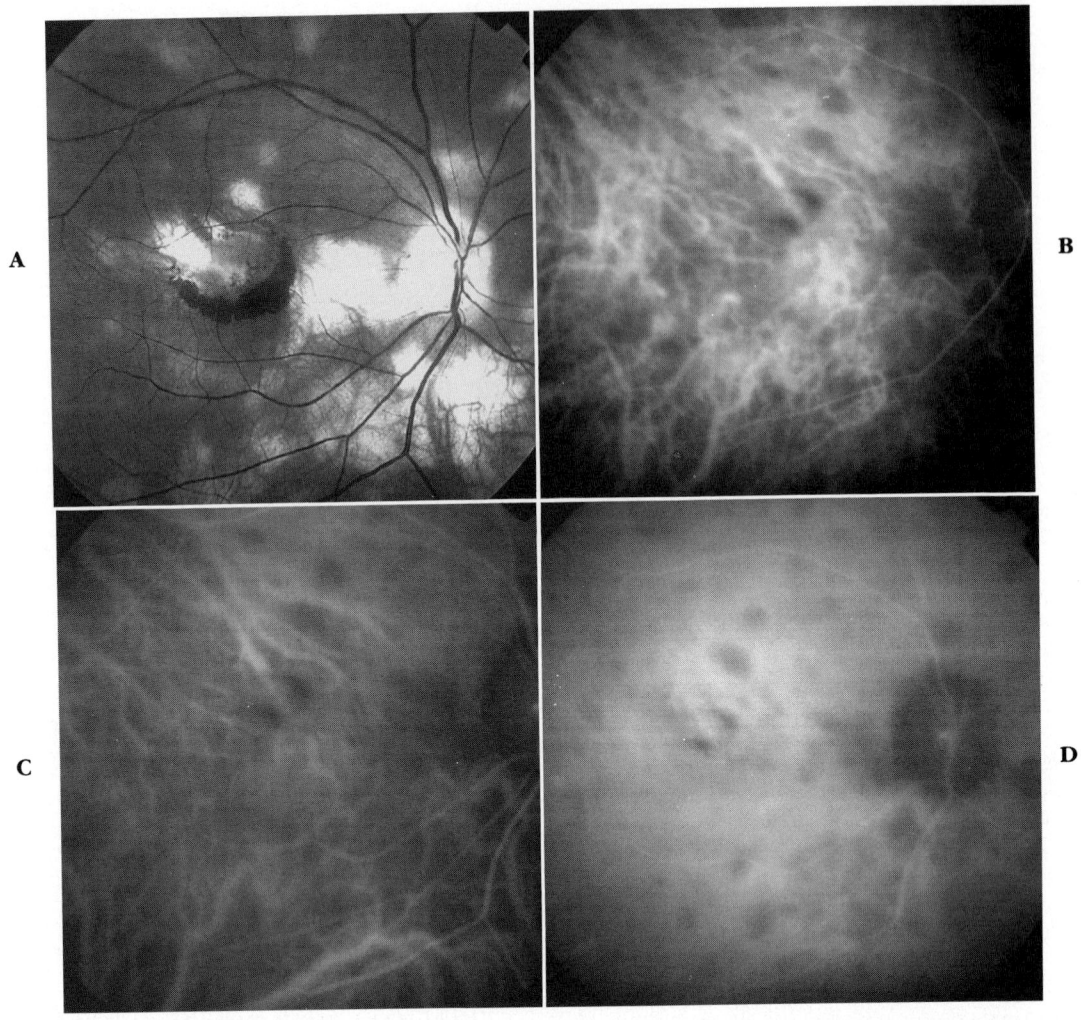


**Fig. 24-4.** Indocyanine green study of patient with birdshot retinochoroidopathy. **A,** Red-free photograph shows blood in macula. **B** to **D,** Areas of hypofluorescence in choroid remain late into study, whereas ICG also demonstrates macular area that suggests subfoveal net.

prolongation. Color-vision alterations can be found, and some patients complain of colors being "washed out" or faded. Others may note a difference in color discrimination between their two eyes.

Because the retinal lesions can be very striking, the diagnosis would appear to be a relatively easy one to make. However, as with all diseases, some cases fall within that "gray" zone. One should consider other diagnoses, such as multifocal choroiditis and panuveitis, described by Nozik and Dorsch[7] and also discussed by Dreyer and Gass.[8] The patients with the condition described by Nozik and Dorsch tend to be younger, more often have unilateral disease, have a greater degree of vitreous inflammation, and are less likely to have night blindness or abnormal electroretinogram (ERG) findings.[8] Further, the lesions in this entity tend to become pigmented, smaller, and better defined than those seen in birdshot retinochoroidopathy. Sarcoidosis has been often considered as an alternative diagnosis in the patients we have seen and evaluated.[9] Brinkman and Rothova[10] reported on six patients with neurosarcoidosis who demonstrated multifocal chorioretinal lesions, as well as optic nerve disease and a periphlebitis. In addition, the multiple evanescent white-dot syndrome, described by Jampol and colleagues,[11] as well as reticulum cell sarcoma, needs to be considered (see Chapter 29). In a report of 11 patients with birdshot retinochoroidopathy, 3 had antibodies against *Borrelia burgdorferi.*[12] It is not known whether these were examples of false-positive reactions or whether in some patients the organism of Lyme disease may play a causative role.

The physician should particularly consider an alternative diagnosis to birdshot retinochoroidopathy in the nonwhite patient, because these cases appear to be rare, if they occur at all. Recently we saw an African-American patient who had been diagnosed with birdshot chorioretinopathy, who, after an extensive evaluation, was found to have intraocular pseudotumor (see Chapter 29).

## TESTS, HISTOLOGY, AND ETIOLOGY

The exact cause of birdshot retinochoroidopathy is unknown. However, recent observations have made for provocative hypotheses. We have found a strong correlation between birdshot retinochoroidopathy and HLA-A29 in white patients.[13] Of the patients tested 80% showed HLA-A29 within their genetic makeup whereas only 7% of control subjects bore this antigen. This unusually high correlation yielded a relative risk of almost 50 (see HLA discussion). This finding suggests a strong genetic predisposition for this disease. Several studies have demonstrated the same strong association with HLA-A29[14-16] (Table 24-1). Le Hoang and coworkers[17] reported that 54 of 58 French patients with birdshot retinochoroidopathy showed HLA-A29 positivity (93.1%, relative risk 157.3), and that subtyping results of 33 of these patients showed the HLA-A29.2 subtype in all. This absence of the HLA-A29.1 subtype raised questions about a possible "resistance motif" in the HLA-A29.1 molecule. Work by Tabary and coworkers[18] showed that the sequence of HLA-A29.2 was identical in both patients and healthy control subjects. A single difference was found in the extracellular domain between the two HLA-A29 subtypes (i.e., A29.1 vs. A29.2). Because the HLA-A29.1 subtype contains a unique mutation, it was conjectured by these authors that the ancestral type was HLA-A29.2 and that the HLA-A29.1 mutation came later and conferred resistance to birdshot retinochoroidopathy. The position of the HLA-A29.1 mutation would not permit it to interact with the T-cell receptor but rather with an accessory molecule, such as CD8.

De Waal and colleagues[19] examined the question of HLA-A29 subtypes and found that in a white population from The Netherlands and Belgium, the HLA-A29.2 was the more common subtype, found in 90% of control subjects. They found that the distribution of HLA-A29.2 versus HLA-A29.1 did not differ among the patients with birdshot retinochoroidopathy whom they examined. Both subtypes were found, but HLA-A29.2 predominated because it is almost 10 times more commonly seen, at least in this population. In contradistinction to the northern European and American experience, some Japanese and Brazilian observers are not sure that they have seen a classic case.[20]

**Table 24-1.** Immunologic parameters in patients with birdshot retinochoroidopathy

| | Nussenblatt et al.[13] | Le Hoang et al.[17] |
|---|---|---|
| Number of cases | 20 | 21 |
| HLA-A29 | | |
| Patients (%) | 80 | 90.5 |
| Control subjects (%) | 7.4 | 7.9 |
| In vitro cellular responses to S-antigen | | |
| Number tested | 13 | 18 |
| Patients positive | 12 (92.3%) | 11 (61%) |
| Basophil degranulation to the S-antigen | | |
| Number tested | – | 18 |
| Patients positive | – | 8 (44%) |

Additional information to support the notion that endogenous immune mechanisms play a role is the finding that patients' lymphocytes demonstrate an in vitro, cell-mediated response to retinal antigens, most notably the retinal S-antigen[13] (Fig. 24-5 and Table 24-1). Jobin and coworkers,[21] using either a lymphocyte proliferation assay or basophil degranulation, found that in vitro positivity to S-antigen appeared more frequently in the period preceding a relapse of ocular inflammation. Further, we have reported that the inflammatory response seen in one eye with birdshot retinochoroidopathy seemed directed to the photoreceptor region, the area from which the retinal S-antigen is isolated.[13] The striking number of patients with birdshot retinochoroidopathy who demonstrate evidence of retinal autoimmunity suggests that this mechanism is an important one in this disease. Further, the disease elicited in monkeys immunized with the retinal S-antigen can take on certain characteristics not dissimilar to that seen in the human condition. The strong HLA association would further add support to the notion of an inbred error of immune regulation. In this disease, HLA-A29 positivity can be used as strong corroborative evidence to support the clinical diagnosis.

Long-term studies of patients with retinal vasculitis have yielded interesting observations. In two patients with retinal vasculitis, Soubrane and colleagues[22] reported the appearance of typical lesions of birdshot retinochoroidopathy 7 and 8 years after the first symptoms. They suggest evaluating patients for the presence of HLA-A29 even late in the course of a retinal vasculitis. A similar evolution of clinical findings was reported by Godel and coworkers.[23] An additional provocative observation was that of Bloch-Michel and Frau[24] who reviewed the records of 20 patients with birdshot retinochoroidopathy and 36 patients with idiopathic retinal vasculitis. Those with the HLA-A29 phenotype were 95% in the birdshot group as opposed to 61% in the other. Long-term follow-up of vasculitis showed only one patient who developed lesions compatible with birdshot. However, the HLA-A29 phenotype in the idiopathic vasculitis group was associated with more posterior pole involvement, a more severe course, and a poorer visual prognosis than in those without this phenotype. The authors suggest that the presence of this gene portends ill for its bearer, with or without lesions typical of birdshot.

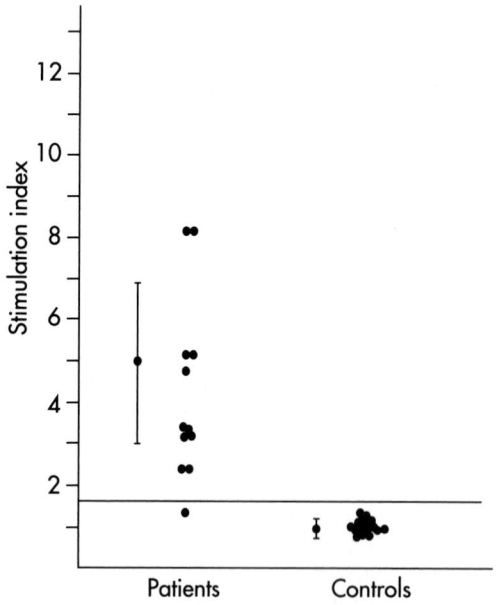


**Fig. 24-5.** Lymphocytes of patient with birdshot retinochoroidopathy demonstrate in vitro proliferative response to retinal S-antigen whereas those of control subjects do not. This in vitro anamnestic response is thought to parallel what occurs in vitro when T cells (and other immune cells) become activated. (From *Am J Ophthalmol* 94:147-158, 1982. Copyright by The Ophthalmic Publishing Company.)

Humoral studies have not been particularly useful in defining further any underlying immunologic abnormality. This includes the absence of circulating anticardiolipin antibodies associated with thromboses and diseases with a significant vascular component.[25] Kuhne and coworkers[26] reported two cases of retinal vasculitis associated with Q fever, induced by *Coxiella burnetii.* One patient showed HLA-A29 positivity; although the authors speculate on the role of this agent in birdshot retinochoroidopathy, they are unable to definitively show a determinate role for this organism.

It is worth noting that we have had at least two cases of an HLA laboratory reporting the HLA typing falsely negative for HLA-A29. One should consider repeating the HLA typing if the clinical picture strongly suggests a diagnosis of birdshot retinochoroidopathy and the HLA report does not show the presence of HLA-A29.

## THERAPY

A well-planned therapeutic plan for the treatment of patients with birdshot retinochoroidopathy still needs to be devised. Three quarters of those we have seen received either periocular or systemic steroids as part of their therapeutic regimen, and this still is the mainstay of therapy. Some patients' visual acuities will linger around the 20/30 to 20/40 range, and we elect not to treat these persons. We will not institute systemic therapy unless there is a significant drop in visual acuity (below 20/40) in both eyes, with the most common reason for decreased visual acuity being cystoid macular edema (Fig. 24-6); rarely one will see subretinal neovascular nets that need prompt attention, with consideration of laser photocoagulation (Fig. 24-7). If steroid therapy is initiated, a slow taper of systemic steroids should be considered followed by low-dose maintenance steroids. Others[27] have suggested using nonsteroidal antiinflammatory agents, but we have not found them helpful and they are not usually within our armamentarium for the treatment of this entity. Periocular steroid is used for the cases in which disease severity is asymmetric or for treatment of exacerbations occuring while patients receive systemic therapy. In the patients with relatively good visual acuities but who need occasional therapy, we really do not know whether these therapeutic approaches have a significant effect on the final visual outcome. It has been the belief of some that these patients' visual prognosis over the long term is guarded, yet others have thought that the disease has a tendency to stabilize. We have seen both extremes occur and are unable to distinguish who will go on to develop severe visual problems.

As with many uveitic entities, we do not know the natural history of this entity. A disconcerting, continued decrease in retinal function and opthalmoscopically evident alterations, such as retinal thinning and attenuation of the retinal vasculature, may be seen even if the ocular inflammatory activity stabilizes. This may be due to the triggering of apoptosis, programmed cell death, of the cells that constitute the retina. Because of these observations, the notion that cytotoxic agents should be given early in the disease has been entertained. We have seen patients who have undergone such therapy, and there does not seem to be a difference in their clinical course. Further, these patients often require long-term immunosuppressive therapy, which is usually difficult to attain with cytotoxic agents. Hesse and colleagues[3] described a patient with birdshot retinochoroidopathy suffering from psoriasis in whom treatment with aromatic retinoids led to resolution of both the ocular and dermatologic problems.

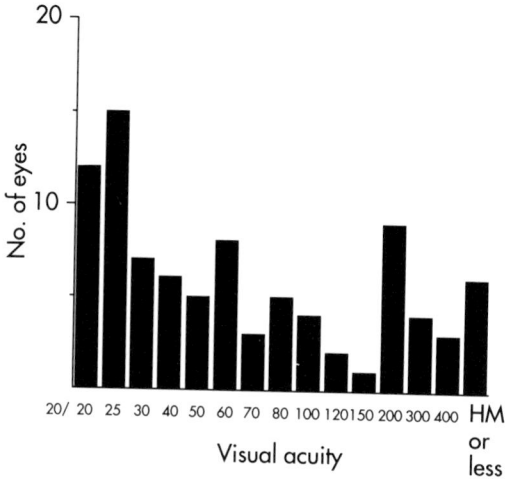


**Fig. 24-6.** Distribution of visual acuities of eyes with birdshot retinochoroidopathy when first seen at our clinic. (Average visual acuity [VA], 20/100-20/125; median VA, 20/50.)

Cyclosporine has been used in some patients, and we have seen good responses.[28] This has been corroborated by Le Hoang and associates.[29] A recent report by Vitale and colleagues[30] corroborates these earlier observations; however, they administered lower doses of the drug (2.5-5 mg/kg/day) because of the concern of renal toxicity. Some patients needed an addition of azathioprine (1.5-2 mg/kg/day). The investigators found that vitreous inflammation was controlled in 23 (88.5%) eyes treated, and a stabilization or improve-

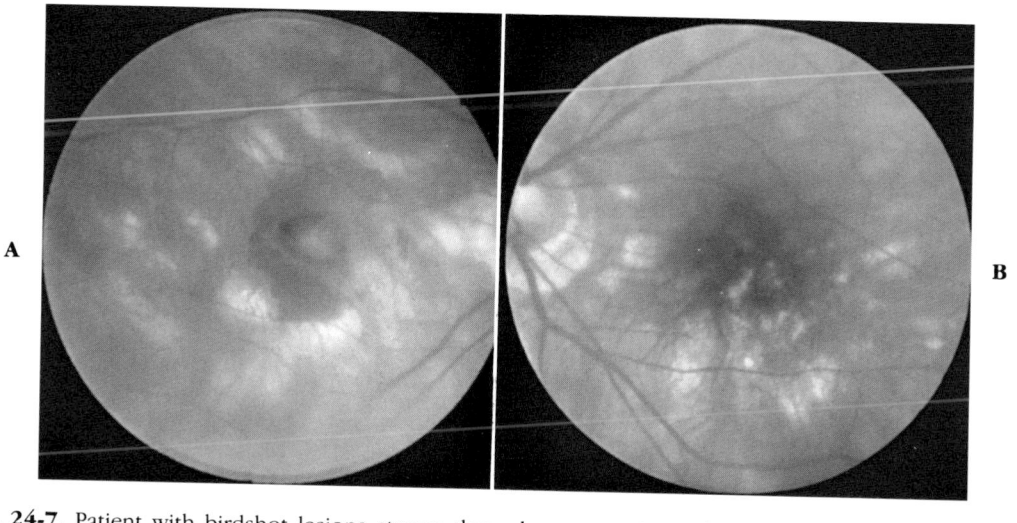


**Fig. 24-7.** Patient with birdshot lesions strewn throughout posterior pole of both eyes. **A,** Right eye has subfoveal net that has bled and raised macula. **B,** Left eye has lesion in macula. (See Color Plate 40.)

ment in visual acuity occurred in 20 (83.3%) eyes. These results are to be expected because this disorder appears mediated by T cells, and therefore an anti–T-cell agent should have a significant effect on the disease course. If need be, cataract surgery can be performed on these patients, with adequate perioperative antiinflammatory therapy, which should result in an abatement of ocular inflammatory activity for at least 3 months.

### Case 24-1

A 54-year-old white man was referred to the National Eye Institute with a complaint of increased floaters and shimmering. He was in good general health. His visual acuity was 20/32 OD, 20/32-1 OS. The anterior chambers both had an occasional cell, and the tensions were normal. The media had 1+ cells and 1+ haze OU. Scattered yellow-white lesions were strewn throughout the fundus, more concentrated in the posterior pole. They appeared deep, probably at the level of the retinal pigment epithelium or photoreceptor region. There were occasional superficial retinal hemorrhages and possibly cystoid edema in the left eye. There was no snowbanking.

A fluorescein angiogram demonstrated rather diffuse retinal vascular leakage, with staining of the disc in both eyes as well, with evidence of mild cystoid edema in the left eye. Goldmann fields were full, but there were patches of nonabsolute scotomas. HLA typing demonstrated the presence of HLA-A29. In vitro cell culturing showed an anamestic response to the retinal S-antigen.

Our diagnosis was that of birdshot retinochoroidopathy. We elected not to treat the patient. After a follow-up period of more than 5 years the patient continues to have good central vision. He complains of an occasional increase in floaters, that his vision varies from day to day, and that his night vision is not as good as it used to be. We believed that prolonged therapy would carry more risk than no therapy.

### Case 24-2

A 47-year-old white man had symptoms for 2 years before coming to the National Eye Institute. Although he had no anterior segment inflammatory disease, vitritis without snowbanking was noted. He had cream-colored lesions typical of birdshot retinochoroidopathy throughout the fundus, as well as a subretinal neovascular net in the right eye. His vision was 20/400 OD, 20/70 OS. The left eye had evidence of cystoid macular edema, and testing revealed HLA-A29 positivity. The subretinal net had formed in spite of a trial of oral steroids. It was our belief that the duration of steroid use was not sufficiently long, and the patient was placed on a regimen of prednisone, 80 mg/day, with a slow taper that brought him to a maintenance dose of 20 mg/day by 3 months. The patient had a slow improvement of vision to 20/32 OS and continued to receive 20 mg/day of prednisone for 6 months, which was tapered to 15 mg/day. This regimen maintains his vision, with minimal systemic secondary effects.

## REFERENCES


1. Ryan SJ, Maumenee AE: Birdshot retinochoroidopathy, *Am J Ophthalmol* 89:31-45, 1980.
2. Gass JDM: Vitiliginous chorioretinitis, *Arch Ophthalmol* 99:1778-1787, 1981.
3. Hesse S, Berbis P, Chemila JF et al: Psoriasis and birdshot chorioretinopathy: response to aromatic retinoids, *Dermatology* 187:137-139, 1993.
4. Heaton JM, Mills RP: Sensorineural hearing loss associated with birdshot retinochoroidopathy, *Arch Otolaryngol Head Neck Surg* 119:680-681, 1993.
5. Fuerst DJ, Tessler HH, Fishman GA et al: Birdshot retinochoroidopathy, *Arch Ophthalmol* 102:214-219, 1984.
6. Lommatzsch PK, Ulrich WD, Ulrich C et al: Birdshot retinochoroidopathy: case report, *Fortschr Ophthalmol* 87:562-566, 1990.
7. Nozik RA, Dorsch W: A new chorioretinopathy associated with anterior uveitis, *Am J Ophthalmol* 76:758-762, 1973.
8. Dreyer RF, Gass JDM: Multifocal choroiditis and panuveitis, *Arch Ophthalmol* 102:1776-1784, 1984.
9. Brod RD: Presumed sarcoid choroidopathy mimicking birdshot retinochoroidopathy, *Am J Ophthalmol*109: 357-358, 1990.
10. Brinkman CJ, Rothova A: Fundus pathology in neurosarcoidosis, *Int Ophthalmol* 17:23-26, 1993.
11. Jampol LE, Sieving PA, Pugh D et al: Multiple evanescent white dot syndrome, *Arch Ophthalmol* 102:671-679, 1984.
12. Suttorp-Schulten MS, Luyendijk L, van Dam AP et al: Birdshot chorioretinopathy and Lyme borreliosis, *Am J Ophthalmol* 115:149-153, 1993.
13. Nussenblatt RB, Mittal KK, Ryan S et al: Birdshot retinochoroidopathy associated with HLA-A29 antigen and immune responsiveness to retinal S-antigen, *Am J Ophthalmol* 94:147-158, 1982.
14. Baarsma GS, Kijlstra A, Oosterhuis JA et al: Association of birdshot retinochoroidopathy and HLA-A29 antigen, *Doc Ophthalmol* 61:267-269, 1986.
15. Le Hoang P, Donnefort N, Foucault C et al: Association between HLA-A29 antigen and birdshot retinochoroidopathy *(Proceedings of the twenty-fifth International Congress of Ophthalmology)*, Amsterdam, 1987, Kugler & Ghedini.
16. Baarsma GS, Priem HA, Kijlstra A: Association of birdshot retinochoroidopathy and HLA-A29 antigen, *Curr Eye Res* 9(suppl):63-68, 1990.
17. LeHoang P, Ozdemir N, Benhamou A et al: HLA-A29.2 subtype associated with birdshot retinochoroidopathy, *Am J Ophthalmol* 113:33-35, 1992.

18. Tabary T, Prochnicka-Chalufour A, Cornillet P et al: HLA-A29 sub-types and "birdshot" choroidoretinopathy susceptibility: a possible "resistance motif" in the HLA-As29.1 molecule, *C R Acad Sci [III]* 313:599-605, 1991.
19. de Waal LP, Lardy NM, van der Horst AR et al: HLA-A29 subtypes and birdshot retinochoroidopathy, *Immunogenetics* 35:51-53, 1992.
20. Mochizuki M, MD, Tokyo, Japan, and Belfort R, MD, Saõ Paulo, Brazil: Personal communications, 1990.
21. Jobin D, Thillaye B, de Kozak Y et al: Severe retinochoroidopathy: variations of humoral and cellular immunity to S-antigen in a longitudinal study, *Curr Eye Res* 9(suppl):91-96, 1990.
22. Soubrane G, Bokobza R, Coscas G: Late developing lesions in birdshot retinochoroidopathy, *Am J Ophthalmol* 109:204-210, 1990.
23. Godel V, Baruch E, Lazar M: Late development of chorioretinal lesions in birdshot retinochoroidopathy, *Ann Ophthalmol* 21:49-52, 1989.
24. Bloch-Michel E, Frau E: Birdshot retinochoroidopathy and HLA-A29+ and HLA-A29− idiopathic retinal vasculitis: comparative study of 56 cases, *Can J Ophthalmol* 26:361-366, 1991.
25. Klok AM, Geertzen R, Rothova A et al: Anticardiolipin antibodies in uveitis, *Curr Eye Res* 11(suppl):209-213, 1992.
26. Kuhne F, Morlat P, Riss I et al: Is A29, B12 vasculitis caused by the Q fever agent? *Coxiella burnetii, J Fr Ophthalmol* 15:315-321, 1992.
27. Hofmann HM, Feicht B: Birdshot chorioretinopathy: systemic therapy with corticosteroids and nonsteroidal antiinflammatory drugs, *Klin Monatsbl Augenheilkd* 197:159-161, 1990.
28. Nussenblatt RB, Palestine AG, Chan CC: Cyclosporin A therapy in the treatment of intraocular inflammatory disease resistant to systemic corticosteroids and cytotoxic agents, *Am J Ophthalmol* 96:275-282, 1983.
29. Le Hoang P, Girard B, Deray G et al: Cyclosporine in the treatment of birdshot retinochoroidopathy (Second International Congress on Cyclosporine, Washington DC, Nov 1987), *Transplant Proc* 20(3 suppl 4):128-130, 1988.
30. Vitale AT, Rodriguez A, Foster CS: Low-dose cyclosporine therapy in the treatment of birdshot retinochoroidopathy, *Ophthalmology* 101:822-831, 1994.

# CHAPTER 25

# Behçet's Disease

Retinal vascular involvement is a common finding in many cases of posterior and intermediate uveitis. Behçet's disease may the best example of a disorder characterized mainly by its retinal vascular involvement, often with devastating effects on the patient's eyesight.

Behçet's disease is a multisystem disorder that is named after the Turkish dermatologist, Hulûsi Behçet (1889-1948),[1] who recognized and reported in 1937 a triad of symptoms, that of recurrent intraocular inflammatory episodes as well as oral and mucosal ulcerations. These observations were based on three patients, two of whom had ocular symptoms atypical of the disorder we recognize today. It should be noted that in the twentieth century at least two other clinicians reported cases with similar findings earlier than did Professor Behçet, Dr. Adamantiades in 1931 (publishing in the French literature)[2] and Dr. Shigeta from Japan in 1924.[3] However, their reports did not stimulate the rather universal interest that Dr. Behçet's in fact did. The disease is one that was known to the ancients, with Hippocrates probably the first to describe an association between ocular inflammation and oral and genital lesions.[4]

The disease has been noted to be especially common in the Far East and in the Mediterranean basin and very frequently noted between 30° and 45° north latitude in Asian and European populations.[5] This corresponds to the old Silk Route used for centuries by traders making the dangerous passage from the East to the West (Fig. 25-1). Japan appears to have the greatest frequency of this disorder,[6] with an overall prevalence of 7 to 8.5 cases/1,000,000 population as calculated in the late 1970s.[7] More recently, it was estimated that there was

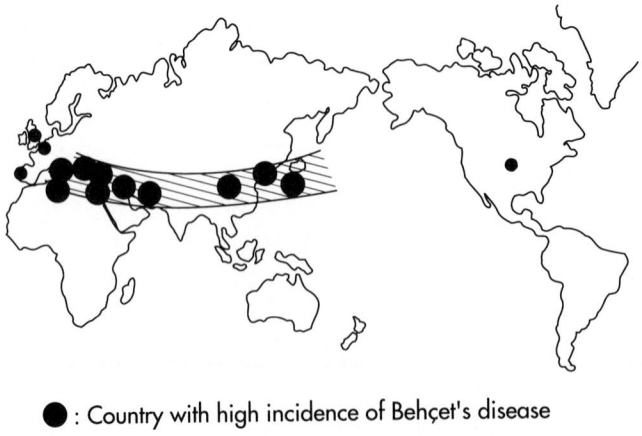


**Fig. 25-1.** Map of broad band through Asia and Europe where Behçet's disease is common. This coincides with old Silk Route. (Courtesy S. Ohno, M.D.)

a total of 16,750 patients with this disease in Japan, with a prevalence rate of 135/million population.[8] However, the northern portions of Japan have a higher incidence than do the southern areas. In 1986, the estimated 15,000 patients in Japan with Behçet's disease, 11,000 of them are under treatment.[5] This diagnosis was applied to more than 20% of the patients with uveitis seen in the uveitis clinic of the University of Tokyo's Department of Ophthalmology from 1965-1977.[7]

This disorder may have devastating consequences to the eyes, and thus it is a disease that has attracted a great deal of attention. Insight into its mechanisms has led to an improvement in our treatment of this disorder.

## CLINICAL MANIFESTATIONS

The diagnosis of Behçet's disease is firmly based on the presence of a constellation of clinical findings. Therefore clinical criteria have been established that help the clinician decide whether a patient has the disease. At least nine sets of clinical criteria have been proposed for the diagnosis of Behçet's disease.[9] For the diagnosis of the disorder on our service, we have adapted the criteria established by the Behçet's disease Research Committee of Japan (see Box 25-1). As can be seen, the criteria add an additional major finding to the original three, that of skin lesions. Further, the presence of ocular inflammatory disease is given greater weight in the diagnosis of the disease. It should also be noted that the minor criteria are not considered in this grading system. The Behçet's Disease Research Committee of Japan recognizes three special cases of Behçet's disease: intestinal Behçet's, vasculo-Behçet's, and neuro-Behçet's disease (essentially the minor criteria). It has also specifically included three laboratory tests: a pathergy test (a skin-prick test), HLA testing for HLA-B51, and a screening for nonspecific factors indicative of immune system activation, such as an elevated erythrocyte sedimentation rate (ESR), positive C-reactive protein, and an increase in peripheral blood leukocytes.

Another system that the reader should be familiar with is the one suggested by the International Study Group for Behçet's Disease,[10] which requires the presence of oral aphthous ulcers in all patients (see Box 25-2). The investigators emphasize the importance of oral aphthous ulcers as a sign of this disease on the basis of data collection from a large number of patients and control subjects, in which they found that 97% of patients with Behçet's disease had oral aphtha.[11]

Other systems have used the minor criteria by equating two of those to one major criterion. There is no question that some degree of uncertainty is built into any system, because the various criteria may manifest at different times during the clinical course. Until we have a better way to diagnose this disease, we have

**Box 25-1**
**Criteria for diagnosis of Behçet's disease**

**MAJOR CRITERIA**

**Recurrent aphthous ulcers of oral mucosa**

Skin lesions
- Erythema nodosum, acne, cutaneous hypersensitivity thrombophlebitis

Genital ulcers

Ocular inflammatory disease
- Recurrent anterior and posterior

**MINOR CRITERIA**

Arthritis

Intestinal ulcers

Epididymitis

Vascular disease
- Obliteration, occlusion, aneurysm

Neuropsychiatric symptoms

**Complete type**

Four major symptoms simultaneously or at different times

**Incomplete type**

Three major symptoms simultaneously or at different times

*or*

Typical recurrent ocular disease with one other major criterion

**Suspect type**

Two major symptoms, excluding ocular

**Possible type**

One main symptom

Modified from Behçet's Disease Research Committee: Clinical research section recommendations, *Jpn J Ophthalmol* 18:291-294, 1974.

**Box 25-2**
**Diagnostic criteria of International Study Group for Behçet's Disease**

**RECURRENT ORAL ULCERATION**

Occurrence of minor or major aphthous lesions, or herpetiform-like lesions, need to have been observed by the physician or patient at least three times within a 12-month period.

**PRESENCE OF TWO OTHER CRITERIA**

**Recurrent genital ulceration**

Observation by the physician or patient of the aphthous ulceration or scar is required.

**Eye lesions**

The ocular disease can include anterior and/or posterior uveitis, cells in the vitreous, or the presence of a retinal vasculitis.

**Skin lesions**

These changes, noted by the physician or patient, include erythema nodosum, pseudofolliculitis, and papulopustular lesions. In addition, lesions would include an acneiform nodule in postadolescent patients not receiving corticosteroid therapy.

**Positive pathergy test result**

Read by physician at 24 to 48 hours.

Modified from International Study Group for Behçet's Disease: Criteria for diagnosis of Behçet's disease, *Lancet* 335:1078-1080, 1990.

**Table 25-1.** Percentage of cases manifesting criteria of Behçet's disease*

| | Men | Women | Total |
|---|---|---|---|
| Major | | | |
| Ocular | 86.2 | 67.8 | 78.6 |
| Aphtha | 97.9 | 98.8 | 98.3 |
| Skin | 89.8 | 91.3 | 90.4 |
| Genital | 76.8 | 83.8 | 79.8 |
| Minor | | | |
| Arthritis | 56.1 | 62.6 | 58.9 |
| Intestinal | 27.7 | 25.9 | 26.9 |
| Vascular | 8.7 | 6.3 | 7.7 |
| Psychiatric | 10.3 | 6.4 | 8.6 |

Data from Mishima S, Masuda K, Izawa Y, et al: Behçet disease in Japan: ophthalmologic aspects, *Trans Am Ophthalmol Soc* 76:225-229, 1979.
*At least 1700 patients were analyzed for each criterion.

**Table 25-2.** Incidence (%) of major criteria as initial manifestation

| | Japan* | | | Israel† |
|---|---|---|---|---|
| Criteria | Men $n = 139$ | Women $n = 70$ | Total $n = 209$ | Total $n = 54$ |
| Ocular | 25.4 | 8.6 | 19.7 | 9 |
| Oral aphtha | 59.4 | 84.3 | 67.8 | 80 |
| Genital ulcers | 14.5 | 25.7 | 18.3 | 2 |
| Skin lesions | 41.7 | 34.3 | 39.2 | 2 |

*Data from Mishima S, Masuda K, Izawa Y, et al: Behçet disease in Japan: ophthalmologic aspects, *Trans Am Ophthalmol Soc* 76:225-229, 1979.
†Data from Chajek T, Fairanu M: Behçet's disease. Report of 41 cases and a review of the literature, *Medicine* 54:179-196, 1975.

favored a strict adherence to the Japanese criteria inasmuch as the patients whom we have thus diagnosed are therefore fairly homogeneous in their clinical findings.

In a 1991 survey of 3316 patients with Behçet's disease in Japan, oral aphtha was the most frequently seen major criterion, occurring in 97.7% of the cases.[12] Other commonly seen problems were skin lesions (90.4%), with genital ulcers and ocular attacks having a similar incidence (79.8% and 78.6%, respectively)[7] (Table 25-1). Oral aphthae are by far the most common presenting major criterion[7] (Table 25-2). After the oral aphthae, the order of appearance of the major criteria is skin lesions, ocular symptoms (25.4% in males), genital ulceration in males, and ocular lesions in females (8.6%). Of the minor criteria the most frequently seen in Japan was that of arthritis (see Table 25-1). The number of males to females with this disease in Japan was 1.2:1 in 1972, whereas in 1981 this had changed to 0.77:1.[5] Differences over 20 years have been noted in the various aspects of the disease and their presence in men and women (Table 25-3). In Turkey, however, the male-to-female ratio is 3.3:1.[5] More males have the complete form of the disease than do females. Although it is a disease with onset during early adulthood, childhood onset has been reported to occur in rare cases.[13,14]

We have reviewed the records of 113 patients with Behçet's disease whom we followed up and found that 64 were male. An earlier review of 49 cases also revealed a male propensity (27 men, 22 women) (Fig. 25-2). The ethnic distri-

**Table 25-3.** Epidemiologic changes in Behçet's disease in Japan from 1972-1991

| Disease type | No. male 1972 | No. female 1991 | Sex 1972 | Ratio 1991 |
|---|---|---|---|---|
| **COMPLETE TYPE** | 594/334 | 588/551 | 1.78 | 1.07 |
| **INCOMPLETE TYPE** | | | | |
| With ocular disease | 403/230 | 750/402 | 1.75 | 1.87 |
| Without ocular disease | 172/298 | 300/725 | 0.58 | 0.41 |
| **INCOMPLETE TYPE** | | | | |
| With genital ulcers | 260/352 | 338/806 | 0.74 | 0.42 |
| Without genital ulcers | 315/176 | 712/321 | 1.79 | 2.22 |
| **INCOMPLETE TYPE** | | | | |
| With both ocular and genital | 88/54 | 73/104 | 1.63 | 0.7 |
| Ocular without genital | 315/176 | 674/298 | 1.79 | 2.26 |
| Genital without ocular | 172/298 | 300/725 | 0.58 | 0.41 |

From Nakae K, Masaki F, Hashimoto T et al: Recent epidemiological features of Behçet's disease in Japan. In Godeau P, Wechsler B, editors: *Behçet's disease,* Amsterdam, 1993, Elsevier.

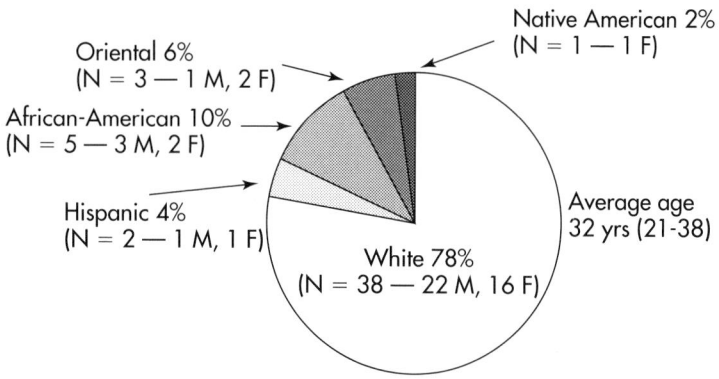


**Fig. 25-2.** Ethnic ratios of patients with Behçet's disease seen at National Eye Institute ($n$ = 49).

bution can be seen as well; 12 of the patients were either of Middle Eastern, Native American, Mediteranean, or Oriental heritage. All the patients had recurrent ocular inflammatory disease. The average visual acuity was between 20/40 to 50 for both males and females. A large number of the eyes (28/98) had vision of 20/400 or worse (Fig. 25-3). Eight of the patients had the complete form of the disease, whereas all the others had three of the major criteria at some point in their clinical course. Three patients had evidence of neuro-Behçet, and all had uveitis. The therapeutic modalities administered to these patients are noted in Fig. 25-4. Barra and colleagues[15] from Brazil reviewed 49 Behçet cases, representing 2% of the total number of uveitis cases they saw over a 16-year period. Of their patients 71% were male with more than three quarters of all the patients being white; in 34.5% the ocular attack was the first symptom of their disease, whereas on the whole it took a little more than 3 years for the ocular symptoms to appear after the first manifestation of disease. In a review of 31 French patients, an ocular manifestation was the first symptom in 29% of the cases.[16]

## Oral aphthous ulcers

An almost universal finding in Behçet's disease is the amount of discomfort the oral lesions can cause. The number of patients with oral aphthae in the general population is quite high. However, in our experience the lesions in patients with Behçet's disease can occur in clusters and may be found not only on the gums but also on the lips, posterior pharynx, uvula, palate, and tongue. They can be small but painful, and they recur (Fig. 25-5). They usually heal in 7 to 10 days without scarring, but scarring occurs when a particu-

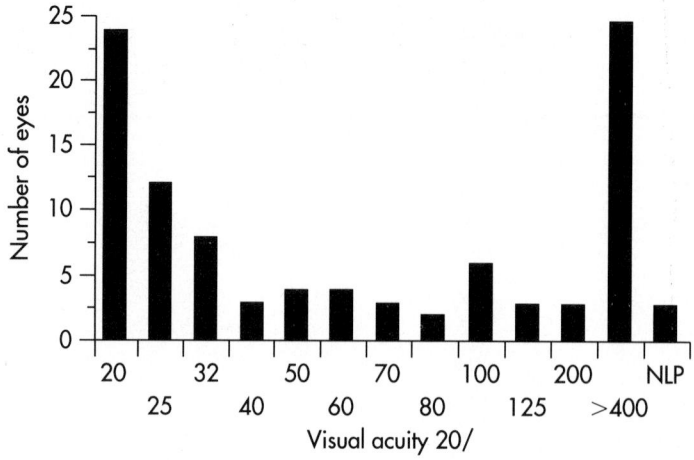


**Fig. 25-3.** Presenting visual acuities of patients with Behçet's disease noted in Fig. 25-2.

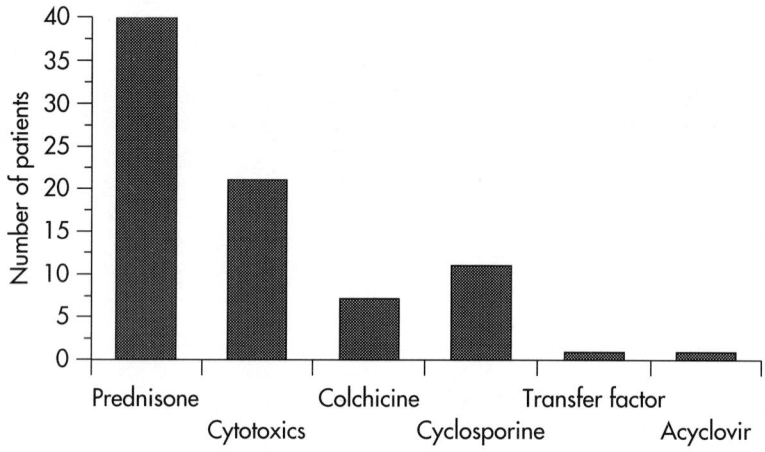


**Fig. 25-4.** Therapeutic modalities used to treat ocular disease of 49 patients with Behçet's disease.

A

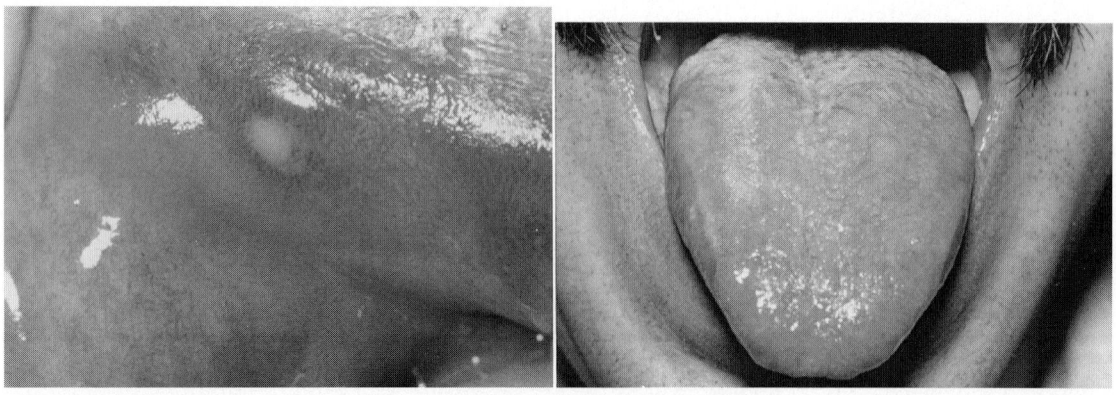

B

**Fig. 25-5.** Aphthous ulcers are common in Behçet's disease. They usually appear several at a time, sometimes on common surfaces such as mucosa of lip **(A)** or on less common regions, such as tonsils and tongue **(B).**

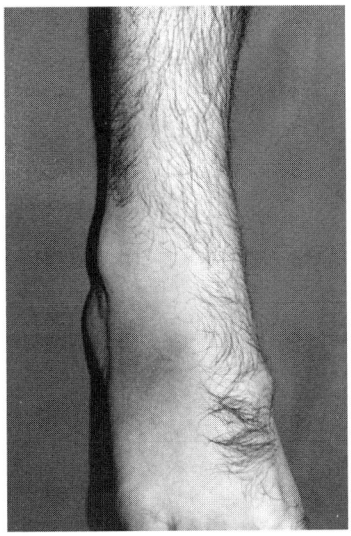

**Fig. 25-6.** Examination of peripheral extremities is important in evaluating patients with Behçet's disease. Just below this patient's ankle (which was painful) is area of erythema nodosum.

larly large ulcer heals. It has been suggested that in contradistinction to the regular flat borders of the aphthae seen in this disorder, the lesions in the Stevens-Johnson syndrome tend to be irregular whereas in Reiter's syndrome, they can have heaped-up edges.[17] Some patients can provoke the appearance of these lesions by eating certain foods, whereas Wray and colleagues[18] have shown that trauma to the oral mucosa can cause these lesions to appear, strikingly reminiscent of the prick test (discussed later).

### Skin lesions

Erythema nodosum–like lesions are noted frequently on the anterior surface of the legs (Fig. 25-6) but can be seen on the face, neck, buttocks, and elsewhere. These lesions involute without ulcerations after several weeks.

Acnelike lesions or folliculitis is another common dermatologic lesion. These acnelike lesions can appear on the back and face and appear histologically identical to the "typical" disorder. Thrombophlebitis is found usually in the extremities. This finding surely denotes a more general vascular disease that can be life-threatening (discussed later). The thrombophlebitis in the extremities can be migratory and can also follow an injection or the taking of a blood sample.

Cutaneous hypersensitivity is a characteristic feature of Behçet's disease. Dermatographia can be observed in one third to one half of the patients. Scratching the skin with a needle or taking a blood sample often results in a pustule at that site. This phenomenon, pathergy, has become the basis for the "prick" test, with some researchers believing that this is an important criterion that can be used in diagnosing the disease (discussed later), first suggested by Curth.[19] In our experience this phenomenon seems to be less common in patients with Behçet's disease seen in our clinic.

### Genital ulcers

The lesions in the male may appear on the scrotum and penis and therefore are quite evident, sending the patient for professional help early in the disease. Female patients usually have their lesions on the vulva or on the vaginal mucosae. Other lesions may be perianal. Kobayashi and colleagues[20] reported that lesions on the vulva occur at the premenstrual portion of the month. It has been suggested that the genital lesions in males are more painful. This has not been our experience. We have seen female patients with particularly painful and distressing genital lesions, frequently diagnosed initially as herpetic in origin.

The genital lesions can be deep and therefore leave scars. Thus an examination of the genital region in a patient with suspected Behçet's disease can be useful inasmuch as signs of old disease may be present.

### Ocular disease

The ocular manifestations in Behçet's disease carry serious implications for the patient. Mamo[21] estimated that vision was lost 3.36 years after the onset of ocular symptoms. The ominous clinical course makes us especially careful in our evaluation of these patients. This has led us to be highly critical in our use of the diagnosis, and the presence of "ocular inflammation" associated with other symptoms does not equate in our minds the diagnosis of Behçet's disease.

The disease can affect both the anterior and posterior portions of the globe, but certain characteristic signs can and should be looked for. Statistically ocular disease manifests some 2 to 3 years after the initial symptoms are noted.[22] The disease is a bilateral one, with rare unilateral cases occurring (see Case 25-1). One important aspect is the recurrent, explosive nature of the ocular disease. Patients do not have "chronic" ocular inflammatory disease,

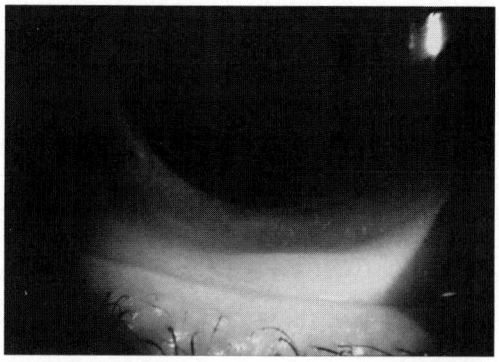

**Fig. 25-7.** Hypopyon is considered classic symptom in Behçet's disease. However, it is not always present during anterior segment inflammation and sometimes will be seen only on gonioscopic examination.

that is, a lingering inflammatory episode that can be chronically noted. Rather the disease will appear floridly active for a set period of time (2-4 weeks), then disappear, with the patient's ocular disease quiescent for some period of time, whether one treats or not. Therefore therapeutic strategies and the evaluation as to whether they are successful must be undertaken with this in mind (see later discussion).

An anterior uveitis or iridocyclitis is seen frequently, with an associated hypopyon in about one third of the cases[7] (Fig. 25-7). The hypopyon may not be visible to the naked eye but seen only with the slit lamp. On occasion a small hypopyon can be seen cradled in the angle when gonioscopic examination is performed. The inflammatory disease has a nongranulomatous appearance. The cells will easily move and slide over the corneal endothelium if the patient's head is tilted in the right direction. When particularly severe, posterior synechiae can obscure the view of the posterior pole. In our experience an isolated vitreous reaction is not characteristic of this disorder. We have observed this when a patient is receiving therapy that is not sufficient to prevent totally the ocular inflammation, and then a smouldering response ensues.

**Retinal disease.** Retinal disease is the most disquieting aspect of the disease and is what ultimately can lead to blindness. It is these recurrent retinal vasoocclusive episodes that ultimately cause irreversible alterations. The fundoscopic examination during the acute attack will, in addition, reveal areas of retinal hemorrhage and edema, accompanied by an inflammatory response in the vitreous. The retinitis often has the appearance of a virally induced lesion, and the decision as to which this may be usually is based on the overall context in which it is being observed (Fig. 25-8). The sequelae of the retinal vasoocclusive episodes can be best seen with use of fluorescein angiography (Fig. 25-9). Some of the changes can be extensive, far more so than imagined on clinical examination alone. Areas of capillary dropout and vascular-tree rearrangement are not uncommon. The loss of a clearly defined capillary free–zone is commonly seen but is not unique to this type of intraocular inflammation. In addition, the angiogram may show diffuse retinal vascular leakage, late staining of the vasculature, leakage from the disc, and neovascularization. It has been thought that the posterior pole disease is essentially that of retinal disease. Rarely one can see evidence of choroidal, outer retinal, or retinal pigment epithelial involvement, raising the question that probably in some patients choroidal involvement is of some importance. An example of this is seen in Fig. 25-10. This patient with Behçet's disease had fluorescein angiographic evidence of a central serous retinopathy associated with retinal edema, further suggesting an occlusion of the choriocapillaris.

Other ocular manifestations include episcleritis, filamentary keratitis, conjunctivitis, and subconjunctival hemorrhages.[23] Extraocular muscle paralysis may be a result of neuro-Behçet's disease.[6]

**Complications.** The complications of repeated inflammatory bouts are of major concern and depend somewhat on where the inflammation is located. Anterior segment inflammation can lead to glaucoma, particularly angle closure. Iris atrophy may be seen as well. Cataract formation is not unusual, due to either the inflammation or the medications added to treat the condition. Iris neovascularization and secondary glaucoma are ominous findings and can accompany the recurrent posterior globe inflammatory episodes. The visual prognosis of a patient with just anterior segment uveitis in Behçet's disease is thought to be good. More women than men in the Japanese experience have this type of disease, and therefore their visual prognosis is less guarded than that for men. We have not seen this subgroup of patients, that is, only anterior segment disease. In our experience the disease most frequently involves both segments of the eye. This has been the

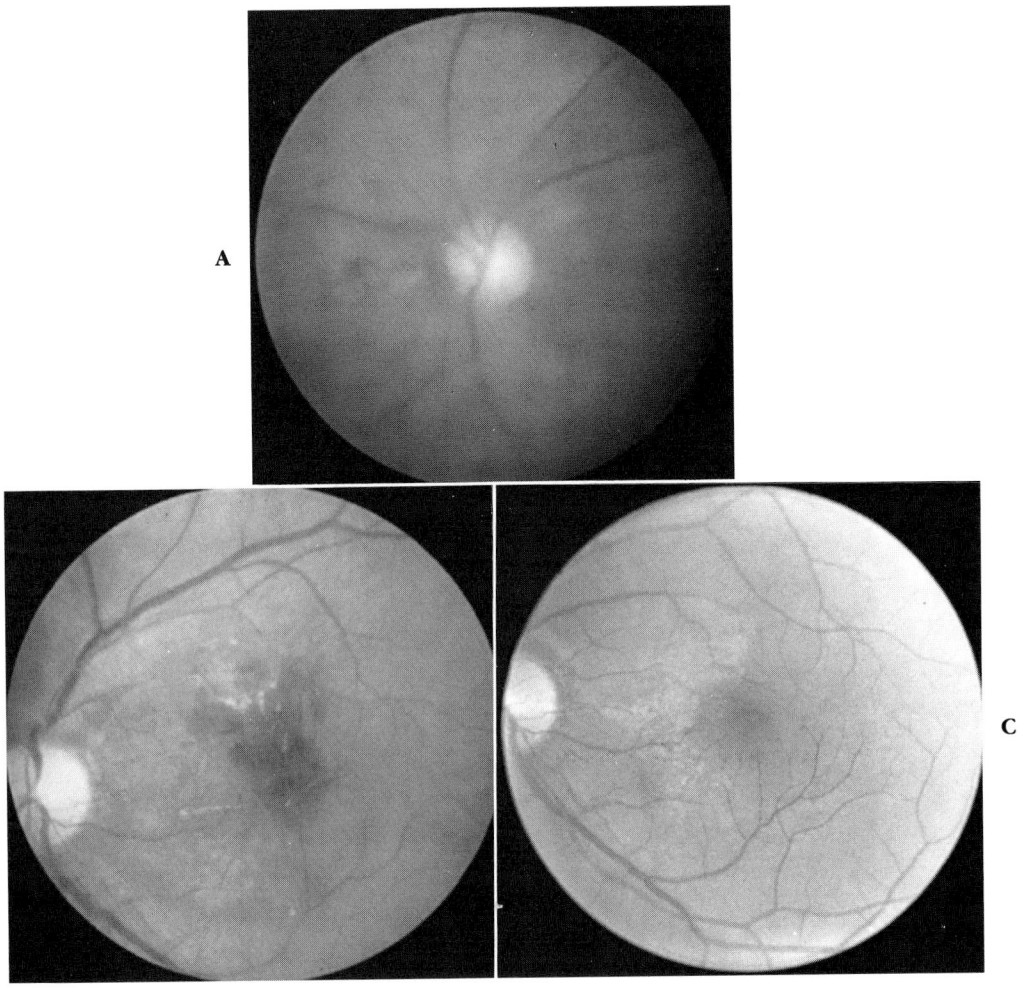


**Fig. 25-8.** Vasoocclusive episodes of posterior pole resulting from Behçet's disease can cause severe visual impairment (**A** and **B**). **C,** Fundus **(B)** after acute episode. Note preretinal membrane that has begun to form.

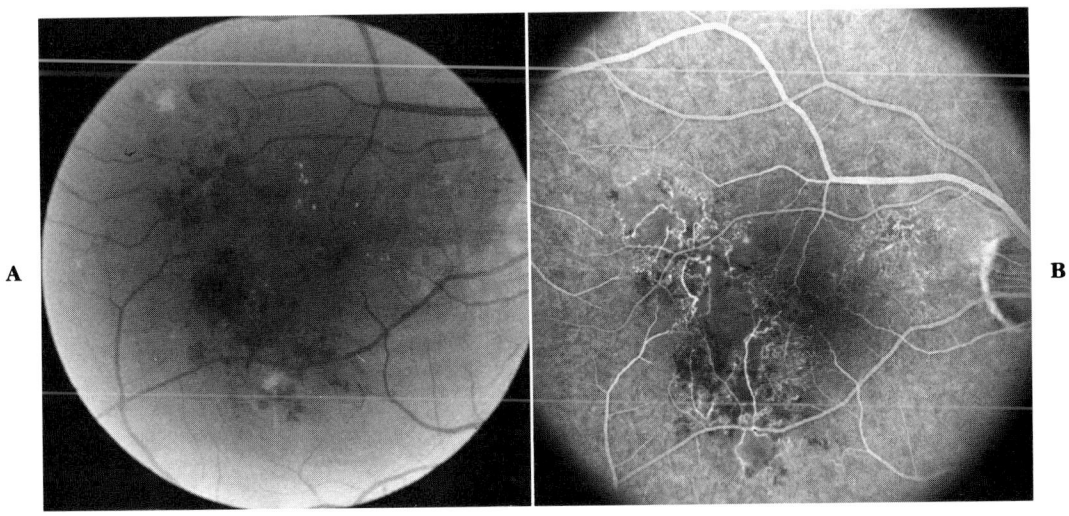


**Fig. 25-9.** Fluorescein angiography can often better show vascular effects that occur with Behçet's disease. This patient has had multiple vasoocclusive attacks of posterior pole **(A),** with fluorescein angiogram showing capillary dropout and vascular remodeling, particularly temporal to macula **(B).**

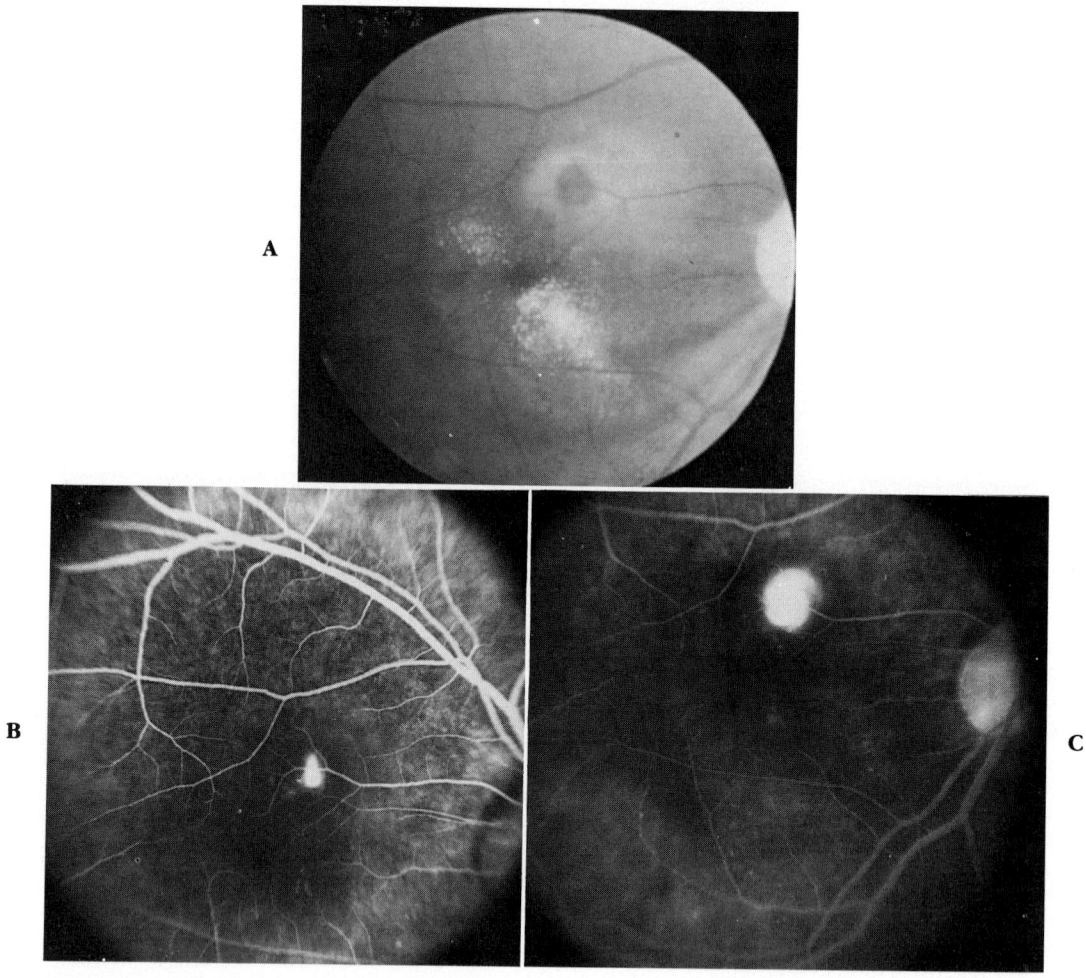


**Fig. 25-10. A** to **C,** Fluorescein angiographic evidence of eccentrically placed serous retinopathy associated with retinal edema and large cyst. These findings suggest occlusion of choriocapillaris rather than retinal disease resulting from this change.

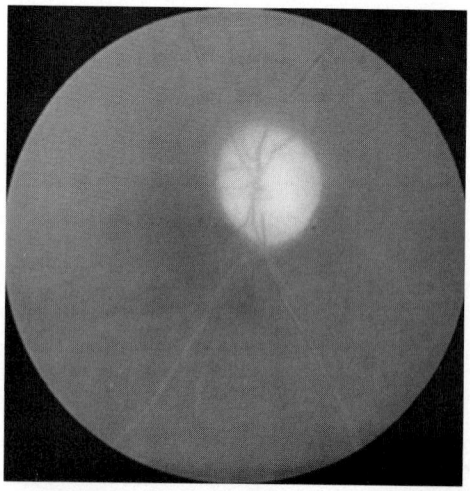

**Fig. 25-11.** End stage of repeat Behçet's disease attacks of posterior pole. Note optic atrophy and sheathed and markedly attenuated vessels. The retina is atrophic.

opinion of Dr. David Ben Ezra in Israel as well (personal communication, 1987).

The posterior segment sequelae of Behçet's disease can lead to serious visual handicap (Fig. 25-11). In a recent report, Sakamoto and colleagues[24] studied 51 patients with Behçet's disease and found that in addition to posterior pole attacks, skin lesions and arthritis were associated with a loss of vision. In women with the disease, anterior segment attacks and increased intervals between attacks were related to retention of vision. Retinal atrophy is the end result of the multiple ocular inflammatory episodes. With this there will be an associated optic atrophy and, often, markedly attenuated retinal vessels. In a percentage of cases there will be an associated neovascular component, leading to recurrent vitreous hemorrhages, subsequent vitreal contraction, and retinal detachment.

In those cases with the full-blown picture, there is little problem in establishing this clinical diagnosis. However, as with all entities, there is overlap in clinical presentation. Further, because parts of the disease spectrum may have occurred some time before and cannot be verified, some uncertainty may arise. The anterior uveitis can mimic almost any severe recurrent process, with the HLA-B27–associated entities particularly so because hypopyon uveitis is seen with these disorders as well. These diseases should be unilateral in their type of presentation whereas in Behçet's disease this presentation occurs only in a small number of cases. Sarcoidosis can mimic some of the posterior pole lesions. However, sarcoidosis is generally more indolent as opposed to the explosive episodes seen in Behçet's disease. The retinitis of Behçet's disease in its most florid form is highly suggestive of a viral retinitis and should certainly be included in the differential diagnosis.

### Minor criteria

As has been alluded to, the associated symptoms of this disorder are legion. As was so aptly emphasized by Geraint James and Spiteri,[25] Behçet's disease can first be seen by many different medical disciplines. Although these symptoms are called "minor," it should be stressed that the term refers only to their import in the determination of the diagnosis. Three of these minor criteria deserve comment.

**Arthritis.** At least half of the patients with Behçet's disease manifest a nonmigrating, nondestructive arthritis, with the knee being the most common joint affected. The arthritis is linked often to a general systemically active state of the disease, accompanied at times by other criteria, such as fever, skin lesions, acute-phase reactants, and, on occasion, ocular lesions. One of our patients could predict an ocular attack when his joints became involved, signaling to him a general activation of his disease. Firestein and colleagues[26] reported the coexistence of relapsing polychondritis and Behçet's disease, in which inflamed cartilage was noted.

**Vascular alterations.** Vessels of all sizes can be involved in this disorder, and angio-Behçet or cardio-Behçet (aortitis) carries a bad prognosis.[27,28] Müftüoglu and coworkers[29] observed vascular involvement in 24% of the 531 cases they reviewed, most being a deep and superficial thrombophlebitis of the legs. These thromboocclusive episodes can cause an elevation of the erythrocyte sedimentation rate. Aneurysms are not uncommon, and their rupture can be the cause of death. Further, deep vessel thrombosis may occur, often involving the large vessels of the body such as the vena cava.[30]

**Neurologic involvement (neuro-Behçet).** This grave complication may affect about 8% of the Japanese patients with Behçet's disease.[7] Of interest was the fact that Inaba[31] reported that most patients with neuro-Behçet did not have ocular disease, with 83.9% of these patients having the incomplete form of the disease and 90.4% having no ocular disease during their clinical course. In 68 autopsy cases, Inaba found that the thalamus, basal ganglia, and the brainstem were involved in 85% to 95% of the cases. In addition to neurologic findings, Behçet's disease can induce frank psychiatric symptoms as well.

In cases of neuro-Behçet, the cerebrospinal fluid shows evidence of pleocytosis. During the acute stage, neutrophils may predominate, leading to a possible diagnosis of aseptic meningitis, whereas in other cases, mononuclear cells may predominate. Inaba[31] has found a predominance of $OKT4^+$ T cells in the cerebrospinal fluid (CSF), and the $\alpha_2$-macroglobulins were markedly increased. Of interest was the fact that the $\beta\text{-}_{1A}$ fraction of C3 was greatly increased during the active stage, suggesting that the alternate pathway of the complement system may be involved. Oligoclonal banding is usually not seen, but Sharief and coworkers[32] have reported the presence of IgA and IgM oligoclonal bands in the CSF of patients with active neuro-Behçet disease and documented the disappearance of the bands with the remission of neurologic disease. Wang and colleagues[33] found that antiocardiolipin antibodies (particularly the IgM isotype) and IL-6 were elevated in the CSF of patients with neuro-Behçet and fell as disease activity abated.

Computed tomographic examination of the brain shows defects in a large number of patients, as will the electroencephalogram (EEG), but some lesions may not be well seen using these types of studies. The use of gadolinium-DTPA—enhanced magnetic resonance imaging (MRI) studies is another approach that appears to provide good definition of central nervous system (CNS) lesions. Of interest were the reports by Ogawa and Sawada,[34] as well as those

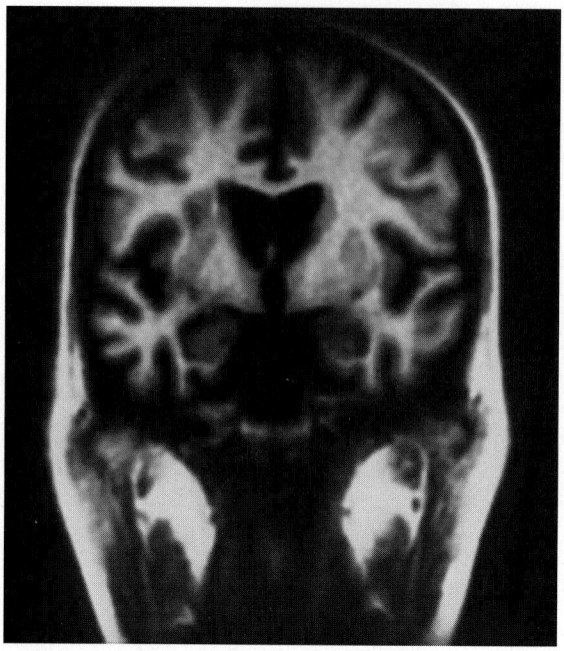

**Fig. 25-12.** MRI of brain of patient with neuro-Behçet. Gray-matter lesions are interpreted to be evidence of CNS activity of disease.

of Edem and coworkers,[35] that the unenhanced MRI images continued to show lesions even after therapy initiation and resolution of clinical disease, whereas the enhanced images showed resolution (Fig. 25-12). Kobayashi and colleagues,[36] using MRI's $T_2$-weighted images, were able to detect a hemorrhagic focus located in the right pontine base.

## IMMUNOLOGIC AND HISTOLOGIC CONSIDERATIONS

The histopathology of the lesions seen in Behçet's disease is that of a perivasculitis associated with tissue destruction (Fig. 25-13). The notion has been that the underlying mechanism leading to this histologic alteration was that of immune complex deposition.[17] Indeed, the deposition of complement components has been reported in some lesions.[37] To support this notion has been the presence of circulating immune complexes in patients with Behçet's disease,[38] as well as neutrophils in the aqueous of eyes with hypopyon uveitis. Increased chemotactic activity of neutrophils has been observed in Behçet's disease.[39,40]

Some observations have suggested that other mechanisms may be at play in this disorder. Kasp and coworkers[41] noted that in 32 patients with Behçet's disease, only one third had elevated circulating immune complex (CIC) levels. Further, the presence of CIC was associated with quiescent periods, which suggested that the CIC may play a beneficial role in the course of the disease (see Chapter 2).

The neurologic lesions include perivascular cuffing with mononuclear cells, focal necrosis, demyelinization, and gliosis.[42] A small number of eyes with this disorder have been examined, particularly with newer immunohistologic techniques. In one report Winter and Yukins[43] believed the underlying lesion was that of an obliterative vasculitis. Mullaney and Collum[44] noted that in an eye they examined there was a necrotizing arteriolitis and phlebitis with thromboses. Mural IgG, IgA, and C3 deposits were noted in the episclera and some choroidal veins but not in the retina.

### Role of T cells

The role of T cells in the underlying mechanism of Behçet's disease appears to be stressed by many observers. Recent immunohistologic studies of the recurrent mouth ulcers of this disorder demonstrated that most of the lymphocytes infiltrating into the lesion were DR-negative T cells, whereas the macrophages were DR-positive.[45] We have seen a predominance of T cells rather than neutrophils in the recurrent hypopyon uveitis of a patient with Behçet's disease. The late David Cogan re-

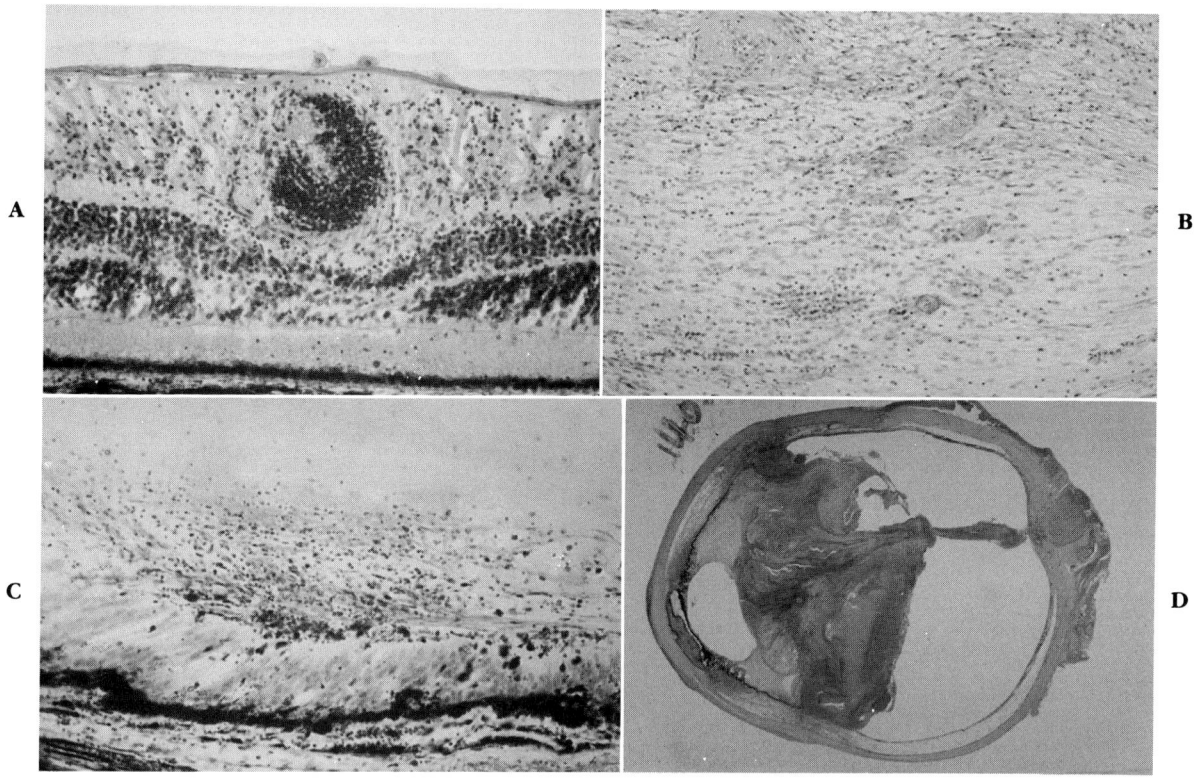


**Fig. 25-13. A,** Retinal vasculitis in Behçet's disease. Note periarteriolar infiltrate and other lymphocytes diffusely spread throughout inner layer of retina. **B,** Occlusive retinitis in retinal vessels of 37-year-old with long-standing complete type of Behçet's disease. **C,** Early stage of ocular disease of patient with neuro-Behçet, with severe pars plana inflammation, macrophages and lymphocytes, and fibrous proliferation. **D,** Enucleated eye of 37-year-old patient with complete type of Behçet's disease shows complete detachment of sensory retina with preretinal and subretinal granulation tissue. (Courtesy Professor J. Inomata, Fukuoka, Japan. From Vasculitis and intraocular neovascularization in Behçet's disease: histopathology of the early and advanced late stages. In Dernouchamps JP, Verougstraete C, Caspers-Velu L, et al, editors: *Recent advance in uveitis.* [Proceedings of the Third International Symposium on Uveitis, Brussels, Belgium, May 24-27, 1992], Amsterdam, 1993, Kugler.)

viewed some 18 Behçet eyes for a joint Japanese-American workshop on Behçet's disease in 1982. Although a perivasculitis was noted, evidence of typical fibrinoid changes associated with immune complex–mediated disease was not present (personal communication, 1984). Charteris and colleagues[46] examined the eyes postmortem of a Behçet patient who suffered from severe recurrent retinal vasculitis. They found a hyaline thickening of the retinal vessels, with a perivascular infiltrate made up of mostly $CD4^+$ T cells bearing large numbers of IL-2 receptors. In another study of five enucleated eyes from Behçet patients, Charteris and coworkers[47] found again a predominance of $CD4^+$ T cells, with no complement or immunoglobulin deposits. We have found essentially the same type of T-cell infiltrate in an eye that we have examined.

Indeed, perturbations of the systemic T-cell circuitry can be found in patients with Behçet's disease. Valesini and coworkers[48] noted an increase in the number of $T6^+$ cells in the blood of Behçet patients with ocular disease, as well as an elevated T8 fraction, thereby lowering the T4/T8 ratio, a finding we have noted in other ocular inflammatory conditions. Essentially the same observations have been noted in Japan by Kikkawa and Shirotsuki[49] studying 11 Behçet patients with uveitis. Other evidence for an intrinsic T-cell problem includes the work of Sakane and colleagues,[50] in which they noted a defect in a T cell mediated–suppressor system. Further, interferon-γ, a T-cell product, was detected at a higher level in the sera of Behçet patients than in control subjects,[51] particularly during the convalescent stage of the disease. Serum IL-2 levels of Behçet patients with ocular involvement were elevated when compared with control subjects and with patients with intermediate uveitis.[52] As with other patients whose uveitis involves the posterior segment, Behçet patients demonstrate evidence of cell-mediated responses to uveitogenic antigens and to their fragments.[53]

Our experience, and now that of others, with cyclosporine further supports the role of T cells in this disease inasmuch as the disease appears effectively controlled in many patients with this anti–T-cell medication (see later discussion). Although the evidence overwhelming incriminates the T cell in this disease, it is clear that there is a rather general and severe immune alteration. Perhaps under T-cell control in the beginning, it seems that the immune system's delicate checks and balances have gone almost universally awry. A full elaboration of all the immune alterations that have been reported in Behçet's disease is beyond the scope of this chapter. The interested reader is referred to the list of selected titles at the end of this chapter.

### HLA typing

HLA typing has proved to be helpful in the diagnosis of Behçet's disease. HLA-B51, a split product of HLA-B5, has been found to be associated with the disease in Japanese patients,[54] with a calculated relative risk of 9.4. The frequency of this antigen in control subjects was 12%, whereas in patients it was 57% (58% in patients with the complete form of the disease vs. 54% in those with the incomplete form). A more recent study using polymerase chain reaction–restriction fragment length polymorphism methodology in evaluating 90 Japanese patients yielded a relative risk for HLA-B51 of 7.9.[55] Some disagreement has arisen as to the strength of these observations when applied to non-Japanese patients. Most of these studies have been performed before the "B5" antigen was split. Godeau and colleagues[56] found an incidence of 54% of HLA-B5 in patients with Behçet's disease (most of Mediterranean origin) versus 13% in the control population. Several other studies, from Israel,[30] Turkey,[57] and Greece,[58] have supported the HLA-B5 association. A further support of the association of HLA-B51 and this disorder came with a recent publication by Villanueva and colleagues.[59] These investigators reported on three siblings, all females, with Behçet's disease, including the ocular manifestations. They all bore the same HLA phenotype, which included HLA-B51.

However, O'Duffy and coworkers[60] found no such association in the 26 patients they typed in the United States, nor did Ohno and colleagues[61] when they typed six white patients. Of course the reason for this may be due to the lack of association. On the other hand, it may reflect the different criteria for diagnosis used in these American studies as opposed to those of the Japanese studies. In Ohno and coworkers' very small group, "atypical" cases were studied, so that the diagnosis was not presumptive in only two of these cases.

Various investigators have attempted to identify an exogenous cause to this disease, particularly a viral one. The incidence of the disease is greater in the northern portions of Japan, although there is no known genetic difference, such as a higher incidence of HLA-B51, between the people in the north as opposed to those in the south of Japan. A somewhat dated report emphasized that there had not been any documented cases of the disease in Nisei living in Hawaii,[62] suggesting that an exogenous source may indeed act as at least a triggering mechanism. Indeed, the search for the presence of live virus in the retina has not been successful, and therapeutic approaches with this concept as its underlying logic have not been rewarding (see later discussion). Denman and colleagues[63] offer a more provocative theory as to the role of virus in this disorder. They have noted that mononuclear cells from these patients have a high concentration of the interferon-induced enzyme, 2′-5′ oligoadenylate synthetase, which is suggestive, but not confirmatory, of a viral infection.[64] They speculate that the virus may act as a "promoter" by stimulating the expansion of clones of abnormal lymphocytes that will induce disease. Bonass and coworkers,[65] using DNA dot-blotting techniques, found evidence of the presence of herpes simplex virus type 1 (HSV-1)–DNA in a high percentage of patients with Behçet's disease. More recent work has centered on the possible role of streptococcal-related antigens as an etiologic agent of this disease. Hirohata and colleagues[66] showed that when *Streptococcus sanguis*–related antigen (RRE KTH-1 antigens) were added to T cells of Behçet's patients in in vitro cultures, the amount of IL-6, an "inflammatory" cytokine, is produced in higher amounts than by T cells from control subjects stimulated in a similar fashion. This suggests that a hypersensitivity response to these bacterial antigens could be a triggering mechanism for this disease. Recently, Pervin and colleagues[67] demonstrated a responsiveness of T-cell clones from patients with Behçet's disease to four peptide determinants within the 65-kd heat shock proteins derived from *Mycobacterium tuberculosis*. Although these are attractive notions, they are far from being proved.

No truly specific tests for the diagnosis of Behçet's disease exist. The "prick" test of the skin, looking for evidence of pathergy, has been suggested as being highly suggestive for the diagnosis of Behçet's disease by some, particularly the Turkish. Skin hyperreactivity has not been a markedly striking feature in the patients we have seen in the United States. Wechsler and colleagues[68] have applied immunofluorescence techniques to skin from which biopsy specimens were obtained after an intradermal injection of distilled water. About 60% of those thought to have Behçet's disease had complement and or IgM deposition as opposed to 14% of control subjects. There was no concordance with HLA-B5. Dogan and colleagues[69] found that total serum sialic acid levels, as well as the proportion of total serum sialic acid to total protein levels, can help to distinguish Behçet's disease from other uveitic entities. Michaelson and coworkers[70] investigated the presence of anticytoplasmic antibodies in this disease by means of an indirect immunofluorescence technique, using guinea pig lip as the tissue substrate. Although 8 of 8 American patients with Behçet's disease had positive test reactions, only 10 of 16 Turkish patients showed positivity. This test awaits further evaluation with larger patient numbers. Recently anticardiolipin antibodies have been observed in several cases of lupus accompanied by retinal vascular disease and were reported to be present in high serum titers in one patient with neuro-Behçet.[71] These antibodies were looked for in Behçet's disease patients with uveitis, and no correlation could be made by Efthimiou and coworkers,[72] but Bergman and colleagues[73] claimed that they (IgM isotype) were increased in these patients. However, Aydintug and coworkers[74] did not find any evidence of anticardiolipin nor antineutrophil cytoplasmic antibodies in 72 Turkish patients they screened. Rather they found that 18% had evidence of antiendothelial cell antibodies (AECA), which did not induce complement-mediated cytotoxicity; neither was the binding due to immune complexes. However, they did find that those with positive AECA were more apt to develop acute thrombotic events and retinal vasculitis.

## THERAPY

The responsibility of the ophthalmologist in the treatment of Behçet's disease is a heavy one. The visual course of the patient is often a major deciding factor as to whether therapy is successful, should be altered, or stopped. Because of the difficulty in treating the posterior pole aspects of this disorder, a litany of therapies has been proposed. In spite of these sometimes intensive therapeutic attempts, loss of useful visual acuity may occur in about three quarters of the eyes 6 to 10 years after the initiation of ocular symptoms.[75]

The most commonly used agents to date have been (1) systemic corticosteroids, (2) cytotoxic agents (alkylating agents), (3) colchicine, and (4) cyclosporine and FK506.

### Systemic corticosteroids

Although Behçet's disease may initially respond to systemic corticosteroids, it will invariably become "resistant," with a further drop in vision and the need for additional therapeutic modes.[75] Some Japanese observers never give corticosteroids for this disease because they believe that in the long run the addition of this agent will result in an even worse visual prognosis.

### Cytotoxic and antimetabolic agents

Several reports from the Mediterranean basin have reported the efficacy of cytotoxic agents (particularly alkylating agents) in the treatment of the ocular component of Behçet's disease.[76-78] Mamo[76] noted no ocular recurrences in most patients treated. Pivetti Pezzi and coworkers[79] found, in a retrospective clinical study, that the visual prognosis of patients treated early on with chlorambucil was considerably better than those treated early with steroid. A reappraisal by Tabbara[80] of the role of chlorambucil in the treatment of this disorder was considerably less favorable. He underlined the significant side effects seen with the drug and noted that three quarters of the eyes studied had a visual acuity of 20/200 or less when chlorambucil was used as the sole therapeutic agent. Kazokoglu and coworkers[81] evaluated the long-term effects of cyclophosphamide and colchicine; and they concluded that in their 64 patients there was no statistically significant positive change in visual acuity nor in the attack rate when compared with the posttreatment period. These observations essentially corroborate those of BenEzra and colleagues,[75] and ours as well. A disturbing report by Takeuchi and Takeuchi[82] found an increased frequency of chromosomal aberrations (dicentrics) in patients with Behçet's disease treated with cytotoxic agents as well as colchicine. A new approach has been to use intravenous pulse cyclophosphamide (which may have less side effects) to treat Behçet's disease, an approach similar to that used for severe renal disease. Our experience has not been especially promising with this method, whereas Hamza and colleagues[83] reported some advantage of this method over pulse steroid therapy. Yazici and colleagues[84] reported that azathioprine was superior to placebo in the treatment of this disease. Although any controlled trial deserves attention, it has been noted that maintenance of visual acuity was a goal that was met with only modest success.[85,86]

### Colchicine

Because results of the leukocyte migration studies showed abnormalities, the use of colchicine was thought ideal inasmuch as it would inhibit such migration. The intent of its use by most practitioners is to prevent recurrences, not to treat the active disease. Hijikata and colleagues[78] found that the visual prognosis for patients receiving colchicine was better than those receiving steroid. A masked randomized study in Turkey, in which patients received colchicine or placebo, demonstrated no differences between the groups.[87]

### Cyclosporine and FK506

Our observation early on in using cyclosporine suggested clearly that patients with Behçet's disease appeared to have a particularly positive therapeutic response to this agent.[88] These observations were confirmed in a randomized double-masked multicenter study in Japan, in which cyclosporine was found to be superior to the original standard therapy.[89] Observations have been made in Israel, where the drug was compared with cytotoxic agents in a masked study,[90] as well as in Turkey.[91] Özyazgan and colleagues,[92] in a single masked study, compared 5 mg/kg/day of cyclosporine with intravenous administration of 1 g cytoxan per month. In this small study of 23 patients, they found that the cyclosporine group had a significantly marked improvement of their vision compared with the other group, but at 24 months it was not clear if this improvement was sustained, leaving the observers with the call for further long-term studies. Kotake and colleagues[93] treated 20 Japanese Behçet patients with low doses of cyclosporine (5 mg/kg/day), finding it effective in 70% of cases. Chavis and coworkers[94] in Saudi Arabia reported a salutary effect of cyclosporine on loss of vision due to papillitis, optic neuritis, macular neuroretinitis, and retinal phlebitis, but not with retinal arteritis. Their approach to therapy is different from the one we have outlined here, with a taper of cyclosporine therapy once clinical improvement is seen; this is thus intermittent low-dose therapy as opposed to continuous low-dose cyclosporine therapy as described by us. We have recently reported our long-term results with cyclosporine in 19 patients with Behçet's disease.[95] We found that combined cyclosporine and prednisone therapy appeared to be an effective means to treat this disorder. The combination permits the use of lower doses of both medications, thus helping to reduce the possibility of untoward secondary effects. Of interest as well was the positive therapeutic effect of cyclosporine therapy reported by Elidan and colleagues[96] on the hearing loss that occurred during Behçet's disease.

With a mechanism that is essentially the same as cyclosporine, it is logical to assume that FK506 would be a useful therapy for this disorder. It has been used in the treatment of presumed pulmonary vasculitis due to Behçet's disease, with resolution of the pulmonary lesion, as well as amelioration of the uveitis.[97]

### Other approaches

Comment should be briefly made about some of the other therapeutic approaches suggested. The use of agents that augment the immune response appears not to be based on any recent information dealing with potential mechanisms for this disease. The use of plasmapheresis may a useful adjunct in an emergency situation, but in our mind is not practical for long-term use and usually must be accompanied by immunosuppressive therapy. The use of antiviral agents cannot be supported by information in the literature at this time. Bonnet and colleagues[98] treated seven patients with plasma exchanges to remove circulating immune complexes and simultaneously gave high doses of acyclovir, with most discouraging results. Some centers both inside and outside the United States have used thalidomide in treating various components of Behçet's disease. Although some aspects of the disease may respond positively to this approach,[99] the ocular lesions do not seem particularly amenable to this agent.[100] An interesting observation has been the use of thalidomide in the treatment of a patient with neuro-Behçet, in whom no relapses were seen when this agent was added to chlorambucil and prednisone.[101] We are not aware of thalidomide being used for the treatment of neovascularization due to Behçet's disease. Oral prostaglandin $E_1$, a potent vasodilator, has been used to treat the leg ulcers sometimes seen associated with the peripheral vascular complications of Behçet's disease.[102]

The approach in our clinic to the Behçet patient with severe ocular involvement is as follows (Fig. 25-14). For patients with bilateral disease and their first attack, we usually use systemically administered prednisone and then slowly taper. We know that long-term therapy of this nature will not protect the patient, but our diagnosis may still be wrong or the patient may indeed have only one attack, albeit very rarely. In some cases it might be useful to observe the patient, particularly if one has not witnessed the attack at its peak, and see only minimal residua. If the attacks become repetitive, or if the initial attack is particularly severe, then alternative therapeutic agents should be considered. We believe, based on our experience and now those of several groups worldwide, that cyclosporine is the initial drug to consider for this disorder—but only after an evaluation determining the feasibility of its use. The goal of therapy is to prevent the recurrent explosive episodes affecting the posterior portion of the globe.

It must be stressed that as of this writing, cyclosporine is not approved for the treatment of this disorder in the United States (but it is in Japan). Therefore appropriate arrangements

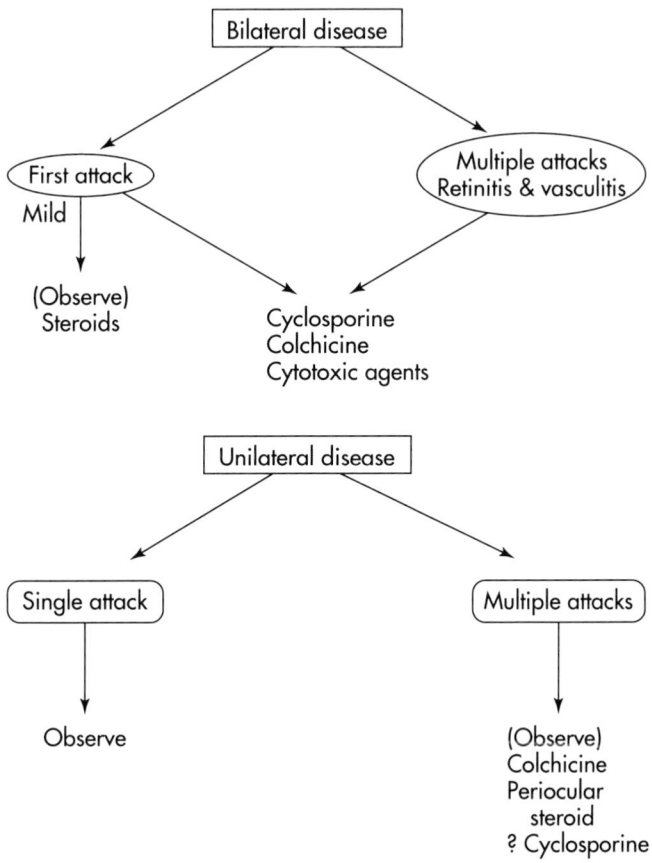


**Fig. 25-14.** General outline for treatment of ocular complications of Behçet's disease.

must be made to use the drug on a compassionate basis. The patient must fully know about the side effects and particularly the renal toxicity, which one hopes can be minimized. If good control is achieved, it may be that the patient needs to be treated for an extended period of time, that is, 1 to 4 years. There can certainly be an attempt to slowly taper the medication during that period. An additional secondary effect of cyclosporine therapy needs to be mentioned here—to date one that has been noted only in Behçet patients in Japan. In those patients, CNS symptoms, including pleocytosis in the spinal fluid, have been noted. Because uveitis and neuro-Behçet are not commonly seen together, these findings are thought to be due to the cyclosporine. We have not, to date, recognized this in the patients we have treated.

If an alternative therapeutic approach is needed, the practitioner might consider the use of colchicine. The usefulness of this medication for this disorder is still in doubt, and strict criteria for its continuation or stoppage must be established. We have not used it for bilateral, sight-threatening disease. Alternatively, cytotoxic agents should be considered as well. The vast bulk of the literature supports the use of alkylating agents (chlorambucil or cyclophosphamide), both for the uveitis and CNS findings in this disease.[103] Once again, patients need to know about the potential side effects of these drugs, and the appropriate authorities, if necessary, need to be apprised of the situation.

In the rare patient with unilateral disease, we usually observe the patient with just one attack. If it becomes unilaterally recurrent, we might continue to observe if the vision were already markedly diminished because of previous attacks. However, if intervention appears indicated, we would consider using either periocular steroid or colchicine. For the rare patient with unilateral disease, we have decided not to use cyclosporine until we feel secure that the renal toxicity can be totally avoided or at least have available exquisitely sensitive methods to permit monitoring. The alternative argument is that most patients will develop bilateral disease, and the eye initially involved may ultimately be the better one. These are difficult questions that the practitioner and patient must wrestle with on an individual basis.

**Case 25-1**

A 38-year-old Korean man had a 2-year history of symptoms supporting the diagnosis of Behçet's disease. He has had biopsy-proved erythema nodosum, as well as several episodes of painful and tender joints, including the knee, ankle, and foot. He had several mouth ulcers present simultaneously, as well as a penile ulcer. He showed HLA-B5 positivity. For the past year he has noticed that the vision in his left eye is blurry. Attempts were made to treat the condition with eyedrops, but the problem appeared to wax and wane in spite of therapy. The patient seemed to average an attack only in the left eye once a month. When we first saw him, visual acuity was 20/12.5 OD, 5/125 OS. The right eye showed no evidence of present or prior uveitic episodes. The left eye had trace flare and cell in the anterior segment. There were 3+ cells and 2+ haze in the vitreous. The retina had areas of gliosis, with diffuse sheathing and markedly attenuated retinal vessels. Because the patient had unilateral disease and was ending a recent recurrence, he was placed on a regimen of 0.6 mg of colchicine three times daily. He was able to tolerate this schedule, and repeat complete blood cell counts showed no alterations. The number of ocular attacks in the left eye decreased from once a month to one every 7 to 9 months. He has remained on this regimen.

**Case 25-2**

A 39-year-old man of Scotch-Irish ancestry had a 6-year history of arthritis, mouth ulcers, acnelike lesions on his back, and penile ulcers. In addition, recurrent anterior and posterior uveitis developed 2 years before he was seen by us. These episodes were treated initially with systemic steroids, but because of the increasing frequency of ocular attacks, he was given chlorambucil. He was maintained on this regimen for 6 months, with some decrease in the number of ocular attacks. However, his white blood cell count began to decrease below 3000/mm$^3$. This medication was discontinued because a dose reduction of chlorambucil did not increase the number of circulating white blood cells, and he began to have increased bouts of uveitis. At this point he was seen by us. His visual acuity was 20/30 OD and 20/60 OS, with mild retinal vascular alterations noted. An electroretinogram showed slightly reduced rod and dark-adapted cone responses in both eyes. The patient was placed on cyclosporine therapy after stopping the cytotoxic agent for more than a month. He has been maintained on cyclosporine therapy for 5 years at ever-decreasing doses, taking 3 mg/kg for an extended period of time. His vision is 20/15 OD, 20/30 OS. There have been no recurrences of his ocular disease. The patient on occasion will develop a mouth ulcer.

**Case 25-3**

A 35-year-old man of Greek extraction developed all four major criteria for Behçet's disease within the span of 1½ years. Initial therapy with chlorambucil and then cyclophosphamide (Cytoxan) resulted in some decrease of his retinal vasoocclusive attacks. The best corrected vision decreased to 20/80 OD, 20/30 OS. Fluorescein angiography findings showed marked areas of capillary dropout, and there was some retinal atrophy, with the optic nerve in the right eye beginning to look pale. The patient was begun on cyclosporine therapy and had a marked resolution of his nonocular symptoms; his ocular attacks dissipated. Over a period of 3 years his vision dropped markedly in both eyes despite the absence of inflammatory disease. When he returned several years later, his vision was confined to hand movements (HM) OD, 20/400 OS. His therapy was stopped.

**Comment 25-3** A most frustrating scenario. It would seem that once retinal alterations due to the uveitis have extensively progressed, the degenerative changes become autonomous from the inflammatory disease that initiated them. We assume that apoptosis-programmed cell death has been initiated. Once this has occurred, even if the uveitis has been controlled, vision will irreversibly decrease.

## REFERENCES


1. Behçet H: Ueber rezideivierende, aphthöse, durch ein Virus verursachte Geschwüre am Mund, am Auge und an den Genitalien, *Dermatol Wochenschr* 46:414-419, 1937.
2. Adamantiadis B: Sur un cas d'iritis à hypopyon recidevante, *Ann Ocul* 168:271-274, 1931.
3. Shigeta T: Recurrent iritis with hypopyon and its pathological findings, *Acta Soc Ophthalmol Jpn* 28:516-521, 1924.
4. Feigenbaum A: Description of Behçet's syndrome in the hippocratic third book of endemic diseases, *Br J Ophthalmol* 40:355-357, 1956.
5. Ohno S: Behçet's disease in the world. In Lehner T, Barnes CG, editors: *Recent advances in Behçet's disease,* London, 1986, Royal Society of Medicine Services.
6. Bietti GB, Bruna F: An ophthalmic report on Behçet's disease. In Monacelli M, Nazzaro P, editors: *Behçet's disease,* Basel, 1966, Karger.
7. Mishima S, Masuda K, Izawa Y et al: Behçet's disease in Japan: ophthalmologic aspects, *Trans Am Ophthalmol Soc* 76:225-279, 1979.
8. Nakae K, Masaki F, Hashimoto T et al: Recent epidemiological features of Behçet's disease in Japan. In Godeau P, Wechsler B, editors: *Behçet's disease,* Amsterdam, 1993, Elsevier.
9. Dilsen N, Koniçe M, Aral O: Our diagnostic criteria of Behçet's disease—an overview. In Lehner T, Barnes CG, editors: *Recent advances in Behçet's disease,* London, 1986, Royal Society of Medicine Services.
10. International Study Group for Behçet's Disease: Criteria for diagnosis of Behçet's disease, *Lancet* 335:1078-1080, 1990.
11. International Study Group for Behçet's Disease: Evaluation of diagnostic ("classification") criteria in Behçet's disease—towards internationally agreed criteria, *Br J Rheumatol* 31:299-308, 1992.
12. Nakae K, Masaki F, Hashimoto T et al: A nation-wide epidemiological survey on Behçet's disease, report 2: association of HLA-B51 with clinico-epidemiological features (Report of Behçet's Disease Research Committee, Japan, Ministry of Health and Welfare, 1992) (in press).
13. Hafner R, Truckenbrodt H: Behçet's syndrome with childhood onset, *Acta Univ Carol [Med] (Praha)* 37:25-30, 1991.
14. Losieau-Corvez MN, de Kerdanet MM, Chevrant-Breton J et al: Phlebothromosis revealing Behçet's disease in a 13 year old adolescent, *Arch Fr Pediatr* 49:815-817, 1992.
15. Barra C, Belfort R Jr, Abreu MT et al: Behçet's disease in Brazil—a review of 49 cases with emphasis on ophthalmic manifestations, *Jpn J Ophthalmol* 35:339-346, 1991.
16. Cochereau-Massin I, Wechsler B, LeHoang P et al: Ocular prognosis in Behçet's disease, *J Fr Ophthalmol* 15:343-347, 1992.
17. Michaelson JB, Chisari FV: Behçet's disease, *Surv Ophthalmol* 26:190-203, 1982.
18. Wray D, Graykowski EA, Notkins AL: Role of mucosal injury in initiating recurrent aphthous stomatitis, *Br Med J [Clin Res]* 283:1569-1570, 1981.
19. Curth HO: Behçet's syndrome, abortive form (?): recurrent aphthous oral lesions and recurrent genital ulcerations, *Arch Derm Syph* 54:179-196, 1946.
20. Kobayashi T, Matsumaya E, Sugimoto T: Gynecological aspect of muco-cutaneous-ocular syndromes, *World Obstet Gynecol* 11:995-999, 1959.
21. Mamo JG: The rate of visual loss in Behçet's disease, *Arch Ophthalmol* 84:451-452, 1970.
22. Imai Y: Studies on prognosis and symptoms of Behçet's disease in long-term observation, *Jpn J Clin Ophthalmol* 25:665-694, 1971.
23. Furusawa T: A clinical study on mucocutaneous ocular syndrome, *Gan Rinsho Ibo* 52:1143-1146, 1958.
24. Sakamoto M, Akazawa K, Nishioka Y et al: Prognostic factors of vision in patients with Behçet's disease, *Ophthalmology* 102:317-321, 1995.
25. Geraint James D, Spiteri MA: Behçet's disease, *Ophthalmology* 89:1279-1284, 1982.
26. Firestein GS, Gruber HE, Weisman MH et al: MAGIC syndrome: mouth and genital ulcers with inflamed cartilage. In Lehner T, Barnes CG, editors: *Recent advances in Behçet's disease,* London, 1986, Royal Society of Medicine Services.
27. Shimizu T, Ehrlich GE, Inaba G et al: Behçet's disease (Behçet's syndrome), *Semin Arthritis Rheum* 8:223-260, 1979.
28. Tai YT, Fong PC, Ng WF et al: Diffuse aortitis complicating Behçet's disease leading to severe aortic regurgitation, *Cardiology* 79:156-160, 1991.
29. Müftüoglu Ü, Yurdakul S, Yazici H et al: Vascular involvement in Behçet's disease—a review of 129 cases. In Lehner T, Barnes CG, editors: *Recent advances in Behçet's disease,* London, 1986, Royal Society of Medicine Services.

30. Chajek T, Fairanu M: Behçet's disease: report of 41 cases and a review of the literature, *Medicine* 54:179-196, 1975.
31. Inaba G: Clinical features of neuro-Behçet's syndrome. In Lehner T, Barnes CG, editors: *Recent advances in Behçet's disease,* London, 1986, Royal Society of Medicine Services.
32. Sharief MK, Hentges R, Thomas E: Significance of CSF immunoglobulins in monitoring neurologic disease activity in Behçet's disease, *Neurology* 41:1398-1401, 1991.
33. Wang CR, Chuang CY, Chen CY: Anticardiolipin antibodies and interleukin-6 in cerebrospinal fluid and blood of Chinese patients with neuro-Behçet's syndrome, *Clin Exp Rheumatol* 10:599-602, 1992.
34. Ogawa M, Sawada T: Sequential gadolinium-DTPA enhanced MRI studies in neuro-Behçet's disease, *Neuroradiology* 33:136-139, 1991.
35. Edem E, Carlier R, Idir AB et al: Gadolinium-enhanced MRI in central nervous system Behçet's disease, *Neuroradiology* 35:142-144, 1993.
36. Kobayashi H, Saito Y, Kaneko Y et al: A case of neuro-Behçet's disease with hemorrhagic brain stem lesion detected by MRI, *Rinsho Shinkeigaku* 32:763-766, 1992.
37. Gamble CN, Wiesner KB, Shapiro RF et al: The immune complex pathogenesis of glomerulonephritis and pulmonary vasculitis in Behçet's disease, *Am J Med* 66:1031-1039, 1979.
38. Levinsky RJ, Lehner T: Circulating soluble immune complexes in recurrent oral ulceration and Behçet's syndrome, *Clin Exp Immunol* 32:193-198, 1978.
39. Matsumura N, Mizushima Y: Leukocyte movement and colchicine treatment in Behçet's disease, *Lancet* 2:813, 1975.
40. Sobel JD, Haim S, Obedeanu N et al: Polymorphonuclear leukocyte function in Behçet's disease, *J Clin Pathol* 30:250-253, 1977.
41. Kasp E, Graham EM, Stanford MR et al: Retinal autoimmunity and circulating immune complexes in ocular Behçet's disease. In Lehner T, Barnes CG, editors: *Recent advances in Behçet's disease,* London, 1986, Royal Society of Medicine Services.
42. Fukuda Y, Hayashi H: Pathologic studies on neuro-Behçet's disease. In *Annual Report of Behçet's Disease Research Committee,* Tokyo, Japan, 1980.
43. Winter FC, Yukins RE: The ocular pathology of Behçet's disease, *Am J Ophthalmol* 62:257-262, 1966.
44. Mullaney J, Collum LM: Ocular vasculitis in Behçet's disease: a pathological and immunohistochemical study, *Int Ophthalmol* 7:183-191, 1985.
45. Poulter LW, Lehner T, Duke O: Immunohistological investigation of recurrent oral ulcers and Behçet's disease. In Lehner T, Barnes CG, editors: *Recent advances in Behçet's disease,* London, 1986, Royal Society of Medicine Services.
46. Charteris DG, Champ C, Rosenthal AR et al: Behçet's disease: activated T lymphocytes in retinal perivasculitis, *Br J Ophthalmol* 76:499-501, 1992.
47. Charteris DG, Barton K, McCartney AC et al: CD4+ lymphocyte involvement in ocular Behçet's disease, *Autoimmunity* 12:201-206, 1992.
48. Valesini G, Pivetti-Pezzi P, Mastrandrea F et al: Evaluation of T cell subsets in Behçet's syndrome using anti–T cell monoclonal antibodies, *Clin Exp Immunol* 60:55-60, 1985.
49. Kikkawa T, Shirotsuki H: Imbalance in T lymphocyte subsets in panuveitis type of Behçet's disease, *J Eye* 1:1007-1010, 1984.
50. Sakane T, Kotani H, Takada S et al: Functional aberration of T cell subsets in patients with Behçet's disease, Arthritis Rheum 25:1343-1351, 1982.
51. Ohno S, Kato F, Matsuda H et al: Studies on spontaneous production of gamma-interferon in Behçet's disease, *Ophthalmologica* 185:187-192, 1982.
52. BenEzra D, Maftzir G, Kalichman I et al: Serum levels of interleukin-2 receptor in ocular Behçet's disease, *Am J Ophthalmol* 115:26-30, 1993.
53. Yamamoto JH, Minami M, Inaba G et al: Cellular autoimmunity to retinal specific antigens in patients with Behçet's disease, *Br J Ophthalmol* 77:584-589, 1993.
54. Ohno S, Matsuda H: Studies of HLA antigens in Behçet's disease in Japan. In Lehner T, Barnes CG, editors: *Recent advances in Behçet's disease,* London, 1986, Royal Society of Medicine Services.
55. Mizuki N, Tanaka H, Kera J et al: Human leukocyte antigen serologic and DNA typing of Behçet's disease and its primary association with B51, *Invest Ophthalmol Vis Sci* 33:3332-3340, 1992.
56. Godeau P, Torre D, Campanchi R et al: HLA-B5 and Behçet's disease. In Dausset J, Svejgaard A, editors: *HLA and disease,* Baltimore, 1977, Williams & Wilkins.
57. Ersoy F, Berkel AI, Firat T et al: HLA antigens associated with Behçet's disease. In Dausset J, Svejgaard A, editors: *HLA and disease,* Paris, 1976, PUB.
58. Palimeris G, Papakonstantinoy P, Mantas M: The Adamantiadis-Behçet's syndrome in Greece. In Saari KM, editor: *Uveitis update,* Amsterdam, 1984, Excerpta Medica.
59. Villaneuva JL, Gonzalez-Dominguez J, Gonzalez-Dominguez R et al: HLA antigen familial study in complete Behçet's syndrome affecting three sisters, *Ann Rheum Dis* 52:155-157, 1993.
60. O'Duffy JD, Taswell HF, Elveback LR: HL-A antigens in Behçet's disease, *J Rheumatol* 3:1-3, 1976.
61. Ohno S, Char DH, Kimura SJ et al: Studies on HLA antigens in American patients with Behçet's disease, *Jpn J Ophthalmol* 22:58-61, 1978.
62. Hirohata T, Kuratsume M, Nomura A: Prevalence of Behçet's syndrome in Hawaii, *Hawaii Med J* 34:244-246, 1975.
63. Denman AM, Hylton W, Pelton BK et al: The viral aetiology of Behçet's disease. In Lehner T, Barnes CG, editors: *Recent advances in Behçet's disease,* London, 1986, Royal Society of Medicine Services.
64. Hylton W, Cayley J, Dore C et al: 2′5′-Oligoadenylate synthetase induction in lymphocytes of patients with connective tissue diseases, *Ann Rheum Dis* 45:220-224, 1986.
65. Bonass WA, Bird-Stewart JA, Chamberlain MA et al: Molecular studies in Behçet's syndrome. In Lehner T, Barnes CG, editors: *Recent advances in Behçet's disease,* London, 1986, Royal Society of Medicine Services.
66. Hirohata S, Oka H, Mizushima Y: Streptococcal-related antigens stimulate production of IL6 and interferon gamma by T cells from patients with Behçet's disease, *Cell Immunol* 140:410-419, 1992.
67. Pervin K, Chiderstone A, Shinnick T et al: T cell epitope expression of mycobacterial and homologous human 65-kilodalton heat shock protein peptides in

short term cell lines from patients with Behçet's disease, *J Immunol* 151:2273-2282, 1993.
68. Wechsler J, Wechsler B, Herreman G et al: Behçet's disease: an immunofluorescent study of intradermal distilled water injection by studying 48 patients' value for diagnosis. Paper presented at the International Academy of Pathology, Paris, France, 1980.
69. Dogan H, Pasaoglu H, Ekinciler OF et al: A comparative study of total protein, total and lipid associated serum sialic acid levels in patients with Behçet's disease and control groups, *Acta Ophthalmol (Copenh)* 70:790-794, 1992.
70. Michaelson JB, Chisari FV, Kansu T: Antibodies to oral mucosa in patients with ocular Behçet's disease, *Ophthalmology* 92:1277-1281, 1985.
71. Salvarani C, Massai G, Macchioni P et al: Anticardiolipin antibodies in a case of neuro-Behçet with superior vena caval obstruction, *Clin Rheumatol* 6:88-91, 1987.
72. Efthimiou J, Cambridge G, Harris EN et al: Anticardiolipin antibodies and vascular complications in Behçet's syndrome. In Lehner T, Barnes CG, editors: *Recent advances in Behçet's disease,* London, 1986, Royal Society of Medicine Services.
73. Bergman R, Lorber M, Lerner M et al: Anticardiolipin antibodies in Behçet's disease, *J Dermatol* 17:164-167, 1990.
74. Aydintug AO, Tokgoz G, D'Cruz DP et al: Antibodies to endothelial cells in patients with Behçet's disease, *Clin Immunol Immunopathol* 67:157-162, 1993.
75. BenEzra D, Cohen E: Treatment and visual prognosis in Behçet's disease, *Br J Ophthalmol* 70:589-592, 1986.
76. Mamo JG: Treatment of Behçet's disease with chlorambucil, *Arch Ophthalmol* 94:580-583, 1976.
77. Tricoulis D: Treatment of Behçet's disease with chlorambucil, *Br J Ophthalmol* 60:55-57, 1976.
78. Hijikata K, Masuda K: Visual prognosis in Behçet's disease: effects of cyclophosphamide and colchicine, *Jpn J Ophthalmol* 22:506-519, 1978.
79. Pivetti Pezzi P, Gasparri V, De Liso P et al: Prognosis in Behçet's disease, *Ann Ophthalmol* 17:20-25, 1985.
80. Tabbara KF: Chlorambucil in Behçet disease: a reappraisal, *Ophthalmology* 90:906-908, 1983.
81. Kazokoglu H, Saatci O, Cuhadaroglu H et al: Long-term effects of cyclophosphamide and colchicine treatment in Behçet's disease, *Ann Ophthalmol* 23:148-151, 1991.
82. Takeuchi F, Takeuchi A: Chromosome aberration in lymphocytes from Behçet's disease, *J Rheumatol* 18:1207-1210, 1991.
83. Hamza M, Meddeb S, Mili I et al: Bolus of cyclophosphamide and methylprednisolone in uveitis in Behçet's disease: preliminary results with the use of new criteria of evaluation, *Ann Med Interne (Paris)* 143:438-441, 1992.
84. Yazici H, Pazarli H, Barnes CG et al: A controlled trial of azathioprine in Behçet's syndrome, *N Engl J Med* 322:281-285, 1990.
85. O'Duffy JD: *N Engl J Med* 322:326-328, 1990 (comment).
86. Tabbara K: *N Engl J Med* 323:195, 1990 (comment).
87. Aktulga E, Altaç M, Müftüoglu A et al: A double blind study of colchicine in Behçet's disease, *Haematologica (Budap)* 65:399-402, 1980.
88. Nussenblatt RB, Palestine AG, Chan CC et al: Effectiveness of cyclosporine therapy for Behçet's disease, *Arthritis Rheum* 28:671-679, 1985.
89. Masuda K, Nakajima A, Urayama A et al: Double-masked trial of cyclosporin versus colchicine and long-term open study of cyclosporin in Behçet's disease, *Lancet* 1:1093-1096, 1989.
90. BenEzra D, Brodsky M, Peér J et al: Ciclosporin (CyA) versus conventional therapy in Behçet's disease: preliminary observations of a masked study. In Schindler R, editor: *Ciclosporin in autoimmune diseases,* Berlin, 1985, Springer-Verlag.
91. Assuman Ü, Müftüoglu H, Pazarli S et al: Treatment of ocular involvement in Behçet's disease with ciclosporin A (preliminary report). In Schindler R, editor: *Ciclosporin in autoimmune diseases,* Berlin, 1985, Springer-Verlag.
92. Özyazgan Y, Yurdakul S, Yazici H et al: Low dose cyclosporin A versus pulsed cyclophosphamide in Behçet's syndrome: a single masked trial, *Br J Ophthalmol* 76:241-243, 1992.
93. Kotake S, Ichiishi A, Kosaka S et al: Low dose cyclosporin treatment for ocular lesions of Behçet's disease, *Nippon Ganka Gakkai Zasshi* 96:1290-1294, 1992.
94. Chavis PS, Antonio SR, Tabbara KF: Cyclosporine effects on optic nerve and retinal vasculitis in Behçet's disease, *Doc Ophthalmol* 80:133-142, 1992.
95. Whitcup SM, Salvo EC Jr, Nussenblatt RB: Combined cyclosporine and corticosteroid therapy for sight threatening uveitis in Behçet's disease, *Am J Ophthalmol* 118:39-45, 1994.
96. Elidan J, Levi H, Cohen E et al: Effect of cyclosporine A on the hearing loss in Behçet's disease, *Ann Otol Rhinol Laryngol* 100:464-468, 1991.
97. Koga T, Yano T, Ichikawa Y et al: Pulmonary infiltrates recovered by FK506 in a patient with Behçet's disease, *Chest* 104:309-311, 1993.
98. Bonnet M, Ouzan D, Trepo C: Plasma exchange and acyclovir in Behçet's disease, *J Fr Ophthalmol* 9:15-22, 1986.
99. Allen BR: The use of thalidomide in orogenital ulceration: an overview. In Lehner T, Barnes CG, editors: *Recent advances in Behçet's disease,* London, 1986, Royal Society of Medicine Services.
100. Hamza MH: Treatment of Behçet's disease with thalidomide, *Clin Rheumatol* 5:365-371, 1986.
101. Ranselaar CG, Boone RM, Kluin-Nelemans HC: Thalidomide in the treatment of neuro-Behçet's syndrome, *Br J Dermatol* 115:367-370, 1986.
102. Takeuchi A, Hashimoto T: Oral prostaglandin $E_1$ as therapeutic modality for leg ulcers in Behçet's disease, *Int J Clin Pharmacol Res* 7:283-289, 1987.
103. O'Duffy JD, Robertson DM, Goldstein NP: Chlorambucil in the treatment of uveitis and menngoencephalitis of Behçet's disease, *Am J Med* 76:75-84, 1984.

## SELECTED READINGS

Dilsen N, Koniçe M, Övöl C, editors: *Behçet's disease,* Amsterdam, 1979, Excerpta Medica.

Inaba G, editor: *Behçet's disease: pathogenetic, mechanism, and clinical feature,* Tokyo, 1982, University of Tokyo Press.

Wechsler B, Godeau P, editors: *Behçet's disease,* Amsterdam, 1993, Excerpta Medica.

# CHAPTER 26

# Retinal Vasculitis

Retinal vascular involvement in many cases of posterior and intermediate uveitis is a common occurrence. The use of the term *vasculitis* is somewhat of a misnomer, because it suggests that the underlying mechanism leading to these alterations is that of a type III hypersensitivity reaction—that is, that of immune complexes. We simply do not know that to be true. Indeed, the evidence available in experimental models, as well as from eyes that have been evaluated, suggests that this is rather not the case. The meager pathologic data available indicate that probably the most accurate term for these entities is a *perivasculitis* and, in most cases, *phlebitis*. Although there are conditions in which the retinal vascular component is the predominant feature of the ocular disease, the ubiquitous nature of these retinal vascular alterations indicates that "retinal vasculitis" can also be a clinical sign. Behçet's disease is perhaps the sine qua non of retinal vasculitis (see Chapter 25); however, myriad disorders can have the same presentation.

## CLINICAL CHARACTERISTICS

Although this chapter deals with multiple mechanisms, patients with retinal vasculitis most often report a painless decrease or marked loss of vision, which may at times be accompanied by floaters. There can also be large areas of scotomata relating to the areas of ischemia. If the retinal vascular changes are in the periphery of the fundus, then patients may report minimal symptoms or none at all, even in light of marked changes noted on ocular examination.

An examination of the retina shows striking vascular alterations, sometimes best seen with use of fluorescein angiography. Active vascular disease is characterized by sheathing of the vessels or in some cases, such as in sarcoidosis, an immense inflammatory response around the vessels that has been described as "candle-wax drippings." Sheathing can skip along the length of a vessel. Although we can only presume what is occurring histologically, it is thought that a perivasculitis is underlying what we describe clinically as sheathing: large numbers of cells either leaving or entering the vessels. What is drawing them there? The simple answer is that it is not known. Speculation easily abounds. It could be due to the expression of vascular endothelial antigens, adhesion molecules, or simple passage of immune cells through the vessel wall to reach the retina and its uveitogenic antigens, or a mixture of all.

Another characteristic of retinal vasculitis is the occlusive retinopathy that can be prominent in some cases. Large areas of capillary dropout are commonly seen. In many inflammatory conditions of the retina, the capillary free zone takes on a markedly jagged and enlarged appearance. Often, in addition to capillary dropout, one sees vascular architectural alterations just temporal to the macula, sometimes manifesting as arteriolar/venule anastomoses and crossing of vessels over the horizontal raphe.

The involvement of primarily the retinal vasculature in an inflammatory disorder is rather commonly seen, the best example being Behçet's disease, discussed in Chapter 25.

However, other well-recognized entities, such as birdshot retinochoroidopathy (see Chapter 24) and sarcoidosis (see Chapter 21), as well as infectious processes, have or can have marked involvement of the retinal vasculature, although we frequently do not think of these diseases in that sense. Indeed, the list of entities with a significant retinal vasculature component is noted in Box 26-1. It is important to note that noninflammatory conditions can also lead to what appears to be a retinal vasculitis. Venous obstruction, Coats' disease, and diabetes mellitus can mimic the changes seen in an inflammatorily driven process.

**Box 26-1**
**Disorders with retinal vasculitis as common finding**

**SYSTEMIC DISORDERS**

- Behçet's disease
- Sarcoidosis
- Systemic lupus erythematosus
- Postvaccination
- Multiple sclerosis
- Wegener's granulomatosis
- Takayasu's disease
- Buerger's disease
- Polyarteritis nodosa
- Polymyositis
- Dermatomyositis
- Whipple's disease
- Crohn's disease
- Sjögren's A antigen

**INFECTIOUS DISORDERS**

- Syphilis
- Toxoplasmosis
- Toxocariasis
- Coccidiomycosis
- Tuberculosis
- Cytomegalovirus
- Herpes simplex
- Herpes zoster
- ARN Acute retinal necrosis
- Candidiasis
- Leptospirosis
- Rickettsia
- Brucellosis
- Amebiasis
- Mononucleosis
- Lyme disease
- Hepatitis

**OCULAR DISORDERS**

- Birdshot retinochoroidopathy
- Pars planitis
- Eales' disease
- Chorioditis
- Retinal arteritis and aneurysms
- Behçet retina sine systemic disease
- Vein occlusion

## OCULAR VASCULITIC DISORDERS WITHOUT SYSTEMIC DISEASE

We have seen patients with ocular findings that make them indistinguishable from patients with Behçet's disease. These patients have none of the systemic findings typical of retinal vasculitis but yet will have recurrent episodes. In addition, some of these persons show HLA-B51 positivity. The possibility that they may develop Behçet's disease certainly exists. However, on a statistical basis, one would expect other features of the disorder to develop within 3 years of the first criteria, and this has not been the case. The recurrent episodes of retinal vasculitis (and retinitis) are frequently difficult to control and may require other immunosuppressive agents in addition to prednisone. Lueck and coworkers[1] reported the case of a patient with recurrent steroid-sensitive uveitis and central nervous system (CNS) disease thought to be due to sarcoidosis. Postmortem examination revealed a histologic picture compatible with Behçet's disease, despite the patient's lack of any of the systemic stigmata associated with this diagnosis. The authors have called this entity the *Behçet MINUS syndrome* (multifocal intermittent neurologic and uveitic syndrome).

We have seen other patients with severe retinal vasculitis that appears unassociated with systemic disease; often attempts to identify an underlying abnormality (e.g., immune complexes, sedimentation rate) prove fruitless. The disorder frequently may continue in spite of aggressive immunotherapy.

### Eales' disease

Although Eales' disease had been discussed by others, the disorder carries the name of Henry Eales who, in 1882,[2] described five young men with recurring vitreal and retinal hemorrhages that were associated with constipation and epistaxis. The definition of the condition has varied considerably over the years. Our group defines Eales' disease as an idiopathic condition that manifests as an obliterative perivasculitis (particularly involving the venule side) affecting the retina in multiple quadrants, starting at or anterior to the equator and progressing posteriorly. The disease sometimes is accompanied by neovascularization, without vitritis, obvious uveal inflammation, or obvious systemic disease. It is in essence a diagnosis of exclusion and probably includes a heterogeneous patient population. There is a strong association with purified protein derivative (PPD) skin positivity,[3] and Pahwa and colleagues[4] reported that strongly positive Mantoux test results were found in 87% of 141 cases. The disease has been estimated to affect 1% of the adult males in India and usually occurs in patients younger than 40 years of age. The process has minimal inflammation associated with it.

The disorder may start with retinal edema, followed by a progressive cuffing of the venules (periphlebitis), followed by peripheral retinal vascular nonperfusion and retinal neovascularization.[5] The condition is one of the retinal periphery, but on occasion it can begin at the optic nerve head, mimicking a vein occlusion. Only with the more characteristic peripheral retinal signs will the diagnosis become clear. The arteries are not involved. Unlike occlusions that result from arteriosclerotic plaques, the occlusion that may occur does not have a propensity to take place at an arteriovenous crossing. The periphlebitis may occlude substantial portions of a vein but in an irregular fashion. Unlike vein occlusions in the posterior pole, those in the periphery will not cause cotton-wool spots.[6] The development of neovascularization may be rapid. Fluorescein angiography examination of the retinal vasculature may show nonperfusion, arteriovenous shunting, and neovascularization (Fig. 26-1). Recurrent vitreous hemorrhage, with ensuing vitreous contraction and retinal detachment, is a serious risk in this disorder.

Although the disease may proceed with its full-blown picture as described, in some patients the disease process may spontaneously reverse itself. The visual prognosis in these patients is not totally hopeless. Elliot[7] reported that 25 of 46 eyes he followed for an average of 6 years had a visual acuity of 20/50 or better, whereas 26% had a vision of 20/200 or worse.

That this is an immune-driven process is still speculative. Part of the definition calls for minimal or no evidence of inflammatory disease. Muthukkaruppan and associates[8] found circulating immune complexes in these patients. Rennie and associates[9] have also noted vestibuloauditory problems associated with the ocular condition, suggesting that this is indeed a systemic ailment. The notion that the disease is due to tuberculosis hypersensitivity is difficult to support because the disease does not seem to be noted in greater number in countries that actively immunize their populace with bacille Calmette-Guérin (BCG) vaccine. It may be that mycobacterial antigens are particularly good initiators of a still-undefined disease mechanism but that other antigens probably are capable of producing the same effect.

Therapy is problematic. For patients with capillary dropout and neovascularization, laser

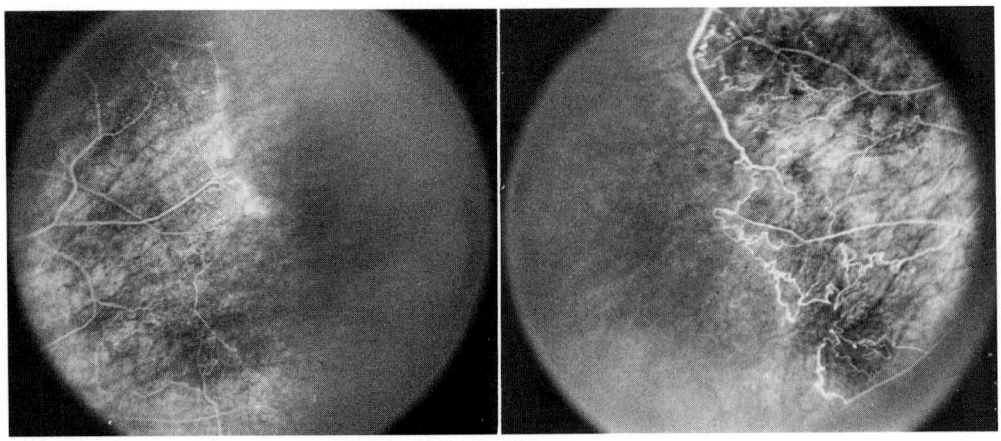


**Fig. 26-1. A** and **B,** Peripheral retinal vasoocclusive disease with neovascularization due to Eales' disease. (Courtesy R. Murphy, M.D.)

ablation could be contemplated. Vitrectomy certainly plays a role in the management of these patients who have recurrent vitreous hemorrhages. Immunosuppressive therapy has not seemed particularly effective in treating the disorder, but it is frequently used as a last resort.

### Retinal aneurysms with arteritis

A rare condition in which multiple sacular and fusiform aneurysms involving the larger arterioles, combined with peripheral vascular nonperfusion and uveitis, has been reported.[10,11] The degree of nonperfusion can be quite profound (Fig. 26-2). A neuroretinitis, as well as retinal neovascularization, optic nerve head swelling, and anterior uveitis, can be associated with this disorder. The disorder occurs in younger persons. It is not clear whether immunosuppressive agents provide beneficial therapy for this condition. Laser photocoagulation has been shown to benefit only a very small number of patients. The underlying nature of the disorder remains in doubt.

Jampol and colleagues[12] reported a case of occlusive retinal arteriolitis with neovascularization. Although the course of the 34-year-white woman whose case is reported had some similarities to the entity just described, no aneurysms were noted.

### Frosted-branch angiitis

Frosted-branch angiitis was first reported in a 6-year-old boy with vessels resembling frosted branches.[13] The disorder usually results in a severe drop in visual acuity, at least during the acute period of the disease. Although both arteries and veins may be involved, the venules tend to be more commonly affected (Fig. 26-3). No specific etiologic factors have been found.

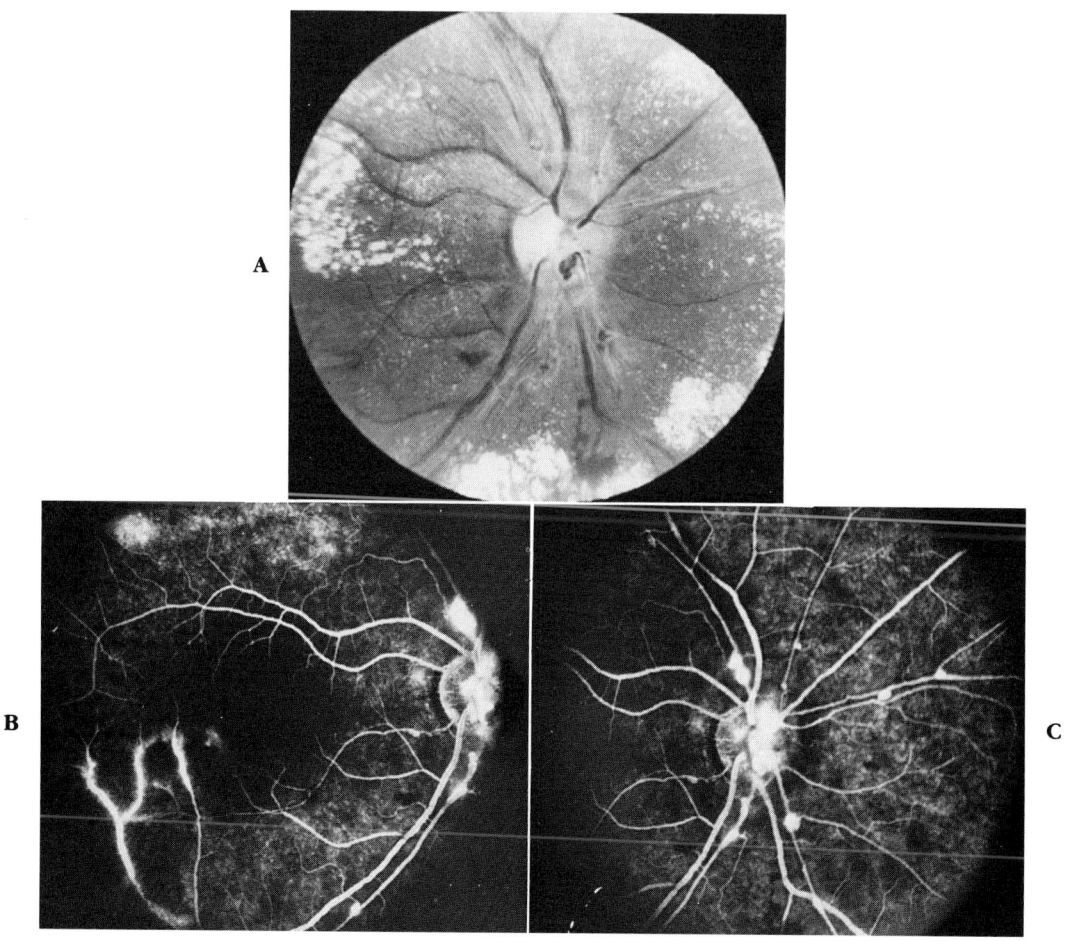


**Fig. 26-2. A** to **C,** Patient with retinal aneurysms and arteritis. Note extensive exudate and hemorrhage, sheathing of vessels, and macroaneurysms. Extensive capillary dropout was seen just beyond these areas of exudate.

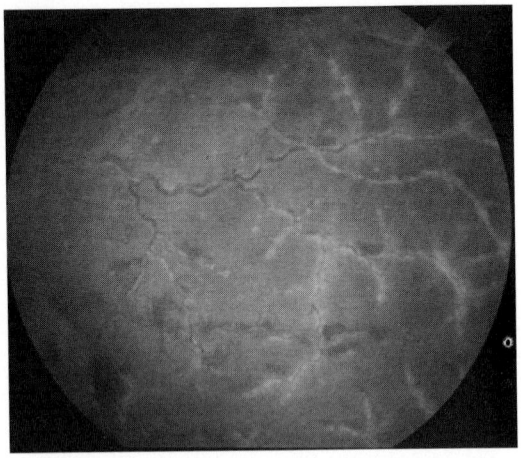

**Fig. 26-3.** Fundus of young boy with idiopathic frosted-branch angiitis. Yannuzzi has suggested that angiitis is seen in children whereas periphlebitis generally is noted in young adults. (Courtesy L. A. Yannuzzi, M.D.) (See Color Plate 41.)

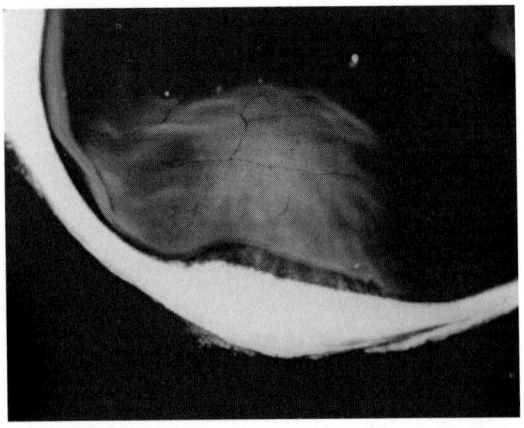

**Fig. 26-4.** Although not retinal vasculitis, posterior scleritis should be considered in patients with poor vision, pain, uveitis, and striae of choroid. (Courtesy David Cogan, M.D.)

One can speculate that it is an extreme example of a diffuse perivasculitis. The "frosting" around the vessels could be in fact thousands (millions?) of cells that are moving through the vascular wall into the retina. It is a condition that will disappear with proper and aggressive therapy. This disorder usually responds to steroids, with treatment advocated in the literature as 1 to 1½ mg/kg prednisone for 10 days.

Similar retinal vascular changes have been described in several conditions. Some of the disorders that need to be considered include sarcoidosis, multiple sclerosis, pars planitis, tuberculosis, syphilis, and systemic lupus erythematosus (SLE) and AIDS-related retinopathies.

### Scleritis

Although scleritis certainly is not a disease of the retinal vasculature, it seems important to discuss it and how it may relate to intraocular inflammatory disease. The vasculature near the scleritis appear to be integrally involved in the inflammatory/pathologic process, with medial necrosis, perivasculitis, or thrombosis often seen.[14,15] The inflammatory reaction associated with an anterior scleritis can spill over into the eye, leading to anterior or even intermediate uveitis. Posterior scleritis is an entity that is frequently not included in the differential diagnosis of posterior pole lesions[16] (Fig. 26-4). This disorder may not be associated with anterior segment changes. Patients frequently report ocular pain, although the eye does not appear inflamed. At times the conjunctiva may be slightly boggy. There may be a mild vitreous inflammatory response associated with a drop in visual acuity. Careful examination of the posterior segment may reveal choroidal folds or even a thickening of the retina, although these processes are often subtle and difficult to determine. Ultrasound examination of the globe is a very useful tool to help in the diagnosis. In many cases the disease responds to corticosteroid therapy, although relapse may occur once the dosage is decreased.

One note of caution. Although most cases of posterior scleritis are not associated with a systemic disorder, it is fitting to consider this caveat. The ophthalmologist needs to be always aware of the fact that this entity can manifest as a systemic disorder, and a careful rheumatologic evaluation seems warranted in most cases.

## OCULAR VASCULITIC DISORDERS WITH SYSTEMIC DISEASE

Perhaps the most common systemic entities that we see with a marked vascular component are sarcoidosis, Behçet's disease, and multiple sclerosis. Although sarcoidosis is usually not thought of as the basis for a retinal vasculitis, it can cause myriad ocular manifestations, including a severe involvement of the retinal vasculature (see Chapter 21). Multiple sclerosis was first associated with ocular inflammatory disease at the turn of this century. In an early article Rucker[17] suggested that perhaps 20% of patients with multiple sclerosis may have retinal sheathing (i.e., vasculitis); others, such as Breger and Leopold,[18] have reported an even higher percentage (14 of 52 patients, or 27%). It would seem that generally fewer than 5% to 8% of these patients have this complication. Behçet's disease, the sine qua non of vasculitis, is discussed in detail in Chapter 25.

Apart from the more common ocular entities, retinal vasculitis can be associated with several systemic entities, many of these among the collagen-vascular group of disorders. A key point to consider in making these diagnoses is that usually the patient's complaints are associated with a subacute chronic disorder. The findings include malaise, weight loss, arthritis, fever, and rash. An important finding is that of mononeuritis multiplex. Mononeuritis multiplex is an acute neuropathy that begins at one named nerve root and then progresses to one or more other nerve roots, one at a time. It more commonly affects the nerve roots of the lower extremities and can have an abrupt painful onset, with the patient reporting deep muscle pain. It is a common presenting sign in polyarteritis nodosa and occurs in a significant number of patients with SLE and rheumatoid arthritis later in the course of their disease. The ophthalmologist should be aware that other disorders can cause mononeuritis multiplex, including diabetes, paraneoplastic syndromes, and even jellyfish stings.[19,20]

Some of the diseases that need to be considered in the search for a systemic cause for retinal vasculitis include the following conditions.

### Systemic lupus erythematosus

SLE is a common systemic disorder that is diagnosed by use of a combination of clinical and laboratory criteria. Thought to be the classic immune complex disorder, it affects the eye with severe intraocular complications in a relatively small number of cases. However, when it does, it can be extremely problematic because it is sometimes difficult to establish adequate therapy. Jabs and coworkers[21] reported on 11 patients with severe retinal vasoocclusive disease and poor visual outcome often associated with CNS lupus (Figs. 26-5 and 26-6). Proliferative retinopathy can be a serious problem as well.[22] This condition raises the intellectually interesting but also practically important question as to whether therapy should consist of laser photocoagulation or systemic immunotherapy to turn off the underlying inflammatory process that presumably induces the retinal vascular alterations.

### Polyarteritis nodosa

Polyarteritis nodosa was first described by Kussmaul and Maier in 1866. It is a necrotizing vasculitis that involves the medium-sized muscular arteries and smaller arterioles. It can present as a bilateral iritis, vitritis, and retinal vasculitis involving both the veins and arteries.[23] It has been estimated that up to 20% of these patients may have ocular involvement.[24] Mononeuritis multiplex, an acute neuropathy described before, has been estimated to develop in two thirds of patients with polyarteritis nodosa. The most common sites are those in the lower extremities. This is a potentially fatal disorder, and current therapy usually consists of corticosteroids and cyclophosphamide.

### Wegener's granulomatosis

Wegener's granulomatosis is characterized by a necrotizing granulomatous vasculitis of the upper and lower respiratory tract, systemic small vessel vasculitis that can involve multiple organs, and a focal necrotizing glomerulonephritis. Ocular complications, including uveitis, scleritis, and retinal vasculitis, can occur in 16% of patients.[25,26] It is important to remember that the anti–neutrophil cytoplasmic antibody (cANCA) test is highly specific for this disease. Soukasian and coworkers[27] reported that the ANCA test result was positive in seven patients with scleritis due to Wegener's granulomatosis but was negative in 54 patients with ocular inflammatory disease due to other causes. Others have reported the usefulness of this test not only for diagnosing but also for following the course of the disease.[28,29]

Two caveats should be kept in mind for the eye care physician. Two patterns of ANCA are reported—a cytoplasmic pattern (cANCA), which is believed to be more specific for Wegener's granulomatosis, and a peripheral pattern (pANCA), which is less useful in making the diagnosis. Young,[30] in testing patients with uveitis, used the ANCA test and found positive results in cases of chronic uveitis of various underlying causes. Because the interpretation of this test is performed manually and there can

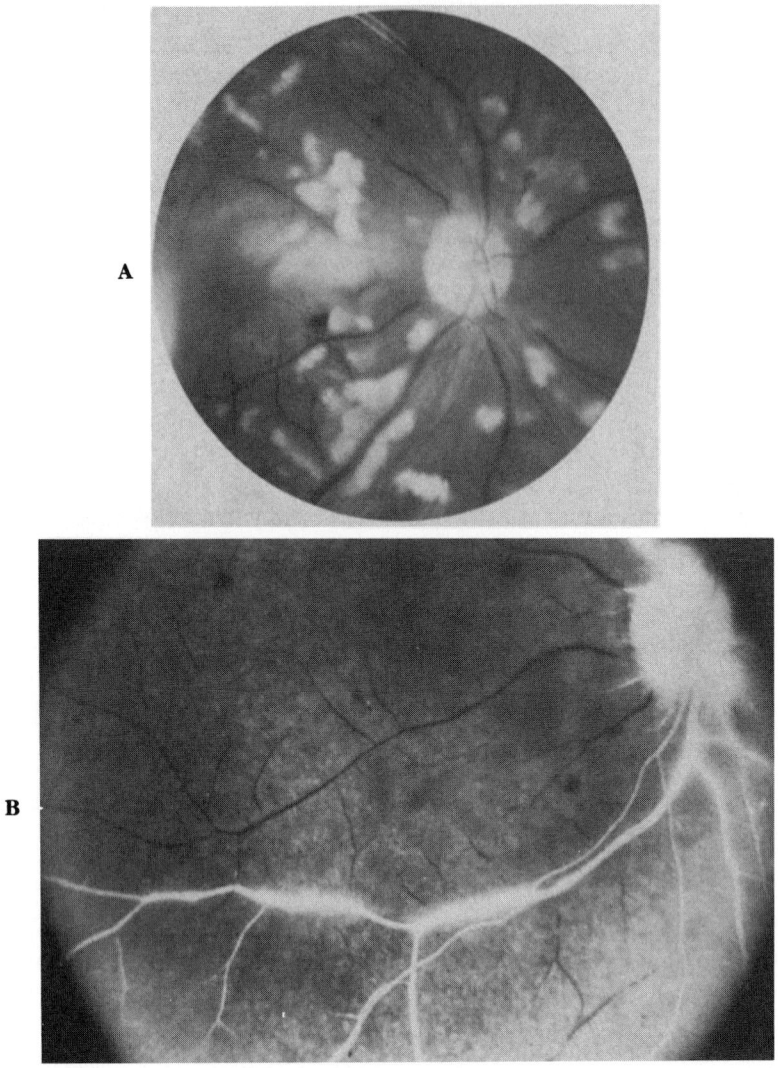


**Fig. 26-5.** Systemic lupus erythematosus. **A,** Fundus shows multiple cotton-wool spots, arterial occlusion, vascular sheathing, and intraretinal hemorrhage. **B,** Extensive nonperfusion, with staining of retinal vessels walls. (Courtesy D. A. Jabs, M.D.; from Jabs DA, Fine SL, Hochberg MC et al: Severe retinal vaso-occlusive disease in systemic lupus erythematosus, *Arch Ophthalmol* 104:558-563, 1986.)

be great variation in results, an enzyme-linked immunosorbent assay (ELISA), directed toward proteinase 3, is now being used. The second caveat is that if a high suspicion remains in the physician's mind, it is useful to repeat the cANCA, because results may initially be negative in Wegener's granulomatosis localized to the orbit or eye but they will become positive with time.

### Whipple's disease

Whipple's disease is a multisystem disorder usually manifesting by malabsorption, diarrhea, and polyarthritis. It has been estimated that less than 5% of cases will have uveitis. The disease is believed due to the Whipple's disease bacillus *(Tropheryma whippelii),* which can be found in vitreous specimens using electron microscopy and the polymerase chain reaction (PCR), along with foamy macrophages.[30a]

In a small number of cases reported, fluorescein angiography results show diffuse vasculitis with hemorrhages, exudates, retinal capillary occlusion, and choroidal folds.[31]

### Crohn's disease

Crohn's disease commonly affects the eye in several ways, including uveitis (pars planitis), retinitis, scleritis, and keratitis. However, Duker and colleagues[32] reported the case of a patient

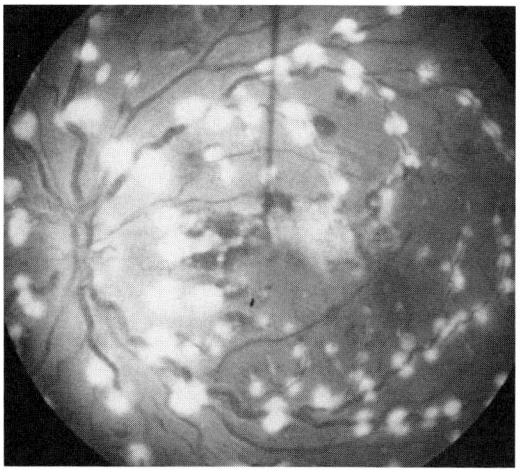

**Fig. 26-6.** Fundus of young woman with difficult-to-control systemic lupus erythematosus. Extensive nerve fiber infarcts and hemorrhage create dramatic picture, with maintenance of good visual acuity. Retinopathy cleared after disease was controlled. (See Color Plate 42.)

with a severe bilateral, obliterative, retinal arteritis and phlebitis. The disorder appeared to respond to systemic corticosteroid and cyclophosphamide therapy. Ruby and Jampol[33] reported on the cases of two patients with retinal vascular disease, one of which had disease involving both the retinal arteries and veins, with an apparent branch retinal artery occlusion.

### Autoantibodies to Sjögren's syndrome A antigen

This systemic lupus–like illness may be systemically mild, but retinal arteriolitis that leads to retinal ischemia, optic disc, and retinal neovascularization may occur.[34]

### Retinal vein occlusion

It is important to note that putative nonimmune mechanisms may lead to ophthalmoscopic findings that mimic an immune-driven pathologic condition[35] such as retinal vein occlusion. After thrombosis, the vein occlusion can develop a secondary perivasculitis.

### Relapsing polychondritis

Relapsing polychondritis is a systemic inflammatory disease of connective tissue that may have associated ocular manifestations. The diagnosis is characteristically made by observation of inflammation of the cartilage of the nose, earlobes, or trachea. Two of these sites suffice for the diagnosis. Alternately, one such site combined with two of the following associated signs is consistent with a diagnosis of polychondritis: hearing loss, vestibular imbalance, ocular inflammation, or rheumatoid factor–negative arthritis. In a review of 112 patients, Isaak and colleagues[36] found ocular signs or symptoms in 21 at the time of diagnosis. Ocular involvement occurred in 57 of these patients at some time during their course. The most common ocular findings were episcleritis (39%) and scleritis (14%). Iridocyclitis has been observed in as many as 30% of patients with this disease[37] but was found in only 9% in the series by Isaak and coworkers. Retinopathy, primarily exudates and hemorrhages, were seen in 9% as well. Occasionally retinal vascular occlusions, serous retinal detachments, and optic neuropathy develop. A systemic vasculitis was reported in 9% of the patients,[36] demonstrating the systemic inflammatory nature of this syndrome. Vessels of any caliber may be involved. It is possible that although the episcleral and scleral involvement in this disease is immunologically similar to the mechanisms that lead to inflammation of the cartilage, the other ocular manifestations that are seen are not tissue-specific but are part of the varied accompanying systemic vascular involvement.

### Viral diseases

The exact role of virus in the development of a vasculitis of the retinal vasculature with no overt destruction of the retina itself still remains to be defined. It is clear that viruses can cause vascular endothelial cells to express receptors that might make them more susceptible to involvement in an immune event. Iwase and coworkers[38] reported on a 6-year-old child who first developed a dendritic corneal ulcer and iritis due to herpes simplex virus type 1, followed by a drop in vision due to a retinal periphlebitis and vitreal inflammatory reaction that responded to acyclovir therapy.

### Tuberculosis

Central retinal artery vasculitis leading to occlusion[39] (see Chapter 10) has been noted.

### Rheumatoid arthritis

In a report by Giordano and colleagues,[40] 11 of 60 patients (18.3%) with rheumatoid arthritis had fluorescein angiographic evidence of retinal vasculitis.

The induction of an experimental autoimmune type of vasculitis in the lungs and brain, as well as elsewhere has been noted in mice after mice lymphocytes were co-cultured with a mouse endothelial cell line.[41]

• • •

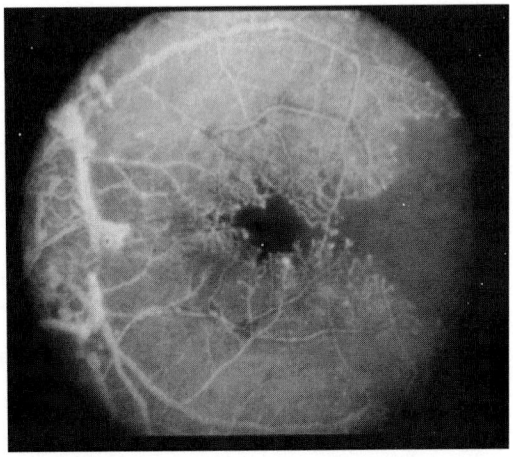

**Fig. 26-7.** Fluorescein angiogram of left eye of 16-year-old woman with decreased vision who suffered from recurrent vitreous hemorrhages. Extensive work-up failed to demonstrate any systemic disorder. High-dose oral prednisone was not successful in preventing progression of disorder.

In summary, this group of disorders that primarily affects the retinal vasculature frequently presents great challenges to treating physicians. In the case of well-defined disorders such as Behçet's disease, aggressive therapy is known to be imperative, with various immunosuppressive avenues open. However, some cases of retinal vascular disease may be quite severe but are neither associated with a systemic disorder nor are well-characterized in the literature. Therefore their natural history is unknown, and they frequently are not associated with impressive inflammatory disease (Figs. 26-7 and 26-8). The therapeutic approach to these cases is problematic and often compounded by the presence of neovascularization. On the basis of purely anecdotal evidence, we have become more convinced that aggressive panretinal photocoagulation (PRP) may have a beneficial effect on the course of the retinal vascular disease, even with no evidence of neovascularization. Indeed, this therapy has seemed to be the only modality that has stabilized some severe cases of retinal vasculitis. It should be added that we have seen severe inflammatory episodes apparently provoked by such an intervention. However, even with that risk, it still may be the indicated approach—clearly if there is evidence of capillary dropout on the angiogram, but perhaps even if there is not.

A

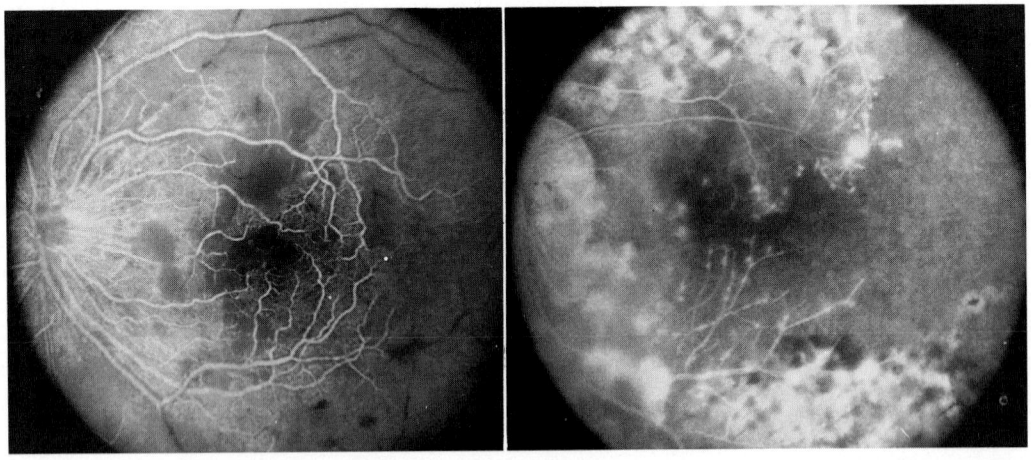

B

**Fig. 26-8. A,** Fluorescein angiogram of 46-year-old man who developed poor vision associated initially with low-grade intraocular inflammatory response. Extensive systemic evaluation revealed no abnormalities. Note extensive capillary loss involving significant portion of posterior pole, as well as nonperfusion of larger vessels. Aggressive immunosuppression to point of toxicity was initiated with no therapeutic effect noted. **B,** Angiogram obtained 9 months after **A** shows further loss of retinal vasculature. Areas of circular hyperfluorescence are from panretinal photocoagulation (PRP), which had been recently initiated, resulting in some stabilization of disorder. However, with such extensive loss already taken place, long-term visual prospects are most guarded.

## REFERENCES


1. Lueck CJ, Pires M, McCartney AC et al: Ocular and neurological Behçet's disease without orogenital ulceration? *J Neurol Neurosurg Psychiatry* 56:505-508, 1993.
2. Eales H: Cases of retinal hemorrhage associated with epistaxis and constipation, *Birmingham Med Rev* 9:262-273, 1880.
3. Ashton N: Pathogenesis and aetiology of Eales's disease. In Pandit YK, editor: *Nineteenth International Congress of Ophthalmology,* Bombay, 1962, The Time of India Press.
4. Moura RA, Oréfice F: Retinal vasculitis. In Oréfice F, Belfort R Jr, editors: *Uveítes,* São Paulo, 1987, Roca.
5. Das T, Biswas J, Kumar A et al: Eales' disease, *Indian J Ophthalmol* 42:3-18, 1994.
6. Wise GN, Dollery CT, Henkind P: *The retinal circulation,* New York, 1971, Harper & Row.
7. Elliot AJ: Recurrent intraocular hemorrhage in young adults (Eales' disease), *Trans Am Ophthalmol Soc* 52:811, 1954.
8. Muthukkaruppan V, Rengarajan K, Chakkalath HR et al: Immunological status of patients of Eales' disease, *Indian J Med Res* 90:351-359, 1989.
9. Rennie WA, Murphy RP, Anderson KC et al: The evaluation of patients with Eales' disease, *Retina* 3:243-247, 1983.
10. Karel I, Peleska M, Divisová G: Fluorescence angiography in retinal vasculitis in children's uveitis, *Ophthalmologica* 166:251-264, 1973.
11. Kincaid J, Schatz H: Bilateral retinal arteritis with multiple aneurysmal dilations, *Retina* 3:171-178, 1983.
12. Jampol LM, Isenberg SJ, Goldberg MF: Occlusive retinal arteriolitis with neovascularization, *Am J Ophthalmol* 81:583-589, 1978.
13. Ito Y, Nakano M, Kyu N et al: Frosted branch angiitis in a child, *Jpn J Clin Ophthalmol* 30:797-803, 1976.
14. Watson PG: The nature and treatment of scleral inflammation, *Trans Ophthalmol Soc UK* 102:257-281, 1982.
15. Watson PG: Diseases of the sclera and episclera. In Duane TD, Jaeger EA, editors: Clinical ophthalmology, vol 4, Philadelphia, 1987, Harper & Row.
16. Benson WE: Posterior scleritis, *Surv Ophthalmol* 32: 297-316, 1988.
17. Rucker CW: Sheathing of the retinal veins in multiple sclerosis, *JAMA* 127:970-973, 1945.
18. Breger BC, Leopold IH: The incidence of uveitis in multiple sclerosis, *Am J Ophthalmol* 62:540-545, 1966.
19. Hellman DB, Laing TJ, Petri M et al: Mononeuritis multiplex: the yield of evaluations for occult rheumatic diseases, *Medicine* 67:145-153, 1988.
20. Hellmann DB: Mononeuritis multiplex. In Klippel J, Dieppe P, editors: *Rheumatology,* Mosby, 1991.
21. Jabs DA, Fine SL, Hochberg MC et al: Severe retinal vaso-occlusive disease in systemic lupus erythematosus, *Arch Ophthalmol* 104:558-563, 1986.
22. Vine AK, Barr CC: Proliferative lupus retinopathy, *Arch Ophthalmol* 102:852-854, 1984.
23. Morgan CM, Foster CS, Gragoudas ES: Retinal vasculitis in polyarteritis nodosa, *Retina* 6:205-209, 1986.
24. Stillermen ML: Ocular manifestations of diffuse collagen disease, *Arch Ophthalmol* 45:239-250, 1951.
25. Fauci AS, Haynes BF, Katz P et al: Wegener's granulomatosis: prospective clinical and therapeutic experience with 85 patients for 21 years, *Ann Intern Med* 98:76-85, 1983.
26. Mangouritsas G, Ulbig M: Cotton-wool spots as the initial ocular manifestation in Wegener's granulomatosis, *German J Ophthalmol* 3:68-70, 1994.
27. Soukasian SH, Foster CS, Niles JL et al: Diagnostic value of anti-neutrophil cytoplasmic antibodies in scleritis associated with Wegener's granulomatosis, *Ophthalmology* 99:125-132, 1992.
28. Nolle B, Specks U, Ludemann J et al: Anticytoplasmic autoantibodies: their immunodiagnostic value in Wegener's granulomatosis and anticytoplasmic antibodies, *Ann Intern Med* 111:28-40, 1989.
29. Cohen Tervaert JW, van der Woude FJ, Fauci AS et al: Association between active Wegener's granulomatosis and anticytoplasmic antibodies, *Arch Intern Med* 149:2461-2465, 1989.
30. Young DW: The antineutrophil antibody in uveitis, *Br J Ophthalmol* 75:208-211, 1991.

30a. Rickman LS, Freeman WR, Green WR et al: Brief report: uveitis caused by *Tropheryma whippelli* (Whipple's bacillus), N Engl J Med 332:363-366, 1995.

31. Avila MP, Jalkh AE, Feldman E et al: Manifestations of Whipple's disease in the posterior segment of the eye, *Arch Ophthalmol* 102:384-390, 1984.
32. Duker JS, Brown GC, Brooks L: Retinal vasculitis in Crohn's disease, *Am J Ophthalmol* 103:664-668, 1987.
33. Ruby AJ, Jampol LM: Crohn's disease and retinal vascular disease, *Am J Ophthalmol* 110:349-353, 1990.
34. Farmer SG, Kinyoun JL, Nelson JL et al: Retinal vasculitis associated with autoantibodies to Sjögren's syndrome A antigen, *Am J Ophthalmol* 100:814-821, 1985.
35. Green WR, Chan CC, Hutchins GM et al: Central retinal vein occlusion: a prospective histopathologic study of 29 eyes in 28 cases, *Trans Am Ophthalmol Soc* 79:371-422, 1981.
36. Issak BL, Liesegang TJ, Michet CJ: Ocular and systemic findings in relapsing polychondritis, *Ophthalmology* 93:681-689, 1986.
37. Matas BR: Iridocyclitis associated with relapsing polychondritis, *Arch Ophthalmol* 84:474-476, 1970.
38. Iwase K, Murao M, Komuro Y et al: A case of dendritic corneal ulcer associated with retinal periphlebitis and uveitis: a new diagnostic method and treatment, *Rinsho Ganka* 40:403-407, 1986.
39. Fountain JA, Wemer RB: Tuberculosis retinal vasculitis, *Retina* 4:48-50, 1984.
40. Giordano N, D'Ettorre M, Biasi G et al: Retinal vasculitis in rheumatoid arthritis: an angiographic study, *Clin Exp Rheumatol* 8:121-125, 1990.
41. Hart MN, Sadewasser KL, Cancilla PA et al: Experimental autoimmune type of vasculitis resulting from activation of mouse lymphocytes to cultured endothelium, *Lab Invest* 48:419-427, 1983.

# CHAPTER 27

# Serpiginous Choroidopathy

Serpiginous choroidopathy is a clinically defined disorder characterized by destruction of the inner choroid and the retinal pigment epithelium (RPE), as well as secondary involvement of the retina. This entity has been known by a multitude of names, including serpiginous choroiditis, geographic choroiditis, geographic choroidopathy, geographic helicoid peripapillary choroidopathy, and macular geographic helicoid choroidopathy.[1-4] Although it was recognized as a distinct but poorly defined entity by the early part of this century, our understanding of this disease remains limited. We still are not sure whether the retinal destruction seen in serpiginous choroidopathy is predominantly mediated by an inflammatory process or by an abiotrophy. In fact, the clinical spectrum of serpiginous choroidopathy may represent several different diseases.

## CLINICAL FEATURES

The typical patient with serpiginous choroidopathy is middle-aged without any major underlying medical problems. Although the disease has been reported in patients of varying ethnic backgrounds, it may more commonly involve white persons. In some series there is a slight preponderance of males with this disorder.[5]

Patients usually report blurred vision or a central or pericentral scotoma in one eye, although examination usually reveals bilateral disease. Serpiginous choroidopathy primarily affects the choroid, choriocapillaris, and RPE. The terms *serpiginous, helicoid,* and *geographic* describe the appearance of the chorioretinal disease, which progresses in a serpentine fashion, usually starting at the optic disc and winding through the posterior pole (Fig. 27-1). Acute lesions appear gray-white or yellow and involve the choriocapillaris and RPE. On careful examination these new lesions appear to have "substance," and they subtly elevate the overlying retina. Acute lesions last up to several months, but with time, lesions becomes atrophic, with disappearance of the choriocapillaris and involvement of the underlying large choroidal vessels.[6] Thinning of the overlying neurosensory retina usually follows disease of the choroid and RPE, and scarring with clumps of RPE are common late in the course of the disease.

Patients rarely have a solitary active lesion involving the posterior pole. Much more commonly, active lesions occur adjacent to an area of choroidal and RPE atrophy. An area of chorioretinal atrophy usually can be found next to the optic disc in symptom-free contralateral eye.

Reports in the literature concerning the inflammatory component associated with the choroidal and RPE lesions of serpiginous choroidopathy vary greatly. Hamilton and Bird,[7] for example, observed no inflammatory disease in the patients they studied. In our experience,

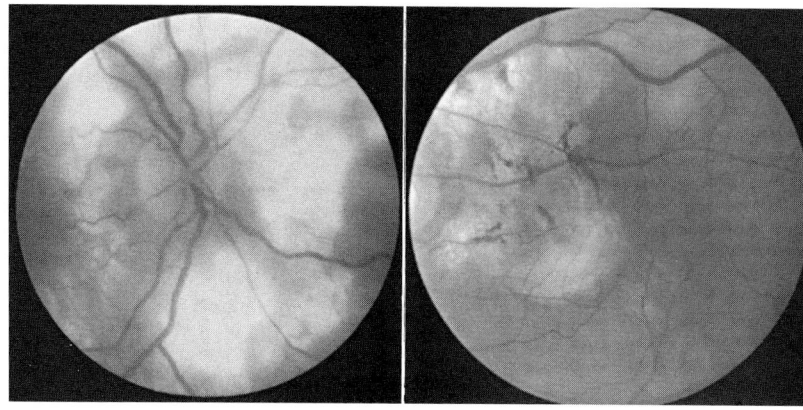


**Fig. 27-1. A,** Large serpiginous lesion surrounding optic disc. Active lesion is seen inferior to disc. Older, atrophic regions can be seen both to right and left of active lesion. Some choroidal vessels can be noted through lesion. **B,** White active lesion, seen at edge of old atrophic area.

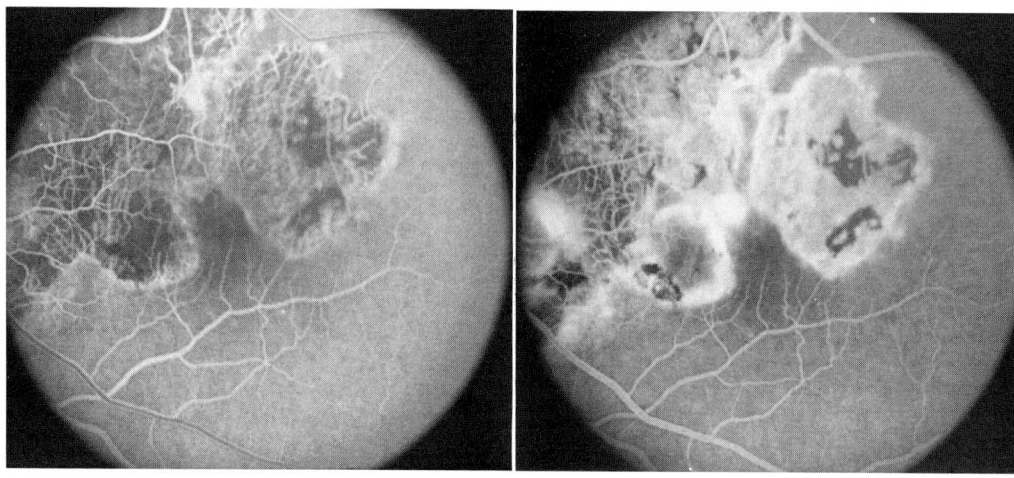


**Fig. 27-2.** Fluorescein angiogram showing choroidal neovascular membrane in patient with serpiginous choroidopathy. **A,** Early frame showing lacy hyperfluorescence. **B,** Late frame showing late leakage in area of choroidal neovascular membrane.

however, cellular reaction in the posterior vitreous can occur, especially in patients with acute lesions, and mild vitritis has been reported in about one third of cases.[8,9] Anterior uveitis has also been described in patients with serpiginous choroidopathy but is more rare.[10] It is important to look for evidence of inflammatory disease, because this finding may help in deciding whether a therapeutic intervention with antiinflammatory agents has a reasonable chance for success (see Chapter 8).

Choroidal neovascularization can also occur in serpiginous choroidopathy. Gass[11] states that choroidal neovascularization occurs in as many as 25% of patients, although we have observed this complication in fewer than 10% of our patients at the National Eye Institute. Blumenkranz and coworkers[5] reported active choroidal neovascularization in 7 of 53 patients with the disease. Choroidal neovascularization may be seen at the time the disease is diagnosed and when located in the macula, may cause a visual disturbance (Fig. 27-2). Although the choroidal neovascularization may regress spontaneously in some cases,[12] we have treated membranes threatening the fovea with laser photocoagulation. Serous detachments of the neurosensory retina, as well as RPE detachments, have been reported in patients with serpiginous choroidopathy.[10,13] Retinal vasculitis may also occur, and branch vein occlusions have been reported.[10,14]

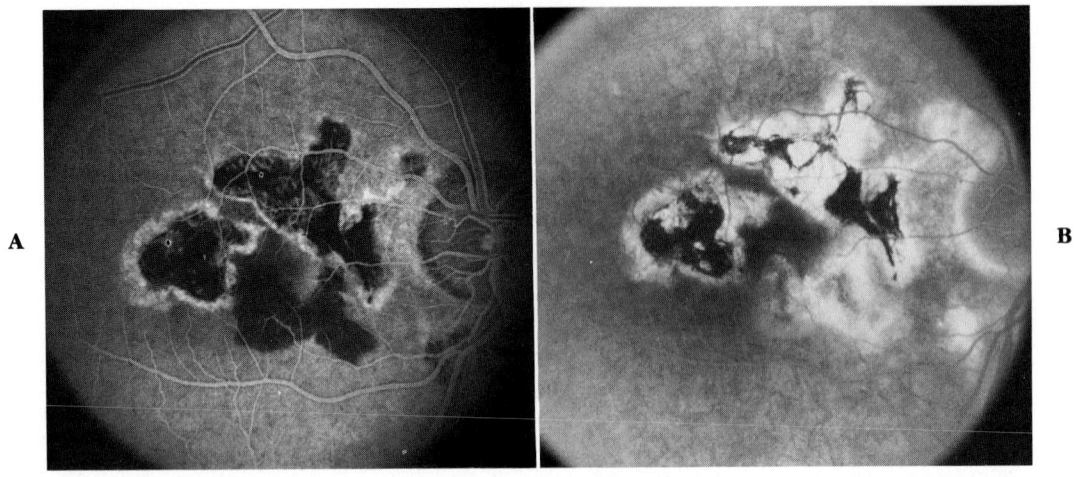


**Fig. 27-3.** Fluorescein angiogram of serpiginous lesion showing **(A)** early phase of angiogram with central blockage and **(B)** late phase, showing more diffuse hyperfluorescence. Areas that continue to block had overlying RPE clumping.

**Box 27-1**
**Findings supporting diagnosis of serpiginous choroiditis**

- Patient
  - White
  - Both sexes
  - Late teens to 60s
- Ocular examination
  - Inflammatory response in the anterior chamber or vitreous sometimes occurs
  - Lesion begins in peripapillary region; centripedal or helicoid progression, giving "geographic" distribution
  - New white-yellow lesions begin at edge of old ones
  - Bilateral involvement
- Additional tests
  - Fluorescein angiography
  - Serial fundus photographs

The disorder usually begins near the disc, with new areas of activity evident at the margin of old lesions. This centripetal or helicoid extension can continue for years. Laatikainen and Erkkilä[15] followed up 15 patients for a mean of 4.9 years and noted new lesions in 8. These acute lesions can cause a decrease in visual acuity that may return after a long recovery period. Weiss and coworkers[9] observed that visual acuity decreased in 9 of 17 eyes after an acute episode and that the visual acuity returned to the preattack level once the acute lesions resolved, although this could take a number of months. They further noted that 15 of 17 eyes ultimately developed lesions involving the fovea, although Laatikainen and Erkkilä[15] noted a loss of central vision in only 6 of 28 eyes.

The diagnosis of serpiginous choroidopathy is made purely on clinical grounds, with the major criteria listed in Box 27-1. Fluorescein angiography and serial fundus photographs are also helpful in following the disease. Fluorescein angiography examinationof an active lesion will show early blockage with late staining manifested by hyperfluorescent borders that spread toward the center of the lesion (Fig. 27-3). The early hypofluorescence of active lesions may be due to blockage of the underlying choroidal fluorescence by swollen RPE cells but more likely represents the impaired choroidal vasculature. Old atrophic lesions will show diffuse staining, and hyperfluorescence is noted in areas of RPE clumping. Late staining of the retinal vessels is seen in patients with a vasculitis or perivasculitis.

As stated earlier, most patients with serpiginous choroidopathy have no associated medical illnesses. Although scattered case reports of diseases associated with this condition exist, they most probably represent chance associations.

## PATHOLOGY

Unfortunately, few eyes with serpiginous choroidopathy have been studied in the pathology laboratory. Histologic examination

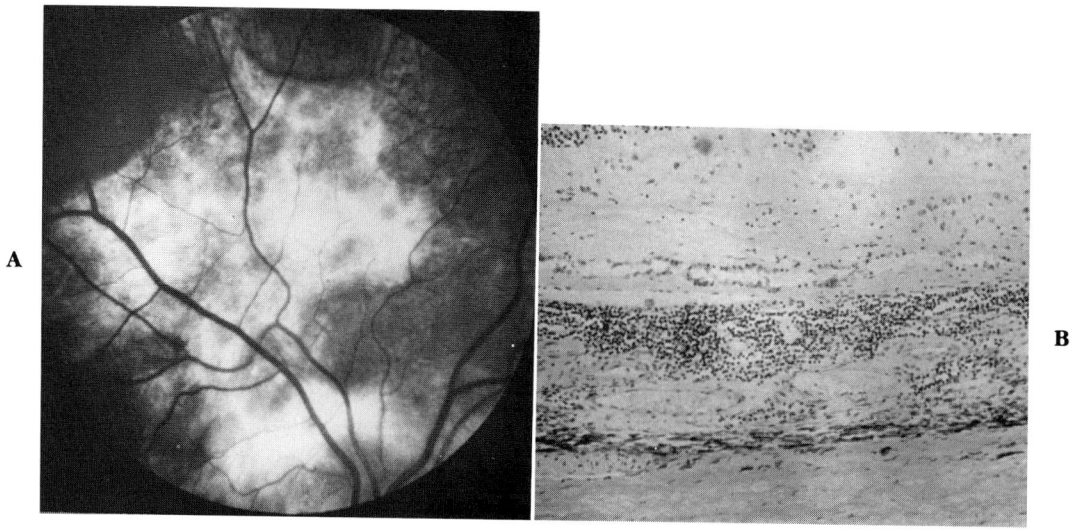


**Fig. 27-4.** Clinical **(A)** and histologic **(B)** photographs of eye of young man with serpiginous choroiditis. Note marked lymphocytic infiltrate into choroid. (Courtesy J.D.M. Gass, M.D.)

shows an extensive loss of the RPE and destruction of the overlying retina. Portions of the choriocapillaris and part of the choroid are filled with a lymphocytic infiltrate, suggesting an inflammatory component to the disease (Fig. 27-4).[16] Areas of RPE hypertrophy and subretinal scarring have also been described.

## ETIOLOGY

The cause of serpiginous choroidopathy is unknown. Maumenee has suggested that the disorder is the result of a vascular abiotrophy and should therefore be considered a degenerative disorder. Laatikainen and Erkkilä[15] indicated that an immune-mediated vasculitis might induce occlusion of the choroidal vessels. The finding of a lymphocytic infiltrate in the choroid and an accompanying vitritis suggests an inflammatory etiologic factor. In one study the incidence of HLA-B7 was higher in 15 Finnish patients with serpiginous choroiditis than in the control group (54.5% vs. 24.3%, $p < 0.05$).[17] In addition, increased antibacterial antibodies, such as antistreptolysin O, were found in eight of the patients with serpiginous choroiditis. The clinical course of the disease, characterized by multiple recurrent inflammatory episodes, is compatible with an infectious disease process such as herpesvirus infection. Serpiginous choroidopathy has been reported after viral meningitis, and some clinicians give anecdotal reports of improvement after treatment with acyclovir. Nevertheless, firm evidence suggesting an infectious cause is lacking. In fact, the inflammatory disease may be a secondary phenomenon unrelated to previous infection. Retinal degeneration after the impairment of the choroidal vasculature could release potentially antigenic moieties, which in genetically prone persons leads to an inflammatory response.

## DIFFERENTIAL DIAGNOSIS

A number of disorders should be considered in the differential diagnosis of serpiginous choroidopathy. The bilateral lesions of acute posterior multifocal placoid pigment epitheliopathy (APMPPE) may appear similar to those of serpiginous choroidopathy. Acute lesions in both diseases may be yellowish and involve the choroid and retina at the level of the RPE, and RPE clumping can be seen late in the course of both diseases (see Fig. 28-4). Acute lesions of both APMPPE and serpiginous choroidopathy show early blockage of fluorescence and late hyperfluorescence. However, the acute lesions of APMPPE resolve within 2 weeks, and recurrence is uncommon. In addition, choroidal atrophy and choroidal neovascularization are atypical in APMPPE but common in serpiginous choroidopathy, and the prognosis for good visual outcome is far better for patients with APMPPE. Nevertheless, we have seen a number of patients with a disease that falls between the classic findings of serpiginous choroidopathy and APMPPE. We have informally termed this condition *APPMPiginous choroidopathy* because these patients have fundus lesions typical of APMPPE but develop recurrent disease more typical for the patient with serpiginous choroidopathy. They do, however, maintain relatively good central vision and do not have the relentless, helical progression characteristic of serpiginous choroidopathy.

Other diseases that cause peripapillary chorioretinal scarring can be confused with serpiginous choroidopathy. Age-related macular degeneration, angioid streaks, idiopathic choroidal neovascularization, toxoplasmosis, the presumed ocular histoplasmosis syndrome, and previous retinal laser photocoagulation are other entities to be considered in the evaluation of patients suspected of having serpiginous choroidopathy.

## THERAPY

Many ophthalmologists would argue that therapeutic interventions do not favorably alter the course of serpiginous choroidopathy. Antituberculous medications have been tried for patients with this disease but with little definitive proof of efficacy.[6] Other antiinflammatory regimens, including corticosteroids and cytotoxic agents, have been used but have never been evaluated in controlled clinical trials.[6] Hooper and Kaplan[18] used the combination of azathioprine (1.5 mg/kg body weight/day), cyclosporine (5 mg/kg/day), and prednisone (1 mg/kg/day) to treat patients with serpiginous choroidopathy and observed a rapid remission of active disease in five patients. Disease in two patients recurred immediately after discontinuation of low-dose therapy but was arrested when therapy was resumed. However, because the clinical course of serpiginous choroidopathy is often characterized by a sporadic course of remissions and recurrence, it is impossible to determine the therapeutic efficacy of any regimen reported to date. Laser photocoagulation appears warranted in some cases of choroidal neovascularization. Sometimes a serous detachment of the retina may occur adjacent to an area of inflammatory activity, and these detachments tend to resolve with corticosteroid therapy.

In our experience, patients with a significant inflammatory response, manifested by vitritis and acute yellowish lesions, appear to have a beneficial response to corticosteroids. We have observed improvement in visual acuity in patients treated with oral prednisone, but again, these data are anecdotal. Nevertheless, it appears logical to treat serpiginous eyes with evidence of inflammatory disease with a trial of corticosteroids as long as one predetermines the definition of a therapeutic response and the length that therapy will be continued before this response is reached. We have also used cyclosporine in combination with corticosteroids to treat some patients with serpiginous choroidopathy, but its therapeutic effects for this condition remain unclear.[19,20] In addition, we have treated one patient—in whom an active lesion was threatening the fovea—with pulse intravenous methylprednisolone at a dose of 1 g/day for 3 days. Finally, some uveitis specialists are using acyclovir to treat this disorder, but its use is based on anecdotal reports of a possible therapeutic effect in a very small number of patients. What is clear is that the ideal therapeutic approach to this disease remains to be discerned, but with so few patients affected, a randomized clinical trial with appropriate statistic power will be difficult to conduct.

### Case 27-1

A 64-year-old white man was referred to the National Eye Institute in 1983 because of a gradual loss of vision in the right eye over the previous 6 months. The left eye was amblyopic. The visual acuity was 20/100 OD and 20/200 OS. There were 1+ cells and flare in both eyes, and the vitreous of each eye had 1+ cells, with some strands. There were choroidal lesions in both eyes compatible with the diagnosis of serpiginous choroiditis, and these were perifoveal in both eyes. The patient was placed on a regimen of 50 mg of prednisone for 1 week, with a slow taper to 20 mg/day over several months' time. His vision improved to 20/25 OD after 3 weeks. We elected to keep the patient on low-dose prednisone (10-15 mg/day) for 1 year. A repeat fluorescein angiogram did not show any further progression of the lesion in that eye. The patient maintains good vision in that eye 3 years after prednisone was discontinued.

### Case 27-2

A 49-year-old white man had first noted blurring of vision in his right eye in 1977. He was noted to have a peripapillary lesion extending into the macular region, giving him poor vision in that eye. An inactive "scar" had been noted inferonasally in the left eye. The patient had a past history of possible tuberculosis. In late 1980 he noted changes in the vision in his left eye, and subsequently he was begun on prednisone therapy (80 mg/day), as well as antituberculous medication. His vision in both eyes varied dramatically, sometimes being as good as 20/25 to

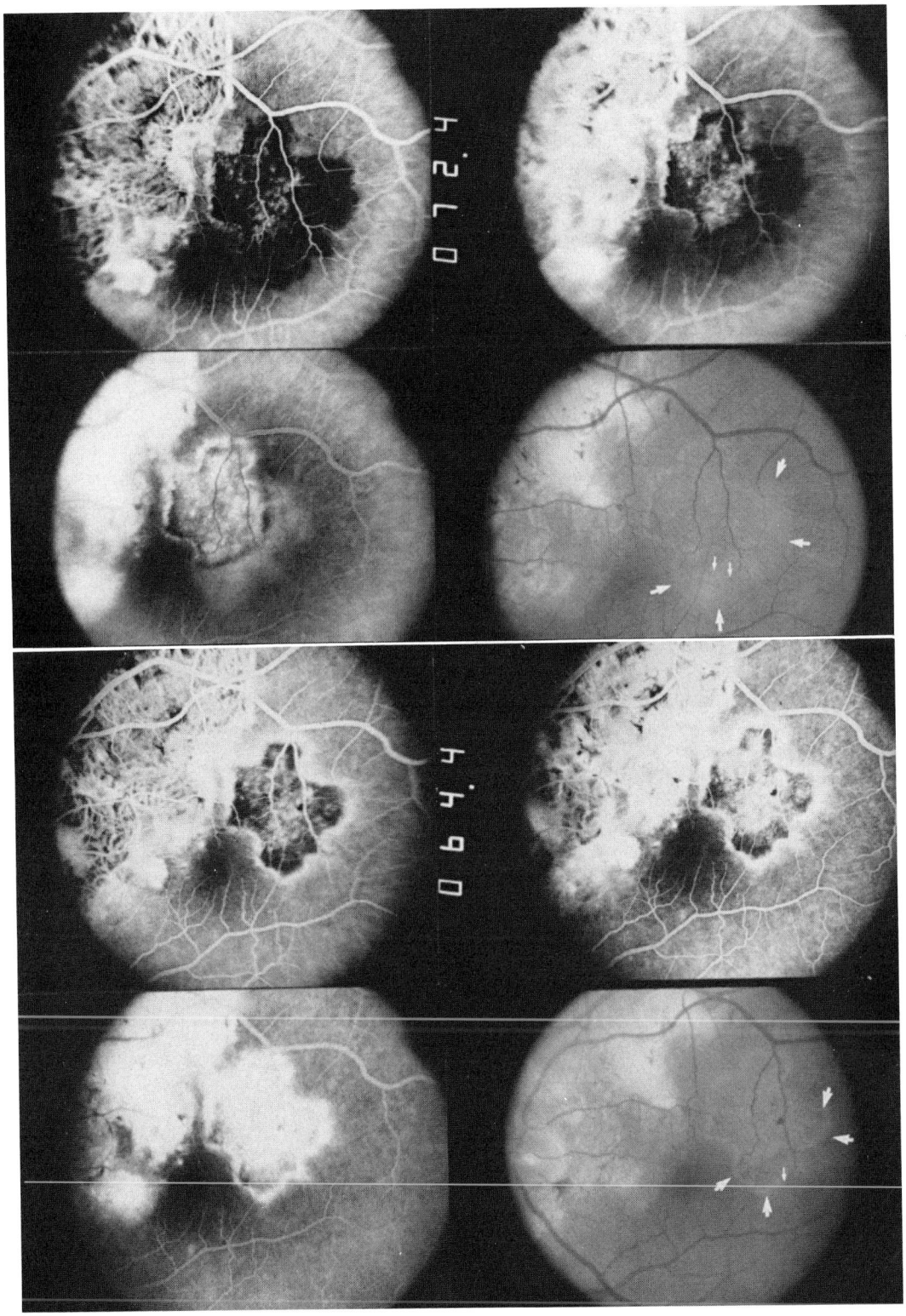


**Fig. 27-5. A,** Fluorescein angiogram and fundus photograph of patient with serpiginous choroiditis, complaints of slightly decreased visual acuity, and metamorphopsia in left eye. Early blocked fluorescence and late leakage are seen at borders of active lesions. Late frame also shows late leakage compatible with serous detachment of adjacent retina *(arrows)*. **B,** Fluorescein angiogram and fundus photograph of same patient 9 days after pulse intravenous methylprednisolone. Patient had noted decreased metamorphopsia. Early blocked fluorescence is no longer seen at border of lesion, and serous retinal detachment has resolved *(arrows)*. (From *Ophthalmology* 98:952, 1991.) (See Color Plate 43.)

20/40 OU. However, with continued prednisone therapy, his vision began to fail in both eyes, with extension of the lesions toward the fovea. When seen at the National Eye Institute in late 1982, his fluorescein angiogram showed central involvement in both eyes and a vision of 20/200 OU. There was no inflammatory response. The patient was begun on cyclosporine, therapy, and no improvement of his vision was seen after 3 months. At this point the cyclosporine therapy was discontinued.

### Case 27-3

A 43-year-old man, diagnosed with bilateral serpiginous choroiditis in 1978, had decreased vision that was worse in the right eye. He lost good central vision in the right eye despite medical and laser therapy. He had exacerbations of inflammatory disease in his left eye in 1986 and 1988, each resolving after periocular injections of betamethasone (Celestone). He was first seen at the National Eye Institute in April 1989 and returned with a flare-up of his disease in September and complaints of metamorphopsia and changes on Amsler grid testing. Although his visual acuity remained 20/20, he was treated with periocular and systemic corticosteroids and his vision returned to baseline. Ten months later, he returned with similar complaints of metamorphopsia. An active lesion with a cream-colored and slightly elevated border was noted on fundus examination. Fluorescein angiogram showed blocked fluorescence in the early frames with late hyperfluorescence. Hyperfluorescence suggestive of a serous detachment of the retina adjacent to the lesion was also noted in the late frames (Fig. 27-5, *A*).

The patient was treated with pulse intravenous methylprednisolone at a dose of 1 g/day for 3 days. He was then placed on a regimen of oral prednisone (20 mg/day) and cyclosporine A (7 mg/kg body weight/day). Within the first 3 to 4 days after therapy the patient noted diminished metamorphopsia, and the angiogram showed resolution of the area of blocked fluorescence (Fig. 27-5, *B*). The patient's subsequent course has been marked by development of a choroidal neovascular membrane (see Fig. 27-2), which was treated with laser photocoagulation. Recently the patient has developed inflammatory activity despite therapy with oral prednisone (60 mg/day) and cyclosporine A (6 mg/kg body weight/day). We have therefore added azathioprine to his therapeutic regimen.

## REFERENCES


1. LM, Orth D, Daily MJ, Babb MF: Subretinal neovascularization with geographic (serpiginous) choroiditis, *Am J Ophthalmol* 88:683-689, 1979.
2. Bock CJ, Jampol LM: Serpiginous choroiditis. In Albert DM, Jocobiec FA, editors: *Principles and practice of ophthalmology,* Philadelphia, 1994, Mosby, pp 517-523.
3. Schatz H, McDonald HR: Geographic helicoid peripapillary choroidopathy (serpiginous choroiditis). In Ryan SJ, Ogden TE, Schachat AP, et al, editors: *Retina,* St Louis, 1989, Mosby.
4. Hardy RA, Schatz H: Macular geographic helicoid choroidopathy, *Arch Ophthalmol* 105:1237-1242, 1987.
5. Blumenkranz MS, Gass JDM, Clarkson JG: Atypical serpiginous choroiditis, *Arch Ophthalmol* 100:1773-1775, 1982.
6. Laatikainen L, Erkkilä H: Serpiginous choroiditis, *Br J Ophthalmol* 58:777-783, 1974.
7. Hamilton AM, Bird AC: Geographical choroidopathy, *Br J Ophthalmol* 58:784-797, 1974.
8. Gass JDM: *Stereoscopic atlas of macular diseases: diagnosis and treatment,* ed 3, St Louis, 1987, Mosby, p 136.
9. Weiss H, Annesley WH Jr, Shields JA et al: The clinical course of serpiginous choroidopathy, *Am J Ophthalmol* 87:133-142, 1979.
10. Masi RJ, O'Connor R, Kimura SJ: Anterior uveitis in geographic or serpiginous choroiditis, *Am J Ophthalmol* 86:228-232, 1978.
11. Gass JDM: *Stereoscopic atlas of macular diseases: diagnosis and treatment,* ed 3, St Louis, 1987, Mosby, p 138.
12. Laatikainen L, Erkkilä H: Subretinal and disc neovascularisation in serpiginous choroiditis, *Br J Ophthalmol* 66:326-331, 1982.
13. Wojno T, Meredith TA: Unusual findings in serpiginous choroiditis, *Am J Ophthalmol* 94:650-655, 1982.
14. Gass JDM: *Stereoscopic atlas of macular diseases: diagnosis and treatment,* ed 3, St Louis, 1987, Mosby, p 140.
15. Laatikainen L, Erkkilä H: A follow-up study on serpiginous choroiditis, *Acta Ophthalmol (Copenh)* 59:707-718, 1981.
16. Gass JDM: *Stereoscopic atlas of macular diseases: diagnosis and treatment,* ed 3, St Louis, 1987, Mosby, p 142.
17. Erkkilä H, Laatikainen L, Jokinen E: Immunological studies on serpiginous choroiditis, *Graefes Arch Clin Exp Ophthalmol* 219:131-134, 1982.
18. Hooper PL, Kaplan HJ: Triple agent immunosuppression in serpiginous choroiditis, *Ophthalmology* 98:948-952, 1991.
19. Nussenblatt RB, Palestine AG, Chan CC: Cyclosporine A therapy in the treatment of intraocular inflammatory disease resistant to systemic corticosteroids and cytotoxic agents, *Am J Ophthalmol* 96:275-282, 1983.
20. Laatikainen L, Tarkkanen A: Failure of cyclosporin A in serpiginous choroiditis, *J Ocular Ther Surg* 3:280-283, 1984.

# CHAPTER 28

# White-Dot Syndromes

Localized, well-circumscribed areas of inflammatory disease in the fundus are certainly a common manifestation of many intraocular inflammatory disorders (see Chapters 14, 21, 22, and 24). In addition, several entities have been noted to occur at times with multiple white dots in the fundus, usually in the deeper layers of the posterior segment. They are grouped here because of their sometimes overlapping features and the belief by some that these disorders may represent the broad spectrum of one underlying entity. Most are acute, sometimes leaving minimal or no permanent long-term visual loss. An infectious cause has been suggested for some, although more recent evidence does not support this theory.

## MULTIPLE EVANESCENT WHITE-DOT SYNDROME

### Clinical findings

Jampol and colleagues[1] reported on 11 patients in whom similar fundoscopic changes were noted. The alterations are unilateral, predominantly seen in young women. Numerous small (100-200 μm), discrete white lesions are noted deep in the retina or at the level of the retinal pigment epithelium (RPE) (Fig. 28-1)—thus the term *multiple evanescent white-dot syndrome (MEWDS)*. The lesions appear in the posterior pole and extend to the midperiphery. They tend to be concentrated in the perifoveal region but seem usually to spare the fovea itself. In addition, there is often a granular appearance to the macula. The granularity may take the appearance of tiny white or orange specks, in no way approaching the size of the deeper circular lesions. The macular changes cause an irregularity to the internal limiting membrane reflex. Other ocular findings include vitreous cells and occasional sheathing of the retinal venules (see Box 28-1). There is usually no significant anterior chamber reaction.

Patients with MEWDS usually do not report an antecedent flulike episode. The mean age of onset of symptoms is about 28 years.[1,2] The decrease in visual acuity is usually quite sudden. The disease may cause a marked drop in visual acuity even to the level of 20/200, and an afferent pupillary defect may be noted. The

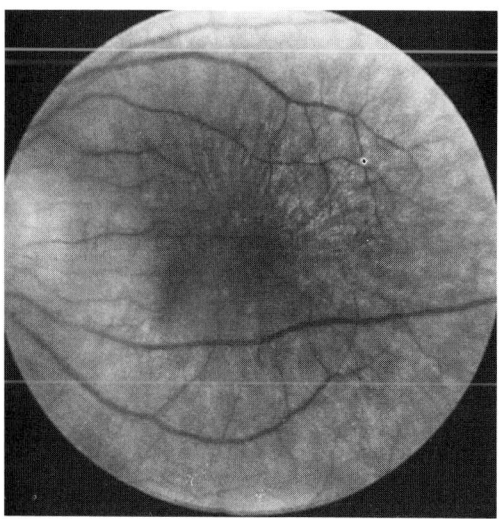

**Fig. 28-1.** Fundus photograph showing alterations noted in MEWDS.

**Box 28-1**
**Clinical findings in multiple evanescent white-dot syndrome**

Sudden drop in visual acuity
Mostly young females
Small discrete white dots at RPE level
"Grainy" macula
ERG changes that reverse after episode
Minimal RPE perturbation after episode
Rarely recurs
Vision returns without medication

disease runs its course after an average of 7 weeks, after which a return to a visual acuity of between 20/20 and 20/40 usually ensues. The white lesions and macular granularity will fade with time, but subtle RPE alterations can be noted. Recurrences of the disorder are only rarely seen.[3,4] Aaberg and colleagues[3] reported a recurrence in a previously affected eye 3 years after the initial visual loss, as well as recurrences in the contralateral eye. Although most reports have come from North America, this disorder has been seen in Europe.[5]

### Laboratory findings

Although no formal evaluation of these patients has been undertaken, there appears to be neither systemic manifestations of this disorder nor characteristic blood test results. Jampol and colleagues[1] reported taking acute and convalescent sera for viral titers in one patient, but no antibody to a specific virus was identified.

Findings on electroretinogram (ERG), early receptor potential (ERP), and visual pig-ment regeneration tests have been noted to be abnormal in these patients during the acute stage, with a return to normal during the recovery phase.[6] Indeed, during the acute phase it was the a wave of the ERG and the ERP amplitudes that were markedly affected. The electrophysiologic data suggest that the disease is primarily that of the RPE. Van Meel and colleagues[7] performed scanning laser densitometry on a patient with MEWDS. Test results noted small areas of absent visual pigment that did not correspond to the white fundic spots. Even with recovery, these abnormal areas of pigment loss were still faintly noted. The authors believe that this study supports the notion that this disorder is the result of a metabolic disturbance at the level of the RPE.

Fluorescein angiography results frequently show early hyperfluorescence with late staining. This is unlike the angiographic findings associated with acute posterior multifocal placoid pigment epitheliopathy (APMPPE) (see later discussion). There is staining as well of the macula and late staining of the disc. In a recent study, indocyanine green angiography showed hypofluorescent lesions throughout the posterior pole, which were more visible on the indocyanine green angiogram than were apparent on clinical examination.[8]

Several entities have ocular manifestations similar to those seen in MEWDS. APMPPE is usually a bilateral disease that has lesions that are considerably larger. With resolution, there is often considerable RPE perturbation in this disorder, whereas in MEWDS the changes are more subtle. In APMPPE, the fluorescein angiographic picture is one of initial blockage with late staining, unlike that seen in MEWDS. Multifocal choroiditis, as first reported by Nozik and Dorsch,[9] and acute retinal pigment epitheliitis are reviewed in the next sections. They can be distinguished from MEWDS by the more severe inflammatory response in the vitreous, long-standing lesions, and cystoid edema in the former, as well as the different evolution of the spots and probable normal electrophysiologic results in the latter. Birdshot retinochoroidopathy has ERG and electrooculogram (EOG) changes that do not improve with time, and the involvement of the retinal vasculature with cystoid edema is quite striking (see Chapter 24). Sarcoidosis should be ruled out in MEWDS patients, because lesions similar to this can be seen. Usually, however, the lesions of sarcoidosis are bilateral, have more vitreous involvement, and can cause far more RPE alterations than is seen in MEWDS. Callanan and Gass[10] have stressed that there may be an overlap of symptoms in the white-dot syndromes.

### Therapy

To date the cases of MEWDS that have been reported have not needed to be treated. Sequelae to the acute episode seem to be minimal, with an expected return to near-preattack vision in about 7 weeks on average.[1]

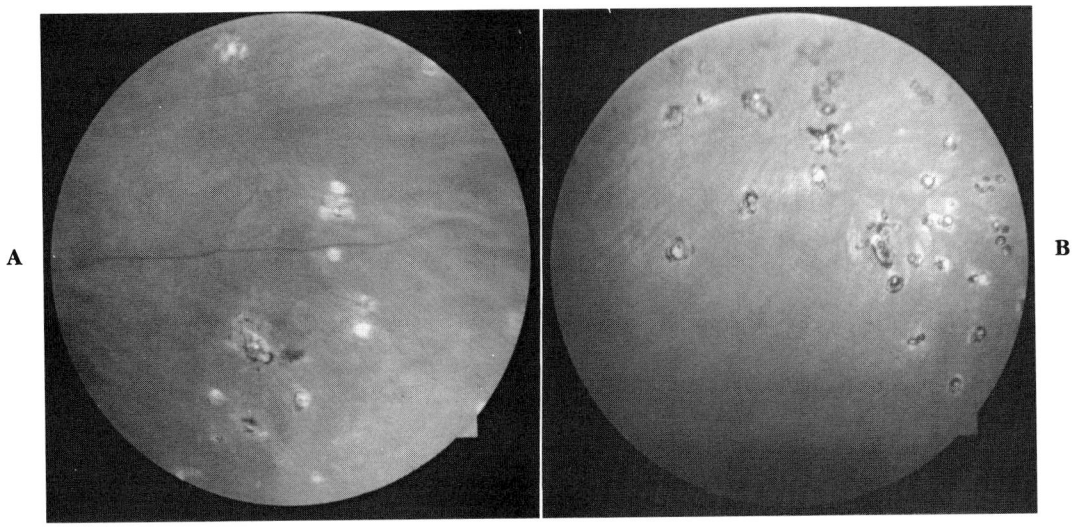


**Fig. 28-2. A** and **B,** Multiple histoplasmosis-like lesions in periphery of patients with focal choroiditis and uveitis. These eyes, unlike those with ocular histoplasmosis syndrome, have a profound vitreous inflammatory response and cystoid macular edema. Both conditions carry risk of subretinal neovascularization of fovea.

## MULTIFOCAL CHOROIDITIS AND PANUVEITIS

Several investigators have reported a fundic condition with characteristics of presumed ocular histoplasmosis syndrome (POHS). This began with Nozik and Dorsch's report[9] of two cases of bilateral uveitis associated with a distinctive chorioretinopathy. The identification of these patients is relevant because of the associated sequelae that may lead to irreversible visual handicap.

### Clinical findings

Patients have a multifocal choroiditis that strongly suggests the ocular histoplasmosis syndrome (Fig. 28-2). However, they also have a significant vitritis and often an anterior uveitis. The lesions, 50 to 200 μm in diameter, can be strewn throughout the fundus but in our experience are posterior to the equator. They have a punched-out appearance and appear to be at the level of the RPE or inner choroid. At times pigment is heaped around the edge of the lesion. The pigmentary changes around the disc that is associated with the histoplasmosis syndrome can be seen here as well. The disorder is bilateral and occurs more frequently in women. In Dreyer and Gass' review[11] the median age was 33 years and in the group reported by Morgan and Schatz, 28 years.[12] Our group of 24 patients (19 female, 5 males) came to us after most had a long, chronic inflammatory course, and averaged 52 years. Morgan and Schatz found that all but one of the patients they examined had myopia. Patients with this disorder do not necessary come from an area that is endemic for histoplasmosis, and a relatively low percentage of them respond to the histoplasmin skin test.[11]

The inflammatory activity in the virteous is marked, and retinal involvement can be noted on close examination. Cystoid macular edema has been found in 14% of the eyes studied by Dreyer and Gass,[11] whereas 41% of our patients had this disorder's sequela. At least one third of the eyes will ultimately have a subretinal neovascular net in the macula.[11] Mild disc edema can also be seen. However, acute and symptomatic blind-spot enlargements with no signs of optic nerve abnormalities have been reported by Khorram and coworkers,[13] who conjecture that this is a manifestation of peripapillary retinal dysfunction. Callanan and Gass[10] reported as well an acutely enlarged blind spot in seven of their patients. Also, in four of these patients, white dots similar to those of MEWDS were transiently noted, suggesting a similar cause for these two disorders. Peripheral chorioretinal streaks, once thought to be seen only in the ocular histoplasmosis syndrome, were noted in 3 of 47 eyes with multifocal choroiditis.[14]

### Punctate inner choroidopathy

Watzke and colleagues[15] described a group of patients with a condition they termed *punc-*

*tate inner choroidopathy (PIC)* which is perhaps a variant of multifocal choroiditis. In their report of 10 moderately myopic women, the ocular changes noted were essentially the same as those already described except that there were no signs of ocular inflammation. The women had blurred vision associated with light flashes and paracentral scotomas. The lesions were 100 to 300 μm in diameter and initially appeared yellow. Reddy and Folk[16] believe that PIC and multifocal choroiditis, although quite similar, can be distinguished. In multifocal choroiditis there is vitreous inflammation and the retinal lesions are less discrete and shallower, whereas PIC lesions are deep, punched out, and cylindric. As well, new lesions can appear with multifocal choroiditis, which is unusual in PIC. In our mind these distinctions blur, and we generally consider this a subgroup of multifocal choroiditis. Although macular edema may be somewhat less common with PIC, both PIC and multifocal choroiditis carry the real risk of subretinal membranes.

### Laboratory findings

Patients with multifocal choroiditis do not appear to originate from areas that are endemic for histoplasmosis. Some patients, however, give a history of an antecedent febrile illness.

Fluorescein angiographic evaluation of the punched-out lesions show early hyperfluorescence, typical of an RPE window defect. Morgan and Schatz[12] noted in some lesions a fuzzy hyperfluorescent leakage late in the angiogram. Electrophysiologic testing does not demonstrate typical findings in multifocal choroiditis. Indeed, the ERG will tend to be normal or borderline in most cases.[11]

The disorders that need to be excluded when diagnosing this condition include many of those mentioned for MEWDS. Of particular note is that of birdshot retinochoroidopathy (see Chapter 24). HLA typing has not been performed on many of these patients, and no information to date suggests any linkage, whereas HLA-A29 is strongly associated with birdshot retinochoroidopathy (see Chapter 24). In addition, the lesions in this entity tend to be smaller and more punched out or discrete in appearance than in birdshot. Birdshot tends to occur in older persons, who have less anterior segment inflammatory disease, more optic nerve involvement, and problems with night vision and color discrimination. The presence of cystoid macular edema appears to be as common in our experience with both entities, but the incidence of subretinal foveal nets is higher in this condition. In ocular histoplasmosis, vitreous cells should not be present, and the lesions are generally larger. The incidence of subfoveal neovascular nets is higher in ocular histoplasmosis. Deutsch and Tessler[17] reported their observations in 28 patients with a pseudohistoplasmosis syndrome; 43% were African-American and 32% had disciform scars. Further, 32% of the patients were presumed to have sarcoidosis, 29% tuberculosis, and 11% syphilis. Multifocal creamy choroidal infiltrates in older patients can be due to a masquerade syndrome (see Chapter 29).[18]

A provocative hypothesis is that this disorder is virally induced. Grutzmacher and coworkers[19] ascribed RPE punched–out lesions to herpes retinitis in an otherwise healthy patient. Tiedeman[20] evaluated 10 patients with the multifocal choroiditis and panuveitis syndrome for evidence of Epstein-Barr virus–specific antibodies. The 10 patients were noted to have antibodies directed against the viral capsid antigen (IgM) or the Epstein-Barr early antigen. None of the control subjects tested were found to have these antibodies, but most did have viral capsid antigen IgG or Epstein-Barr nuclear antigen antibodies, indicating previous exposure to this virus. Viral capsid IgM followed by IgG responses will rise during an incubation period of 4 to 5 weeks, whereas the early antigen increases with the appearance of clinical findings 5 to 10 weeks after exposure. The nuclear antigen increases slowly after 2 months and stays for life, but the IgM anti–viral capsid antigen decreases over a period of 6 to 12 months. Although none of the patients had overt systemic disease, Tiedeman hypothesized that these responses suggested an active or persistent state of viral infection and that the patients may be immunologically unable to clear the virus. Because we know that the ocular disease can continue for years, this suggests that such persons would in theory have a higher risk of developing the systemic complications of Epstein-Barr virus, an association to date not made. Further, chronic Epstein-Barr infection has been reported by Wong and coworkers[21] to manifest a different intraocular inflammatory disease picture that responds to acyclovir. More recent observations have not borne out these observations. Spaide and colleagues[22] evaluated 11 patients with multifocal choroiditis whom they compared with 11 sex- and age-matched control subjects for the presence of anti-EBV antibodies. They found that neither the antiviral capsid antigen IgG nor the antinuclear antigen antibody titers were significantly different between the two groups. None of the patients in either group had IgM antibodies to the antiviral capsid antigen. One patient with multifocal choroiditis and three control subjects had positive anti–early antigen antibody titers.

Chorioretinal biopsies of the lesions in multifocal choroiditis have shown the presence not of virus (see Case 28-2) but of a large number of B cells in the choroid.[23] This is in contradistinction to Nölle and Eckardt's report[24] that in nine vitrectomy specimens from patients with this disorder there was a large number of T cells—about one third of the cell population being macrophages—and only rare B cells. Charteris and Lee[25] reported the necropsy results of eyes from a 59-year-old woman with this disorder. They noted that 70% to 80% of the lymphocytes were identified as T cells; less than 20% were B cells. In situ hybridization for identification of herpes simplex virus showed negative results. The finding of a large number of T cells, presumably in the choroid, in this study reflects that different underlying mechanisms will result in similar clinical entities, as we as well had seen in this entity[23] (see Case 28-2).

Therapy for multifocal choroiditis has centered on the use of immunosuppressive agents (see following discussion), with varying success. An interesting hypothesis is that an initial viral disorder may have triggered an immune response that no longer requires the presence of the virus but rather needs immunosuppressive therapy to be controlled.

For those patients with the PIC subgroup of disease, a novel mechanistic explanation has been recently offered by Scheider.[26] He hypothesized that young myopic women are more prone to develop this syndrome because of their tendency to have bacteremia, which, coupled with the attenuated choroidal vessels of myopia, would increase their risk of infectious thromboses.

### Therapy

Periocular or systemic corticosteroids have been used to treat multifocal choroiditis. In Dreyer and Gass' report,[11] 6 of 18 patients had improvement of vision with steroid therapy, whereas 9 had no change and in 2 it was thought that this form of therapy halted a rapid decline in vision. Morgan and Schatz[12] reported that in their patients the inflammatory disease responded very well to steroid therapy and that most patients were left with good vision. Of our 24 patients to date, of the 17 who needed steroid therapy, 10 had cystoid macula edema. Our experience has shown a moderately good patient response to steroid therapy, but the disorder can be stubbornly chronic, requiring at least the consideration of the addition of other immunosuppressive agents. In our experience the visual prognosis is guardedly optimistic. Of great interest was Morgan and Schatz' observation[12] that subretinal neovascular lesions regressed with steroid therapy. This was not Dreyer and Gass' observation[11] in one patient. We have not observed regression in our patients. Laser ablation of the subretinal net appears to be indicated—however, with several caveats. The first is that there is the potential for an increase in the inflammatory response after such an intervention, something to avoid if we theorize that the inflammatory response is the underlying "initiator" of the neovascular net. Second, the experience of Dreyer and Gass suggests that laser ablation has not been particularly successful in preventing a further deterioration of vision.

Nölle and Eckardt[24] saw no impressive therapeutic effect of vitrectomy in nine patients with this disease. We have limited experience with the removal of submacular neovascular nets in such patients. Often these cases, unlike those of histoplasmosis syndrome, have a great deal of fibrosis associated with the net, making the removal most difficult, if at all possible.

## ACUTE RETINAL PIGMENT EPITHELIITIS

### Clinical findings

Acute retinal pigment epitheliitis was first reported by Krill and Deutman,[27] who described a group of relatively young patients with fairly subtle alterations at the level of the RPE. The condition resulted in an acute drop in visual acuity, or metamorphopsia. Some of the changes may be so mild as to not bring the patient to the physician. Clusters of lesions, usually in the posterior pole, are noted. The lesions themselves are deep, fine, dark-gray or black spots, which in their acute stage are surrounded by a yellow halo. With resolution the halo may disappear and the lesions may appear darker in color. Central serous retinopathy has been noted in this entity, presumably due to the perturbation of the RPE. Retinopathy may be either bilateral or unilateral and can affect both men and women. A gradual resolution with complete or near-complete return to good vision occurs in 6 to 12 weeks.

### Laboratory findings

The fluorescein angiogram will demonstrate an area of hypofluorescence surrounded by an area of hyperfluorescence. As the disorder progresses, it leaves a somewhat depigmented background, and a "lacy" hyperfluorescence may be noted. Central serous retinopathy may also be documented on angiographic examination.

Electrophysiologic testing may show an abnormal EOG during the acute phase of the disease, which will return toward normal as the disorder wanes. The finding does, however, strongly suggest that the disorder affects the RPE in a far more widespread manner than is appreciated on the basis of ophthalmoscopic observations. The ERG and visually evoked cortical responses have been reported as being normal.[28]

Because of the acute nature of the illness, it has been assumed that it is of viral origin. To date no studies have corroborated this hypothesis.

### Therapy

No therapy is generally called for because the disease should resolve spontaneously.

## ACUTE POSTERIOR MULTIFOCAL PLACOID PIGMENT EPITHELIOPATHY

Acute posterior multifocal placoid pigment epitheliopathy (APMPPE) is a term first used by Gass in 1968[29] to describe a syndrome of multiple, large, plaquelike lesions at the level of the RPE that are associated with temporary visual loss. Although there is no histologic confirmation that this is an inflammatory disease, the transient nature of the lesions and a possible association with a viral prodrome have led most authors to consider APMPPE as a manifestation of inflammation or infection at the level of the RPE or superficial choroid. It is probable that the clinical entity of benign diffuse external exudative retinitis first described by Scuderi and colleagues[30] in 1948 represents part of the clinical spectrum that we now include in the diagnosis of APMPPE.

### Clinical findings

The disease usually manifests with a sudden onset of visual blurring or flashing lights in a patient younger than 30 years of age.[31-33] There is no gender predilection. Older patients have occasionally been reported. In some patients, flashing lights precede the visual loss by several weeks. Most cases are bilateral and simultaneously appear in both eyes. However, unilateral cases and a delay of the appearance of the disease in the second eye by several weeks have also been noted. The anterior segments may have no significant inflammation or there may be a 1 to 2+ nongranulomatous inflammation. The vitreous may also have a mild to moderate inflammatory response. The characteristic clinical finding is that of multiple, flat, yellow-white (cream-colored) plaques at the level of the RPE (Fig. 28-3). These plaques are of varying sizes and are clearly defined. The placoid lesions typically begin in the macula or posterior pole, with later developing lesions noted more peripherally. The lesions do not extend beyond the equator. Cystoid macular edema is not a prominent part of this syndrome and is rarely, if ever, seen. In the acute phase the vision is often moderately decreased but rarely falls below 20/400. Some patients may have only a mild decrease, with vision in the 20/25 to 20/40 range. Visual field testing will demonstrate a central or pericentral scotoma.[34]

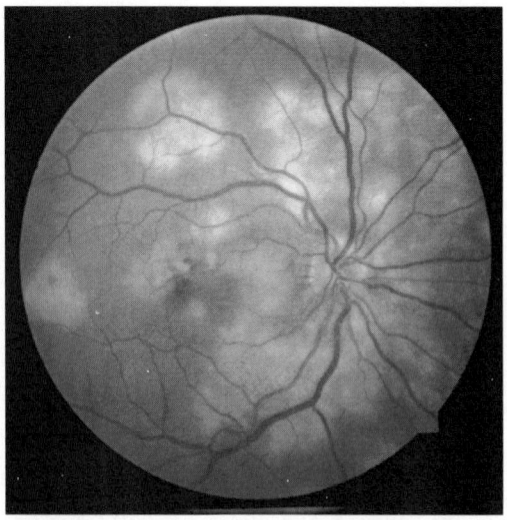

**Fig. 28-3.** Acute lesions of APMPPE. (See Color Plate 44.)

Papillitis is occasionally seen in association with this disease.[35] Characteristically the vision begins to improve spontaneously within a few weeks after the onset of symptoms but may be somewhat slower in resolving.[31-34] Usually preceding the visual improvement by a few weeks is the initial resolution of the cream-colored placoid lesions. As the fundus lesions resolve, they lose their cream-colored appearance. Older lesions may resolve while new lesions are still appearing. There is often a residual RPE stippling, mottling, and depigmentation (Fig. 28-4). Vision usually returns to near normal, but some patients may have mild residual visual deficits. Snellen acuity returns rapidly in most patients, but residual defects in visual fields, color vision, and the Stiles-Crawford effect may persist for 1 year.[34] Some few patients will have significant residual visual loss.[36]

Although APMPPE is thought to be a nonrecurrent disorder and the prognosis has been considered favorable, there are reports of recurrences. Of 13 patients in one study 5 had late recurrences in previously unaffected eyes.[36] We have observed one patient who had recurrent episodes of APMPPE leading to significant visual loss.

APMPPE occurs in otherwise healthy persons. Many authors have noted a viral prodrome in some patients.[31-33] Occasional reports of erythema nodosum,[37] episcleritis,[33] neurosensory hearing loss[38] and cerebral vasculitis[39] associated with APMPPE have reinforced the concept that this is an immune-driven vascular alteration. However, there is no coherent explanation for the development of this disease. APMPPE may not be a specific disease but rather a response of the RPE or choroid to various disease processes.

In addition to the striking clinical fundus appearance, the fluorescein angiogram findings are characteristic in APMPPE[31-33,40] (Fig. 28-5). In the acute stage of the disease, during which there are active cream-colored lesions, the choroidal fluorescence is blocked in the early phases of the angiogram. In the late stages there is staining of the lesions that had previously blocked fluorescence. Hypofluorescence followed by hyperfluorescence in combination with appropriately sized and colored fundic lesions is diagnostic of APMPPE. Fluorescein angiography findings in the late or resolved stage of the disease are less characteristic and demonstrate transmission defects in the RPE without leakage.

Usually the disorder is limited to the eye. However, there have been several cases of APMPPE that have been associated with cerebral vasculitis.[41] This can occur at the time of the ocular disease or months later. A pleocytosis may be seen in the cerebrospinal fluid. In one report,[42] multifocal white-matter lesions were seen on magnetic resonance imaging, with the neurologic symptoms disappearing with steroid therapy.

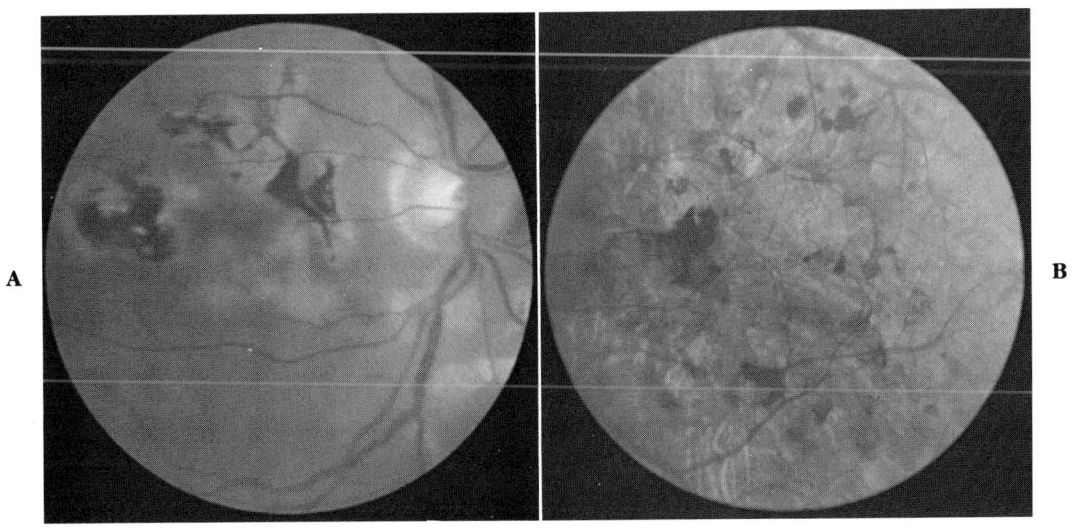


**Fig. 28-4. A,** Reparative phase with RPE clumping. **B,** Late phase of disease, showing profound amount of RPE perturbation.

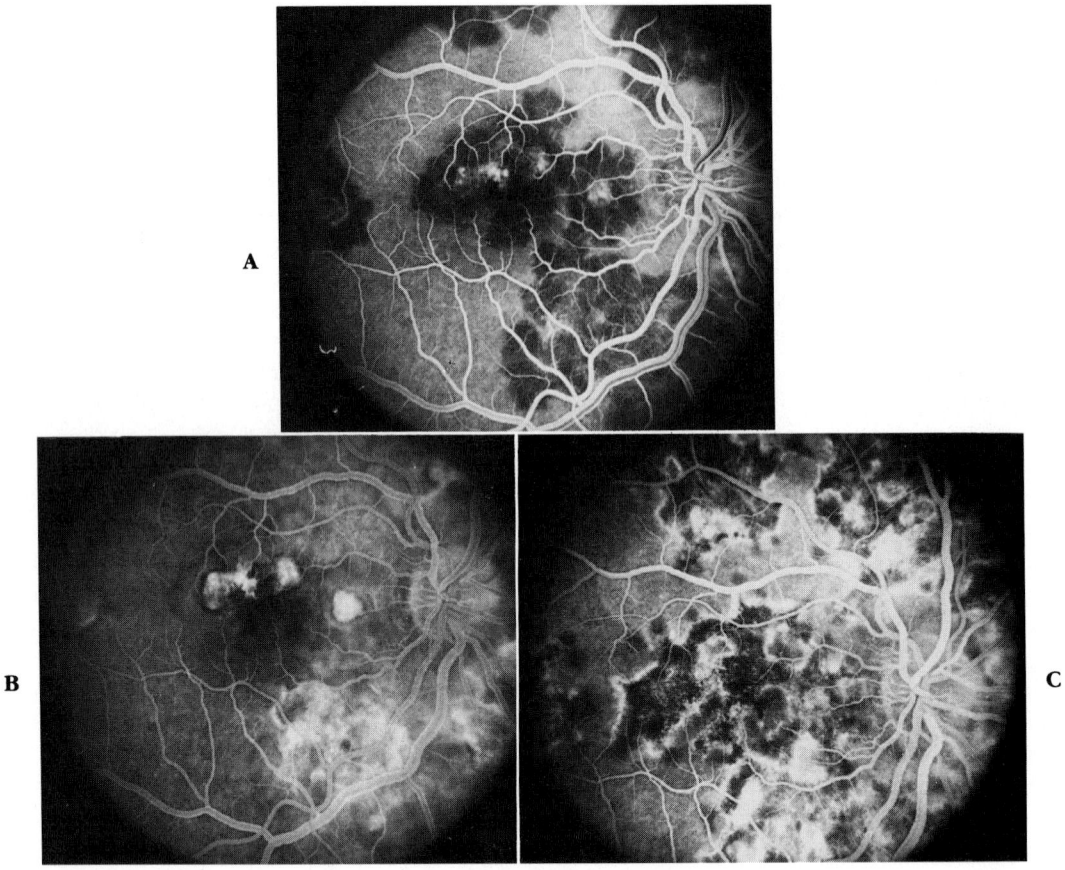


**Fig. 28-5. A,** Early blockage of lesions seen on fluorescein angiogram. **B,** Late hyperfluorescence seen in inferior portion of same lesion. **C,** Extensive hyperfluorescence seen in angiogram of eye with old APMMPE.

## Etiology

In his initial description Gass[29] believed that the site of the lesion in APMPPE was at the level of the RPE or was due to an abnormality in choroidal perfusion with secondary involvement of the RPE.[29] The EOG is markedly impaired during the acute phase of the disease, supporting the concept of RPE involvement.[34] Isolated areas of choroidal nonperfusion inside placoid lesions suggest that the primary lesion is impaired filling of the choroid[40] perhaps due to a choroidal vasculitis.[43] It is now thought that the choroidal vasculature is obstructed at the level of the precapillary arterioles. It is interesting to note that a true vasculitis such as Wegener's granulomatosis can produce ocular lesions that resemble the lesions of APMPPE.[44] The varying size of the APMPPE lesions could support a choroidal hypoperfusion hypothesis. It is possible that APMPPE is part of a spectrum of choroidal perfusion abnormalities, and, as Young and colleagues[40] suggest, patients with more confluent lesions may have less a favorable clinical course than patients with APMPPE; yet the lesions appear to have the same root cause—that of choroidal ischemia with secondary involvement of the RPE.[40] The photoreceptors are most likely involved by this ischemic process, accounting for the visual loss and the slow recovery of sensitive measures of photoreceptor function such as the Stiles-Crawford effect.[34] Patients with unilateral lesions but bilateral perfusion abnormalities have been described, further supporting the choroidal location of the disease process. The variability in the degree of choroidal ischemia may explain some of the unusual sequelae of APMPPE, such as subretinal neovascular membranes. Preceding viral illnesses are certainly often reported and raise the possibility of a localized viral infection. Bodine and colleagues[45] reported one case they believe was associated with Lyme disease.

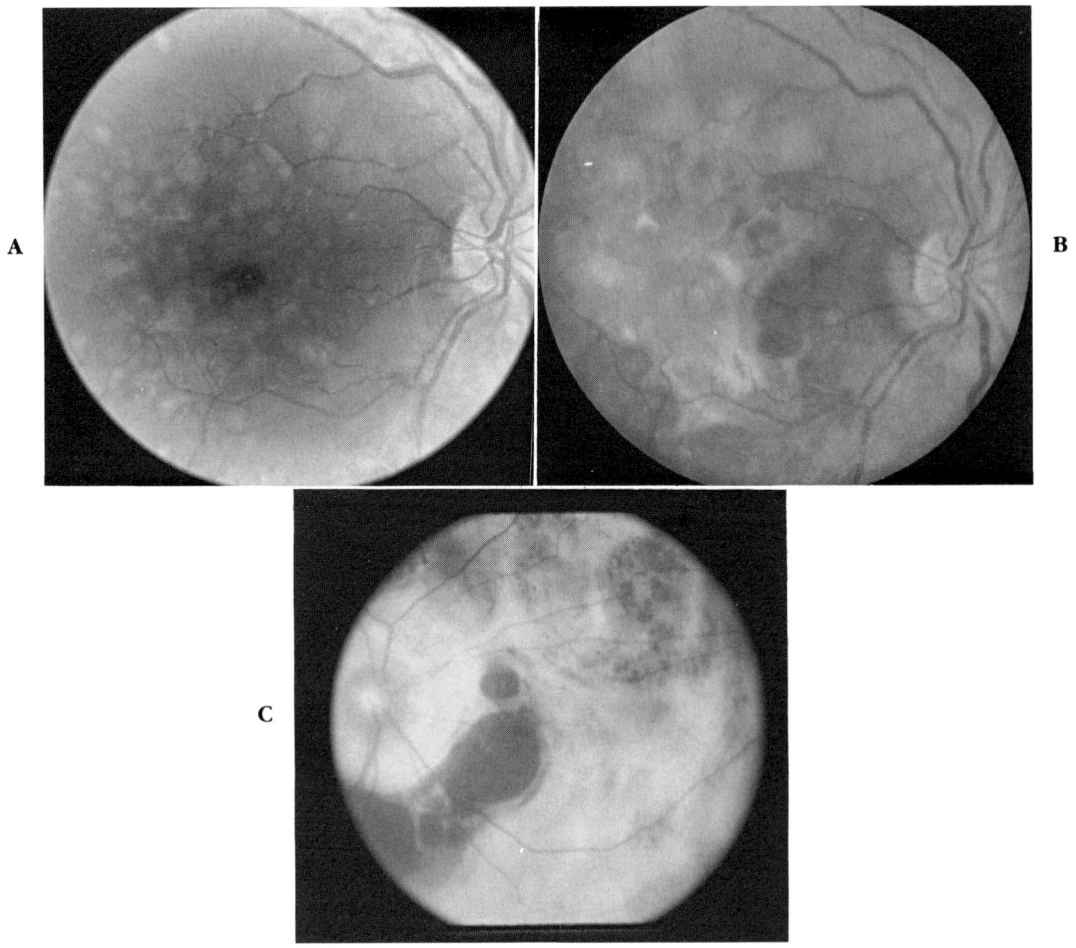


**Fig. 28-6. A,** Early changes of subretinal fibrosis syndrome and uveitis. With time these changes coalesced to form picture seen in **B. C,** Extensive subretinal fibrosis involving disc and then extending into macula region. (See Color Plate 45.)

### Therapy

Most patients with APMPPE have a good visual prognosis and do not require therapy. Some authors have used systemic corticosteroid therapy, but it is difficult to assess its value in view of the overall favorable prognosis (see Case 28-2).

## SUBRETINAL FIBROSIS AND UVEITIS SYNDROME

### Clinical findings

We reported on the first three patients with this disorder.[46] The entity is characterized by a chronic inflammation in the vitreous with whitish-yellow subretinal lesions that appear to be gliotic or fibrotic (Fig. 28-6, *A* and *B*). These lesions can coalesce to form a large sheet of this fibrotic-appearing material. The lesion can progress to encompass the whole posterior pole, with loss of vision. However, in some cases the progression may not continue and a steady state may be reached. In some cases the lesion may encircle but not encroach the macula (Fig. 28-6, *C*). In some cases, although the macula is not directly involved, cystoid macular edema may result, with a subsequent drop in visual acuity. The vitreal inflammatory response may be quite marked, and there may be a low to moderate anterior chamber response. In our experience the patients have all been young females, the most African-Americans, and in all but one instance the disease has been bilateral. Others have reported this entity in males.[47] The number of cases followed is still too small to define the ultimate visual outcome in these patients.

It is interesting to note that the entity may

have been reported by Adalbert Fuchs in his 1949 atlas of the ocular fundus.[48] In it he described an "extremely rare" bilateral condition in which there were large areas of connective-tissue formation under the retina that led to a severe drop in visual acuity.*

## Laboratory findings

In more advanced cases, the ERG and EOG show marked diminishment. The ERG may show changes of both rod and cone function.[46] The fluorescein angiogram shows predominantly subretinal alterations. In the early phase of the angiogram one may see multiple areas of blockage of choroidal fluorescence as well as hyperfluorescence. In the later phase of the angiogram, staining of the lesions without leakage can be noted.

Laboratory testing does not appear to be contributory. Culturing of peripheral lymphocytes has not demonstrated an in vitro anamnestic response to retinal antigens, such as the S-antigen.

We performed an immunohistochemical evaluation of two eyes with this entity[49,50] (Fig. 28-7). These studies revealed a markedly inflamed choroid with a predominance of B cells and plasma cells. Complement and IgG were deposited above Bruch's membrane. In one eye a granulomatous lymphocytic infiltrate was present in the choroid. Of the T-cell subpopulations, there was a predominance of the helper/inducer subset. Müller cells expressed class II antigens. There were no circulating antiretinal antibodies, and virus could not be cultured from the specimen. The subretinal fibrosis contained islands of cells that were interpreted as originating from the RPE. The impression was that a dysregulation leading to a B-cell disorder with antibody and complement deposition occurs. This leads to retinal and RPE damage, as well as the development of fibrosis. Without any data to date, one can speculate what is at the basis of this B-cell dysregulation and whether the B cells are the cause of the fibrosis. One possible explanation is that the two are not related but rather the cause of a shift in T-cell subsets, from a Th1 response to a Th2 profile. Whereas Th1 cells would produce interferon and IL-2, the Th2 inducer cells would produce a lymphokine cascade rich in IL-4, which could stimulate B cells, and transforming growth factor–beta (TGF-β), a lymphokine associated with scarring and fibrosis.

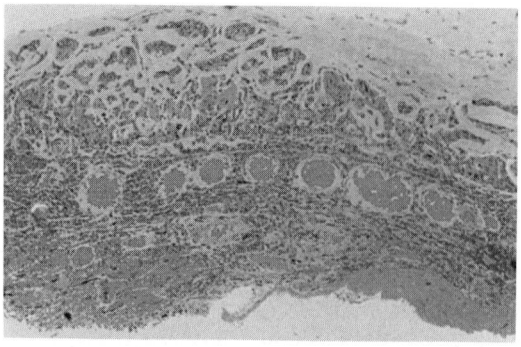

**Fig. 28-7.** Chorioretinal biopsy specimen from patient with subretinal fibrosis and uveitis syndrome. There is marked choroidal infiltration by lymphocytes, as well as replacement of normal retinal structures by islands of irregular cells and amorphous connective tissue. Electron microscopy examination revealed that the connective tissue consisted of collagen fibrils and these islands of cells had characteristics suggestive of RPE. Both T and B lymphocytes were seen, but differential increase in number of B cells as compared with peripheral blood was noted. No virus or other organisms were found either by culture or by electron microscopy examination. (From Palestine AG, Nussenblatt RB, Chan CC, et al: Histopathology of the subretinal fibrosis and uveitis syndrome, *Ophthalmology* 92:838-844, 1985.)

Although we believe that this entity is a distinct one, as do Cantrill and Folk,[51] several other conditions could mimic its clinical features. A long-standing retinal detachment can lead to subretinal fibrosis. Ocular inflammatory conditions to consider include sarcoidosis, ocular histoplasmosis syndrome, APMPPE, syphilis, tuberculosis, birdshot retinochoroidopathy, and toxoplasmosis.

## Therapy

Therapeutic interventions to date have not been particularly successful. One exception to this is cystoid macular edema, in which the edema seems to respond to corticosteroid therapy, resulting in an increase in visual acuity. However, we have not been impressed that our therapeutic intervention has slowed or altered in any way the fibrotic changes. Fortunately for some persons, the progression of the disease can be very slow or stop altogether for reasons that are not known. Corticosteroid therapy would seem appropriate in light of the B-cell nature of the disease. However, it is known that the factors stimulating fibroblast proliferation

*We are indebted to Dr. Nassim Calixto of Belo Horizonte, Brazil, for bringing this to our attention.

may not be affected by this kind of therapy. One patient has been treated with aggressive cytotoxic therapy[50] (cyclosphosphamide), and the course of the disease was not altered. The disease of one of our patients seems to have been controlled with methotrexate.

## ACUTE ZONAL OCCULT OUTER RETINOPATHY

Gass[52] recently reported on 13 patients, predominantly young women (77%), with a group of findings that he has named acute zonal occult outer retinopathy (AZOOR). These changes include a rapid loss of one or more large zones of outer retinal function, as well as photopsia, with minimal fundoscopic changes. There is little or no clinical evidence of inflammatory disease. The disorder is characterized by the development of one or more scotomas (readily documented with visual field testing), usually associated with photopsia, in one or both eyes. There are initially minimal fundoscopic changes, but the electroretinogram findings will be abnormal. With time there are striking RPE changes (Fig. 28-8). During the early phase of the disease a large number of disorders need to be excluded, including retrobulbar neuritis, a pituitary or intracranial tumor, and cancer-associated retinopathy (CAR). In the later phases of the disease, the differential diagnosis turns to those disorders that cause retinal vascular narrowing and RPE alterations, including syphilis, retinal vasculitis, and diffuse unilateral subacute neuroretinitis (DUSN). Gass believes that the visual prognosis is good, with a stabilization of the scotomas and retinal changes. Steroid therapy has been given to date to six of these patients, with only one having a noticeable improvement.

• • •

In summary, the several entities discussed here are believed by some to be essentially one entity that expresses itself clinically in multiple ways. It is our belief that they can be clinically differentiated. Further, until we learn more about the underlying mechanisms, we cannot really speculate as to whether these are all separate entities or just variations on a theme. However, there are strong reasons to distinguish them on the basis of their clinical findings, because doing so is helpful in predicting the ultimate visual outcome in an individual patient. Inasmuch as we are dealing with a range of disorders—from those that are not sight-threatening and that resolve without therapy to others for which we have no effective therapy and which carry potential for severe visual handicap—it would seem that their recognition on clinical grounds and their very different natural histories would justify our noting them as separate conditions. It is, however, important to remember that many believe that these disorders represent a spectrum of basically the same underlying disorder. Gass,[52] for instance, would place such disorders as MEWDS, multifocal choroiditis, and geographic atrophy of the RPE under the rubric of AZOOR with focal fundus lesions. Time will tell.

**Case 28-1**

A 24-year-old Hispanic woman came to the eye clinic because of poor vision in the right eye for 3 months. Testing revealed OD HM, OS 20/20.

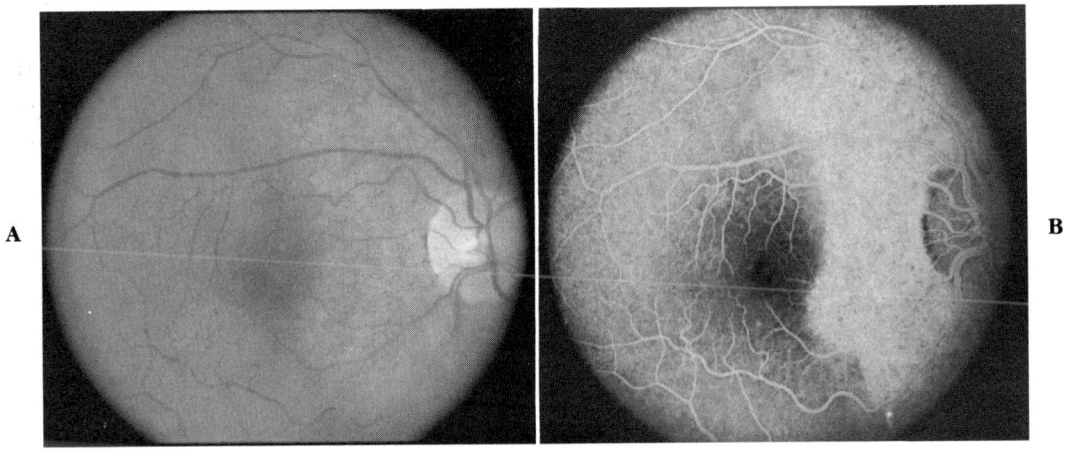


**Fig. 28-8. A,** Fundus photograph. **B,** Fluorescein angiogram of patient with AZOOR. (See Color Plate 46.)

Examination of the right eye showed extensive subretinal fibrosis, extending from around the disc and encompassing essentially all of the posterior pole. The left eye was normal. A work-up was begun to rule out several disorders, including syphilis, tuberculosis, and sarcoid, and testing results supported none of these diagnoses. The patient's toxoplasmosis titer was positive. It was thought that she had subretinal fibrosis with uveitis syndrome. Because the right eye had such poor vision, it was elected not to treat her. She returned 3 months later with a complaint of decreased vision in the left eye. The visual acuity was OD HM, OS 20/200. Patches of white subretinal fibrosis associated with a vitreal response was noted. The patient was placed on a regimen of 80 mg of prednisone daily, but her vision continued to decrease and new lesions were noted. An alkylating agent was begun along with the prednisone. In spite of this therapy the vision continued to decrease in the left eye until it reached that of the right.

**Comment 28-1** Many cases will not proceed inexorably to poor vision. We have noted patients whose vision will stabilize and a few with unilateral disease. However, the ideal therapy for this potentially sight-threatening, predominantly B-cell disease, is lacking.

### Case 28-2

A 27-year-old white man was treated with laser therapy 2 years before being seen for a small retinal hole in the periphery of the right eye. He came for an ophthalmologic evaluation because of a 1-month history of scotomas and flashing lights in the left eye, with the same findings now in the right eye. This was treated with prednisone (60 mg/day) but with no change in the symptoms. He is in good health, was taking no medication, and had no significant past medical history. When seen, his visual acuity was OD 20/20, OS 20/200. There was no anterior segment inflammation, but there were 1+ cells in the vitreous of both eyes. There were white-yellow subretinal infiltrates in both the posterior pole and the retinal periphery. These became more yellowish in appearance with time. Some areas had subretinal scarring and RPE pigment clumping. The fluorescein angiogram showed that some lesions showed initial blockage with late staining, typical of APMPPE. There was no macular edema. The EOG findings were OD 188%, OS 142%. The ERG showed diminished oscillatory potentials. Hardy-Rand-Rittler (HRR) plates showed that color vision testing was highly abnormal in the left eye. As the disease progressed, new lesions appeared in the right eye, and the central vision seemed to be threatened. Cyclosporine was added to the patient's therapeutic regimen for 3 months. Although there appeared to be resolution of the lesions, the disease now resembled that of serpiginous choroiditis (Fig. 28-9). The patient has been followed up for 10 years, with his vision maintained at OD 20/32, OS 20/63. He has had no recurrences. The fundus in both eyes shows marked RPE clumping extending out to the retinal periphery.

**Comment 28-2** Those who have followed up this patient coined his retinopathy as being a case of "ampiginous" chorioretinopathy. Did our therapy play any role in maintaining his vision? We of course do not know. He did not suffer a recurrence, typical of APMPPE. The retinal appearance was not typical of this disease, however; the extensive changes and scar-

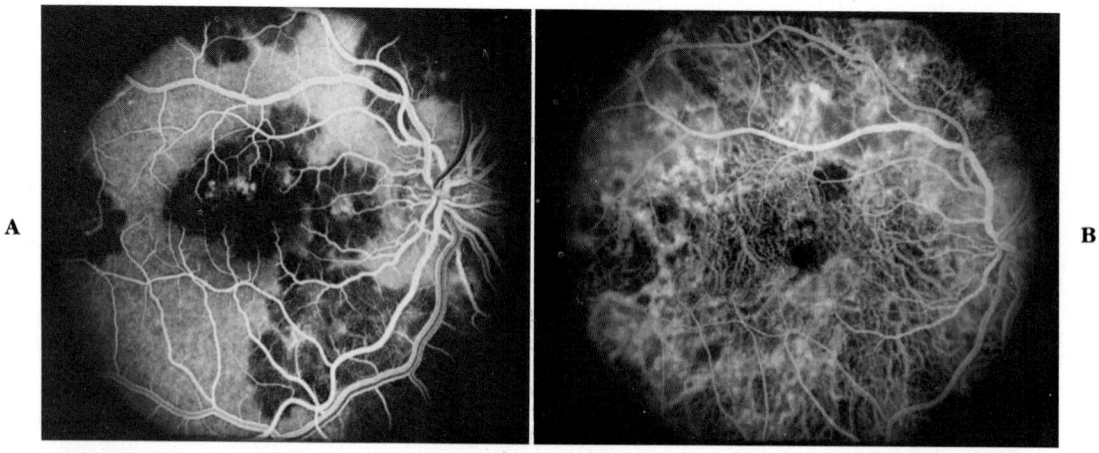


**Fig. 28-9.** Fluorescein angiogram of patient with "ampiginous" chorioretinopathy. **A,** Clinical picture of APMPPE confirmed by angiogram. **B,** Angiogram (taken about 1½ years later) is more typical of serpiginous choroiditis.

ring were more typical of serpiginous chorioretinopathy.

### Case 28-3

A 53-year-old myopic Japanese-American woman had a small symptomatic retinal hole noted on a routine ocular examination. This was treated with laser therapy. Some months later, she noted floaters and decreased visual acuity. She was noted to have in the right eye 1+ vitreal cells and multiple creamy-white lesions strewn throughout the posterior pole and extending toward the equator. Despite prednisone therapy, her vision continued to decline in that eye. Her vision dropped to 20/400 after a macular hemorrhage and subsequent fibrosis ensued. Some months later the same problem developed in her left eye. Her vision decreased somewhat to 20/30, with multiple creamy-white lesions in the fundus. She underwent an extensive evaluation to uncover an underlying problem for what was diagnosed as a multifocal choroiditis. Results of a lumbar puncture were normal, as were a gallium scan and conjunctival biopsy. Of interest was the finding of elevated serum titers for herpes simplex 1 (1:2560), herpes simplex 2 (1:320), and herpes zoster (1:640). Because of this finding, the patient was begun on a short course of acyclovir, but the lesions continued to evolve, and new lesions were seen. The progression in the left eye continued along the same course as that seen in the right, and both antiviral and immunosuppressive therapy was not effective in altering the course of the disease.

Thus the disease presented the ophthalmologists with a diagnostic dilemna, and with the macula in the left eye threatened, it was decided to perform a chorioretinal biopsy. There was mild atrophy of the inner retinal layers. The choroid was filled with B cells and plasma cells. There were nodules at the level of the RPE that resembled Dalen-Fuchs nodules but were made up predominantly of B cells. Virus could not be detected using immunofluorescence, electron microscopy, and culture. It was decided to treat the patient with cyclophosphamide. The logic of the decision was that (1) there was no evidence of active infection and (2) with a predominantly B-cell infiltrate, cyclosporine—with its effect essentially on the T-cell arm of the immune response—would not be indicated. The patient's ocular disease responded rapidly to cyclophosphamide (initial dose, 2 mg/kg, then lowered) combined with 17.5 mg of prednisone. The lesions involuted, and cytotoxic medication was stopped after about 1 year's time. Her eyes have shown no inflammatory activity for more than 3 years after stopping therapy. The patient required a cataract extraction in the right eye, from which a biopsy specimen was obtained, but she maintains a visual acuity of 20/400, 20/30.

**Comment 28-3** The white-dot syndromes still remain problematic. The chorioretinal biopsy helped enormously in determining a therapeutic approach. In addition, the finding of B cells in this disease was quite unexpected. We have seen a similar finding in a biopsy specimen of another patient with this disorder. It is interesting to note that T-cell infiltrates at this level of the eye can look clinically essentially the same.[21]

## REFERENCES


1. Jampol LM, Sieving PA, Pugh D et al: Multiple evanescent white dot syndrome. I. Clinical findings, *Arch Ophthalmol* 102:671-674, 1984.
2. Mamalis N, Daily MJ: Multiple evanescent white-dot syndrome: a report of eight cases, *Ophthalmology* 94:1209-1212, 1987.
3. Aaberg TM, Campo RV, Joffe L: Recurrences and bilaterality in the multiple evanescent white-dot syndrome, *Am J Ophthalmol* 100:29-37, 1985.
4. Meyer RJ, Jampol LM: Recurrences and bilaterality in the multiple evanescent white-dot syndrome, *Am J Ophthalmol* 101:388-389, 1986.
5. Borruat FX, Othenin-Girard P, Safran AB: Multiple evanescent white dot syndrome, *Klin Monatsbl Augenheilkd* 198:453-456, 1991.
6. Sieving PA, Fishman GA, Jampol LM et al: Multiple evanescent white dot syndrome. II. Electrophysiology of the photoreceptors during retinal pigment epithelial disease, *Arch Ophthalmol* 102:675-679, 1984.
7. van Meel GJ, Keunen JE, van Norren D et al: Scanning laser densitometry in multiple evanescent white dot syndrome, *Retina* 13:29-35, 1993.
8. Ie D, Glaser BM, Murphy RP et al: Indocyanine green angiography in multiple evanescent white-dot syndrome, *Am J Ophthalmol* 117:7-12, 1994.
9. Nozik RA, Dorsch W: A new chorioretinopathy associated with anterior uveitis, *Am J Ophthalmol* 76:758-762, 1973.
10. Callanan D, Gass JD; Multifocal choroiditis and choroidal neovascularization associated with the multiple evanescent white dot syndrome and acute idiopathic blind spot enlargement syndrome. *Ophthalmology* 99:1678-1685, 1992.
11. Dreyer RF, Gass JDM: Multifocal choroiditis and panuveitis: a syndrome that mimics ocular histoplasmosis, *Arch Ophthalmol* 102:1776-1784, 1984.
12. Morgan CM, Schatz H: Recurrent multifocal choroiditis, *Ophthalmology* 93:1138-1147, 1986.
13. Khorram KD, Jampol LM, Rosenberg MA: Blind spot enlargement as a manifestation of multifocal choroiditis, *Arch Ophthalmol* 109:1403-1407, 1991.
14. Spaide RF, Yannuzzi LA, Freund KB: Linear streaks in multifocal choroiditis and panuveitis, *Retina* 11:229-231, 1991.
15. Watzke RC, Packer AJ, Folk JC et al: Punctate inner choroidopathy, *Am J Ophthalmol* 98:572-584, 1984.
16. Reddy CV, Folk JC: Multifocal choroiditis with panuveitis, diffuse subretinal fibrosis, and punctate inner choroidopathy. In Ryan SJ, editor: *Retina,* ed 2, St Louis, 1994, Mosby.

17. Deutsch TA, Tessler HH: Inflammatory pseudohistoplasmosis, *Ann Ophthalmol* 17:461-465, 1985.
18. Jakobiec FA, Sacks E, Kronish JW et al: Multifocal static creamy choroidal infiltrates: an early sign of lymphoid neoplasia, *Ophthalmology* 94:397-406, 1987.
19. Grutzmacher RD, Henderson D, McDonald PJ et al: Herpes simplex chorioretinitis in a healthy adult, *Am J Ophthalmol* 96:788-794, 1983.
20. Tiedeman JS: Epstein-Barr viral antibodies in multifocal choroiditis and panuveitis, *Am J Ophthalmol* 103:659-663, 1987.
21. Wong KW, D'Amico DJ, Hedges TR II et al: Ocular involvement associated with chronic Epstein-Barr virus disease, *Arch Ophthalmol* 105:788-792, 1987.
22. Spaide RF, Sugin S, Yannuzzi LA et al: Epstein-Barr virus antibodies in multifocal choroiditis and panuveitis, *Am J Ophthalmol* 112:410-413, 1991.
23. Martin D, Chan CC, de Smet MD et al: The role of chorioretinal biopsy in the management of posterior uveitis, *Ophthalmology* 100:705-714, 1993.
24. Nölle B, Eckardt C: Vitrectomy in multifocal choroiditis, *Ger J Ophthalmol* 2:14-19, 1993.
25. Charteris DG, Lee WR: Multifocalposterior uveitis: clinical and pathological findings, *Br J Ophthalmol* 74:688-693, 1990.
26. Scheider A: Multifocal inner choroiditis, *Ger J Ophthalmol* 2:1-9, 1993.
27. Krill AE, Deutman AF: Acute retinal pigment epitheliitis, *Am J Ophthalmol* 74:193-205, 1972.
28. Deutman AF: Acute retinal pigment epitheliitis, *Am J Ophthalmol* 78:571-578, 1974.
29. Gass JDM: Acute posterior multifocal placoid pigment epitheliopathy, *Arch Ophthalmol* 80:177-185, 1968.
30. Scuderi G, Recupero SM, Valvo A: Acute posterior multifocal placoid pigment epitheliopathy, *Ann Ophthalmol* 9:189-194, 1977.
31. Ryan SJ, Maumenee AE: Acute posterior multifocal placoid pigment epitheliopathy, *Am J Ophthalmol* 74:1066-1074, 1972.
32. Holt WS, Regan ADJ, Trempe C: Acute posterior multifocal placoid pigment epitheliopathy, *Am J Ophthalmol* 81:403-412, 1976.
33. Savino PJ, Weinberg RJ, Yassin JC et al: Diverse manifestations of acute posterior multifocal placoid pigment epitheliopathy, *Am J Ophthalmol* 77:659-662, 1974.
34. Smith VC, Porkorny J, Ernest JT et al: Visual function in acute posterior multifocal placoid pigment epitheliopathy, *Am J Ophthalmol* 85:192-199, 1978.
35. Kirkham TH, ffytche TJ, Sanders MD: Placoid pigment epitheliopathy with retinal vasculitis and papillitis, *Br J Ophthalmol* 56:875-880, 1972.
36. Damato BE, Nanjiani M, Foulds WS: Acute posterior multifocal placoid pigment epitheliopathy: a followup study, *Trans Ophthalmol Soc UK* 103:517-522, 1983.
37. Deutman AF, Oosterhuis JA, Boen-tan TN et al: Acute posterior multifocal placoid pigment epitheliopathy, *Br J Ophthalmol* 56:863-874, 1972.
38. Clearkin LG, Hung SO: Acute posterior multifocal placoid pigment epitheliopathy associated with transient hearing loss, *Trans Ophthalmol Soc UK* 103:562-564, 1983.
39. Kersten DH, Lessell S, Carlow TJ: Acute posterior multifocal placoid pigment epitheliopathy and late-onset meningo-encephalitis, *Ophthalmology* 94:393-396, 1987.
40. Young NJA, Bird AC, Sehmi K: Pigment epithelial diseases with abnormal choroidal perfusion, *Am J Ophthalmol* 90:607-618, 1980.
41. Althaus C, Unsöld R, Figge C et al: Cerebral complications in acute posterior multifocal placoid pigment epitheliopathy, *Ger J Ophthalmol* 2:150-154, 1993.
42. Stoll G, Reiners K, Schwartz A et al: Acute posterior multifocal placoid pigment epitheliopathy with cerebral involvement, *J Neurol Neurosurg Psychiatry* 54:77-79, 1991.
43. Spaide RF, Yannuzzi LA, Slakter J: Choroidal vasculitis in acute posterior multifocal placoid epitheliopathy. *Br J Ophthalmol* 75:685-687, 1991.
44. Kinyoun JL, Kalina RE, Klein ML: Choroidal involvement in systemic necrotizing vasculitis, *Arch Ophthalmol* 105:939-942, 1987.
45. Bodine SR, Marino J, Camisa TJ et al: Multifocal choroiditis with evidence of Lyme disease, *Ann Ophthalmol* 24:169-173, 1992.
46. Palestine AG, Nussenblatt RB, Parver LM et al: Progressive subretinal fibrosis and uveitis, *Br J Ophthalmol* 68:667-673, 1984.
47. Rubens Belfort, Jr, MD: Personal communication.
48. Fuchs A: *Diseases of the fundus oculi with atlas,* Philadelphia, 1949, Blakiston.
49. Palestine AG, Nussenblatt RB, Chan CC et al: Histopathology of the subretinal fibrosis and uveitis syndrome, *Ophthalmology* 92:838-844, 1985.
50. Kim MK, Chan CC, Belfort R Jr et al: Histopathologic and immunohistopathologic features of subretinal fibrosis and uveitis syndrome, *Am J Ophthalmol* 104:15-23, 1987.
51. Cantrill HL, Folk JC: Multifocal choroiditis associated with progressive subretinal fibrosis, *Am J Ophthalmol* 101:170-180, 1986.
52. Gass JD: Acute zonal occult outer retinopathy. (Donders lecture: The Netherlands Ophthalmological Society, Maastricht, Holland, June 19, 1992), *J Clin Neuro Ophthalmol* 13:79-97, 1993.

# CHAPTER 29

# Masquerade Syndromes

The masquerade syndromes comprise a group of disorders that occur with intraocular inflammation and are often misdiagnosed as a chronic idiopathic uveitis. The term *masquerade syndrome* was first used in the ophthalmic literature in 1967 to describe a conjunctival carcinoma manifesting as a case of chronic conjunctivitis[1]; today, however, the term most commonly is used to describe disorders simulating chronic uveitis. Because many of the masquerade syndromes are malignant processes, early diagnosis and prompt treatment are critical (see Box 29-1). Other disorders such as retinal degenerations and intraocular foreign body can also masquerade as a uveitis, and again, misdiagnosis frequently leads to inappropriate therapy. This chapter focuses on the malignant conditions that can masquerade as uveitis but also discusses nonmalignant disorders often misdiagnosed as chronic idiopathic ocular inflammatory disease.

## INTRAOCULAR LYMPHOMA

Although intraocular lymphoma is a lethal disease, early diagnosis and treatment can improve the prognosis. This disease was previously misnamed reticulum-cell sarcoma because the large malignant cells resembled sarcoma cells. However, these tumors are more appropriately classified as intraocular large-cell lymphomas.

Several types of lymphoma can involve the eye and mimic uveitis. Hodgkin's disease, characterized by painless lymphadenopathy, fever, night sweats, weight loss, and the presence of Reed-Sternberg cells on histologic examination, can involve the eye. Ocular involvement in Hodgkin's lymphoma is relatively rare and usually occurs late in the course of the disease.[2] There is one case in the ophthalmic literature in which a patient with Hodgkin's disease had retinal periphlebitis as the initial clinical finding.[3] Other ocular manifestations include iritis or chorioretinitis with associated vitritis.

Two clinically distinct forms of non-Hodgkin's lymphoma more frequently involve the eye: (1) non-Hodgkin's lymphoma of the central nervous system (NHL-CNS), and (2) systemic non-Hodgkin's lymphoma that metastasizes to the eye. Patients with systemic non-Hodgkin's lymphoma metastatic to the eye are usually quite sick with fever, lymphadenopathy, and weight loss. Diagnosis in these cases is rarely puzzling. In contrast, the patient with NHL-CNS that first manifests ocular findings is often a diagnostic dilemma.

### Non-Hodgkin's lymphoma of central nervous system

NHL-CNS, also known as primary CNS lymphoma, arises from the brain, spinal cord, leptomeninges, or the eye and then may spread throughout the CNS.[4-6] Systemic spread outside the CNS occurs more rarely and has been reported in fewer than 10% of autopsies.[7,8] Although this is a rare tumor, the incidence of

**Box 29-1**
**Ophthalmic conditions masquerading as idiopathic uveitis**

**MALIGNANT DISORDERS**

- Intraocular lymphomas
  - Non-Hodgkin's lymphoma of central nervous system
  - Systemic non-Hodgkin's lymphomas metastatic to eye
  - Hodgkin's lymphoma
- Carcinoma metastatic to eye
  - Lung
  - Renal
  - Lung
- Uveal melanoma
- Childhood carcinomas
  - Retinoblastoma
  - Leukemia
  - Medulloepithelioma
  - Juvenile xanthogranuloma
- Paraneoplastic syndromes
  - Cancer-associated retinopathy
  - Bilateral diffuse uveal melanocytic proliferation (BDUMP)

**NON-MALIGNANT DISORDERS**

- Intraocular foreign body
- Retinal detachment
- Myopic degeneration
- Pigment dispersion syndrome
- Retinal degenerations
- Postoperative infections
  - Fungal
  - *Proprionibacterium acnes*
- Postvaccination disorders and drug reactions
  - Rifabutin
  - Didanosine (ddl)

NHL-CNS has trebled over the last 10 years, an increase that cannot be fully explained by acquired immunodeficiency syndrome (AIDS) or other causes of immunosuppression.[9] The median age for patients with NHL-CNS is between 50 and 60 years with a slight male predominance.[4,9] However, cases in children have been reported,[10,11] and the two youngest patients with reported cases of intraocular lymphoma occurred in 15- and 27-year-old persons.[12,13] As in NHL-CNS, immunosuppression appears to be a risk factor for the development of ocular lymphoma. Ocular lymphoma has now been

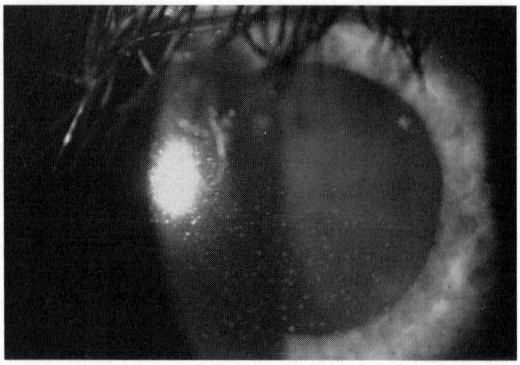

**Fig. 29-1.** Anterior segment of eye of patient with biopsy-proved intraocular large-cell lymphoma demonstrating corneal keratitic precipitates (KP).

associated with AIDS.[14] In addition, ocular lymphoma has been reported in a number of patients undergoing immunosuppression after organ transplantation.[15]

In a large case series by Hochberg and Miller,[9] patients with NHL-CNS showed four distinct clinical profiles: (1) solitary or multiple discrete intracranial nodules, (2) diffuse meningeal or periventricular lesions, (3) subretinal infiltrates or vitritis, and (4) localized intradural spinal masses. Ocular involvement may precede detectable disease in other parts of the CNS, although the percentage of cases in which this occurs may be overestimated in the ophthalmic literature, in which there is a selection bias for patients who have ocular disease. In a study performed at the National Eye Institute, two thirds of the patients with ocular disease had undiagnosed CNS disease at the time of their diagnosis.[16] The mean time between the onset of ocular symptoms and the onset of CNS symptoms in one study was 29 months (range, 7-108 months).[17] In this study, systemic spread outside the CNS was noted in 6% of patients and disease was limited to the eye in 22%.

The most common ocular symptoms associated with intraocular lymphoma are blurred vision and floaters; redness and pain are rare. Patients have decreased visual acuity, although the vision is usually better than one would expect from the clinical examination. Slit-lamp biomicroscopy often reveals mild anterior segment inflammation with aqueous cells and flare and keratic precipitates on the corneal endothelium (Fig. 29-1).[6,12,16-18] Vitreous cells, occurring in sheets, are typical of the disease (Fig. 29-2), and examination of the fundus usually

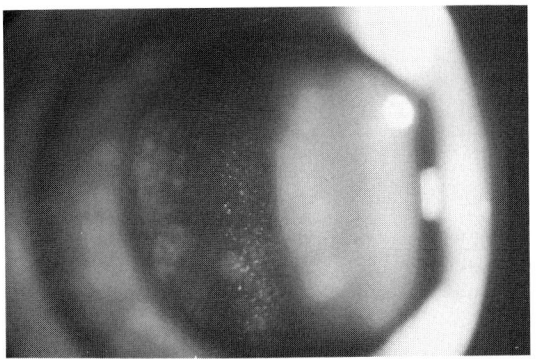

**Fig. 29-2.** Slit-lamp biomicroscopy examination revealing sheets of vitreous cells characteristic of intraocular lymphoma. (See Color Plate 47.)

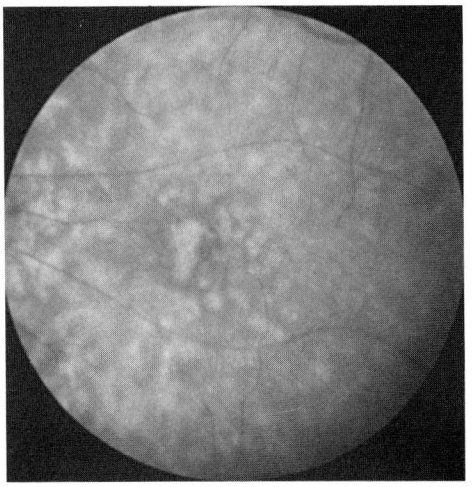

**Fig. 29-3.** Retinal photograph of patient with biopsy-proved intraocular lymphoma demonstrating multiple yellow lesions deep to retina.

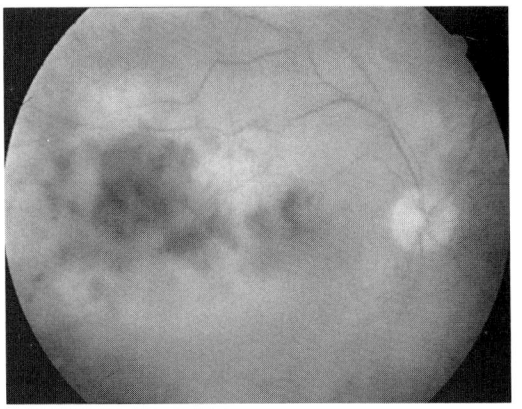

**Fig. 29-4.** Fundus photograph of patient with intraocular lymphoma showing retinal infiltrates and hemorrhage mimicking cytomegalovirus retinitis. Findings resolved with therapy for lymphoma. (See Color Plate 48.)

shows subretinal yellow infiltrates through a hazy vitreous (Fig. 29-3). Atypical presentations have been reported, including a hemorrhagic retinal vasculitis that resembled a viral retinitis (Fig. 29-4).[19] In some cases the fundus may appear normal, and subretinal lesions may be noted only with use of fluorescein angiography. Although the disease may start in one eye, bilateral disease is common after several months.[12,16]

**Diagnosis.** Many patients with intraocular lymphoma have CNS disease at the time of presentation, and a thorough history and neurologic examination are warranted. CNS findings such as headaches, focal weakness, sensory deficits, confusion, and difficulty with gait are common findings. A history of recent seizure is also a strong indication of CNS involvement. Magnetic resonance imaging (MRI) and a lumbar puncture should be performed on all patients suspected of having an intraocular lymphoma, even if neurologic symptoms are absent (Fig. 29-5). Because lymphoma cells can be fragile, samples should be immediately hand carried to the cytology laboratory for processing, and at least 5 to 10 ml of cerebrospinal fluid (CSF) should be sent for cytologic examination. A repeat lumbar puncture may be necessary for the diagnosis.

If the CSF shows no malignant cells, we perform a vitrectomy in an attempt to make the diagnosis of lymphoma. A standard three-port pars plana vitrectomy is performed. Tissue culture medium (RPMI-1640, Rosewell Park Memorial Institute, Mediatech, Inc., Herndon, Va.) enriched with 10% fetal calf serum is added to the collection chamber of the vitrectomy machine to improve cell viability. An initial 10-ml sample of core vitreous is also obtained at the start of the vitrectomy and taken immediately to the cytology laboratory for processing.

The methods used to process vitreous specimens have been delineated previously.[20,21] Briefly, the vitreous specimen is centrifuged at 1000 rpm for 8 minutes at 4° C. The cell pellet is resuspended in 4 ml of fresh tissue culture medium and cytocentrifuged for 10 minutes. The machine places centrifuged specimens directly onto gelatinized slides. Giemsa-, Gram-, or Diff Quick–stained slides are prepared, and additional slides are prepared for immunohistochemical staining for B- and

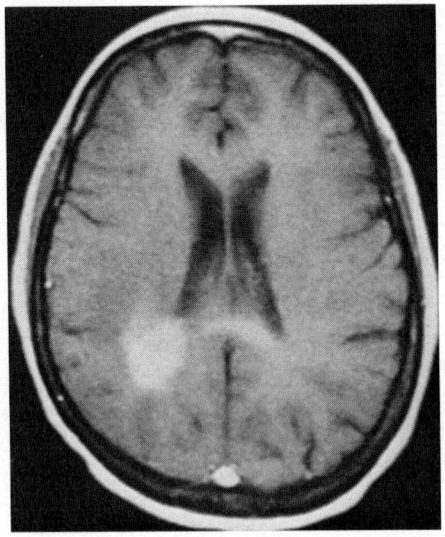

**Fig. 29-5.** MRI scan showing mass lesion in temporal lobe of patient with intraocular lymphoma.

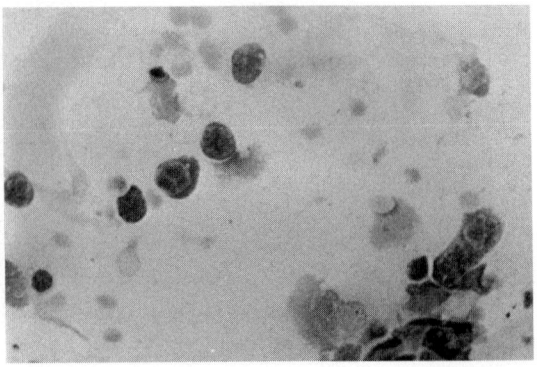

**Fig. 29-6.** Cells obtained from vitrectomy specimen from patient with large-cell lymphoma demonstrating large cells with hyperchromatic, pleomorphic nuclei. (Original magnification × 400; Diff Quick stain.)

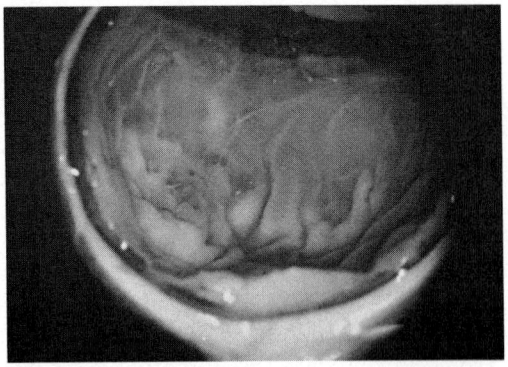

**Fig. 29-7.** Enucleation specimen of patient with intraocular lymphoma shows multiple white areas of retinal and subretinal tumor infiltration with adjacent areas of retinal hemorrhage. (See Color Plate 49.)

T-cell markers and for kappa and lambda light chains.

Multiple vitreous specimens may be needed to make the diagnosis of intraocular lymphoma. Char and colleagues[22] reported that 3 of 14 patients in whom ocular lymphoma was later diagnosed required that more than one vitreous specimen be obtained, and we found that multiple samples were needed to make the correct diagnosis in 3 of 10 patients.[16] Mishandling of vitreous samples partially accounts for some of the difficulty in making the correct diagnosis. In addition, treatment with corticosteroids may obscure the diagnosis of intraocular lymphoma. Corticosteroids can be cytolytic in CNS lymphoma, and this exquisite sensitivity of tumor cells appears to be unique to NHL-CNS. In a number of cases, corticosteroids caused CNS lymphoma lesions to decrease in size or disappear, hindering the ability to make the correct diagnosis. Because many patients with intraocular lymphoma are treated with corticosteroids at the time of vitrectomy, the viability of tumor cells in the samples may be diminished, which may contribute to the difficulty in diagnosing this disease. Finally, because the number of malignant cells in a vitreous specimen may be few, it is critical that the cytologist be experienced in the diagnosis of lymphoma. The diagnosis of intraocular lymphoma can easily be missed by pathologists with little experience in reviewing vitreous specimens for lymphoma.

Typical lymphoma cells are large and pleomorphic with scanty cytoplasm, and hypersegmented nuclei with prominent nucleoli are often diagnostic (Fig. 29-6). However, only a few of these characteristic cells are present in any specimen, and most vitreous samples predominantly contain reactive lymphocytes, histiocytes, necrotic debris, and fibrinous material. The diagnosis of NHL-CNS is usually confirmed by the finding of malignant cells showing B-cell markers with either a kappa or lambda light chain monoclonal response. Gross examination of eyes with NHL-CNS show large gray patches of subretinal and retinal infiltration above a thickened choroid (Fig. 29-7).

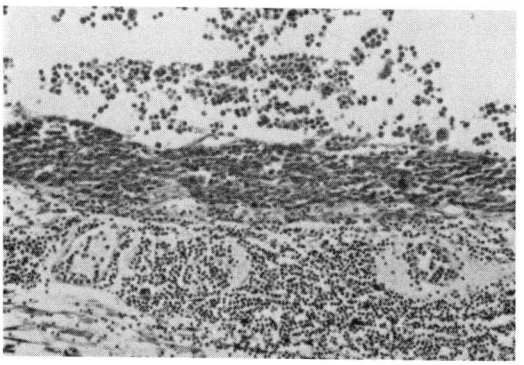

**Fig. 29-8.** Photomicrograph of enucleated globe shown in Fig. 29-7 reveals tumor infiltration between Bruch's membrane and retinal pigment epithelium. Reactive lymphocytes and some tumor cells are seen in overlying vitreous. (Original magnification × 200; hematoxylin-eosin stain.) (See Color Plate 50.)

Collections of lymphoma cells are characteristically found between Bruch's membrane and the retinal pigment epithelium (RPE) (Fig. 29-8). Reactive T lymphocytes can be seen in the retina and choroid in areas surrounding the tumor cells.

The differential diagnosis for patients suspected of having an intraocular lymphoma often includes sarcoidosis. Therefore evaluation of these patients should include a chest x-ray examination, angiotensin-converting enzyme level, serum and urine calcium level, and pulmonary function testing to rule out this diagnosis. A limited gallium scan of the chest and lacrimal glands may also be use-ful. If patients have a diminished diffusing capacity on pulmonary function testing, we often obtain a pulmonary consultation and consider bronchoscopic examination to make the diagnosis of sarcoidosis. Other diseases to consider include syphilis, tuberculosis, acute retinal necrosis, and cytomegalovirus retinitis.

## Treatment

The treatment of NHL-CNS is controversial and the ideal therapy unproved. Radiation therapy was first proposed for the treatment of a chronic uveitis in 1911,[23] and historically, radiotherapy has been recommended as the initial therapy for NHL-CNS.[24] In patients with detectable lymphoma limited to the eyes, controversy centers around whether to limit therapy to the eye or to treat the CNS prophylactically. Char and colleagues[22] reported on two patients with isolated ocular involvement treated with only ocular radiation who had no recurrent disease 24 and 109 months after treatment. NHL-CNS tends to be quite radiosensitive and responds well to 1500 to 4500 rads. However, many researchers recommend cranial irradiation (4500 rads to the whole brain) in addition to orbital radiation in cases of isolated ocular involvement, inasmuch as many patients have subclinical CNS involvement by the time intraocular lymphoma manifests.[22,25] In the series by Peterson and colleagues,[13] 10 of 11 patients with lymphoma limited to the eyes at initial presentation later developed CNS disease. In fact, Rouwen and colleagues[25] advise a combination of chemotherapy and radiotherapy for intraocular lymphoma even if CNS disease cannot be documented on MRI or lumbar puncture. Chemotherapy is recommended to treat possible CNS disease, and radiotherapy is given because penetration of the blood-retinal barrier by chemotherapeutic agents is uncertain. If CNS disease is documented, there is less controversy surrounding the treatment of intraocular lymphoma. In these patients, combined radiotherapy and chemotherapy are more frequently recommended, although this therapeutic approach may not be ideal because of induced CNS toxicity.

A number of chemotherapy regimens have been employed for the treatment of intraocular lymphoma. High-dose Ara-C can lead to therapeutic drug levels in the CSF, and there have been reports of successful treatment of intraocular lymphomas with this therapy alone.[26] However, some studies indicate that CSF levels of systemically administered chemotherapeutic agents may be variable and short-lived.[27] We therefore recommend placement of an Ommaya reservoir for delivery of intrathecal methotrexate to ensure adequate drug levels in the CSF. A number of researchers have employed intrathecal methotrexate for the treatment of intraocular lymphoma but always in combination with radiotherapy.[22] DeAngelis and colleagues[4] recently showed that the addition of chemotherapy to cranial radiotherapy significantly improved disease-free survival and contributed to overall survival of patients with primary CNS lymphoma.

However, combined radiotherapy and chemotherapy can cause significant toxicity. Cranial radiotherapy produces significant CNS toxicity in long-term survivors. Furthermore, Bleyer[28] and DeAngelis and colleagues[4] emphasize that chemotherapy can exacerbate the toxicity produced by radiotherapy, especially with methotrexate. In contrast to the usual sequence of therapy for intraocular lymphoma, in which radiotherapy is administered before chemotherapy, the use of chemotherapy before radiotherapy may reduce the risk of leukoencephalopathy and protect against late toxicity.[28,29] Further research is obviously needed to determine the best therapeutic regimen for this lethal disease. The National Cancer Institute and the National Eye Institute are investigating a treatment protocol employing systemic and intrathecal chemotherapy for the treatment of NHL-CNS.[30] Nine patients with NHL-CNS involving the eye or brain were treated with high-dose intravenous methotrexate with leucovorin rescue, thiotepa, dexamethasone, and intraventricular cytarabine. Cycles were repeated every 21 days to complete response or best response. To date, a complete response was achieved in eight of nine patients, with a mean follow-up of more than 1 year. In an attempt to treat the lymphoma in both the eye and the CNS but avoid the toxicity of combined therapy, radiotherapy is used after chemotherapy only for recurrent disease.

Although most patients with NHL-CNS have a good initial response to therapy, recurrence is common and the 5-year survival is less than 5%. Hochberg and Miller[9] reported an overall median survival time from diagnosis of 13.5 months in patients with primary CNS lymphoma, and Freeman and colleagues[17] reported a mean survival time of 26 months for patients with intraocular lymphoma. How-ever, some reports suggest that intrathecal chemotherapy combined with radiotherapy of the orbits and whole brain may improve survival.[22]

### Systemic non-Hodgkin's lymphoma metastatic to eye

Systemic NHL can metastasize to the eye and cause an anterior or a posterior uveitis. Unlike the location of NHL-CNS cells between the RPE and Bruch's membrane, lymphoma cells in patients with systemic NHL characteristically infiltrate the choroid and may be mistaken for an ocular melanoma.[31] Metastatic lymphoma may also cause a hypopyon or hyphema in an otherwise uninflamed eye.[32] Although most patients with NHL have symptoms of lymphadenopathy, fever, and weight loss, ocular involvement may be the initial presentation of the disease.[31]

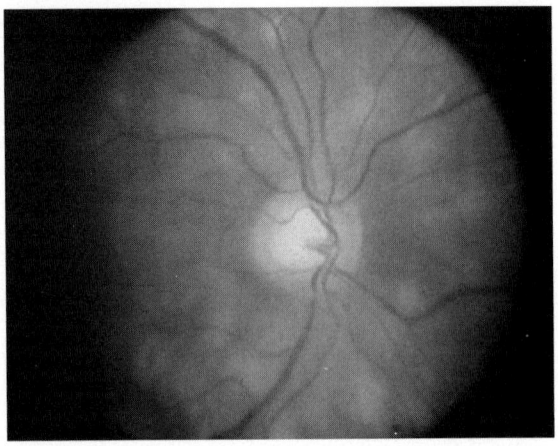

**Fig. 29-9.** Multiple yellow choroidal infiltrates in patient with lymphoid hyperplasia of uvea. (See Color Plate 51.)

## LYMPHOID HYPERPLASIA OF UVEA

Lymphoid hyperplasia of the uvea is a disorder characterized by infiltration of the uveal tract by well-differentiated small lymphocytes. The disease was initially referred to as inflammatory pseudotumors of the uveal tract, or intraocular pseudotumor.[33,34] Although the disease is usually unilateral, bilateral cases have been reported. Clinical features include anterior uveitis, vitritis, choroidal infiltrates, and iris heterochromia (Fig. 29-9).[34,35] Extraocular extension may occur, leading to conjunctival salmon-colored lesions, as well as orbital masses that cause proptosis and diplopia.[34,36] The disease is usually painless unless severe glaucoma develops.

Diagnosis has been based on histologic findings in enucleation specimens or biopsy specimens obtained from extraocular extensions of the tumor. We recently were able to make the diagnosis on the basis of a chorioretinal biopsy specimen in a 39-year-old man with painless choroidal thickening.[37] A number of pathologists believe that lymphoid hyperplasia of the uvea is probably a low-grade lymphoid neoplasia. The tumor often responds to therapy with corticosteroids, although some cases warrant the use of moderate doses of radiotherapy; unlike patients with NHL-CNS, the long-term prognosis for these patients is quite favorable.[35,36]

## OTHER MALIGNANT PROCESSES MANIFESTING AS UVEITIS

A uveal melanoma can manifest as a unilateral uveitis. Melanomas involving the ciliary body can produce dilated episcleral vessels called *sentinel vessels,* which may be misdiagnosed as an episcleritis. Melanomas of the iris can produce anterior chamber cells and flare,[38] and choroidal melanomas are often associated with cataract and a focal choroidal mass that may be mistaken for a sarcoid or tuberculous granuloma, or a posterior scleritis.[39]

Choroidal metastases can produce signs and symptoms of uveitis. In some case series, up to half of the ocular metastases are recognized before the diagnosis of an underlying malignant process.[40] Renal and lung carcinomas are the malignant conditions most likely to manifest with ocular metastases. Although breast carcinomas frequently metastasize to the eye, in more than 90% of cases the primary lesion is known at the time the ocular lesion is noted. Patients with possible metastatic disease to the eye should undergo a thorough medical evaluation to determine the underlying primary cancer. In some cases, needle aspiration of the ocular tumor may be helpful in the diagnosis.[41]

In children, retinoblastoma may manifest with tumor cells floating in the anterior chamber and be mistaken for iritis.[42] Because retinoblastoma is the most common intraocular malignant process in childhood, any young child with leukokoria, strabismus, or an undiagnosed uveitis should have the possibility of retinoblastoma excluded. Acute myelogenous leukemia can also manifest as uveitis in children, and in some cases, an anterior chamber paracentesis can be diagnostic.[43,44] Other tumors such as medulloepitheliomas and benign lesions such as juvenile xanthogranuloma can masquerade as idiopathic uveitis.[45]

Paraneoplastic syndromes may also cause intraocular inflammation and masquerade as a uveitis. Cancer-associated retinopathy (CAR) is a paraneoplastic syndrome that was initially described in three patients with oat cell carcinoma of the lung[46] but has now been reported with a number of malignant conditions. Patients usually have loss of vision, and although the fundus can appear normal early in the course of the disease, vascular sheathing, disturbances of the RPE, and optic disc pallor may ensue. Histologic studies show destruction of the photoreceptors.[47] Thirkill and coworkers[48] have identified retinal autoantibodies in patients with CAR, and some patients have responded favorably to corticosteroid therapy. These findings suggest that the retinal destruction may be partly immune-mediated.

Another paraneoplastic disorder that can masquerade as an iodiopathic uveitis has recently been named bilateral diffuse uveal melanocytic proliferation (BDUMP). Machemer[49] first reported bilateral diffuse uveal melanocytic tumors in a patient with a large retroperitoneal mass thought to be pancreatic carcinoma, and Barr and colleagues[50] reported on four similar patients with bilateral diffuse melanocytic uveal tumors in patients with an associated systemic malignant process diagnosed by biopsy or at autopsy. Although the condition occurs in patients with carcinomas, the underlying malignant processes are often occult.[51] Gass and Glatzer[52] characterize the ocular findings by the presence of multiple subtle round and oval subretinal red patches that demonstrate early hyperfluorescence on angiographic examination; multiple, slightly elevated, pigmented and nonpigmented uveal melanocytic tumors with evidence of diffuse thickening of the uveal tract; exudative retinal detachment; and the rapid development of cataracts. Episcleral injection, vitreous cells, and other signs of mild ocular inflammation can be seen.

Histopathologic findings in the ocular lesions show diffuse uveal tract infiltrates with apparently benign, spindle-shaped melanocytic cells. Some of these cells have vesiculated nuclei with prominent nucleoli, and many of the cells have foamy cytoplasm, but mitotic figures are not characteristic.[50] BDUMP should be suspected in patients with bilateral diffuse melanocytic uveal tumors, serous retinal detachments, and cataract. It is important to recognize this condition so that patients can be evaluated for underlying malignant conditions that may warrant immediate therapy to improve prognosis.

## MULTIPLE SCLEROSIS

Ocular inflammatory disease may occur in patients with multiple sclerosis. Although some authors classify multiple sclerosis in a list of masquerade syndromes, we prefer to consider multiple sclerosis as a cause of uveitis—like other uveitides with both CNS and ocular manifestations such as Vogt-Koyanagi-Harada disease. Optic neuritis is a frequent finding in patients with multiple sclerosis, and Rizzo and Lessell[53] showed that within 15 years multiple sclerosis develops in more than 50% of patients with optic neuritis. Multiple sclerosis was first associated with inflammatory eye disease in the early 1900s, and Breger and Leopold[54] found uveitis in 14 of 52 patients with multiple sclerosis. The most common ocular findings in patients with multiple sclerosis include intermediate uveitis and periphlebitis, and the uveitis may precede or follow the development of multiple sclerosis. Ohguro and colleagues[55] recently showed that 8 of 14 patients with multiple sclerosis had serum antibodies to arrestin (retinal S-antigen), although none of these patients had uveitis. In addition, antibody titers were higher during relapses than during remissions. These findings suggest that antibodies reactive with arrestin may be related to the clinical course of multiple sclerosis. Also, because arrestin is found in the eye, antiarrestin antibodies may explain the development of uveitis in some patients with multiple sclerosis.

## OTHER NONMALIGNANT CONDITIONS

A number of nonmalignant conditions can masquerade as idiopathic uveitis. An intraocular foreign body may elicit an anterior or a posterior uveitis. Patients with uniocular uveitis should be questioned about possible antecedent trauma. Gonioscopic examination should be performed to rule out a foreign body in the angle, and patients at high risk for an intraocular foreign body, such as construction workers, may require an ultrasound or CT scan to make the diagnosis. Retinal detachment can sometimes produce enough intraocular inflammation to be misdiagnosed as a uveitis, and myopic degeneration can produce cream-colored atrophic lesions that may be confused as a focal choroiditis.

Mydriatic agents can cause pigmented cells in the aqueous humor and may lead to improper grading of anterior chamber inflammation. Pigment dispersion syndrome is characterized by accumulation of pigment on the posterior surface of the central cornea in a vertical, spindle-shaped pattern (Krukenberg's spindle) (Fig. 29-10). Pigment granules may also be deposited on the anterior surface of the lens and on the iris, leading to heterochromia. Pigment dispersion may be associated with glaucoma, and in some cases may be mistaken for a uveitis.[56] Patients with retinal degenerations, such as retinitis pigmentosa (RP), may have a number of signs consistent with underlying inflammatory disease. Vitreous cells, posterior subcapsular cataract, and cystoid macular edema may occur,[57-59] and in patients in whom the characteristic bone spicule pigment is minimal, the underlying diagnosis of RP may be missed. It is of interest that some have suggested that the ocular inflammation in these cases may be due to a secondary immunologic reaction against retinal antigens released into the vitreous as the retina degenerates. Thirkill and colleagues[60] showed that sera from 11 of 52 patients with RP (21%) exhibited a minimum of twice the clinically normal reactivity with retinal antigens when assayed by ELISA, and 8 of these 11 patients possessed antibodies to the retinal S-antigen. The authors concluded that patients with RP who have indications of immunologic hypersensitivity to known uveitopathogenic retinal antigens are at higher risk for autoimmune retinopathies. Williams and coworkers[61] demonstrated that activated RP peripheral lymphocytes adhered to and altered cultured human RPE cells, suggesting that immune-mediated cytopathologic effects

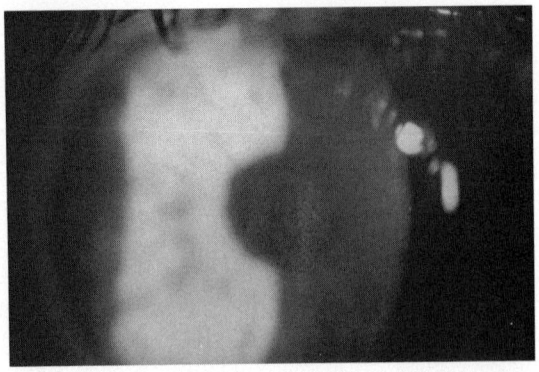

**Fig. 29-10.** Kruckenberg's spindle in patient with pigment dispersion syndrome that masqueraded as anterior uveitis. (Courtesy Muriel Kaiser-Kupfer, M.D.)

**Table 29-1.** Uveitis associated with medications

| Medication | Uveitis |
|---|---|
| Anticholinesterases and direct-acting agonists | Anterior uveitis |
| Hydralazine | Lupuslike syndrome with episcleritis and retinal vasculitis |
| Nitrogen mustard | Necrotizing uveitis with retinal vasculitis |
| Rifabutin | Hypopyon uveitis |
| Procainamide | Lupuslike syndrome with episcleritis |
| Intraocular gases | |
| Air | Anterior uveitis |
| Perfluorocarbons | Fibrinous anterior uveitis |
| Silicone oil | Anterior uveitis |
| Alpha-chymotrypsin | Severe vitritis |

may contribute to the retinal degeneration in RP.[61] If this secondary immunologic response contributes to the deterioration of visual function in patients with RP, immunosuppressive therapy may have a role in the treatment of some patients with retinal degeneration, although this hypothesis needs to be tested in controlled studies.

Indolent ocular infections may mimic a chronic idiopathic uveitis, and they are discussed in detail in Chapter 10. Fungal infections of the choroid, retina, and vitreous may occur in immunosuppressed patients, in patients with systemic fungal infections, or in patients in the postsurgical period. *Propionibacterium acnes*, a pathogen that has recently been recognized as a cause of uveitis, may not appear clinically for months after cataract surgery. *P. acnes* endophthalmitis is discussed in detail in Chapter 18.

Finally, uveitis may occur after vaccination and has also been associated with a vast number of medications, some which are listed in Table 29-1. Even topical administration of corticosteroids has been associated with the development of an anterior uveitis.[62] Of course, many of the associations between uveitis and medications may not represent a direct causal effect. Nevertheless, patients with an anterior uveitis should be asked whether they have recently started any new medications.

It is clear that a number of entities cause intraocular inflammation, and in the absence of a correct diagnosis, inappropriate therapy may be prescribed. A list of the diseases that can masquerade as a chronic idiopathic uveitis should be considered in the evaluation of all patients with undiagnosed inflammatory eye disease.

## REFERENCES


1. Theodore FH: Conjunctival carcinoma masquerading as chronic conjunctivitis, *Eye Ear Nose Throat Monthly* 46:1419-1420, 1967.
2. Kamellin S: Uveitis associated with Hodgkin's disease: report of a case, *Arch Ophthalmol* 31:517-519, 1944.
3. Barr CC, Joondeph HC: Retinal periphlebitis as the initial clinical finding in a patient with Hodgkin's disease, *Retina* 3:253-257, 1983.
4. DeAngelis LM, Yahalom J, Thaler H et al: Combined modality therapy for primary CNS lymphoma, *J Clin Oncol* 10:635-643, 1992.
5. Appen RE: Posterior uveitis and primary cerebral reticulum cell sarcoma, *Arch Ophthalmol* 93:123-124, 1975.
6. Rockwood EJ, Zakov ZN, Bay JW: Combined malignant lymphoma of the eye and CNS (reticulum-cell sarcoma), *J Neurosurg* 61:369-374, 1984.
7. Henry JM, Heffner RR Jr, Dillard SH et al: Primary malignant lymphomas of the central nervous system, *Cancer* 34:1293-1302, 1974.
8. Murray K, Kun L, Cox J: Primary malignant lymphoma of the central nervous system: results of treatment of 11 cases and review of the literature, *J Neurosurg* 65:600-607, 1986.
9. Hochberg FH, Miller DC: Primary central nervous system lymphoma, *J Neurosurg* 68:835-853, 1988.
10. Helle TL, Britt RH, Colby TV: Primary lymphoma of the central nervous system: clinicopathological study of experience at Stanford, *J Neurosurg* 60:94-103, 1984.
11. Cohen IJ, Vogel R, Matz S et al: Successful non-neurotoxic therapy (without radiation) of a multifocal primary brain lymphoma with methotexate, vincristine, and BCNY protocol (DEMOB), *Cancer* 57:6-11, 1986.
12. Qualman SJ, Mendelsohn G, Mann RB et al: Intraocular lymphomas: natural history based on a clinicopathologic study of eight cases and review of the literature, *Cancer* 52:878-886, 1983.
13. Peterson K, Gordon KB, Heinemann M-H et al: The clinical spectrum of ocular lymphoma, *Cancer* 72:843-849, 1993.
14. Schanzer CM, Font RL, O'Malley RE: Primary ocular malignant lymphoma associated with the acquired immune deficiency syndrome, *Ophthalmology* 98:88-91, 1991.
15. Johnson BL: Intraocular and central nervous system lymphoma in a cardiac transplant recipient, *Ophthalmology* 99:987-992, 1992.
16. Whitcup SM, de Smet MD, Rubin BI et al: Intraocular lymphoma: clinical and histopathologic diagnosis, *Ophthalmology* 100:1399-1406, 1993.
17. Freeman LN, Schachat AP, Knox DL et al: Clinical features, laboratory investigations, and survival in ocular reticulum cell sarcoma, *Ophthalmology* 94:1631-1639, 1987.

18. Barr CC, Green WR, Payne JW et al: Intraocular reticulum-cell sarcoma: clinicopathologic study of four cases and review of the literature, *Surv Ophthalmol* 19:224-239, 1975.
19. de Smet MD, Nussenblatt RB, Davis JL et al: Large cell lymphoma masquerading as a viral retinitis, *Int Ophthalmol* 14:413-417, 1990.
20. Davis JL, Solomon D, Nussenblatt RB et al: Immunocytochemical staining of vitreous cells: indications, techniques, and results, *Ophthalmology* 99:250-256, 1992.
21. Ljung BM, Char D, Miller TR et al: Intraocular lymphoma: cytologic diagnosis and the role of immunologic markers, *Acta Cytol* 32:840-847, 1988.
22. Char DH, Ljung B-M, Miller T et al: Primary intraocular lymphoma (ocular reticulum cell sarcoma): diagnosis and management, *Ophthalmology* 95:625-630, 1988.
23. Koster W: Über die Direkte Behandlung von Augenerkrankungen mit Radium und Metothorium, *Strahlentherapie* 3:1913.
24. Margolis L, Fraser R, Lichter A et al: The role of radiation therapy in the management of ocular reticulum cell sarcoma, *Cancer* 45:688-692, 1980.
25. Rouwen AJP, Wijermans PW, Boen-Tan TN et al: Intraocular non-Hodgkin's lymphoma treated with systemic and intrathecal chemotherapy and radiotherapy: a case report and review of the literature, *Graefes Arch Clin Exp Ophthalmol* 227:355-359, 1989.
26. Baumann MA, Ritch PS, Hande KR et al: Treatment of intraocular lymphoma with high-dose Ara-C, *Cancer* 57:1273-1275, 1986.
27. Shapiro WR, Young DF, Tehta BM: Methotrexate: distribution in cerebrospinal fluid after intravenous, intraventricular and lumbar injections, *N Engl J Med* 293:161-166, 1975.
28. Bleyer WA: Neurologic sequelae of methotrexate and ionizing radiation: a new classification, *Cancer Treat Rep* 65(suppl 1):89-98, 1981.
29. Geyer JR, Taylor EM, Milstein JM: Radiation, methotrexate, and white matter necrosis: laboratory evidence for neural radioprotection with pre-irradiation methotrexate, *Int J Radiat Oncol Biol Phys* 15:373-375, 1988.
30. Stark-Vancs V, Whitcup SM, Nussenblatt RB et al: Chemotherapy for the treatment of primary central nervous system lymphoma (PCNSL) involving the eye or brain, *Ophthalmology* 101(suppl):132, 1994.
31. Fredrick DR, Char DH, Ljung BM et al: Solitary intraocular lymphoma as an initial presentation of widespread disease, *Arch Ophthalmol* 107:395-397, 1989.
32. Guzak SV: Lymphoma as a cause of hyphema, *Arch Ophthalmol* 84:229-231, 1970.
33. Ryan SJ, Frank RN, Green WR: Bilateral inflammatory pseudotumors of the ciliary body, *Am J Ophthalmol* 72:586-591, 1971.
34. Ryan SJ, Zimmerman LE, King FM: Reactive lymphoid hyperplasia: an unusual form of intraocular pseudotumor, *Trans Am Acad Ophthalmol Otolaryngol* 76:652-671, 1972.
35. Jakobiec FA, Sacks E, Kronish JW et al: Multifocal static creamy choroidal infiltrates: an early sign of lymphoid neoplasia, *Ophthalmology* 94:397-406, 1987.
36. Desroches G, Abrams GW, Gass JDM: Reactive lymphoid hyperplasia of the uvea: a case with ultrasonographic and computed tomographic studies, *Arch Ophthalmol* 101:725-728, 1983.
37. Cheung MK, Martin DF, Chan CC et al: Diagnosis of reactive lymphoid hyperplasia by chorioretinal biopsy, *Am J Ophthalmol* 118:457-462, 1994.
38. Litricin O: Diffuse malignant ring melanoma of the iris and ciliary body, *Ophthalmologica* 178:235-238, 1979.
39. Char DH, Schwartz A, Miller TR et al: Ocular metastases from systemic malignant melanoma, *Am J Ophthalmol* 90:702-707, 1980.
40. Ferry AP, Font RL: Carcinoma metastatic to the eye and orbit. I. A clinicopathologic study of 227 cases, *Arch Ophthalmol* 92:276-286, 1974.
41. Shields JA, Shields CL, Ehya H et al: Fine-needle aspiration biopsy of suspected intraocular tumors (the 1992 Urwick lecture), *Ophthalmology* 100:1677-1684, 1993.
42. Croxatto JO, Fernandez MR, Malbran ES: Retinoblastoma masquerading as ocular inflammation, *Ophthalmologica* 186:48-53, 1983.
43. Kincaid MC, Green WR: Ocular and orbital involvement in leukemia, *Surv Ophthalmol* 27:211-232, 1983.
44. Rosenthal AR: Ocular manifestations of leukemia: a review, *Ophthalmology* 90:899-905, 1983.
45. DeBarge LR, Chan CC, Greenberg S et al: Chorioretinal, iris, and ciliary body infiltration by juvenile xanthogranuloma masquerading as uveitis, *Am J Ophthalmol* 39:65-71, 1994.
46. Sawyer RA, Selhorst JB, Zimmerman LE et al: Blindness caused by photoreceptor degeneration as a remote effect of cancer, *Am J Ophthalmol* 81:606-613, 1976.
47. Buchanan TAS, Gardiner TA, Archer DB: An ultrastructural study of retinal photoreceptor degeneration associated with bronchial carcinoma, *Am J Ophthalmol* 97:277-287, 1984.
48. Thirkill CE, Roth AM, Keltner JL: Cancer-associated retinopathy, *Arch Ophthalmol* 105:372-375, 1987.
49. Machemer R: Zur Pathogenese des flächenhaften malignen Melanoms, *Klin Monatsbl Augenheilkd* 148: 641-652, 1966.
50. Barr CC, Zimmerman LE, Curtin VT et al: Bilateral diffuse melanocytic uveal tumors associated with systemic malignant neoplasms: a recently recognized syndrome, *Arch Ophthalmol* 100:249-255, 1982.
51. Ryll DL, Campbell RJ, Robertson DM et al: Pseudometastatic lesions of the choroid, *Ophthalmology* 87:1181-1186, 1980.
52. Gass JDM, Glatzer RJ: Acquired pigmentation simulating Peutz-Jeghers syndrome: initial manifestation of diffuse uveal melanocytic proliferation, *Br J Ophthalmol* 75:693-695, 1991.
53. Rizzo JF, Lessell S: Risk of developing multiple sclerosis after uncomplicated optic neuritis, *Neurology* 38:185-190, 1988.
54. Breger BC, Leopold IH: The incidence of uveitis in multiple sclerosis, *Am J Ophthalmol* 62:540-545, 1966.
55. Ohguro H, Chiba S, Igarashi Y et al: β-Arrestin and arrestin are recognized by autoantibodies in sera from multiple sclerosis patients, *Proc Natl Acad Sci USA* 90:3241-3245, 1993.

56. Char DH: Intraocular masquerade syndromes. In Tasman W, Jaeger EA, editors: *Duane's clinical ophthalmology,* Philadelphia, 1989, JB Lippincott.
57. Heckenlively JR: The frequency of posterior subcapsular cataract in the hereditary retinal degenerations, *Am J Ophthalmol* 93:733-738, 1982.
58. Fetkenhour CL, Choromokos E, Weinstein J et al: Cystoid macular edema in retinitis pigmentosa, *Trans Am Acad Ophthalmol Otolaryngol* 83:515-521, 1977.
59. Fishman GA, Maggiero JM, Fishman M: Foveal lesions seen in retinitis pigmentosa, *Arch Ophthalmol* 95: 1993-1996, 1977.
60. Thirkill CE, Roth AM, Takemoto DJ et al: Antibody indications of secondary and superimposed retinal hypersensitivity in retinitis pigmentosa, *Am J Ophthalmol* 112:132-137, 1991.
61. Williams LL, Lew HM, Shannon BT et al: Activated retinitis pigmentosa peripheral lymphocytes adhere to and alter cultured human retinal pigment epithelial cells, *Invest Ophthalmol Vis Sci* 33:2848-2860, 1992.
62. Krupin T, LeBlanc RP, Becker B et al: Uveitis in association with topically administered corticosteroid, *Am J Ophthalmol* 70:883-885, 1970.

# Index


**A**

Acetyltrimethylcolchicine, 125-126
Acquired immunodeficiency syndrome, 186-196; *see also* Human immunodeficiency virus infection
Acute bacterial endophthalmitis, 256-257
Acute posterior multifocal placoid pigment epitheliopathy
  serpiginous choroidopathy versus, 367-368
  as white-dot syndrome, 376-379
Acute retinal necrosis, 198-203
Acute zonal occult outer retinopathy, 381
Acyclovir
  action and indications of, 122-124
  herpes simplex keratitis and, 207-208
  herpes zoster infection and, 194, 208-209
  retinal necrosis and, 202
Adhesion molecules
  monoclonal antibody therapy and, 120-121
  pathogenesis and, 38-40
Age, planning of therapy and, 99
Agglutination test, leptospirosis and, 177
AIDS; *see* Human immunodeficiency virus infection
AIDS-related complex, 187
*Alaria mesocercaria*, 252
Alkylating agent, 106-110
  Behçet's disease and, 347, 348
  dosage of, 105
  indications and dosages for, 108-109
  mode of action of, 106-108
  secondary effects of, 109-110
Allergy testing, 84
Allograft rejection, 61
Alternate-day therapy, steroid, 104-105
Amebiasis, 251
Amocarzine, for onchocerciasis, 248
Amoxicillin, Lyme disease and, 174
Amphotericin B
  candidal infection and, 180
  for fungal endophthalmitis, 259
  histoplasmosis and, 233
Ampicillin, for leptospirosis, 177
Anergy, skin testing and, 84
Anesthetic, steroids with, 103
Aneurysm, retinal, 357
Angiography
  fluorescein; *see* Fluorescein angiography
  indocyanine green, 87-88, 149
  birdshot retinochoroidopathy and, 323
Angiotensin-converting enzyme inhibitor, 294, 295-296
Angiitis, frosted-branch, 357-358
Anicteric leptospirosis, 177
Ankylosing spondylitis, 268-269
Anterior chamber
  cataract extraction and, 138
  immune response in, 19
  paracentesis of, 146-147
  parasitic infection of, 245
  slit-lamp examination of, 61-64
  tuberculosis and, 159
Anterior chamber tube shunt to encircling band procedure, 143
Anterior chamber–acquired immune deviation, 19
Anterior segment
  Behçet's disease and, 339-340
  ischemia of, 276
Anterior uveitis, 265-277
  Behçet's disease and, 339-340
  causes of, 75
  clinical description of, 265-266
  differential diagnosis of, 71
  epidemiology of, 265
  Fuchs' heterochromic iridocyclitis and, 273-275
  HLA-B27–associated, 267-273
    ankylosing spondylitis and, 268-269
    inflammatory bowel disease and, 273
    juvenile rheumatoid arthritis and, 270-273
    psoriatic arthropathy and, 273
    Reiter's syndrome and, 269-270
    Whipple's disease and, 273
  idiopathic, 266-273
  sarcoidosis and, 290-291
Antibiotic
  leptospirosis and, 177
  Lyme disease and, 174
  syphilis and, 166-167

Antibody
anticardiolipin, 347
anticytoplasmic, 343
antiendothelial, 343
aqueous humor tested for, 84
Behçet's disease and, 343
to CD4 antigen, 7
to CD8 antigen, 7
histoplasmosis, 232
human immunodeficiency virus, 186
Lyme disease and, 173
multifocal choroiditis and, 375
onchocerciasis and, 247
serpiginous choroidopathy and, 367
toxoplasmosis, 219, 221
Vogt-Koyanagi-Harada disease and, 318
Antibody-dependent cell-mediated cytotoxicity, 16
Antifungal therapy, for endophthalmitis, 259
Antigen
anterior chamber response to, 19
antinuclear, 272
autoimmunity and
ocular, 32-38
T-cell response and, 29
B cells and, 10
Behçet's disease and, 346
CD4, antibodies to, 7
classes of, 21-27
histocompatibility lymphocyte, 23-27
histoplasmin, 232
human immunodeficiency virus, 186
human leukocyte; *see* Human leukocyte antigen
Kveim, 296
multifocal choroiditis and, 374
oral tolerance and, 121-122
S-, 32-38
sarcoidosis and, 289
Sjögren's syndrome A, 361
sympathetic ophthalmia and, 305
toxoplasmosis, 212-213, 218-219
Vogt-Koyanagi-Harada disease and, 318-319
Antigen-presenting cell, 4
Antihelminthic agent, *Toxocara canis* and, 241
Anti-Mac-1 antibody, 120-121
Antimetabolite, 110-112; *see also* Azathioprine; Methotrexate
Behçet's disease and, 347-348
dosage of, 105
Antineutrophil cytoplasmic antibody
testing for, 83
Wegener's granulomatosis and, 359-360
Anti–T-cell monoclonal antibody, 120-121
Antinuclear antigen, 272
Antitoxoplasmosis therapy, 127-128
Antituberculous agent, for serpiginous choroidopathy, 368
Antiviral agent, 122-126; *see also* Acyclovir; Ganciclovir
for cytomegalovirus retinitis, 191-194
for herpes simplex virus, 207-208
Aphthous ulcer, 337-339
APMPPE; *see* Acute posterior multifocal placoid pigment epitheliopathy
Aqueous
anterior chamber paracentesis and, 146-147
Aqueous—cont'd
toxoplasmosis and, 221
Aqueous drainage device, glaucoma and, 143
Aqueous humor, antibody testing of, 84
Argyll Robertson pupil, 165
Arrestin, 32-33; *see also* S-antigen
Arteritis; *see* Retinal artery; Retinal vasculitis
Arthritis
Behçet's disease and, 343
Lyme disease and, 171, 173
rheumatoid
azathioprine for, 110
juvenile, 142
retinal vasculitis and, 361-362
sarcoidosis and, 293-294
Arthropathy, psoriatic, 273
Ascarid infestation, 238-242
Aspergillosis, 180
Asteroid body, sarcoidosis and, 294
Atovaquone, 127-128, 223-224
Auditory disorder, 313
Autoimmune disease
azathioprine for, 110
birdshot retinochoroidopathy and, 325
cyclosporine and, 116-117
infection versus, 85
intermediate uveitis and, 280, 285
sympathetic ophthalmia and, 206, 305
toxoplasmosis and, 218-219
Autoimmunity
ocular, 32-38
antigens in, 32-38
immunology and histopathology of, 34-38
T-cell response and, 29-32
Azathioprine
action and effects of, 110-111
cyclosporine with, 118
dosage of, 105
for serpiginous choroidopathy, 368
structure of, 107

## B

B cell
characteristics of, 8-13
histoplasmosis, 233
subretinal fibrosis and, 380
B1 lymphocyte, function of, 10
Bacterial infection, 155-181; *see also* Infection
Band keratopathy, 136-137
Barrier, blood-ocular, 285
Bayes' theorem, 80
*Baylisascaris procyonis*, 252
Behçet's disease, 334-351
alkylating agents for, 108-109
azathioprine for, 110
clinical manifestations of, 335-344
genital ulcers and, 339
minor criteria in, 343-344
ocular, 339-340
oral aphthous ulcers and, 337-339
skin lesions and, 339
colchicine for, 126
cytomegalovirus retinitis and, 146
epidemiology of, 334-335, 337

Behçet's disease—cont'd
FK506 for, 118-119
immune system in, 344-347
laser treatment for, 145
methotrexate for, 111
retinal necrosis and, 202
retinal vasculitis and, 355
steroids and, 102
testing for, 84
therapy for, 347-351
Behçet's minus syndrome, 355
Bejel, 168-169
Benzimidazole, 248
Betamethasone, 102
Biomicroscopy, slit-lamp, 60-64
Biopsy
chorioretinal, 85, 147-148
conjunctival, 85
multifocal choroiditis and, 375
sarcoidosis and, 295
subretinal fibrosis and, 380
Birdshot retinochoroidopathy, 325-332
clinical manifestations of, 325-329
HLA haplotypes in, 24, 25
multifocal choroiditis and, 374
testing for, 85, 329-330
therapy for, 330-332
Blackfly, onchocerciasis and, 244-249
Blau syndrome, 294
Blindness; *see also* Vision loss
Behçet's disease and, 340
fungal endophthalmitis causing, 258-259
river, 244-249
Blood cell; *see* Lymphocyte; T cell; White blood cell
Blood-borne infection, toxoplasmosis as, 225-226
Blood-ocular barrier
breakdown of, 62
intermediate uveitis and, 285
Blue cone response, 85
Body, asteroid, 294
Bone, syphilis and, 162, 163
*Borrelia burgdorferi*, 160, 170-174
relapsing fever and, 174-175
Bovine melanin protein, 33
Bowel disease, Crohn's, 360-361
Bowman's membrane, 136-137
Brain, syphilis and, 162
Bromocriptine, 126
Bronchoalveolar lavage, in sarcoidosis, 296
Brucellosis, 178
Bruch's membrane, 292-293
Buckling, scleral, 190
Busacca nodule, 63, 64
BV-ara-U, 125

## C

Calcium hydroxyapatite, 136-137
Calcofluor, 259
CAM (cell-adhesion molecule), 38-40
Cancer-associated retinopathy, 391
*Candida*, 179-180, 258-259
Capsaicin, 209
Capsulotomy, laser, 145
Carcinoma-associated retinopathy, 391
Cardiovascular system
Lyme disease and, 171
syphilis and, 161-162
Cascade, complement, 15
Case report, 91-93
Case-control study, 92
Cataract
Fuchs' heterochromic iridocyclitis and, 275
HIV infection and, 191
intermediate uveitis and, 286
sarcoidosis and, 297
uveitis and, 64
Cataract extraction, 137-142
anterior chamber and, 138
inflammation caused by, 259-260
intracapsular versus extracapsular, 137-138
intraocular lens and, 140-142
pars plana lensectomy for
sarcoidosis and, 297
with vitrectomy, 138-140
preoperative drug therapy for, 136
for sarcoidosis, 297
sympathetic ophthalmia and, 302
Vogt-Koyanagi-Harada disease and, 322
Caterpillar hair, 250-251
CD4 antigen, 7
CD8 antigen, 7
CD4 cell
HIV infection and, 186
cytomegalovirus retinitis and, 189
progressive outer retinal necrosis and, 202
sympathetic ophthalmia and, 304
Vogt-Koyanagi-Harada disease and, 318
$CD4^+$ cell
Behçet's disease and, 345
leprosy and, 157
toxoplasmosis and, 219
Vogt-Koyanagi-Harada disease and, 322
$CD5^+$ cell, 10
$CD8^+$ cell
sympathetic ophthalmia and, 304
toxoplasmosis and, 219
Vogt-Koyanagi-Harada disease and, 318, 322
CD62E, 39
Ceftriaxone, Lyme disease and, 174
Cell
anterior chamber, 61
B; *see* B cell
corticosteroids affecting, 99-102
endothelial, 20
Fuchs' heterochromic iridocyclitis and, 275
of immune system, 3-17; *see also* Immune system, cells of
lymphoma, 388
retinal pigment epithelium, proliferation of, 66
sarcoidosis and, 294-295
sympathetic ophthalmia and, 303-304
T; *see* T cell
Cell-adhesion molecules, 38-40
Cell-mediated cytotoxicity, antibody-dependent, 16
Cell-mediated immune mechanism, 17
Central nervous system; *see* Nervous system
Cerebrospinal fluid
Behçet's disease and, 343

Cerebrospinal fluid—cont'd
leptospirosis and, 176, 177
Lyme disease and, 171
lymphoma and, 387
syphilis and, 162, 168
Vogt-Koyanagi-Harada disease and, 319
Chamber, anterior; *see* Anterior chamber
Chancre, syphilitic, 161
Chelation, for band keratopathy, 136-137
Chemotherapy, lymphoma and, 389-390
Chest x-ray examination, sarcoidosis and, 295
Child
intermediate uveitis in, 280, 286
sarcoidosis in, 294
seasonal hyperacute panuveitis in, 252-253
syphilis in, 162-163
testing for, 166
*Toxocara canis* infection in, 242
toxoplasmosis in, 219, 222-223
vitrectomy in, 144
Chlorambucil
Behçet's disease and, 343
dosage of, 105, 109
structure of, 107
Chorioretinal biopsy, 85, 147-148
subretinal fibrosis and, 380
Chorioretinal scar, 274
Chorioretinitis
*Onchocerca* causing, 246
vitiliginous; *see* Birdshot retinochoroidopathy
Choroid
anatomy of, 21
examination of, 67
metastasis to, 391
parasitic infection of, 245
sympathetic ophthalmia and, 300
tuberculosis and, 158, 159
Choroidal neovascularization
histoplasmosis and, 234-235
toxoplasmosis causing, 215-216
Choroidal nodule, 67
Choroiditis
histoplasmosis, 233
multifocal, 373-375
birdshot retinochoroidopathy versus, 328
as white-dot syndrome, 373-375
*Mycobacterium avium*, 195
*Pneumocystis carinii*, 194-195
Choroidopathy; *see also* Birdshot retinochoroidopathy
"APMPPiginous," 367-368
punctate inner, 373-374
serpiginous, 364-370
Chronic cyclitis; *see* Intermediate uveitis
Chronic granulomatous disease, 178-179
Cidofovir, 194
Ciliary process, swelling in, 314
Circulating immune complex; *see* Immune complex
Clindamycin, for toxoplasmosis, 127, 223
Clinical studies of uveitis, 91-93
Clofazimine, leprosy and, 157
Cohort study, 92
Colchicine
action and indications for, 125-126
Behçet's disease and, 348
Colony-stimulating factor, 125
Color vision, 327-328
Combined therapy, for cytomegalovirus retinitis, 193-194
Complement, pathways of, 15
Computed tomography, 83
Condylomata lata, syphilis and, 161
Congenital disorder
Lyme disease as, 171
syphilis as, 162-163
testing for, 166
toxoplasmosis as, 213, 214, 219, 222-223
case report of, 224-225
Conjunctiva
biopsy of, 85
sarcoidosis and, 290
tuberculosis and, 158-159
Conjunctival injection, 60
Connective tissue disease
retinal vasculitis and, 358-359
scleritis in, 72-73
Cornea
onchocerciasis and, 244
slit-lamp examination of, 60-61
transplantation of, 137
tuberculosis and, 158-159
Corticosteroid, 99-106
Behçet's disease and, 343, 351
birdshot retinochoroidopathy and, 330-331
Fuchs' heterochromic iridocyclitis and, 275
for fungal endophthalmitis, 258
for herpes simplex keratitis, 207
for herpes zoster infection, 209
histoplasmosis and, 233-234
intermediate uveitis and, 285
Lyme disease and, 174
mode of action of, 99-106
multifocal choroiditis and, 375
preoperative, 136
preparations and dosages of, 102-103
sarcoidosis and, 296-297
secondary effects of, 103
for serpiginous choroidopathy, 368
subretinal fibrosis and, 380
sympathetic ophthalmia and, 307-308
for toxoplasmosis, 128
Vogt-Koyanagi-Harada disease and, 321
Cortisone, 102
Cotton-wool spot
appearance of, 66
HIV infection and, 188-189
Creatinine, cyclosporine and, 117
Crisis, glaucomatous cyclitic, 275
Crohn's disease, 360-361
Cryotherapy
intermediate uveitis and, 286
toxoplasmosis and, 224
*Cryptococcus neoformans*, 180
Culture, anterior chamber paracentesis for, 146-147
Cyclitic crisis, glaucomatous, 275
Cyclitis, chronic; *see* Intermediate uveitis
Cyclocryotherapy, for glaucoma, 143
Cyclogyl, 126-127
Cyclopentolate, 127

Cyclophosphamide
action of, 107
Behçet's disease and, 347-348, 350
dosage of, 105
indications of, 108-109
structure of, 107
Cycloplegic agent, 126-127
Cyclosporine
action and effects of, 113-117
autoimmune disease and, 36
Behçet's disease and, 346, 348, 349-350
birdshot retinochoroidopathy and, 331-332
bromocriptine and, 126
combination therapy with, 118
dosage of, 105, 115
indications for, 115-116
intermediate uveitis and, 286
mode of action of, 113-115
National Eye Institute study of, 93
preoperative, 136
sarcoidosis and, 297
secondary effects of, 116-117
for serpiginous choroidopathy, 368
sympathetic ophthalmia and, 308-309
Vogt-Koyanagi-Harada disease and, 321
Cyclosporine G, 118
Cyclotherapy, sympathetic ophthalmia and, 302
Cyst
of *Toxocara canis*, 238
of *Toxoplasma gondii*, 212, 218
autoimmune response to, 220
Cysticercosis, 250
Cystoid macular edema
examination for, 66
intermediate uveitis and, 281-282, 285, 286
sarcoidosis and, 292
Cytochrome P-450, 113
Cytokine
cell-adhesion molecules and, 40
eye and, 20
networks of, 15
targets and effects of, 6
Cytomegalovirus
Behçet's disease and, 146
foscarnet for, 124
ganciclovir for, 123-124, 125
HIV infection and, 188-194
Cytotoxic agent
Behçet's disease and, 347-348
types of, 106-113
Cytotoxicity, antibody-dependent cell-mediated, 16

## D

Dalen-Fuchs nodule
sarcoidosis and, 291-292, 295
sympathetic ophthalmia and, 300-303
Dapsone, leprosy and, 157-158
Daraprim; *see* Pyrimethamine
Demographics, patient, 73
Dendritic keratitis, 209
Dermatographia, 339
Detachment, retinal; *see* Retinal detachment
Dexamethasone, 102
Diagnostic testing, 79-89
ancillary ophthalmic tests and, 85-88
image analysis and, 83
laboratory, 82-83
likelihood of disease and, 79-81
neurologic, 88
new, 88-89
skin testing and, 83-84
tissue samples and, 84-85
Diethylcabamazine citrate, 247
Diethylcarbamazine, *Toxocara canis* and, 241
Differential diagnosis, development of, 69-78
acute versus chronic disease in, 69-70
case histories in, 75-78
granuloma and, 70
location of inflammation and, 71-73
patient demographics in, 73
response to previous therapy and, 75-78
signs and symptoms in, 73-74
unilateral versus bilateral disease and, 70
Differentiation, macrophage, 4
Diffuse unilateral subacute neuroretinitis, 251-252
Diffuse uveal melanocytic proliferation, 391
Diptera infestation, 249-250
Disc, optic, sarcoidosis and, 293
Disease pathogenesis, 18-42; *see also* Pathogenesis
Dispersion, pigment, 392
DNA testing, 88-89
Doxycycline, 177
Lyme disease and, 174
Drug therapy, 97-129; *see also specific drug*
antitoxoplasmosis, 127-128
antiviral, 122-126; *see also* Acyclovir; Ganciclovir
bromocriptine and, 126
colchicine and, 125-126
corticosteroid; *see* Corticosteroid
FK506 and, 118-119
goals and philosophy of, 97-98
immunostimulators and, 128
immunosuppressive, 99-120
alkylating agents and, 106-110
antimetabolites for, 110-112
corticosteroids and, 99-106
cyclosporine and, 113-118; *see also* Cyclosporine
cytotoxic agents and, 106-113
monoclonal antibodies and, 121-122
mydriatic and cycloplegic agents and, 126-127
nonsteroidal antiinflammatory drugs and, 129
oral tolerance and, 121-122
plasmapheresis and, 128-129
rapamycin and, 119-120
response to, in differential diagnosis, 75-78
Drug-induced disorder
HIV infection and, 196
malignancy as, 110
uveitis as, 393

## E

Eales' disease, 158, 355-357
Edema, cystoid macula; *see* Cystoid macular edema
Egg, *Toxocara canis*, 238
ELAM-1, 39
Electrolytes, corticosteroids affecting, 106

Electrooculography
multiple evanescent white-dot syndrome and, 372
retinal pigment epitheliitis and, 376
subretinal fibrosis and, 380
sympathetic ophthalmia and, 302
Vogt-Koyanagi-Harada disease and, 318
Electrophysiologic testing, 85
Electroretinography
multiple evanescent white-dot syndrome and, 372
retinal pigment epitheliitis and, 376
subretinal fibrosis and, 380
sympathetic ophthalmia and, 302
Vogt-Koyanagi-Harada disease and, 318
Endemic syphilis, 168-169
Endocrine system, corticosteroids affecting, 104
Endophthalmitis
bacterial, 256-257
acute, 256-257
chronic, 257-258
fungal, 179-181, 258-259
*Toxocara canis*, 239
Endothelial cell, 20
Endothelial leukocyte adhesion molecule-1, 39
Endotheliopathy, autoimmune, 280
Endotoxin
autoimmune disease and, 36
bacterial, 155
Endotoxin-induced uveitis, 155
Enucleation, 307
Enzyme-linked immunosorbent assay
Lyme disease and, 173
relapsing fever and, 175
*Toxocara canis* and, 240-241
toxoplasmosis and, 220
Wegener's granulomatosis and, 360
Eosinophils
characteristics of, 14
sympathetic ophthalmia and, 303
Epiretinal membrane, removal of, 145
Epitheliitis, retinal pigment, 375-376
Epitheliopathy, acute posterior multifocal placoid pigment
serpiginous choroidopathy versus, 367-368
as white-dot syndrome, 376-379
Epithelium, retinal pigment; *see* Retinal pigment epithelium
Epstein-Barr virus
choroidal disease and, 198
multifocal choroiditis and, 374-375
Erythema chronicum migrans, 170, 171, 173
Erythema nodosa, sarcoidosis and, 293, 295
Erythema nodosum, Behçet's disease and, 339
Erythromycin, relapsing fever and, 175
E-selectin, 39
ETDRS chart, 59, 85-86
Ethambutol, for tuberculosis, 159
Ethnic differences
Behçet's disease and, 337
birdshot retinochoroidopathy and, 329
HLA antigens and, 25
sympathetic ophthalmia and, 303
Vogt-Koyanagi-Harada disease and, 312, 313, 320
Ethylenediaminetetraacetic acid, 136-137
Evanescent white-dot syndrome, multiple, 371-372
Examination of patient, 58-68
choroid and, 65-67
external, 59
intraocular pressure and, 59-60
optic nerve and, 68
of pupils and extraocular muscles, 59
of retina, 65-67
slit-lamp, 60-64
visual acuity and, 58-59
of vitreous, 64-65
Extracapsular cataract extraction; *see* Cataract extraction
Extraocular muscle, examination of, 59
Exudate, intermediate uveitis and, 280-281, 283
Eyelid
leprosy and, 156
syphilis and, 163-164

## F

Fenestration, optic nerve, 202-203
Fetus
Lyme disease and, 171
syphilis in, 162-163
Fever, relapsing, 174-175
Fibrin, 136
Fibrosis, subretinal, 377
Fibrovascular membrane, 63
55-kd Tac monoclonal antibody, 120
FK506, 118-119
Behçet's disease and, 348
dosage of, 105
Flare, anterior chamber, 62
Floater, patient history of, 51
Flucytosine, 180
Fluid
cerebrospinal; *see* Cerebrospinal fluid
corticosteroids affecting, 106
subretinal, 67
vitreous; *see* Vitreous
Fluorescein angiography
acute posterior multifocal placoid pigment epitheliopathy and, 376, 377
Behçet's disease and, 340, 341, 342
birdshot retinochoroidopathy and, 326, 327
diagnostic, 86, 87
Eales' disease and, 356
intermediate uveitis and, 283
multifocal choroiditis and, 374
retinal vasculitis and, 358
serpiginous choroidopathy and, 365, 366, 369
sympathetic ophthalmia and, 302
toxoplasmosis and, 214
Vogt-Koyanagi-Harada disease and, 316, 318
white-dot syndrome and, 372
Fluorescent treponema antibody absorption test
likelihood of disease and, 82-83
Lyme disease and, 173
syphilis and, 165-166
5-Fluorouracil
glaucoma and, 143
local injection of, 112-113
Foscarnet
action and indications of, 124
cytomegalovirus retinitis and, 192, 193
herpes zoster and, 194

Foscarnet—cont'd
progressive outer retinal necrosis and, 203, 205
Fracture, syphilis and, 162
Frambesia, 169-170
Frosted-branch angiitis, 357-358
Fuchs' heterochromic iridocyclitis
anterior uveitis with, 273-275
toxoplasmosis and, 216-217
Fundus
acute posterior multifocal placoid pigment epitheliopathy and, 377
birdshot retinochoroidopathy and, 326
multifocal choroiditis and panveitis and, 373
multiple evanescent white-dot syndrome and, 371-372
Vogt-Koyanagi-Harada disease and, 315
Fungal infection, 179-181
endophthalmitis caused by, 288-289
histoplasmosis as, 229-235

## G

Gallium scan, sarcoidosis and, 296
Ganciclovir
action and indications of, 123-124
colony-stimulating factor and, 125
cytomegalovirus retinitis and, 191-194
foscarnet with, 124
progressive outer retinal necrosis and, 203-205
Gastrointestinal system, corticosteroids affecting, 106
Genital ulcer, 339
Geographic choroidopathy; *see* Serpiginous choroidopathy
German measles, 209
Giardiasis, 248-249
Glaucoma
Behçet's disease and, 340
examination for, 63-64
herpes simplex virus and, 208
intermediate uveitis and, 280
lens-induced uveitis and, 276
sarcoidosis and, 292, 297
surgery for, 142-144
UGH syndrome and, 260
Vogt-Koyanagi-Harada disease and, 314
Glaucomatous cyclitic crisis, 275
Goniotomy, 142-144
Graft, rejection of, 61
Granulomatous disease
causes of, 71
in differential diagnosis of uveitis, 70
histoplasmosis versus, 232
infection and, 178-179
keratic precipitates and, 60-61
lens-induced, 259
leprosy and, 156, 157
sarcoidosis as, 289-298; *see also* Sarcoidosis
sympathetic ophthalmia as, 299-309; *see also* Sympathetic ophthalmia
tuberculosis as, 158
Wegener's granulomatosis and
testing for, 83
vasculitis with, 359-360
Growth factor, 19
Gumma, of syphilis, 161, 164

## H

Hair, caterpillar, 250-251
Hansen's disease, 156-158
Haplotype, HLA; *see* Human leukocyte antigen
Haze, vitreous, 65
Helicoid choroidopathy; *see* Serpiginous choroidopathy
Helminth infection, onchocerciasis and, 244-249
Helminth infestation
*Taenia solium* and, 250
*Toxocara canis* and, 251-252
Helper T cell
characteristics of, 8, 10
corticosteroids and, 99, 101
Hemorrhage
retinal, 66
vitreous, 281
Hereditary disorder
granulomatous, 178-179
sarcoidosis and, 294
Herpes simplex virus, 207-208
acyclovir for, 122-123
keratitis caused by, 207-208
rapid tests for, 89
retinal necrosis and, 201
retinitis caused by, 207-208
sorivudine for, 125
testing for, 84-85
Herpes zoster
acyclovir for, 122-123
HIV infection and, 191
rapid tests for, 89
retinal necrosis and, 201
Herpes zoster ophthalmicus, 207-208
Herpesvirus hominis, retinal necrosis and, 201
Heterochromic iridocyclitis, Fuchs'
anterior uveitis with, 273-275
toxoplasmosis and, 216-217
Hilar adenopathy, in sarcoidosis, 294, 295
Histamine, 13
Histocompatibility lymphocyte antigen, 23-27
Histology
Behçet's disease and, 344-347
sympathetic ophthalmia and, 302-303
Histoplasmin antigen, 232
Histoplasmosis, 179, 229-235
etiology of, 232-233
ocular appearance of, 229-230
subfoveal neovascular membrane and, 149-150
systemic findings in, 229
therapy for, 233-235
History taking, 51-57
HLA typing; *see* Human leukocyte antigen
Hodgkin's lymphoma, 385
HPMPC
action and indications for, 124-125
for cytomegalovirus retinitis, 194
Hruby lens examination
for cystoid macular edema, 66
grading of vitreous cells with, 64
retinal lesion and, 67
Human immunodeficiency virus infection, 186-196
anterior uveitis with, 276
atovaquone and, 127-128
clinical manifestations of, 186-188

Human immunodeficiency virus infection—cont'd
cytomegalovirus retinitis in, 188-194
drug-related inflammation in, 196
fungal infection in, 181
herpes zoster in, 194
immune response to, 42
immunostimulators and, 128
lymphoma and, 386
*Mycobacterium avium* choroiditis in, 195
*Pneumocystis carinii* choroiditis in, 194-195
progressive outer retinal necrosis and, 203-205
syphilis and, 160, 167, 168
toxoplasmosis and, 217-218
atovaquone for, 224
case report of, 225
treatment of, 224
Human leukocyte antigen
Behçet's disease and, 346
birdshot retinochoroidopathy and, 329
distribution of, 24
histoplasmosis and, 233
intermediate uveitis and, 279-280
pathogenesis and, 23-27
serpiginous choroidopathy and, 367
Vogt-Koyanagi-Harada disease and, 320
Hutchinson's teeth, 163
Hydrocortisone, 102
Hyperacute panuveitis, seasonal, 252-253
Hypermature lens, 259-260
Hyperplasia, lymphoid, 150, 390-391
Hypersensitivity reaction
Behçet's disease and, 339
characteristics of, 15-17
immune complex–mediated, 26-28; *see also* Immune complex
methotrexate causing, 112
testing for, 84
Hypertension, cyclosporine and, 115
Hyphema, UGH syndrome and, 260
Hypopyon
Behçet's disease and, 340
definition of, 63
seasonal hyperacute panuveitis and, 253

## I

ICAM; *see* Intracellular adhesion molecule-1
Imaging, diagnostic, 83
Immune complex
Behçet's disease and, 344
circulating, 83
Eales' disease and, 356
inflammatory response caused by, 16-17
tissue damage caused by, 26-28
toxoplasmosis and, 220
Immune system
Behçet's disease and, 344-347
birdshot retinochoroidopathy and, 329-330
cells of, 3-17
B cells, 8-13
complement system and, 15
eosinophils, 14
hypersensitivity reactions and, 15-17
macrophages and monocytes, 3-5
mast, 13-14
Immune system—cont'd
cells of—cont'd
resident ocular, 14-15
T cells, 3-8
corticosteroids affecting, 99-100
eye and, 18-21
histoplasmosis and, 232-233
intraocular lens and, 259-260
leprosy and, 157
onchocerciasis and, 247
retinal necrosis and, 200-201
sarcoidosis and, 289
subretinal fibrosis and, 380
sympathetic ophthalmia and, 302-307
*Toxocara canis* and, 239-241
toxoplasmosis affecting, 217-218
Vogt-Koyanagi-Harada disease and, 318-320
Immunocompromised patient; *see* Immunosuppression
Immunodeficiency, 186-196; *see also* Human immunodeficiency virus infection
Immunofluorescent assay
Lyme disease and, 173
relapsing fever and, 175
Immunogenetics, 22-27
Immunoglobulin
Behçet's disease and, 343, 344
functions and characteristics of, 10-13
multifocal choroiditis and, 374, 375
Immunostimulator, 128
Immunosuppression, 99-120
alkylating agents for, 106-110
antimetabolites and, 110-112
Behçet's disease and, 348-350
corticosteroid for, 99-106; *see also* Corticosteroid
cyclosporine for, 113-118; *see also* Cyclosporine
cytotoxic agents for, 106-113
intermediate uveitis and, 286
oral tolerance and, 20-21
toxoplasmosis and, 217-218
visual acuity testing and, 85
Implant
ganciclovir, 193
Molteno, glaucoma and, 143-144
Imuran; *see* Azathioprine
Indocyanine green angiography, 87-88, 149
birdshot retinochoroidopathy and, 327
Infant; *see* Neonate
Infection, 155-260
anterior chamber paracentesis for, 146-147
anterior uveitis with, 276-277
endophthalmitis and
acute, 256-257
chronic, 257-258
fungal, 258-259
fungal, 179-181
histoplasmosis as, 229-235
granulomatous disease and, 178-179
immune mechanisms in, 40, 41-42
intermediate uveitis and, 283
leprosy, 156-158
as masquerade syndrome, 393
opportunistic, 117
parasitic, 238-250; *see also* Parasitic infection
serpiginous choroidopathy and, 367

Infection—cont'd
spirochetal, 160-178
brucellosis, 178
leptospirosis, 175-178
Lyme disease, 170-174
pinta, 167-168
relapsing fever, 174-175
syphilis, 160-169
yaws, 169-170
tuberculosis, 158-160
viral
acute retinal necrosis caused by, 198-203
Behçet's disease and, 346
cytomegalovirus; *see* Cytomegalovirus
herpes simplex, 207-208; *see also* Herpes simplex virus
herpes zoster; *see* Herpes zoster
human immunodeficiency, 186-196; *see also* Human immunodeficiency virus infection
immune response to, 41-42
multifocal choroiditis and, 374
progressive outer retinal necrosis and, 203-205
retinal vasculitis and, 361
Infiltration, sympathetic ophthalmia and, 302
Inflammation
Behçet's disease and, 339-340
cataract surgery and, 140-142
corticosteroids for, 97-98
degree and location of, 97-98
keratic precipitates and, 60-61
laser treatment and, 146
leprosy and, 156-158
multifocal choroiditis and, 375
postoperative, 256-260
retinal vasculitis and, 354-355
rifabutin causing, 196
sarcoidosis and, 291
surgery and, 135-136
sympathetic ophthalmia and; *see* Sympathetic ophthalmia
*Toxocara canis* and, 241
toxoplasmosis and, 220
types of reactions to, 16-17
Vogt-Koyanagi-Harada disease and, 313, 316
Injection, periocular
birdshot retinochoroidopathy and, 330-331
method of, 102-103
multifocal choroiditis and, 375
Injury, sympathetic ophthalmia after, 299-309; *see also* Sympathetic ophthalmia
Inner choroidopathy, punctate, 373-374
Interferometry, laser, 85-86
Interferon
toxoplasmosis and, 219
Vogt-Koyanagi-Harada disease and, 319
Interleukins
Behçet's disease and, 345-346
cyclosporine and, 114-115
function of, 8
hypersensitivity reaction and, 16
macrophage and, 5
onchocerciasis and, 247
pro- and antiinflammatory, 20
target and effects of, 6
Intermediate uveitis, 279-287
clinical manifestations of, 280-282
differential diagnosis of, 71-72, 282
epidemiology of, 279-280
etiology of, 284-285
Lyme disease and, 170-171
prognosis of, 282
treatment of, 285-287
Interphotoreceptor retinoid-binding protein
anterior chamber–acquired immune deviation and, 19
autoimmune disease and, 33, 34-36
sympathetic ophthalmia and, 305
Interstitial keratitis
syphilis and, 165
tuberculosis and, 158
Intracapsular cataract extraction, 137
Intracellular adhesion molecule-1, 39
Intraocular fluid, 84
Intraocular lens, 140-142
inflammation from, 259-260
intermediate uveitis and, 287
Intraocular lymphoma, 385-390
Intraocular pressure, 59-60
Iridocyclitis
Behçet's disease and, 340
Fuchs' heterochromic
anterior uveitis with, 273-275
toxoplasmosis and, 216-217
sarcoidosis and, 291
Iridotomy, laser, 145
Iris
glaucoma surgery and, 143
onchocerciasis and, 244
sarcoidosis and, 290-291
tuberculosis and, 158
Vogt-Koyanagi-Harada disease and, 314
Iris nodule, types of, 63
Irradiation, sympathetic ophthalmia and, 302
Ischemia, anterior segment, 276
Isoniazid, tuberculosis and, 159-160
Ivermectin, for onchocerciasis, 248

## J

Jarisch-Herxheimer reaction
relapsing fever and, 175
syphilis and, 168
Juvenile rheumatoid arthritis, 142
anterior uveitis with, 270-273

## K

Kawasaki disease, 275
Keratic precipitates
characteristics of, 60-61
differential diagnosis and, 70
Fuchs' heterochromic iridocyclitis and, 274
herpes simplex virus and, 208
Vogt-Koyanagi-Harada disease and, 313, 314, 322
Keratitis
herpes simplex, 207-208
syphilis and, 163, 164
tuberculosis and, 158
Ketoconazole, 259
Kirisawa's uveitis, 198
Koeppe nodule, 63

KP; *see* Keratic precipitates
Kveim test, 84
  sarcoidosis and, 296

## L

Laboratory tests for uveitis, 82-83
Lacrimal gland, sarcoidosis and, 290, 295
Lactate dehydrogenase, *Toxocara canis*, 239
Larva, *Toxocara canis*, 238
Larval migrans, 238-239
Laser cell/flare meter, 88
Laser interferometry, 85-86
Laser treatment
  for cataract extraction, 138
  histoplasmosis and, 234-235
  indications for, 145-146
  inflammation caused by, 260
  multifocal choroiditis and, 375
  sympathetic ophthalmia and, 302
  types of, 145-146
Latent syphilis, 161
Lavage, bronchoalveolar, 296
Lens
  intraocular, 140-142
    intermediate uveitis and, 287
  *Toxocara canis* in, 239
Lensectomy, toxoplasmosis and, 224
Lens-induced uveitis, 259
  anterior, 276
Leprosy, 156-158
Leptospirosis, 175-178
Leukotriene, 14
Levamisole, 128
Literature evaluation, 91-93
Liver, methotrexate affecting, 111-112
Long-acting thyroid stimulatory antibody, 17
Lumbar puncture, 313
Lupus erythematosus, 359
Lyme disease, 170-174
  clinical manifestations of, 170-172
  diagnosis of, 172-173
  etiology of, 170
  intermediate uveitis and, 283
  pretest likelihood of, 80
  prognosis of, 173-174
  sarcoidosis versus, 294
  treatment of, 174
Lymphadenectomy
  in sarcoidosis, 294, 295
  syphilis and, 161
Lymphatic drainage, 18
Lymphocyte; *see also* CD cell *entries*
  in anterior chamber, 61-62
  B, 8-13
    characteristics of, 8-13
    histoplasmosis, 233
    subretinal fibrosis and, 380
  corticosteroids and, 99
  retinal necrosis and, 200
  sarcoidosis and, 289
  sympathetic ophthalmia and, 304, 305
  T; *see* T cell
  Vogt-Koyanagi-Harada disease and, 319
Lymphoid hyperplasia, 150
Lymphokine, 8
Lymphoma, intraocular, 385-390
Lysozyme, 296

## M

Macrofilaricidal agent, 248
Macrophage, 3-5
Macula
  birdshot retinochoroidopathy and, 327-329
  cystoid edema of; *see* Cystoid macular edema
  cytomegalovirus and, 190
  *Toxocara canis* and, 239
  toxoplasmosis and, 223
Maculopathy, histoplasmosis and, 230-231
Magnetic resonance imaging
  Behçet's disease and, 343-344
  diagnostic, 83
  intermediate uveitis and, 283
  lymphoma and, 387
Major histocompatibility complex, 4
Malignancy
  alkylating agents causing, 110
  masquerade syndromes and, 385-391
  toxoplasmosis and, 221
Malignant melanoma, 302
Marker, cell, on phagocytic cells, 3
Masquerade syndrome, 385-393
  intraocular lymphoma as, 385-390
  lymphoid hyperplasia of uvea and, 390-391
  malignancy and, 385-391
  multiple sclerosis and, 392
  nonmalignant, 392-393
Mast cell, 13-14
Measles, 209
Mediator, synechiae and, 63
Medical history, 51-57
Medical therapy, nonsurgical, 97-129; *see also* Drug therapy
Melanin protein, bovine, 33
Melanocytic proliferation, diffuse uveal, 391
Melanoma, 302
Membrane
  Bruch's, 292-293
  epiretinal, removal of, 145
  fibrovascular, 63
  neovascular; *see also* Neovascularization
    histoplasmosis and, 232
    subfoveal, 149
  pupillary, laser treatment of, 145
Memory B cell, 9-10
Meningovascular syphilis, 162
Mepron; *see* Atovaquone
Metamorphopsia, 231
Metastatic lymphoma, 390
Methotrexate
  action and effects of, 113-117
  cyclosporine with, 118
  dosage of, 105
  structure of, 107
Methylprednisolone
  dosage of, 105
  potency of, 102
  for serpiginous choroidopathy, 368
  Vogt-Koyanagi-Harada disease and, 321

Miconazole, 259
Microfilaria, of *Onchocerca*, 244
Minocycline, 128
Mitomycin, 143
Molteno implant, 143-144
Monoclonal antibody
  cell-adhesion molecules and, 40
  cytomegalovirus-specific, 193
  types of, 121-122
Monocyte, 3-5
Mononeuritis multiplex, 359
Mucocutaneous lymph node syndrome, 275
Müller cells, 19-20
Multifocal choroiditis
  birdshot retinochoroidopathy versus, 328
  as white-dot syndrome, 373-375
Multifocal placoid pigment epitheliopathy, acute posterior
  serpiginous choroidopathy versus, 367-368
  as white-dot syndrome, 376-379
Multiple evanescent white-dot syndrome, 371-372
Multiple sclerosis
  intermediate uveitis and, 280, 285
  masquerade syndromes and, 392
  vasculitis with, 358-359
Muscle, extraocular, examination of, 59
Musculoskeletal system, corticosteroids affecting, 106
*Mycobacterium avium* choroiditis, 195
*Mycobacterium leprae*, 156-158
Mydriatic agent
  indications for, 126-127
  masquerade syndromes and, 392

## N

National Eye Institute cyclosporine study, 93
Nd:YAG laser; *see* Laser treatment
Necrosis, retinal
  acute, 198-203
  progressive outer, 203-205
Nematode, 251-252; *see also* Parasitic infection
Nematode infection, *Toxocara canis* as, 238-242
Neodynium:yttrium-aluminum-garnet laser; *see also* Laser treatment
  cataract extraction and, 138
  indications for, 145-146
  inflammation caused by, 260
  sympathetic ophthalmia and, 302
Neonate
  syphilis in, 162-163
    testing for, 166
  toxoplasmosis in, 219, 222-223
Neoplasia, azathioprine causing, 111
Neovascular membrane, subfoveal, 149
Neovascularization
  choroidal, histoplasmosis and, 234-235
  intermediate uveitis and, 281, 282
  multifocal choroiditis and, 375
  pars planitis and, 284
  serpiginous choroidopathy and, 361
  subretinal
    histoplasmosis and, 232, 234-235
    sarcoidosis and, 292
  toxoplasmosis causing, 215-216
  Vogt-Koyanagi-Harada disease and, 314
Nephrotoxicity, HPMPC causing, 125
Nerve, optic; *see* Optic nerve
Nervous system
  Behçet's disease and, 343-344
  corticosteroids affecting, 106
  leptospirosis and, 177
  Lyme disease and, 172
  lymphoma of, 385-390
  relapsing fever and, 175
  sarcoidosis and, 294
  syphilis and, 162, 168
  toxoplasmosis and, 213
Neurologic deficit
  Behçet's disease and, 343-344
  Lyme disease and, 172
Neurologic test, 88
Neuropathy, optic, retinal necrosis and, 199
Neuroretinitis, parasitic, 251-252
Neurosyphilis, 162
  testing for, 168
Neutropenia, ganciclovir and, 192
Neutrophil, corticosteroids affecting, 100
Night vision, 327-328
Nitrogen mustard, 106-107
*Nocardia*, 181
Nodule
  Busacca, 63, 64
  choroidal, 67
  Dalen-Fuchs
    sarcoidosis and, 291-292, 295
    sympathetic ophthalmia and, 300-303
  iris, 290-291
  Vogt-Koyanagi-Harada disease and, 313, 314
Nodulectomy, for onchocerciasis, 247
Non-Hodgkin's lymphoma, 385-390
Nonsteroidal antiinflammatory drug, 129
  for arthritis, 272

## O

Obliterative perivasculitis, 356
Occlusive retinopathy, 354
Occult outer retinopathy, acute zonal, 381
Ocular cell, resident, 14-15
Ocular examination, 58-68; *see also* Examination of patient
*Oestrus ovis*, 249-250
OKT2 monoclonal antibody, 120
Onchocerciasis, 244-249
Ophthalmia, sympathetic, 299-309; *see also* Sympathetic ophthalmia
Ophthalmomyiasis, 249-250
Opportunistic infection, 117; *see also* Human immunodeficiency virus infection
Opsin, 33
Optic disc, sarcoidosis and, 293
Optic nerve
  examination of, 68
  retinal necrosis and, 200, 202-203
  *Toxocara canis* and, 239
  toxoplasmosis and, 223
  Vogt-Koyanagi-Harada disease and, 315
Oral aphthous ulcer, 337-339
Oral tolerance, 20-21, 121-122
Oral ulceration, Behçet's disease and, 337-339
Outer retinopathy, acute zonal occult, 381

## P


p22 antigen, 212-213
Pain
  relapsing fever and, 174
  relief of, 97
Panencephalitis, subacute sclerosing, 209
Panuveitis
  birdshot retinochoroidopathy versus, 328
  multifocal choroiditis and, 373-375
  seasonal hyperacute, 252-253
Papilledema, sarcoidosis and, 293
Papule, syphilis and, 161, 162
Paracentesis, anterior chamber, 146-147
Paraneoplastic syndrome, 391
Parasitic infection, 238-250
  amebiasis as, 251
  caterpillar hairs causing, 250-251
  cysticercosis as, 250
  giardiasis as, 248-249
  immune response to, 41-42
  neuroretinitis caused by, 251-252
  onchocerciasis as, 244-249
  ophthalmomyiasis as, 249-250
  seasonal hyperacute panuveitis and, 252-253
  *Toxocara canis* and, 238-242
  toxoplasmosis as, 211-226; *see also* Toxoplasmosis
Parenchymatous neurosyphilis, 162
Parodel; *see* Bromocriptine
Pars plana, examination of, 68
Pars plana lensectomy, 138-140
  for sarcoidosis, 297
Pars planitis
  cause of, 284-285
  intermediate uveitis and
    clinical manifestations of, 281
    epidemiology of, 279-280
    prognosis of, 279
  vitrectomy for, 286
Pathogenesis, 18-42
  autoimmunity and
    ocular, 32-38
    T cells and, 29-32
  cell-adhesion molecules and, 38-40
  immune characteristics of eye and, 18-21
  immune complex–mediated disease and, 26-28
  immunogenetics and, 22-27
  T cells and, 29-32
  viral and parasitic disease and, 41-42
Patient examination, 58-68
Patient history, 51-57
  questionnaire for, 53-57
Penetrating trauma, sympathetic ophthalmia after, 299-309; *see also* Sympathetic ophthalmia
Penicillin
  leptospirosis and, 177
  Lyme disease and, 174
  syphilis and, 167-168
Periocular injection
  birdshot retinochoroidopathy and, 330-331
  intermediate uveitis and, 285
  method of, 102-103
  multifocal choroiditis and, 375
  secondary effects of, 103
Peripapillary pigment, histoplasmosis and, 232
Peripheral uveitis; *see* Intermediate uveitis
Peripheral vascular sheathing, 66
Periphlebitis, Eales' disease and, 356
Phacoanaphylaxis, 259, 302
  sympathetic ophthalmia and, 304-305
Phacoantigenic glaucoma, 276
Phagocytosis, 15-17
Phlyctenular keratoconjunctivitis, 158
Phosducin, 33-34
Photocoagulation
  histoplasmosis and, 234-235
  retinal, 145-146
Photophobia
  pain relief and, 97
  relapsing fever and, 174
Phthisis bulbi, 282
Pigment
  peripapillary, histoplasmosis and, 232
  white-dot syndrome and, 371-383
Pigment dispersion syndrome, 392
Pigment epitheliopathy, acute posterior multifocal placoid
  serpiginous choroidopathy versus, 367-368
  as white-dot syndrome, 376-379
Pigment epithelium, retinal; *see* Retinal pigment epithelium
Pinta, 169-170
Placoid pigment epitheliopathy, acute posterior multifocal
  serpiginous choroidopathy versus, 367-368
  as white-dot syndrome, 376-379
Plasma cell, 275
Plasmapheresis
  Behçet's disease and, 348
  effectiveness of, 128-129
*Pneumocystis carinii* choroiditis, 194-195
Pneumonitis, 112
Pole, posterior
  Behçet's disease and, 341
  birdshot retinochoroidopathy and, 326
Polyarteritis nodosa, 359
Polychondritis, relapsing, 361
Polymerase chain reaction, 88-89
  for toxoplasmosis, 221
Posterior multifocal placoid pigment epitheliopathy
  acute, 376-379
  serpiginous choroidopathy versus, 367-368
Posterior pole
  Behçet's disease and, 341
  birdshot retinochoroidopathy and, 326
Posterior scleritis, 358
Posterior segment
  Behçet's disease and, 341, 342
  Fuchs' heterochromic iridocyclitis and, 273-275
  sarcoidosis and, 291-293
Posterior uveitis
  causes of, 75
  differential diagnosis of, 72
  electroretinography and, 85
Postoperative sympathetic ophthalmia, 299-300
Postoperative uveitis, 256-260
Precipitates, keratic; *see* Keratic precipitates
Prednisolone, 102

Prednisone
  Behçet's disease and, 349
  cyclosporine with, 118
  dosage of, 104
  National Eye Institute study of, 93
  potency of, 102
  preoperative, 136
  *Toxocara canis* and, 241
  toxoplasmosis and, 223
  Vogt-Koyanagi-Harada disease and, 321
Pregnancy, toxoplasmosis in, 213, 221
Pressure, intraocular; *see* Intraocular pressure
Pretest likelihood of disease, 79-81
Prick test, in Behçet's disease, 339, 347
Probenecid, HPMPC with, 124-125
Progressive outer retinal necrosis, 203-205
Prolactin, bromocriptine and, 126
Proliferation, diffuse uveal melanocytic, 391
Proliferative vitreoretinopathy, 145
*Propionibacterium acnes*, 257-258
Protease, macrophage and, 5
Protein
  in anterior chamber, 62
  bovine melanin, 33
  interphotoreceptor retinoid-binding
    autoimmune disease and, 33, 34-36
    sympathetic ophthalmia and, 305
Protozoan infection, 248-249; *see also* Parasitic infection
Psoriatic arthropathy, 273
Pulse cyclophosphamide, 109
  Behçet's disease and, 348
Punctate inner choroidopathy, 373-374
Pupil
  Argyll Robertson, 165
  examination of, 59
Pupillary block glaucoma, 143
Pupillary membrane, laser treatment of, 145
Purified protein derivative, 83-84
  ocular tuberculosis and, 158, 159
  tuberculosis and, 159
Purified protein derivative test, reaction to, 17
Pyrimethamine, 127
  toxoplasmosis and, 223

## Q

Questionnaire, patient history, 53-57

## R

Racial differences
  birdshot retinochoroidopathy and, 329
  HLA antigens and, 25
  sympathetic ophthalmia and, 303
  Vogt-Koyanagi-Harada disease and, 312, 313, 320
Radiation therapy
  lymphoma and, 389-390
  sympathetic ophthalmia and, 299
Radiographic evaluation
  diagnostic, 83
  sarcoidosis and, 295
Randomized clinical trial, 92
Rapamycin, 119-120
Rapid plasma reagin test, for syphilis, 165
Reactive lymphoid hyperplasia, 150
Receptor
  autoimmunity and, 32
  corticosteroids and, 99, 100
  function of, 8
Recoverin, 33
Reiter's syndrome, 269-270
Rejection of allograft, 61
Relapsing fever, 174-175
Relapsing polychondritis, 361
Renal system
  anterior uveitis and, 275
  cyclosporine and, 115, 116-117
  HPMPC and, 125
  methotrexate and, 112
Resident ocular cell, 14-15
  pathogenesis of disease and, 19-20
Respiratory sarcoidosis, 295-296
Retina; *see also* Retinal *entries*
  Behçet's disease and, 340
  birdshot retinochoroidopathy and, 325-332
  chorioretinal biopsy and, 147-148
  examination of, 65-67
  leprosy and, 157
  parasitic infection of, 245
  pars planitis and, 284
  pathogenesis of disease and, 21
  photocoagulation of, 145-146
  sympathetic ophthalmia and, 303
  *Toxocara canis* and, 241
  toxoplasmosis and, 213, 215
Retinal artery; *see also* Retinal vasculitis
  alterations in, 66
  aneurysm of, 357
  Behçet's disease and, 334, 340
  giardiasis and, 249
  intermediate uveitis and, 281
  pars planitis and, 284
  *Toxocara canis* and, 239
Retinal detachment
  acute retinal necrosis with, 198
  cytomegalovirus retinitis and, 190
  retinal necrosis and, 202
  rhegmatogenous
    acute retinal necrosis with, 198
    intermediate uveitis and, 281
    Schwartz syndrome and, 275
  sympathetic ophthalmia and, 309
  Vogt-Koyanagi-Harada disease and, 315, 321
Retinal necrosis
  acute
    clinical features of, 199-200
    differential diagnosis of, 201-202
    epidemiology of, 199
    etiology of, 200-201
    treatment of, 202-203
  progressive outer, 203-205
Retinal pigment epitheliitis, 375-376
Retinal pigment epithelium
  in cytomegalovirus retinitis, 189
  epitheliitis of, 375-376
  multiple evanescent white-dot syndrome and, 371-372
  pathogenesis of disease and, 19-20
  proliferation of, 66
  retinal necrosis and, 199

Retinal pigment epithelium—cont'd
sarcoidosis and, 292
serpiginous choroidopathy and, 364-370
Vogt-Koyanagi-Harada disease and, 315
Retinal S-antigen; *see* S-antigen
Retinal vasculitis, 354-362
aneurysm and, 357
birdshot retinochoroidopathy and, 330
clinical manifestations of, 354-355
Eales' disease and, 355-357
examination for, 66
frosted-branch angiitis and, 357-358
retinal necrosis and, 199
scleritis and, 358
systemic disease with, 358-362
Retinal vein, occlusion of, 361
Retinitis
cytomegalovirus; *see also* Cytomegalovirus
Behçet's disease and, 146
HIV infection and, 188-194, 217
herpes simplex, 207-208
histoplasmosis, 232-233
in HIV infection
cytomegalovirus and, 188-194
progressive outer retinal necrosis and, 194
varicella-zoster and, 194
syphilis and, 165
Retinitis pigmentosa, 392
Retinoblastoma, 391
Retinochoroidopathy, birdshot, 325-332
HLA haplotypes in, 24, 25
testing for, 85
Retinoid-binding protein, interphotoreceptor
anterior chamber–acquired immune deviation and, 19
sympathetic ophthalmia and, 305
Retinopathy
acute zonal occult outer, 381
cancer-associated, 391
human immunodeficiency virus, 187
occlusive, 354
Retrovirus, 186; *see also* Human immunodeficiency virus infection
Rhegmatogenous retinal detachment; *see* Retinal detachment
Rheumatoid arthritis
azathioprine for, 110
juvenile, 142
retinal vasculitis and, 361-362
Rhodopsin, 33
Rifabutin, 196
River blindness, 244-249
RNA, corticosteroids and, 99
Rubella, 209

## S

Sabin-Feldman test, 220
S-Ag; *see* S-antigen
Sample size, in clinical trial, 92-93
Sandimmune; *see* Cyclosporine
S-antigen, 32-38
autoimmune disease and, 32-38
birdshot retinochoroidopathy and, 329
oral tolerance and, 21, 121
sympathetic ophthalmia and, 305
S-antigen—cont'd
toxoplasmosis and, 218-219, 220
Sarcoiditis, intermediate uveitis and, 283
Sarcoidosis, 289-298
Behçet's disease versus, 343
birdshot retinochoroidopathy versus, 329
clinical manifestations of, 290-294
diagnosis of, 295-296
epidemiology of, 289
etiology of, 289-290
intraocular lens and, 141-142
keratic precipitates in, 61
lymphoma versus, 389
pathology of, 294-295
postoperative inflammation in, 136
treatment of, 296-298
Scaffolding in vitreous, 214-215
Scar
Fuchs' heterochromic iridocyclitis and, 274
toxoplasmosis causing, 213
Schwartz syndrome, 275
Schwartzman toxin, 155
Sclera, tuberculosis and, 158
Scleral buckling, cytomegalovirus retinitis and, 190
Scleritis, 358
connective tissue disease and, 72-73
slit-lamp examination and, 60
Sclerosing panencephalitis, subacute, 209
Sclerosis, multiple
intermediate uveitis and, 280, 285
masquerade syndromes and, 392
Scotoma, cytomegalovirus and, 190
Seasonal hyperacute panuveitis, 252-253
Secondary malignancy, 110
Sentinel vessel, 391
Serotonin, 13-14
Serpiginous choroidopathy, 364-370
clinical manifestations of, 364-366
differential diagnosis of, 367-368
etiology of, 367
pathology of, 364-370
therapy for, 368, 370
Sex differences
Behçet's disease and, 336-337
Vogt-Koyanagi-Harada disease and, 313
Sexually transmitted disease
human immunodeficiency virus infection as, 186
syphilis as, 160-169
Sheathing, peripheral vascular, 66
Sialic acid, 347
Silicone oil tamponade, 190-191
Sjögren's syndrome A antigen, 357
Skin
Behçet's disease and, 339
corticosteroids affecting, 106
Lyme disease and, 170
sarcoidosis and, 293, 295, 296
syphilis and, 161
Vogt-Koyanagi-Harada disease and, 313
Skin examination, 73
Skin testing, 83-84
histoplasmosis and, 232
Slit-lamp biomicroscopy, 60-64

Snowbank
intermediate uveitis and, 280-281
pars planitis and, 284
Sorivudine, 125
Spiramycin, 128
Spirochetal infection, 160-178
brucellosis as, 178
leptospirosis, 175-178
Lyme disease, 170-174
relapsing fever, 174-175
syphilis, 160-169
yaws and pinta, 169-170
Spleen
anterior chamber–acquired immune deviation and, 19
sarcoidosis and, 294
*Sporotrichum schenckii*, 180
Spot
cotton-wool, 66
"histo," 229-230
Staphylococcal infection, 257
Steroid; *see* Corticosteroid
Stippling of retinal pigment, 189
*Streptococcus sanguis*–related antigen, 346-347
*Streptomyces hygroscopicus*, 119
*Streptomyces tsukubaenis*, 118
Subacute neuroretinitis, diffuse unilateral, 251-252
Subacute sclerosing panencephalitis, 209
Subfoveal neovascular membrane, 149
Submacular surgery, 148-151
Subretinal disorder
fibrosis and, 379-380
Vogt-Koyanagi-Harada disease and, 315
Subretinal neovascularization
histoplasmosis and, 232, 234
laser treatment of, 146
toxoplasmosis causing, 215-216
Subretinal space, 67
Subretinal surgery, 148-151
Sugiura's sign, 313
Sulfadiazine, 127
toxoplasmosis and, 223
Sulfasoxazole, for toxoplasmosis, 128
Sunset glow appearance, 315
Suramin, for onchocerciasis, 248
Surgery, 135-151
band keratopathy and, 136-137
cataract, 137-142; *see also* Cataract extraction
corneal transplantation and, 137
diagnostic, 146-147
anterior chamber paracentesis as, 146-147
chorioretinal biopsy as, 147-148
subretinal, 148-151
glaucoma and, 142-144
for histoplasmosis, 235
for juvenile arthritis, 272-273
laser, 145-146
preoperative steroid therapy and, 136
retinal necrosis and, 202
for sarcoidosis, 297
sympathetic ophthalmia and, 299-300, 307
*Toxocara canis* and, 241
vitreoretinal disease and, 144-145
Sustained-release device, for ganciclovir, 125
Swelling, ciliary, 314
Sympathetic ophthalmia, 299-309
clinical manifestations of, 299-302
immunologic characteristics of, 302-307
therapy for, 307-309
Vogt-Koyanagi-Harada disease versus, 320-321
Syphilis, 160-169
clinical manifestations of, 161-165
endemic, 168-169
etiology of, 160-161
HIV infection and, 181
testing for, 82-83
Systemic lupus erythematosus, 359

## T

T cell
autoimmunity and, 29-32
Behçet's disease and, 344-345
birdshot retinochoroidopathy and, 331
characteristics of, 5-8
corticosteroids and, 99, 101
cyclosporine and, 115
hypersensitivity reaction and, 15-16
leprosy and, 157
multifocal choroiditis and, 375
retinal necrosis and, 200
subretinal fibrosis and, 380
sympathetic ophthalmia and, 304
Vogt-Koyanagi-Harada disease and, 318-319
T-cell receptor
autoimmunity and, 32
function of, 8
Tabes dorsalis, 162
Tachyzoite, toxoplasmosis, 218-219, 220
*Taenia solium*, 250
Tamponade, silicone oil, 190-191
Teeth, Hutchinson's, 163
Tertiary syphilis, 161
Testing, diagnostic, 79-89; *see also* Diagnostic testing
Tetracaine
for relapsing fever, 175
for toxoplasmosis, 128
Tetracycline, Lyme disease and, 174
Thalidomide, for Behçet's disease, 349
Thiabendazole
for neuroretinitis, 252
*Toxocara canis* and, 241
Thrombosis, Behçet's disease and, 343
Tick-borne disease
Lyme disease as, 170-174
relapsing fever and, 174-175
Tissue plasminogen activator, 136
Tongue, Behçet's disease and, 337-339
Topical cyclosporine, 116
Toxicity
of cancer therapy, 389-390
of methotrexate, 111
of rapamycin, 120
renal
of cyclosporine, 116-117
HPMPC causing, 125
Toxin, Schwartzman, 155
*Toxocara canis*, 238-242, 251-252
histopathology of, 239-241

*Toxocara canis*—cont'd
treatment of, 241
Toxoplasmosis, 211-226
clinical manifestations of, 213-218
congenital versus acquired, 222-223
diagnosis of, 220
drugs for, 127-128
Fuchs' heterochromic iridocyclitis and, 274
histopathology of, 218-219
immune response to, 219-220
inflammatory response to, 220
organism causing, 211-212
therapy for, 223-226
TPI test, 166
Trabeculodialysis, 143
Transfer factor, 128
Transforming growth factor-β
anterior chamber–acquired immune deviation and, 19
function of, 8
oral tolerance and, 20-21
Transfusion, toxoplasmosis from, 225-226
Transplacental transmission, of Lyme disease, 171; *see also* Congenital disorder
Transplantation, corneal, 137
Trauma, sympathetic ophthalmia after, 299-309; *see also* Sympathetic ophthalmia
Trematode infestation, 252
*Treponema pallidum*, 160-169
endemic, 168-169
Lyme disease and, 173
Triamcinolone
intermediate uveitis and, 285
potency of, 102
Trifluridine, 207
Trimethoprim-sulfamethoxazole, 223
Trisodium phosphonoformate; *see* Foscarnet
Trophozoite, of *Toxoplasma gondii*, 211
Tropicamide, 126
Tuberculoid form of leprosy, 156
Tuberculosis, testing for, 83-84, 159
Tumor necrosis factor-α
immune complex–mediated disease and, 26
toxoplasmosis and, 219

## U

UGH syndrome, 260
Ulcer, in Behçet's disease, 337-339
Ultrasonography, 283-284
Unilateral subacute neuroretinitis, diffuse, 251-252
Urethritis, in Reiter's syndrome, 269
Uvea, lymphoid hyperplasia of, 390-391
Uveal melanocytic proliferation, diffuse, 391
Uveitis
anterior, 265-277; *see also* Anterior uveitis
lens-induced, 276
causes of, 69-71
differential diagnosis of, 69-78; *see also* Differential diagnosis, development of
infectious; *see* Infection
intermediate, 279-287; *see also* Intermediate uveitis
lens-induced, 259
literature on, 91-93
syndromes masquerading as, 385-393
Uveitogenic antigen
autoimmunity and, 32-38
pathogenesis and, 21
Uveomeningitis; *see* Vogt-Koyanagi-Harada disease

## V

Vaccination, cyclosporine and, 117
Vaccination-induced uveitis, 393
Varicella zoster virus, sorivudine and, 125
Varicella-zoster virus
HIV infection and, 194
reactivation of, 208
Vascular system
Behçet's disease and, 343
retinal; *see* Retinal artery; Retinal vasculitis
sentinel vessel and, 391
Vasculitis
alkylating agents for, 110
retinal, 354-362; *see also* Retinal vasculitis
Vasoocclusion, Behçet's disease and, 343
Vein, retinal, occlusion of, 357
Venereal Disease Research Laboratory test, 165-166
HIV infection and, 168
for syphilis, 82-83
Venereal disease, syphilis as, 160-169
Venule, Eales' disease and, 356
Vidarabine ointment, 207
Viral infection; *see* Infection, viral; *specific virus*
Behçet's disease and, 346
Visceral larval migrans, 238-239
Vision loss
Behçet's disease and, 342
fungal endophthalmitis causing, 258-259
patient history of, 51-52
river blindness and, 244-249
toxoplasmosis causing, 215-216
Visual acuity
birdshot retinochoroidopathy and, 330
histoplasmosis and, 149
intermediate uveitis and, 280
intraocular lens and, 141
planning of therapy and, 98
sarcoidosis and, 294
testing of, 58-59, 85
toxoplasmosis and, 223
Vogt-Koyanagi-Harada disease and, 316
Vitiliginous chorioretinitis; *see* Birdshot retinochoroidopathy
Vitrectomy
diagnostic, 147
Eales' disease and, 357
intermediate uveitis and, 286
pars plana lensectomy with, 138-140
*Toxocara canis* and, 241
toxoplasmosis and, 224
Vitreoretinal disease, surgery for, 144-145
Vitreoretinopathy, proliferative, 145
Vitreous
examination of, 64-65
histoplasmosis and, 232
intermediate uveitis and, 285
lymphoma and, 388
parasitic infection of, 245
*Toxocara canis* and, 241

Vitreous—cont'd
toxoplasmosis and, 214-215
Vitreous hemorrhage, 281
Vitritis, 199
Vogt-Koyanagi-Harada disease, 312-322
azathioprine for, 110
Busacca's nodule and, 63, 64
clinical manifestations of, 312-317
diagnosis of, 317-320
sympathetic ophthalmia and, 304-307, 320-321
therapy for, 317-318

## W

Wegener's granulomatosis
cyclophosphamide for, 109
testing for, 83
vasculitis with, 359-360
Weil's disease, 176
Western blot analysis, for toxoplasmosis, 221
Whipple's disease, 360
White blood cell
B cell
characteristics of, 8-13
histoplasmosis, 233
subretinal fibrosis and, 380
leptospirosis and, 177
lymphocytes; *see* Lymphocyte; T cell
macrophage, 3-5
White blood cell—cont'd
neutrophil, 98
White-dot syndrome, 371-383
acute posterior multifocal placoid pigment epitheliopathy and, 376-379
acute zonal occult outer retinopathy and, 381
multifocal choroiditis and, 373-375
multiple evanescent, 371-372
retinal pigment epitheliitis and, 375-376
subretinal fibrosis and uveitis and, 379-380
Worm infestation
onchocerciasis and, 244-249
*Taenia solium* and, 250-251
*Toxocara canis* as, 238-242, 251-252
Wound, sympathetic ophthalmia after, 299-309

## X

X-linked granulomatous disease, 178-179

## Y

YAG laser; *see* Neodynium:yttrium-aluminum-garnet laser
Yaws, 169-170

## Z

Zidovudine, 128
Zonal occult outer retinopathy, acute, 381
Zoster infection; *see* Herpes zoster